Junqueira's
Basic Histology
TEXT AND ATLAS

Anthony L. Mescher, PhD

Emeritus Professor of Anatomy and Cell Biology

Indiana University School of Medicine

Bloomington, Indiana

New York   Chicago   San Francisco   Athens   London   Madrid   Mexico City
Milan   New Delhi   Singapore   Sydney   Toronto

Junqueira's Basic Histology, Seventeenth Edition

1 2 3 4 5 6 7 8 9   LWI   28 27 26 25 24 23

ISBN 978-1-264-93039-5
MHID 1-264-93039-9
ISSN 0891-2106

Notice

Medicine is an ever-changing science. As new research and clinical experience broaden our knowledge, changes in treatment and drug therapy are required. The author and the publisher of this work have checked with sources believed to be reliable in their efforts to provide information that is complete and generally in accord with the standards accepted at the time of publication. However, in view of the possibility of human error or changes in medical sciences, neither the author nor the publisher nor any other party who has been involved in the preparation or publication of this work warrants that the information contained herein is in every respect accurate or complete, and they disclaim all responsibility for any errors or omissions or for the results obtained from use of the information contained in this work. Readers are encouraged to confirm the information contained herein with other sources. For example and in particular, readers are advised to check the product information sheet included in the package of each drug they plan to administer to be certain that the information contained in this work is accurate and that changes have not been made in the recommended dose or in the contraindications for administration. This recommendation is of particular importance in connection with new or infrequently used drugs.

This book was Minion Pro by KnowledgeWorks Global Ltd.
The editors were Michael Weitz and Christina M. Thomas.
The production supervisor was Catherine H. Saggese.
Project management was provided by Nitesh Sharma of KnowledgeWorks Global Ltd.

This book is printed on acid-free paper.

The Figure Credit section for this book begins on page 527 and is considered an extension of the copyright page.

McGraw Hill books are available at special quantity discounts to use as premiums and sales promotions, or for use in corporate training programs. To contact a representative, please, visit the Contact Us pages at www.mhprofessional.com.

Contents

Preface

This 17th edition of *Junqueira's Basic Histology: Text and* Atlas continues to emphasize the features that have made it a preferred resource for over 50 years, for both students in the health professions and undergraduates internationally. Foremost among these features are (1) its **concise and straightforward text** which provides all information on human histology such students require without unnecessary detail and (2) its **excellent blend of high-quality photomicrographs and clear, uncluttered, well-labeled illustrations**. Each chapter—covering histological methods, fundamentals of cell biology, the biology of the basic tissues, and each of the body's organ systems—maintains a focus on these attributes while also being up-to-date and including other features not found in competing textbooks.

Testifying to its value to students and experts alike, *Junqueira's Basic Histology* is a **perennial best-seller** among histology text and atlases on Amazon and a **"Core Title in the Health Sciences"** by Doody's Medical Book Review Service. It has also been chosen as a **top reference source for histology** content at several online resources for healthcare professionals teaching or learning anatomy and histology. *Junqueira* meets the needs of students and professors throughout the world and has been **published in 18 languages** besides English.

Today's students in the health professions most likely study histology not as a separate course, but as part of larger curricular blocks such as "Human Structure" or "Molecules, Cells and Tissues," or within the context of individual organ systems. *Junqueira's Basic Histology* has long facilitated such integrated approaches to learning by including along with the basic structural features of cells, tissues and organs, an emphasis on how their structures relate to their functions. This allows Junqueira to provide not only a firm foundation for later studies in **pathology** (study of diseased tissues) but also a strong basis in the cell biological aspects of **biochemistry, immunology, endocrinology, and many aspects of physiology, as well as authoritative introductions to** medical specialties such as **hematology, dermatology, dentistry, ophthalmology, urology** and others.

New features in this 17th English edition of *Junqueira* include the following:

- Major portions of the text have been rewritten for still **greater conciseness, simplicity, and readability**, with more important facts repeated in the figure captions.
- Chapters in the online version available with **AccessMedicine** in your medical library's online resources now include **500 multiple-choice questions** for self-assessment of your understanding of the chapter's key points.

- The rewritten text places more emphasis on the **embryonic origins** of tissues and organs where this is useful for understanding structure and function. This **more clearly integrates histology** with the embryological and gross anatomical components of the modern curriculum.
- While revising and shortening each chapter where feasible, I have **updated several specific topics** as needed.

Other features introduced in recent editions unique to *Junqueira's Basic Histology* that are retained and improved include:

- Brilliant, high quality, **full-color illustrations**, rendered with three-dimensional detail and well-labeled, summarize basic aspects of each structure.
- A full-color **photographic atlas**, with all highlights labeled, includes every major cell, tissue type, and organ in the body.
- The standard atlas is supplemented by dozens of **research-generated photos** of cells and other microscopic structures not routinely included in student atlases, but kindly provided for this textbook by researchers from all over the world.
- **Summary Tables** in each chapter organize and condense important information, facilitating efficient learning.
- Comprehensive **"Summaries of Key Points"** at the end of each chapter, briefly recapping fundamental facts from the text and figures.
- Multiple-choice **"Assess Your Knowledge" questions**, including questions with clinical vignettes for framing medical relevance and applications of basic science concepts, allow the learner to gauge how well they comprehend each chapter.
- Selected **"Medical Applications"** boxes are placed throughout each chapter to help learners appreciate the medical relevance of the material being studied.
- The digital version of *Junqueira's Basic Histology: Text and Atlas*, available with McGraw Hill's **AccessMedicine** through most medical libraries, incorporates a detailed **Lab Guide** for that material, including **(1) the learning objectives for that laboratory session, (2) a list of important structures to identify and terms to use and understand, (3) detailed microscopic directions for studying each tissue and locating those structures,** and **(4) self-assessment questions** with each session. These laboratory exercises link to photographic material in the Junqueira textbook and can be used with slides in

any virtual or glass slide collection, making this digital Lab Guide a unique instrument among other histology texts and atlases. ***No other major textbook of tissue biology includes detailed guidance for learners through the microscopic or laboratory portion of the typical undergraduate or medical school coverage of histology.***

■ Included with the digital Lab Guide on AccessMedicine are links to an excellent **collection of scannable and focusable virtual light microscope slides**.

Students who cannot link to AccessMedicine may lack access to this digital Lab Guide but may still utilize the collection of over 150 virtual light microscope slides of human tissues and organs at: **http://medsci.indiana.edu/junqueira/ virtual/junqueira.htm**. This set of virtual slides is available without restrictions for use with any instructor's guide for human histology lab exercises.

To allow additional review of what's been learned or to assist rapid assimilation of the material in *Junqueira's Basic Histology*, I've also authored for McGraw Hill a set of 200 full-color **Lange Basic Histology Flash Cards**. Each card includes images of key structures to identify, a summary of important facts about those structures, and a clinical comment. This valuable learning aid is available from Amazon.com.

With its concise yet authoritative and up-to-date presentations, excellent color micrographs and illustrations, and links with a digital Lab Guide and slide collection, I feel sure that *Junqueira's Basic Histology* will continue as one of the most valued and widely used educational resources in histology worldwide. I thank for you for reading this summary and hope you will appreciate the upcoming tour through the body's microscopic structures. As always, users are invited to provide me with feedback about any aspect of the book's content or features.

Anthony L. Mescher
Indiana University School of Medicine—Bloomington

Acknowledgments

I wish to thank the students at Indiana University School of Medicine and the undergraduates at Indiana University Bloomington with whom I studied histology and cell biology for over 38 years and from whom I have learned much about presenting basic concepts most effectively. Their input has greatly helped in the task of maintaining and updating the presentations in this classic textbook. The help of Sue Childress and Dr. Mark Braun was invaluable in slide preparation and creation of the virtual microscope for human histology, respectively.

As with the last edition, the present text includes multiple-choice questions at the end of each chapter, aimed to test the learner's retention and understanding of important points in that body of material. Many of these questions were used in my courses, but others are taken or modified from a few of the many excellent review books published by McGraw Hill/Lange for students preparing to take the United States Medical Licensing Examination. These include *Histology and Cell Biology: Examination and Board Review*, by Douglas Paulsen; *USMLE Road Map: Histology*, by Harold Sheedlo; and *Anatomy, Histology, & Cell Biology: PreTest Self-Assessment & Review*, by Robert Klein and George Enders. The use here of questions from these valuable resources is gratefully acknowledged. Students are referred to those review books for hundreds of additional self-assessment questions.

I am also grateful to colleagues and reviewers throughout the world who provided specialized expertise or original photographs, as also acknowledged further in these figures' captions. I thank those professors and students in the United States and countries throughout the world who provided useful suggestions that have improved the new edition of *Junqueira's Basic Histology*. Finally, I am pleased to acknowledge the help and collegiality provided by the staff of McGraw Hill, especially editors Michael Weitz and Christina Thomas, whose work made possible publication of this 17th edition of *Junqueira's Basic Histology: Text and Atlas*.

Anthony L. Mescher
Indiana University School of Medicine—Bloomington

1

Histology & Its Methods of Study

Histology explores the body's tissues and how these are arranged to produce functional organs. The subject involves all aspects of tissue biology, from cellular biology to microscopic anatomy, focusing on how cell activities, shapes, and groupings are optimized for specific organ functions.

Tissues have two interacting components: cells and extracellular matrix (ECM). The ECM involves many kinds of macromolecules, most of which form complex structures, such as collagen fibrils. The ECM supports the cells and contains the fluid transporting nutrients to the cells and carrying away their wastes and secretory products. Cells produce the ECM locally and are in turn strongly influenced by matrix molecules. Many matrix components bind to specific cell surface receptors that span the cell membranes and connect to structural components inside the cells, forming a continuum in which cells and the ECM function together in a well-coordinated manner.

During embryonic development, cells and their associated matrix become functionally specialized and give rise to fundamental types of tissues with characteristic structural features. Organs form by an orderly combination of these tissues, and their precise arrangement allows the functioning of each organ and of the organism.

The small size of cells and matrix components makes histology dependent on the use of microscopes and molecular methods of study. Advances in biochemistry, molecular biology, physiology, immunology, and pathology are essential for a better knowledge of tissue biology. Familiarity with the tools and methods of any branch of science is essential for a proper understanding of the subject. This chapter reviews common methods used to study cells and tissues, focusing on microscopic approaches.

PREPARATION OF TISSUES FOR STUDY

The most common procedure used in histologic research is the preparation of tissue slices or "sections" that can be examined visually with transmitted light. Because most tissues and organs are too thick for light to pass through, thin translucent sections are cut from them and placed on glass slides for microscopic examination of their internal structures.

The ideal microscopic preparation is preserved so that the tissue on the slide has the same structural features it had in the body. However, this is often not feasible because the preparation process can remove cellular lipid, with slight distortions of cell structure. Figure 1–1 summarizes the initial steps used in tissue preparation for light microscopy.

Fixation

To preserve tissue structure and prevent degradation by enzymes released from the cells or microorganisms, pieces of

FIGURE 1–1 Sectioning fixed and embedded tissue.

| Fixation | Dehydration | Clearing | Infiltration | Embedding |

52°-60°C

Drive wheel
Block holder
Paraffin block
Tissue
Steel knife

b

Most tissues studied histologically are prepared as shown, with this sequence of steps **(a)**:

- **Fixation:** Small pieces of tissue are placed in chemical solutions that preserve cell and tissue structure by cross-linking proteins and inactivating degradative enzymes.
- **Dehydration:** The tissue is transferred through a series of increasingly concentrated alcohol solutions, ending in 100%, which removes all water.
- **Clearing:** Alcohol is removed in organic solvents in which both alcohol and paraffin are miscible.
- **Infiltration:** The tissue is then placed in melted paraffin until it becomes completely infiltrated with this substance.
- **Embedding:** The paraffin-infiltrated tissue is placed in a small mold with melted paraffin and allowed to harden.
- **Trimming:** The resulting paraffin block is trimmed to expose the tissue for sectioning (slicing) on a microtome.

Similar steps are used in preparing tissue for transmission electron microscopy (TEM), except special fixatives and dehydrating solutions are used with smaller tissue samples and embedding involves epoxy resins which become harder than paraffin to allow very thin sectioning.

(b) A **microtome** is used for sectioning paraffin-embedded tissues for light microscopy. The trimmed tissue specimen is mounted in the paraffin block holder, and each turn of the drive wheel by the histologist advances the holder a controlled distance, generally from 1 to 10 μm. After each forward move, the tissue block passes over the steel knife edge and a section is cut at a thickness equal to the distance the block advanced. The paraffin sections are placed on glass slides and allowed to adhere, deparaffinized, and stained for light microscope study. For TEM, sections less than 1 μm thick are prepared from resin-embedded cells using an ultramicrotome with a glass or diamond knife.

organs are placed as soon as possible after removal from the body in solutions of stabilizing or cross-linking compounds called **fixatives**. Because a fixative must fully diffuse through the tissues to preserve all cells, organs are usually cut into small fragments before fixation to facilitate penetration. To improve cell preservation in large organs, fixatives are often introduced via blood vessels, with vascular perfusion allowing fixation rapidly throughout the tissues.

One widely used fixative for light microscopy is formalin, a buffered isotonic solution of 37% formaldehyde. Both this compound and glutaraldehyde, a fixative used for electron

microscopy, react with the amine groups (NH_2) of proteins, preventing their degradation by common proteases. Glutaraldehyde also cross-links adjacent proteins, reinforcing cell and ECM structures.

Electron microscopy provides much greater magnification and resolution of very small cellular structures, and fixation must be done very carefully to preserve additional "ultrastructural" detail. In these studies glutaraldehyde-treated tissue is then immersed further in buffered osmium tetroxide, which preserves (and stains) cellular lipids as well as proteins.

Embedding & Sectioning

To permit thin sectioning, fixed tissues are infiltrated and embedded in a material that imparts a firm consistency. Embedding materials include paraffin, used routinely for light microscopy, and plastic resins, which are adapted for both light and electron microscopy.

Before infiltration with such media, the fixed tissue must undergo **dehydration** by having its water extracted gradually by transfers through a series of increasing ethanol solutions, ending in 100% ethanol. The ethanol is then replaced by an organic solvent miscible with both alcohol and the embedding medium, a step referred to as **clearing** because infiltration with the reagents used here gives the tissue a translucent appearance.

The fully cleared tissue is then placed in melted paraffin in an oven at 52–60°C, which evaporates the clearing solvent and promotes **infiltration** of the tissue with paraffin, and then **embedded** by allowing it to harden in a small container of paraffin at room temperature. Tissues to be embedded with plastic resin are also dehydrated in ethanol and then infiltrated with plastic solvents that harden when cross-linking polymerizers are added. Plastic embedding avoids the higher temperatures needed with paraffin, helping to avoid tissue distortion.

The hardened block with tissue and surrounding embedding medium is trimmed and placed for sectioning in an instrument called a **microtome** (Figure 1–1). Paraffin sections are typically cut at 3–10 μm thickness for light microscopy, but electron microscopy requires sections less than 1 μm thick. One micrometer (1 μm) equals 1/1000 of a millimeter (mm). Other spatial units commonly used in microscopy are the nanometer (1 nm = 0.001 μm = 10^{-6} mm) and the angstrom (1 Å = 0.1 nm or 10^{-4} μm). The sections are placed on glass slides and stained for light microscopy or on metal grids for electron-microscopic staining and examination.

›› MEDICAL APPLICATION

Biopsies are tissue samples removed during surgery or routine medical procedures. In the operating room, biopsies are fixed in vials of formalin for processing and microscopic analysis in a pathology laboratory. If results of such analyses are required before the medical procedure is completed, for example, to know whether a growth is malignant before the patient is closed, a much more rapid processing method is used. The biopsy is rapidly frozen in liquid nitrogen, preserving cell structures and at the same time making the tissue hard and ready for sectioning. A microtome called a **cryostat** in a cabinet at subfreezing temperature is used to section the block with tissue, and the frozen sections are placed on slides for rapid staining and microscopic examination by a pathologist.

Freezing of tissues is also effective in histochemical studies of very sensitive enzymes or small molecules because freezing, unlike fixation, does not inactivate most enzymes. Finally, because clearing solvents often dissolve cell lipids in fixed tissues, frozen sections are also useful when structures containing lipids are to be studied histologically.

Staining

Most cells and extracellular material are completely colorless, and to be studied microscopically, tissue sections must be stained (dyed). Methods of staining have been devised that make various tissue components not only conspicuous but also distinguishable from one another. Dyes stain material rather selectively, often behaving like acidic or basic compounds and forming electrostatic (salt) linkages with ionizable radicals of macromolecules in tissues. Cell components, such as nucleic acids with a net negative charge (anionic), have an affinity for basic dyes and are thus termed **basophilic**; cationic components, such as proteins with many ionized amino groups, stain more readily with acidic dyes and are termed **acidophilic**.

Examples of basic dyes include toluidine blue, alcian blue, and methylene blue. Hematoxylin also behaves like a basic dye, staining basophilic tissue components. The main tissue components that ionize and react with basic dyes do so because of acids in their composition (eg, DNA, RNA, and glycosaminoglycans). Acidic dyes like eosin, orange G, and acid fuchsin stain acidophilic components of tissues, such as mitochondria, secretory granules, and collagen.

Of all staining methods, the simple combination of **hematoxylin and eosin (H&E)** is the most common. Hematoxylin stains DNA in the cell nucleus, RNA-rich portions of the cytoplasm, and the matrix of cartilage, producing a dark blue or purplish color. In contrast, eosin stains other cytoplasmic structures and collagen pink (Figure 1–2a). In H&E, eosin acts as a **counterstain**, usually a single dye applied separately to distinguish additional features of a tissue. More complex procedures, such as trichrome stains (eg, Masson trichrome), allow greater distinctions among various extracellular tissue components.

The **periodic acid–Schiff (PAS) reaction** utilizes the hexose rings of polysaccharides and other carbohydrate-rich tissue structures and stains such macromolecules distinctly purple or magenta. Figure 1–2b shows an example of cells with carbohydrate-rich areas well-stained by the PAS reaction. The DNA of cell nuclei can be specifically stained using a modification of the PAS procedure called the Feulgen reaction.

Basophilic or PAS-positive material can be further identified by enzyme digestion: pretreatment of a tissue section with an enzyme that specifically digests one substrate. For example, pretreatment with ribonuclease will greatly reduce cytoplasmic basophilia with little overall effect on the nucleus, indicating the importance of RNA for this cytoplasmic staining.

Lipid-rich structures of cells are revealed by avoiding the processing steps that remove lipids, such as treatment with heat and organic solvents, and staining with **lipid-soluble dyes** such as **Sudan black**, which can be useful in diagnosis of metabolic diseases that involve intracellular accumulations of cholesterol, phospholipids, or glycolipids. Less-common methods of staining can employ **metal impregnation** techniques, typically using solutions of silver salts to visualize certain ECM fibers and specific cellular elements in nervous tissue. The Appendix lists important staining procedures used for most of the light micrographs in this book.

FIGURE **1–2** Hematoxylin and eosin (H&E) and periodic acid–Schiff (PAS) staining.

Micrographs of epithelium lining the small intestine, **(a)** stained with H&E, and **(b)** stained with the PAS reaction for glycoproteins. With H&E, basophilic cell nuclei are stained purple, while cytoplasm stains pink. Cell regions with abundant oligosaccharides on glycoproteins, such as the ends of the cells at the lumen (**L**) or the scattered mucus-secreting goblet cells (**G**), are poorly stained by H&E. With PAS, however, cell staining is most intense at the lumen, where projecting microvilli have a prominent layer of glycoproteins at the lumen's lining (**L**), and in the mucin-rich granules of goblet cells. Cell surface glycoproteins and mucin are PAS-positive due to their high content of oligosaccharides and polysaccharides, respectively. The PAS-stained tissue was counterstained with hematoxylin to show the cell nuclei. (a. ×400; b. ×300)

Slide preparation, from tissue fixation to observation with a light microscope, may take from 12 hours to 2½ days, depending on the size of the tissue, the embedding medium, and the method of staining. The final step before microscopic observation is mounting a protective glass coverslip on the slide with clear adhesive.

❯ LIGHT MICROSCOPY

Conventional bright-field microscopy and more specialized applications like fluorescence, phase-contrast, confocal, and polarizing microscopy are all based on the interaction of light with tissue components and are used to reveal tissue features.

Bright-Field Microscopy

With the **bright-field microscope**, stained tissue is examined with ordinary light passing through the preparation. As shown in Figure 1–3, the microscope includes an optical system and mechanisms to move and focus the specimen. The optical components are the **condenser** focusing light on the object to be studied; the **objective** lens enlarging and projecting the image of the object toward the observer; and the **eyepiece** (or **ocular** lens) further magnifying this image and projecting it onto the viewer's retina or a charge-coupled device (CCD) highly sensitive to low light levels with a camera and a monitor. The total magnification is obtained by multiplying the magnifying power of the objective and ocular lenses.

The critical factor in obtaining a crisp, detailed image with a light microscope is its **resolving power**, defined as the smallest distance between two structures at which they can be seen as separate objects. The maximal resolving power of the light microscope is approximately 0.2 μm, which can permit clear images magnified 1000–1500 times. Objects smaller or thinner than 0.2 μm (such as a single ribosome or cytoplasmic microfilament) cannot be distinguished with this instrument. Likewise, two structures such as mitochondria will be seen as only one object if they are separated by less than 0.2 μm. The microscope's resolving power determines the quality of the image, its clarity and richness of detail, and depends mainly on the quality of its objective lens. Magnification is of value only when accompanied by high resolution. Objective lenses providing higher magnification are designed to also have higher resolving power. The ocular lens only enlarges the image obtained by the objective and does not improve resolution.

FIGURE **1–3** Components and light path of a bright-field microscope.

Photograph of a bright-field light microscope showing its mechanical components and the pathway of light from the substage lamp to the eye of the observer. The optical system has three sets of lenses:

- The **condenser** collects and focuses a cone of light that illuminates the tissue slide on the stage.
- **Objective** lenses enlarge and project the illuminated image of the object toward the eyepiece. Interchangeable objectives with different magnifications routinely used in histology include ×4 for observing a large area (field) of the tissue at low magnification; ×10 for medium magnification of a smaller field; and ×40 for high magnification of more detailed areas.
- The two **eyepieces** or oculars magnify this image another ×10 and project it to the viewer, yielding a total magnification of ×40, ×100, or ×400.

Virtual microscopy, typically used for the study of bright-field microscopic preparations, involves the conversion of a stained tissue preparation to high-resolution digital images and permits study of tissues using a computer or other digital device, without an actual stained slide or a microscope. In this technique, regions of a glass-mounted specimen are captured digitally in a grid-like pattern at multiple magnifications using a specialized slide-scanning microscope and saved as thousands of consecutive image files. Software then converts this dataset for storage on a server using a format that allows access, visualization, and navigation of the original slide with common web browsers or other devices. With advantages in cost and ease of use, virtual microscopy is rapidly replacing light microscopes and collections of glass slides in histology laboratories for students.

Fluorescence Microscopy

When certain cellular substances are irradiated by light of a proper wavelength, they emit light with a longer wavelength—a phenomenon called **fluorescence**. In **fluorescence microscopy**, tissue sections are usually irradiated with ultraviolet (UV) light and the emission is in the visible portion of the spectrum. The fluorescent substances appear bright on a dark background. For fluorescent microscopy, the instrument has a source of UV or other light and filters that select rays of different wavelengths emitted by the substances to be visualized.

Fluorescent compounds with affinity for specific cell macromolecules may be used as fluorescent stains. The compounds DAPI and Hoechst stain specifically bind DNA and are widely used to stain cell nuclei, emitting a characteristic blue fluorescence under UV. Acridine orange binds both DNA and RNA but emits different colors with these nucleic acids in fluorescent microscopy, allowing them to be localized separately in cells (Figure 1–4a). Another important application of fluorescence microscopy is achieved by coupling compounds such as fluorescein to molecules that will specifically bind to certain cellular components and thus allow the identification of these structures under the microscope (Figure 1–4b). Antibodies labeled with fluorescent compounds are extremely important in immunohistochemistry. (See the section on Visualizing Specific Molecules.)

Phase-Contrast Microscopy

Unstained cells and tissue sections, which are usually transparent and colorless, can be studied with these modified light microscopes. Cellular detail is normally difficult to see in unstained tissues because all parts of the specimen have roughly similar optical densities. **Phase-contrast microscopy**, however, uses a lens system that produces visible images from transparent objects and, importantly, can be used with living cultured cells (Figure 1–5).

Phase-contrast microscopy is based on the principle that light changes its speed when passing through cellular and extracellular structures with different refractive indices. These changes are used by the phase-contrast system to cause the structures to appear lighter or darker in relation to each other. Without the requirements of tissue fixation and staining, phase-contrast microscopes allow study of live cells and are prominent tools in all cell culture laboratories. A modification of phase-contrast microscopy is **differential interference contrast microscopy** with Nomarski optics, which produces an image of cells with a more apparent three-dimensional (3D) aspect (Figure 1–5c).

Confocal Microscopy

With a regular bright-field microscope, the beam of light is relatively large and fills the specimen. Stray (excess) light reduces contrast within the image and compromises the resolving power of the objective lens. Confocal microscopy (Figure 1–6) avoids these problems and achieves high resolution and sharp

FIGURE **1–4** Appearance of cells with fluorescent microscopy.

Components of cells are often stained with compounds visible by fluorescence microscopy.

(a) Acridine orange binds nucleic acids and causes DNA in cell nuclei (**N**) to emit yellow light and the RNA-rich cytoplasm (**R**) to appear orange in these cells of a kidney tubule.

(b) Cultured cells stained with DAPI (4′,6-diamino-2-phenylindole) that binds DNA and with fluorescein phalloidin that binds actin

filaments show nuclei with blue fluorescence and actin filaments stained green. Important information such as the greater density of microfilaments at the cell periphery is readily apparent. (Both ×500)

(Figure 1–4b, reproduced with permission from Drs Claire E. Walczak and Rania Rizk, Indiana University School of Medicine, Bloomington.)

FIGURE **1–5** Unstained cells' appearance in three types of light microscopies.

Living neural crest cells growing in culture appear differently with various techniques of light microscopy. Here the *same field* of unstained cells, including two differentiating pigment cells, is shown using three different methods (all ×200):

(a) Bright-field microscopy: Without fixation and staining, only the two pigment cells can be seen.

(b) Phase-contrast microscopy: Cell boundaries, nuclei, and cytoplasmic structures with different refractive indices affect

in-phase light differently and produce an image of these features in *all* the cells.

(c) Differential interference contrast microscopy: Cellular details are highlighted in a different manner using Nomarski optics. Phase-contrast microscopy, with or without differential interference, is widely used to observe live cells grown in tissue culture.

(Reproduced with permission from Dr Sherry Rogers, Department of Cell Biology and Physiology, University of New Mexico, Albuquerque, NM.)

FIGURE **1–6** Principle of confocal microscopy.

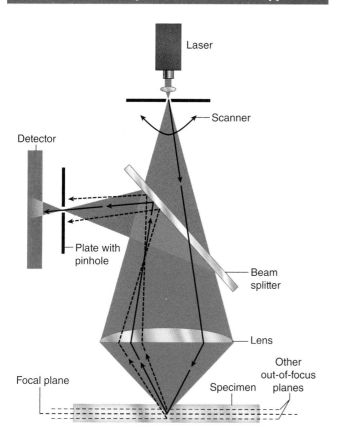

Although a very small spot of light originating from one plane of the section crosses the pinhole and reaches the detector, rays originating from other planes are blocked by the blind. Thus, only one very thin plane of the specimen is focused at a time. The diagram shows the practical arrangement of a confocal microscope. Light from a laser source hits the specimen and is reflected. A beam splitter directs the reflected light to a pinhole and a detector. Light from components of the specimen that are above or below the focused plane is blocked by the blind. The laser scans the specimen so that a larger area of the specimen can be observed.

focus by using (1) a small point of high-intensity light, often from a laser and (2) plate with a pinhole aperture in front of the image detector. The point light source, the focal point of the lens, and the detector's pinpoint aperture are all optically conjugated or aligned to each other in the focal plane (confocal), and unfocused light does not pass through the pinhole. This greatly improves resolution of the object in focus and allows the localization of specimen components with much greater precision than with the bright-field microscope.

Confocal microscopes include a computer-driven mirror system (the beam splitter) to move the point of illumination across the specimen automatically and rapidly. Digital images captured at many individual spots in a very thin plane of focus are used to produce an "optical section" of that plane. Creating such optical sections at a series of focal planes through the specimen allows them to be digitally reconstructed into a 3D image.

Polarizing Microscopy

Polarizing microscopy allows the recognition of stained or unstained structures made of highly organized subunits. When normal light passes through a **polarizing** filter, it exits vibrating in only one direction. If a second filter is placed in the microscope above the first one, with its main axis perpendicular to the first filter, no light passes through. If, however, tissue structures containing oriented macromolecules are located between the two polarizing filters, their repetitive structure rotates the axis of the light emerging from the polarizer and they appear as bright structures against a dark background (Figure 1–7). The ability to rotate the direction of vibration of polarized light is called **birefringence** and is a feature of crystalline substances or substances containing highly oriented molecules, such as cellulose, collagen, microtubules, and actin filaments.

FIGURE **1–7** Tissue appearance with bright-field and polarizing microscopy.

Polarizing light microscopy produces an image only of material having repetitive, periodic macromolecular structure; features without such structure are not seen. Pieces of thin, unsectioned mesentery were stained with red picrosirius, orcein, and hematoxylin, placed on slides and observed by bright-field **(a)** and polarizing **(b)** microscopy.

(a) With bright-field microscopy collagen fibers appear red, with thin elastic fibers and cell nuclei darker. (×40)

(b) With polarizing microscopy only the collagen fibers are visible and exhibit intense yellow or orange birefringence. (a: ×40; b: ×100)

The utility of all light microscopic methods is greatly extended with digital cameras. Many features of digitized histologic images can be analyzed quantitatively using appropriate software. Such images can also be enhanced to allow objects not directly visible through the eyepieces to be examined on a monitor.

› ELECTRON MICROSCOPY

Transmission and scanning electron microscopes are based on the interaction of tissue components with beams of electrons. The wavelength in an electron beam is much shorter than that of light, allowing a 1000-fold increase in resolution.

Transmission Electron Microscopy

The **transmission electron microscope (TEM)** is an imaging system that permits resolution around 3 nm. This high resolution allows isolated particles magnified as much as 400,000 times to be viewed in detail. Very thin (40–90 nm), resin-embedded tissue sections are typically studied by TEM at magnifications up to approximately 120,000 times.

Figure 1–8a indicates the components of a TEM and the basic principles of its operation: a beam of electrons focused using electromagnetic "lenses" passes through the tissue section to produce an image with black, white, and intermediate shades of gray regions. These regions of an electron micrograph correspond to tissue areas through which electrons

---

FIGURE 1–8 Electron microscopes.

(a) Transmission electron microscope

(b) Scanning electron microscope

Electron microscopes are large instruments generally housed in a specialized EM facility.

(a) Schematic view of the major components of a **transmission electron microscope (TEM)**, which is configured rather like an upside-down light microscope. With the microscope column in a vacuum, a metallic (usually tungsten) filament (cathode) at the top emits electrons that travel to an anode with an accelerating voltage between 60 and 120 kV. Electrons passing through a hole in the anode form a beam that is **focused electromagnetically** by circular electric coils in a manner analogous to the effect of optical lenses on light.

The first lens is a condenser focusing the beam on the section. Some electrons interact with atoms in the section, being absorbed or scattered to different extents, while others are simply transmitted through the specimen with no interaction. Electrons reaching the objective lens form an image that is then magnified and finally projected on a fluorescent screen or a charge-coupled device (CCD) monitor and camera.

In a TEM image, areas of the specimen through which electrons passed appear bright (electron lucent), while denser areas or those that bind heavy metal ions during specimen preparation absorb or deflect electrons and appear darker (electron dense). Such images are therefore always black, white, and shades of gray, although TEM images are sometimes colorized later.

(b) With the **scanning electron microscope (SEM)** the focused electron beam does not pass through the specimen, but rather is moved sequentially (scanned) from point to point across its surface. For SEM, specimens are coated with metal atoms with which the electron beam interacts, producing reflected electrons and newly emitted secondary electrons. All of these are captured by a detector, transmitted to amplifiers, and processed to produce a black-and-white image on the monitor. The SEM shows only surface views of the coated specimen but with a striking 3D, shadowed quality. The inside of organs or cells can be analyzed after sectioning to expose their internal surfaces.

passed readily (appearing brighter or electron-lucent) and areas where electrons were absorbed or deflected (appearing darker or more electron-dense). To improve contrast and resolution in TEM, compounds with **heavy metal ions** are often added to the fixative or dehydrating solutions used for tissue preparation. These include osmium tetroxide, lead citrate, and uranyl compounds, which bind cellular macromolecules, increasing their electron density and visibility.

Cryofracture and **freeze etching** are techniques that allow TEM study of cells without fixation or embedding and have been particularly useful in the study of membrane structure. In these methods, very small tissue specimens are rapidly frozen in liquid nitrogen and then cut or fractured with a knife. A replica of the frozen exposed surface is produced in a vacuum by applying thin coats of vaporized platinum or other metal atoms. After removal of the organic material, the replica of the cut surface can be examined by TEM. With membranes, the random fracture planes often split the lipid bilayers, exposing protein components whose size, shape, and distribution are difficult to study by other methods.

Scanning Electron Microscopy

Scanning electron microscopy (SEM) provides a high-resolution view of the surfaces of cells, tissues, and organs. Like the TEM, this microscope produces and focuses a very narrow beam of electrons, but in this instrument, the beam does not pass through the specimen (Figure 1–8b). Instead, the surface of the specimen is first dried and spray-coated with a very thin layer of heavy metal (often gold) that reflects electrons in a beam scanning the specimen. The reflected electrons are captured by a detector, producing signals that are processed to produce a black-and-white image. SEM images are usually easy to interpret because they present a 3D view that appears to be illuminated in the same way that large objects are seen with highlights and shadows caused by light.

❯ AUTORADIOGRAPHY

Microscopic **autoradiography** is a method of localizing newly synthesized macromolecules in cells or tissue sections. Radioactively labeled metabolites (nucleotides, amino acids, sugars) provided to living cells or experimental animals are incorporated into specific macromolecules (DNA, RNA, protein, glycoproteins, and polysaccharides). After tissue fixation, processing, and sectioning only the new, labeled macromolecules continue to emit weak and localized radiation, unincorporated isotope having been washed out during the processing steps. Slides or TEM grids with radiolabeled cells or tissue sections are coated in a darkroom with photographic emulsion in which silver bromide crystals act as microdetectors of the radiation in the same way that they respond to light in photographic film. After an adequate exposure time in lightproof boxes, the slides are developed photographically. Silver bromide crystals reduced by the radiation produce small black grains of metallic silver, which under either the light microscope or TEM indicate the locations of radiolabeled macromolecules in the tissue (Figure 1–9).

Much histological information becomes available by autoradiography. If a radioactive precursor of DNA (such as tritium-labeled thymidine) is used, it is possible to know which

---

FIGURE **1–9** Microscopic autoradiography.

Autoradiographs are tissue preparations in which particles called **silver grains** indicate the cells or regions of cells in which specific macromolecules were synthesized just prior to fixation. Shown here are autoradiographs from the salivary gland of a mouse injected with ³H-fucose 8 hours before tissue fixation. Fucose was incorporated into oligosaccharides, and the free ³H-fucose was removed during fixation and sectioning of the gland. Autoradiographic processing and microscopy reveal locations of newly synthesized glycoproteins containing that sugar.

(a) Black grains of silver from the light-sensitive material coating the specimen are visible over cell regions with secretory granules and the duct indicating glycoprotein locations. (×1500)

(b) The same tissue prepared for TEM autoradiography shows silver grains with a coiled or amorphous appearance again localized mainly over the granules (**G**) and in the gland lumen (**L**). (×7500)

(Figure 1–9b, reproduced with permission from Drs Ticiano G. Lima and A. Antonio Haddad, School of Medicine, Ribeirão Preto, Brazil.)

cells in a tissue (and how many) are replicating DNA and preparing to divide. Dynamic events may also be analyzed. For example, if one wishes to know where in the cell protein is produced, if it is secreted, and its path in the cell before being secreted, several animals are injected with a radioactive amino acid and tissues collected at different times after the injections. Autoradiography of the tissues from the sequential times will indicate the migration of the radioactive proteins.

CELL & TISSUE CULTURE

Live cells and tissues can be maintained and studied outside the body in culture (in vitro). In the organism (in vivo), cells are bathed in fluid derived from blood plasma and containing many different molecules required for survival and growth. Cell culture allows the direct observation of cellular behavior under a phase-contrast microscope, and many experiments technically impossible to perform in the intact animal can be accomplished in vitro.

The cells and tissues are grown in complex solutions of known composition (salts, amino acids, vitamins) to which serum or specific growth factors are added. Cells to be cultured are dispersed mechanically or enzymatically from a tissue or organ and placed with sterile procedures in a clear dish to which they adhere, usually as a single layer (Figure 1–5). Such preparations are called **primary cell cultures**. Some cells can be maintained in vitro for long periods because they become immortalized and constitute a permanent **cell line**. Most cells obtained from normal tissues have a finite, genetically programmed life span. However, certain changes (some related to oncogenes; see Chapter 3) can promote cell immortality, a process called **transformation**, and are similar to the initial changes in a normal cell becoming a cancer cell. Improvements in culture technology and use of specific growth factors now allow most cell types to be maintained in vitro.

As shown in Chapter 2, incubation of living cells in vitro with a variety of new fluorescent compounds that are sequestered and metabolized in specific compartments of the cell provides a new approach to understanding these compartments, both structurally and physiologically. Other histologic techniques applied to cultured cells have been particularly important for understanding the locations and functions of microtubules, microfilaments and other components of the cytoskeleton.

> **>> MEDICAL APPLICATION**
>
> Cell culture is very widely used to study molecular changes that occur in cancer; to analyze infectious viruses, mycoplasma, and some protozoa; and for many routine genetic or chromosomal analyses. Cervical cancer cells from a patient later identified as Henrietta Lacks, who died from the disease in 1951, were used to establish one of the first cell lines, called **HeLa cells**, which are still used in research on cellular structure and function throughout the world.

ENZYME HISTOCHEMISTRY

Enzyme histochemistry (or cytochemistry) is a method for localizing cellular structures using a specific enzymatic activity present in those structures. To preserve the endogenous enzymes, histochemical procedures usually use unfixed or mildly fixed tissue, which is sectioned on a cryostat to avoid adverse effects of heat and organic solvents on enzymatic activity. For enzyme histochemistry: (1) tissue sections are immersed in a buffer containing the substrate of the enzyme to be localized at the appropriate temperature and pH; (2) the enzyme is allowed to act on its substrate; (3) the section is then put in contact with a marker compound that reacts with a product of the enzymatic action on the substrate; and (4) the final product from the marker, which must be insoluble and visible by light or electron microscopy, precipitates over the site of the enzymes, identifying their location.

Examples of enzymes that can be detected histochemically include the following:

- **Phosphatases**, which remove phosphate groups from macromolecules (Figure 1–10)
- **Dehydrogenases**, which transfer hydrogen ions from one substrate to another, such as many enzymes of the citric acid (Krebs) cycle, allowing histochemical identification of such enzymes in mitochondria
- **Peroxidase**, which promotes the oxidation of substrates with the transfer of hydrogen ions to hydrogen peroxide

> **>> MEDICAL APPLICATION**
>
> Many enzyme histochemical procedures are used in the medical laboratory, including Perls' Prussian blue reaction for iron (used to diagnose the iron storage diseases, hemochromatosis and hemosiderosis), the PAS-amylase and alcian blue reactions for polysaccharides (to detect glycogenosis and mucopolysaccharidosis), and reactions for lipids and sphingolipids (to detect sphingolipidosis).

VISUALIZING SPECIFIC MOLECULES

A specific macromolecule present in a tissue section may also be identified by using tagged compounds or macromolecules that bind *specifically* with the molecule of interest. The compounds that interact with the molecule must be visible with the light or electron microscope, often by being tagged with a detectible label. The most common labels are fluorescent compounds, radioactive atoms that can be detected with autoradiography, molecules of peroxidase or other enzymes that can be detected with histochemistry, and metal (usually gold) particles that can be seen with light and electron microscopy. These methods can be used to detect and localize specific sugars, proteins, and nucleic acids.

FIGURE **1–10** Enzyme histochemistry.

(a) Micrograph of cross-sections of kidney tubules treated histochemically to demonstrate alkaline phosphatases (with maximum activity at an alkaline pH) showing strong activity of this enzyme at the apical surfaces of the cells at the lumens (**L**) of the tubules. (×200)

(b) TEM image of a kidney cell in which acid phosphatase has been localized histochemically in three lysosomes (**Ly**) near the nucleus (**N**). The dark material within these structures is lead phosphate that precipitated in places with acid phosphatase activity. (×25,000)

(*Figure 1–10b, reproduced with permission from Dr Eduardo Katchburian, Department of Morphology, Federal University of São Paulo, Brazil.*)

Examples of molecules that interact specifically with other molecules include the following:

- **Phalloidin**, a compound extracted from the mushroom, *Amanita phalloides*, interacts strongly with the actin protein of microfilaments.
- **Protein A**, purified from *Staphylococcus aureus* bacteria, binds to the Fc region of antibody molecules, and can therefore be used to localize naturally occurring or applied antibodies bound to cell structures.
- **Lectins**, glycoproteins derived mainly from plant seeds, bind to carbohydrates with high affinity and specificity. Different lectins bind to specific sugars or sequences of sugar residues, allowing fluorescently labeled lectins to be used to stain specific glycoproteins or other macromolecules bearing specific sequences of sugar residues.

Immunohistochemistry

A highly specific interaction between macromolecules is that between an antigen and its antibody. For this reason, labeled antibodies are routinely used in **immunohistochemistry** to identify and localize many specific proteins, not just those with enzymatic activity that can be demonstrated by histochemistry.

The body's immune cells interact with and produce **antibodies** against other macromolecules—called antigens—that are recognized as "foreign," not a normal part of the organism, and potentially pathogenic. Antibodies belong to the **immunoglobulin** family of glycoproteins and are secreted by lymphocytes. These molecules normally bind specifically to their provoking antigens and help eliminate them.

Widely applied for both research and diagnostic purposes, every immunohistochemical technique requires an antibody against the protein or other antigen that is to be detected. This means that the protein must have been previously purified using biochemical or molecular methods so that antibodies against it can be produced. To produce antibodies against protein x of a certain animal species (eg, a human or a rat), the isolated protein is injected into an animal of another species (eg, a rabbit or a goat). If the protein's amino acid sequence is sufficiently different for this animal to recognize it as foreign—that is, as an antigen—the animal will produce antibodies against the protein.

Different groups (clones) of lymphocytes in the injected animal recognize different parts of protein x and each clone produces an antibody against that part. These antibodies are collected from the animal's plasma and constitute a mixture of **polyclonal antibodies**, each capable of binding a different region of protein x.

It is also possible, however, to inject protein x into a mouse and a few days later isolate the activated lymphocytes and place them into culture. Growth and activity of these cells can be prolonged indefinitely by fusing them with lymphocytic tumor cells to produce hybridoma cells. Different hybridoma clones produce different antibodies against the several parts of protein x, and each clone can be isolated and cultured separately so that the different antibodies against protein x can be collected separately. Each of these antibodies is a **monoclonal antibody**. An advantage of using a monoclonal antibody rather than polyclonal antibodies is that it can be selected to be highly specific and to bind strongly to the protein to be detected, with less nonspecific binding to other proteins that resemble the one of interest.

In immunohistochemistry, a tissue section that one believes contains the protein of interest is incubated in a solution containing antibody (either monoclonal or polyclonal) against this protein. The antibody binds specifically to the protein and after a rinse to remove unbound antibody the protein's location in the tissue or cells can be seen with either the light or electron microscope by visualizing the antibody bound to its specific antigen. Antibodies are commonly tagged with fluorescent compounds, with peroxidase or alkaline phosphatase for histochemical detection, or with electron-dense gold particles for TEM.

As Figure 1–11 indicates, there are **direct and indirect methods of immunocytochemistry**. The direct method just utilizes a labeled antibody that binds the protein of interest.

Indirect immunohistochemistry involves sequential application of two antibodies and additional washing steps. The (primary) antibody specifically binding the protein of interest is not labeled. The detectible tag is conjugated to a **secondary antibody** made in an animal species different ("foreign") from that which made the primary antibody. For example, primary antibodies made by mouse lymphocytes (such as most monoclonal antibodies) are specifically recognized and bound by antibodies made in a rabbit or goat injected with mouse antibody immunoglobulin.

The indirect method is used more widely in research and pathologic tests because it is more sensitive, with the extra level of antibody binding serving to amplify the visible signal. Moreover, the same preparation of labeled secondary antibody can be used in studies with many different primary antibodies (specific for different antigens) if all these are made in the same animal species. There are other indirect methods that involve the use of other intermediate molecules, such as the biotin-avidin technique, which are also used to amplify detection signals.

Examples of indirect immunocytochemistry are shown in Figure 1–12, demonstrating the use of this method with cells in culture or after tissue sectioning for both light microscopy and TEM. Indirect immunohistochemistry has largely replaced autoradiography in studies of localized cell proliferation; by providing bromodeoxyuridine, a thymidine analog, instead of radiolabeled thymidine, nuclei of growing cells can be recognized by antibodies specific for bromodeoxyuridine incorporated into DNA, and the time-consuming steps of photographic processing are eliminated.

❯❯ MEDICAL APPLICATION

Because cells in some diseases, including many cancer cells, often produce proteins unique to their pathologic condition, immunohistochemistry can be used by pathologists to diagnose many diseases, including certain types of tumors and some virus-infected cells. Table 1–1 shows some applications of immunocytochemistry routinely used in clinical practice.

Hybridization Techniques

Hybridization usually implies the specific binding between two single strands of nucleic acid, which occurs under appropriate

---

FIGURE **1–11** Immunocytochemistry techniques.

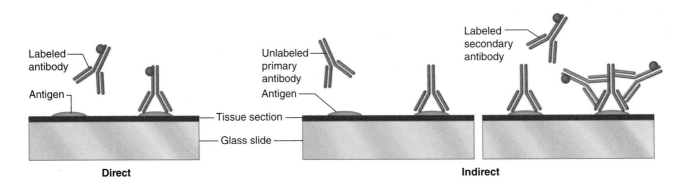

Immunocytochemistry (or immunohistochemistry) can be direct or indirect. **Direct immunocytochemistry** (left) uses an antibody made against the tissue protein of interest and tagged directly with a label such as a fluorescent compound or peroxidase. When placed with the tissue section on a slide, these labeled antibodies bind specifically to the protein (antigen) against which they were produced and can be visualized by the appropriate method. **Indirect immunocytochemistry** (right) uses first a **primary antibody** made against the protein (antigen) of interest and applied to the tissue section to bind its specific antigen. Then a **labeled secondary antibody** is obtained that was (1) made in another species against immunoglobulin proteins (antibodies) from the species in which the primary antibodies were made and (2) labeled with a fluorescent compound or peroxidase. When the labeled secondary antibody is applied to the tissue section, it specifically binds the primary antibodies, indirectly labeling the protein of interest on the slide. Because more than one labeled secondary antibody can bind each primary antibody molecule, labeling of the protein of interest is amplified by the indirect method.

FIGURE **1–12** Cells and tissues stained by immunohistochemistry.

cytoplasm. Primary antibodies against the filament protein desmin and fluorescein isothiocyanate (FITC)-labeled secondary antibodies were used in the indirect staining technique, with the nucleus counterstained blue with DAPI. (×650)

(b) A section of small intestine treated with an antibody against the enzyme lysozyme. The secondary antibody labeled with peroxidase was then applied and the localized brown color produced histochemically with the peroxidase substrate 3,3′-diamino-azobenzidine (DAB). The method demonstrates lysozyme-containing structures in scattered macrophages and in the large clusters of cells. Nuclei were counterstained with hematoxylin. (×100)

(c) A section of pancreatic cells in a TEM preparation incubated with an antibody against the enzyme amylase and then with protein A coupled with gold particles. Protein A has high affinity toward antibody molecules and the resulting image reveals the presence of amylase with the gold particles localized as very small black dots over dense secretory granules and developing granules (left). With specificity for immunoglobulin molecules, labeled protein A can be used to localize any primary antibody. (×5000)

(Figure 1–12c, reproduced with permission from Dr Moise Bendayan, Departments of Pathology and Cell Biology, University of Montreal, Montreal, Canada.)

Immunocytochemical methods to localize specific proteins can be applied to either light microscopic or TEM preparations using a variety of labels.

(a) A single cultured uterine cell stained fluorescently to reveal a meshwork of intermediate filaments (green) throughout the

conditions if the strands are complementary. The greater the similarities of their nucleotide sequences, the more readily the complementary strands form "hybrid" double-strand molecules. Hybridization at stringent conditions allows the specific identification of sequences in genes or RNA. This can occur with cellular DNA or RNA when nucleic acid sequences in solution are applied directly to prepared cells and tissue sections, a procedure called **in situ hybridization** (ISH).

TABLE **1–1** Examples of specific antigens with diagnostic importance.

Antigens	Diagnosis
Specific cytokeratins	Tumors of epithelial origin
Protein and polypeptide hormones	Certain endocrine tumors
Carcinoembryonic antigen (CEA)	Glandular tumors, mainly of the digestive tract and breast
Steroid hormone receptors	Breast duct cell tumors
Antigens produced by viruses	Specific virus infections

This technique is ideal for (1) determining if a cell has a specific sequence of DNA, such as a gene or part of a gene (Figure 1–13), (2) identifying the cells containing specific messenger RNAs (mRNAs) (in which the corresponding gene is being transcribed), or (3) determining the localization of a gene in a specific chromosome. DNA and RNA of the cells must be initially denatured by heat or other agents to become completely single-stranded, and the nucleotide sequences of interest are detected with **probes** consisting of single-stranded complementary DNA (cDNA). The probe may be obtained by cloning, by polymerase chain reaction (PCR) amplification of the target sequence, or by chemical synthesis if the desired sequence is short. The probe is toned with nucleotides containing a radioactive isotope (localized by autoradiography) or modified with a small compound such as digoxigenin (identified by immunocytochemistry). A solution containing the probe is placed over the specimen under conditions allowing hybridization and after the excess unbound probe is washed off, the localization of the hybridized probe is revealed through its label.

FIGURE **1–13** In situ hybridization (ISH).

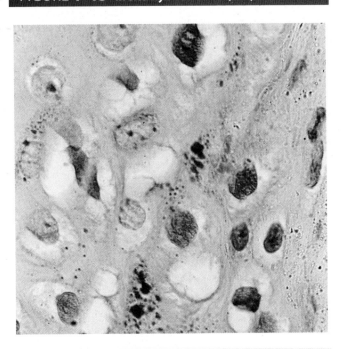

In situ hybridization of this tissue section with probes for the human papillomavirus (HPV) reveals the presence of many cells containing the virus. The section was incubated with a solution containing a digoxigenin-labeled complementary DNA (cDNA) probe for the HPV DNA. The probe was then visualized by direct immunohistochemistry using peroxidase-labeled antibodies against digoxigenin. This procedure stains brown only those cells containing HPV. (×400; H&E)

(*Reproduced with permission from Dr Jose E. Levi, Virology Lab, Institute of Tropical Medicine, University of São Paulo, Brazil.*)

❯ INTERPRETATION OF STRUCTURES IN TISSUE SECTIONS

In studying and interpreting stained tissue sections, it is important to remember that microscopic preparations are the result of a series of processes that began with collecting the tissue and ended with mounting a coverslip on the slide. Certain steps in this procedure may distort the tissues slightly, producing minor structural abnormalities called **artifacts** not present in the living tissue.

One such distortion is minor shrinkage of cells or tissue regions produced by the fixative, by the ethanol or by the heat needed for paraffin embedding. Shrinkage can create artificial spaces between cells and other tissue components. Such spaces can also result from the loss of lipids or low-molecular-weight substances not preserved by the fixative or removed by the dehydrating and clearing fluids. Slight cracks in sections may also appear as large spaces in the tissue.

Other artifacts may include small wrinkles in the section (which the novice may confuse with linear structures in tissue) and precipitates from the stain (which may be confused with cellular structures such as cytoplasmic granules). Students must be aware of the existence of artifacts and able to recognize them.

Another difficulty in the study of histologic sections is the impossibility of differentially staining all tissue components on one slide. A single stain can seldom clearly demonstrate nuclei, mitochondria, lysosomes, basement membranes, elastic fibers, etc. With the light microscope, it is necessary to examine preparations stained by different methods before an idea of the whole composition and structure of a cell or tissue can be obtained. The TEM allows the observation of cells with all its internal structures and surrounding ECM components, but only a few cells in a tissue can be conveniently studied in these very small samples.

Finally, when a structure's **three-dimensional** volume is cut into very thin sections, the sections appear microscopically to have only two dimensions: length and width. When examining a section under the microscope, the viewer must always keep in mind that components are missing in front of and behind what is being seen because many tissue structures are thicker than the section. Round structures seen microscopically may be portions of either spheres or tubes. Because structures in a tissue have different orientations, their two-dimensional (2D) appearance will also vary depending on the plane of section. A single convoluted tube will appear in a tissue section as many separate rounded or oval structures (Figure 1–14).

FIGURE **1–14** Interpretation of 3D structures in 2D sections.

In thin sections, 3D structures appear to have only two dimensions. Such images must be interpreted correctly to understand the actual structure of tissue and organ components. For example, blood vessels and other tubular structures appear in sections as round or oval shapes whose size and shape depend on the transverse or oblique angle of the cut. A highly coiled tube will appear as several round and oval structures. In TEM sections of cells, round structures may represent spherical organelles or transverse cuts through tubular organelles such as mitochondria. It is important to develop such interpretive skills to understand tissue and cell morphology in microscopic preparations.

Histology & Its Methods of Study   SUMMARY OF KEY POINTS

Preparation of Tissues for Study

- Chemical **fixatives** such as formalin are used to preserve tissue structure by cross-linking and denaturing proteins, inactivating enzymes, and preventing cell autolysis or self-digestion.
- **Dehydration** of the fixed tissue in alcohol and **clearing** in organic solvents prepare it for embedding and sectioning.
- **Embedding** in paraffin wax or epoxy resin allows the tissue to be cut into very thin sections (slices) with a microtome.
- Sections are mounted on glass slides for **staining**, which is required to reveal specific cellular and tissue components with the microscope.
- The most used staining method is a combination of the dyes hematoxylin and eosin, **H&E**, which act as basic and acidic stains, respectively.
- Cell substances with a net negative (anionic) charge, such as DNA and RNA, react strongly with hematoxylin and basic stains; such material is said to be "**basophilic.**"
- Cationic substances, such as collagen and many cytoplasmic proteins react with eosin and other acidic stains and are said to be "**acidophilic.**"

Light Microscopy (LM)

- **Bright**-field microscopy, the method usually employed by both students and pathologists, uses **ordinary light**, a system of **glass lenses** (like other LM methods), and stained sections to distinguish tissue components by variously colored stain affinities.
- **Fluorescence microscopy** uses **UV light**, under which only fluorescent molecules are visible, allowing localization of fluorescent probes which can be much more specific than routine stains.
- **Phase-contrast microscopy** uses the **differences in refractive index** of various natural cell and tissue components to produce an image without staining, allowing observation of living cells.
- **Confocal microscopy** involves scanning the specimen at successive focal planes with a focused light beam, often from a laser, and produces a 3D reconstruction from the images.

Electron Microscopy

- **Transmission electron microscopy (TEM)** utilizes ultrathin sections, special "stains" containing **heavy metal salts**, and an electromagnetically focused **electron beam** to produce black & white images with roughly 10-fold better resolution than is possible with LM.
- **Scanning electron microscopy (SEM)** uses tissue coated with heavy metal atoms and an electron beam played across this coated surface, with reflected electrons captured electronically to produce a high-resolution, 3D image of that surface.

Autoradiography

- This process localizes cell components synthesized from **radioactive precursors** by detecting silver grains produced by the radiation in a photographic emulsion coating a tissue section or cells after fixation.
- With either light microscopy or TEM, autoradiography permits unique studies of processes such as tissue growth (using radioactive DNA precursors) or cellular pathways of macromolecular synthesis.

Cell & Tissue Culture

- Cells can be grown in vitro from newly **explanted** tissues (primary cultures) or as long-established cell lines and can be examined in the living state by phase-contrast light microscopy.

Enzyme Histochemistry

- **Histochemical (or cytochemical) techniques** use specific enzymatic activities in lightly fixed or unfixed tissue sections to produce visible products in the specific enzyme locations.
- Fixation and paraffin embedding denatures most enzymes, but histochemistry usually uses **frozen tissue** sectioned with a **cryostat** so that endogenous enzymes can generate the stain.
- Enzyme classes commonly studied by histochemistry include phosphatases, dehydrogenases, and peroxidases, with peroxidase often conjugated to antibodies used in immunohistochemistry.

Visualizing Specific Molecules

- Some substances specifically bind certain targets in cells.
- **Immunohistochemistry** is based on specific reactions between an antigen and antibodies labeled with visible markers, often fluorescent compounds or peroxidase for light microscopy and gold particles for TEM.
- If the cell or tissue antigen of interest is detected by directly binding a labeled **primary antibody** specific for that antigen, the process is considered **direct immunohistochemistry**.
- **Indirect immunohistochemistry** uses an unlabeled primary antibody that is detected bound to its antigen with labeled **secondary antibodies**.
- The indirect immunohistochemical method is more commonly used because the added level of antibody binding amplifies the signal detected and provides greater technical flexibility.

- Specific gene sequences or mRNAs of cells can be detected microscopically using labeled cDNA probes in a technique called **in situ hybridization (ISH)**.

Interpretation of Structures in Tissue Sections

- Many steps in tissue processing, slide preparation, and staining can introduce minor **artifacts** such as spaces and precipitates that are not normally present in the living tissue and must be recognized.
- Sections of cells or tissues are essentially 2D planes through 3D structures, and understanding this fact is important for their correct interpretation and study.

Histology & Its Methods of Study ASSESS YOUR KNOWLEDGE

1. In preparing tissue for routine light microscopic study, which procedure immediately precedes clearing the specimen with an organic solvent?
   a. Dehydration
   b. Fixation
   c. Staining
   d. Clearing
   e. Embedding

2. Which of the following staining procedures relies on the cationic and anionic properties of the material to be stained?
   a. Enzyme histochemistry
   b. PAS reaction
   c. H&E staining
   d. Immunohistochemistry
   e. Metal impregnation techniques

3. In a light microscope used for histology, resolution and magnification of cells are largely dependent on which component?
   a. Condenser
   b. Objective lens
   c. Eyepieces or ocular lenses
   d. Specimen slide
   e. The control for illumination intensity

4. Cellular storage deposits of glycogen, a free polysaccharide, could best be detected histologically using what procedure?
   a. Autoradiography
   b. Electron microscopy
   c. Enzyme histochemistry
   d. H&E staining
   e. PAS reaction

5. Adding heavy metal compounds to the fixative and ultrathin sectioning of the embedded tissue with a glass knife are techniques used for which histologic procedure?
   a. Scanning electron microscopy
   b. Fluorescent microscopy
   c. Enzyme histochemistry
   d. Confocal microscopy
   e. TEM

6. Resolution in electron microscopy greatly exceeds that of light microscopy due to which of the following?
   a. The wavelength of the electrons in the microscope beam is shorter than that of a beam of light.
   b. The lenses of an electron microscope are of greatly improved quality.
   c. For electron microscopy, the tissue specimen does not require staining.
   d. The electron microscope allows much greater magnification of a projected image than a light microscope provides.
   e. An electron microscope can be much more finely controlled than a light microscope.

7. Microscopic autoradiography uses radioactivity and can be employed to study what features in a tissue section?
   a. The types of enzymes found in various cell locations
   b. Cellular sites where various macromolecules are synthesized
   c. The sequences of mRNA made in the cells
   d. The dimensions of structures within the cells
   e. The locations of genes transcribed for specific mRNA

8. To identify and localize a specific protein within cells or the ECM, one would best use what approach?
   a. Autoradiography
   b. Enzyme histochemistry
   c. Immunohistochemistry
   d. TEM
   e. Polarizing microscopy

9. In situ hybridization is a histologic technique used to visualize what type of macromolecule?
   a. Proteins
   b. Carbohydrates
   c. Certain enzymes
   d. Nucleic acids
   e. Lipids

10. Hospital laboratories frequently use unfixed, frozen tissue specimens sectioned with a cryostat for rapid staining, microscopic examination, and diagnosis of pathologic conditions. Besides saving much time by avoiding fixation and procedures required for paraffin embedding, frozen sections retain and allow study of what macromolecules normally lost in the paraffin procedure?
    a. Carbohydrates
    b. Small mRNA
    c. Basic proteins
    d. Acidic proteins
    e. Lipids

Answers: 1a, 2c, 3b, 4e, 5e, 6a, 7b, 8c, 9d, 10e

2 The Cytoplasm

Cells and extracellular material together comprise the tissues that make up animal organs. In all tissues, cells are the basic structural and functional units, the smallest living parts of the body. Animal cells are enclosed by cell membranes and are **eukaryotic**, each with a distinct, membrane-enclosed **nucleus** surrounded by **cytoplasm**, fluid containing a system of membranous organelles, non-membranous macromolecular assemblies, and polymerized cytoskeletal proteins. In contrast, much smaller bacterial cells are prokaryotic, with cell walls but lacking nuclei, membranous cytoplasmic structures, and cytoskeletons.

CELL DIFFERENTIATION

The average adult human body consists of nearly 40 trillion cells, according to the best available estimate. These cells exist as hundreds of histologically distinct cell types, all derived from the zygote, the single cell formed by the merger of a spermatozoon with an oocyte at fertilization. The first zygotic cellular divisions produce cells called **blastomeres**, and as part of the early embryo's inner cell mass blastomeres give rise to all tissue types of the fetus. Explanted to tissue culture cells of the inner cell mass are called **embryonic stem cells**. Most cells of the fetus undergo a specialization process called **differentiation** in which they predominantly express sets of genes that mediate specific cytoplasmic activities, becoming efficiently organized in tissues with specialized functions and usually changing their shape accordingly. For example, muscle cell precursors elongate into long, fiber-like cells containing large arrays of actin and myosin. All animal cells contain actin filaments and myosins, but muscle cells are specialized for using these proteins to convert chemical energy into forceful contractions.

Major cellular functions performed by specialized cells in the body are listed in Table 2–1. It is important to understand that the functions listed there can be performed by most cells of the body; specialized cells have greatly expanded their capacity for one or more of these functions during differentiation. Changes in cells' microenvironments under normal and pathologic conditions can cause the same cell type to have variable features and activities. Cells that appear similar structurally often have different families of receptors for signaling molecules such as hormones and extracellular matrix (ECM) components, causing them to behave differently. For example, because of their diverse arrays of receptors, breast fibroblasts and uterine smooth muscle cells are exceptionally sensitive to female sex hormones, while most other fibroblasts and smooth muscle cells are insensitive.

THE PLASMA MEMBRANE

The **plasma membrane** (**cell membrane** or plasmalemma) that envelops every eukaryotic cell consists of phospholipids, cholesterol, and proteins, with oligosaccharide chains covalently linked to many of the phospholipids and proteins. This limiting membrane functions as a selective barrier regulating the passage of materials into and out of the cell and facilitating the transport of specific molecules. One important role

TABLE **2–1**	Differentiated cells typically specialize in one activity.
General Cellular Activity	**Specialized Cell(s)**
Movement	Muscle and other contractile cells
Form adhesive and tight junctions between cells	Epithelial cells
Synthesize and secrete components of the extracellular matrix	Fibroblasts, cells of bone and cartilage
Convert physical and chemical stimuli into action potentials	Neurons and sensory cells
Synthesis and secretion of degradative enzymes	Cells of digestive glands
Synthesis and secretion of glycoproteins	Cells of mucous glands
Synthesis and secretion of steroids	Certain cells of the adrenal gland, testis, and ovary
Ion transport	Cells of the kidney and salivary gland ducts
Intracellular digestion	Macrophages and neutrophils
Lipid storage	Fat cells
Metabolite absorption	Cells lining the intestine

of the cell membrane is to keep constant the ion content of cytoplasm, which differs from that of the extracellular fluid. Membrane proteins also perform many specific recognition and signaling functions, playing a key role in the interactions of the cell with its environment.

Although the plasma membrane defines the outer limit of the cell, a continuum exists between the interior of the cell and extracellular macromolecules. Certain plasma membrane proteins, the **integrins**, are linked to both the cytoskeleton and ECM components and allow continuous exchange of influences in both directions between the cytoplasm and material in the ECM.

Membranes range from 7.5 to 10 nm in thickness and consequently are visible only in the transmission electron microscope (TEM). The line between adjacent cells sometimes seen faintly with the light microscope consists of plasma membrane proteins plus extracellular material, which together can reach a dimension visible by light microscopy.

Membrane phospholipids are amphipathic, consisting of two nonpolar (hydrophobic or water-repelling) long-chain fatty acids linked to a charged polar (hydrophilic or water-attracting) head that bears a phosphate group (Figure 2–1a). Phospholipids are most stable when organized into a double layer (bilayer) with the hydrophobic fatty acid chains located in a middle region away from water and the hydrophilic polar head groups contacting the water (Figure 2–1b). Molecules of cholesterol, a sterol lipid, insert at varying densities among the closely packed phospholipid fatty acids, restricting their movements and modulating the fluidity of all membrane components. Phospholipids in each half of the bilayer are different. For example, in the well-studied membranes of red blood cells, phosphatidylcholine and sphingomyelin are more abundant in the outer half, while phosphatidylserine and phosphatidylethanolamine are more concentrated in the inner layer. Some of the outer layer's lipids, known as **glycolipids**, include oligosaccharide chains that extend outward from the cell surface and contribute to a delicate cell-surface coating called the **glycocalyx** (Figures 2–1b and 2–2). With the TEM the cell membrane—as well as all cytoplasmic membranes—may exhibit a trilaminar appearance after fixation in osmium tetroxide; osmium binds the polar heads of the phospholipids and the oligosaccharide chains, producing the two dark outer lines that enclose the light band of osmium-free fatty acids (Figure 2–1b).

Proteins are major constituents of membranes (~50% by weight in the plasma membrane). **Integral proteins** are incorporated directly within the lipid bilayer, whereas **peripheral proteins** are bound to one of the two membrane surfaces, particularly on the cytoplasmic side (Figure 2–2). Peripheral proteins can be extracted from cell membranes with salt solutions, whereas integral proteins can be extracted only by using detergents to disrupt the lipids. The polypeptide chains of many integral proteins span the membrane, from one side to the other, several times and are accordingly called **multipass proteins**. Integration of the proteins within the lipid bilayer is mainly the result of hydrophobic interactions between the lipids and nonpolar amino acids of the proteins.

Freeze-fracture electron-microscope studies of membranes show that parts of many integral proteins protrude from both the outer and inner membrane surface (Figure 2–2b). Like those of glycolipids the carbohydrate moieties of glycoproteins project from the external surface of the plasma membrane and contribute to the glycocalyx (Figure 2–3). They are important components of proteins acting as **receptors**, which participate in important interactions such as cell adhesion, cell recognition, and the response to protein hormones. As with lipids the distribution of membrane polypeptides is different in the two surfaces of the cell membranes, making all membranes in the cell asymmetric.

Studies with labeled membrane proteins of cultured cells reveal that many such proteins are not bound rigidly in place and are able to move laterally (Figure 2–4). Such observations as well as data from biochemical, electron microscopic, and other studies showed that membrane proteins comprise a moveable mosaic within the fluid lipid bilayer, the well-established **fluid mosaic model** for membrane structure (Figure 2–2a). Unlike the lipids, however, lateral diffusion of many membrane proteins is often restricted by their cytoskeletal attachments. Moreover, in most epithelial cells tight junctions between the cells (see Chapter 4) also restrict lateral diffusion of unattached transmembrane proteins and outer layer lipids, producing different domains within the cells' membranes.

FIGURE **2–1** Lipids in membrane structure.

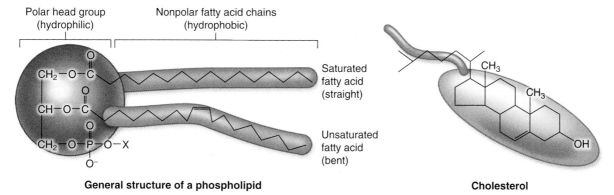

General structure of a phospholipid

Cholesterol

a

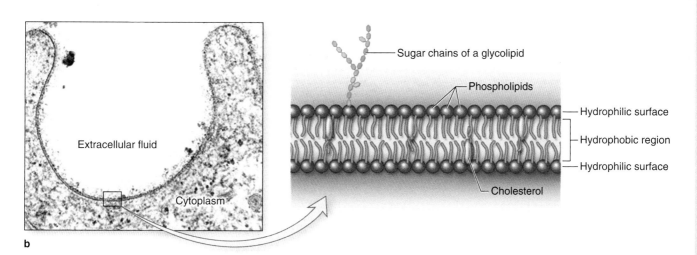

b

(a) Membranes of animal cells have as their major lipid components **phospholipids** and **cholesterol**. A phospholipid is amphipathic, with a phosphate group charge on the polar head and two long, nonpolar fatty acid chains, which can be straight (saturated) or kinked (at an unsaturated bond). Membrane cholesterol is present in about the same amount as phospholipid.

(b) The amphipathic nature of phospholipids produces the bilayer structure of membranes as the charged (hydrophilic) polar heads spontaneously form each membrane surface, in direct contact with water, and the hydrophobic nonpolar fatty acid chains are buried in the membrane's middle, away from water. Cholesterol molecules are also amphipathic and are interspersed less evenly

throughout the lipid bilayer; cholesterol affects the packing of the fatty acid chains, with a major effect on membrane fluidity. The outer layer of the cell membrane also contains **glycolipids** with extended carbohydrate chains.

Sectioned, osmium-fixed cell membrane may have a faint trilaminar appearance with the transmission electron microscope (TEM), showing two dark (electron-dense) lines enclosing a clear (electron-lucent) band. Reduced osmium accumulates on the hydrophilic phosphate groups present on each side of the internal region of fatty acid chains where osmium is not deposited. The "fuzzy" material on the outer surface of the membrane represents the **glycocalyx** of oligosaccharides of glycolipids and glycoproteins. (×100,000)

Membrane proteins that are components of large enzyme complexes are also usually less mobile, especially those involved in the transduction of signals from outside the cell. Such protein complexes occur in specialized membrane patches termed **lipid rafts** with higher concentrations of cholesterol and saturated fatty acids reducing lipid fluidity. This together with the presence of scaffold proteins, that maintain spatial relationships between enzymes and signaling proteins, allows the proteins assembled within lipid rafts to remain close and interact more efficiently.

Transmembrane Proteins & Membrane Transport

The plasma membrane is the site where materials are exchanged between the cell and its environment. Most small molecules cross the membrane by the general mechanisms shown schematically in Figure 2–5 and explained as follows:

▪ **Diffusion** transports small, nonpolar molecules directly through the lipid bilayer. Lipophilic (fat-soluble) molecules diffuse through membranes readily, water very slowly.

FIGURE **2–2** Proteins associated with the membrane lipid bilayer.

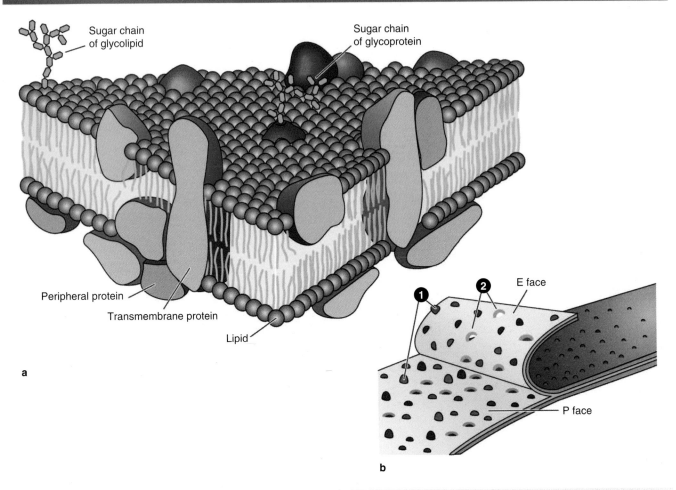

Sugar chain of glycolipid

Sugar chain of glycoprotein

Peripheral protein

Transmembrane protein

Lipid

a

E face

P face

b

(a) The fluid mosaic model of membrane structure emphasizes that the phospholipid bilayer of a membrane also contains proteins inserted in it or associated with its surface (peripheral proteins) and that these proteins can move within the fluid lipid phase. **Integral proteins** are firmly embedded in the lipid layers, with those that completely span the bilayer called **transmembrane proteins**. Hydrophobic amino acids of these proteins interact with the hydrophobic fatty acid portions of the membrane lipids. Both the proteins and lipids may have externally exposed oligosaccharide chains.

(b) When cells are frozen and fractured (**cryofracture**) the lipid bilayer of membranes often splits along the hydrophobic center, at the line of weakness formed by the fatty acid tails of phospholipids. Electron microscopy of such cryofracture preparation replicas provides a useful method for studying membrane structures. Most of the protruding membrane particles seen (1) are proteins or aggregates of proteins that remain attached to the half of the membrane adjacent to the cytoplasm (P or protoplasmic face). Fewer particles are found attached to the outer half of the membrane (E or extracellular face). Each protein bulging on one surface has a corresponding depression (2) on the opposite surface.

■ **Channels** are multipass proteins forming transmembrane pores through which ions or small molecules pass selectively. Cells open and close specific channels for Na^+, K^+, Ca^{2+}, and other ions in response to various physiological stimuli. Water molecules usually cross the plasma membrane through channel proteins called **aquaporins**.

■ **Carriers** are transmembrane proteins that bind small molecules and translocate them across the membrane via conformational changes in the proteins.

Diffusion, channels, and carrier proteins operate passively, allowing movement of substances across membranes down a concentration gradient due to its kinetic energy. In contrast, membrane **pumps** are enzymes engaged in **active transport**, utilizing energy from the hydrolysis of adenosine triphosphate (ATP) to move ions and other solutes across membranes, against often steep concentration gradients. Because they consume ATP pumps are also called **ATPases**.

These transport mechanisms are summarized with additional detail in Table 2–2.

FIGURE **2–3** Membrane proteins.

Phospholipid

Glycolipid

Carbohydrate

Interstitial fluid

Polar head of
phospholipid
molecule

Phospholipid
bilayer

Glycoprotein

Protein

Nonpolar tails
of phospholipid
molecule

Cholesterol

Integral protein

Peripheral protein

Filaments of
cytoskeleton

Cytosol

Functions of Plasma Membrane

1. **Physical barrier:** Establishes a flexible boundary, protects cellular contents, and supports cell structure. Phospholipid bilayer separates substances inside and outside the cell.
2. **Selective permeability:** Regulates entry and exit of ions, nutrients, and waste molecules through the membrane.
3. **Electrochemical gradients:** Establishes and maintains an electrical charge difference across the plasma membrane.
4. **Communication:** Contains receptors that recognize and respond to molecular signals.

Both protein and lipid components often have covalently attached oligosaccharide chains exposed at the external membrane surface. These contribute to the cell's **glycocalyx**, which provides important antigenic and functional properties to the cell surface. Membrane proteins serve as receptors for various signals coming from outside cells, as parts of intercellular connections, and as selective gateways for molecules entering the cell.

Transmembrane proteins often have multiple hydrophobic regions buried within the lipid bilayer to produce a channel or other active site for specific transfer of substances through the membrane.

Transport by Vesicles: Endocytosis & Exocytosis

Macromolecules normally enter cells by being enclosed within folds of plasma membrane (often after binding specific membrane receptors) which fuse and pinch off internally as spherical cytoplasmic **vesicles** (or vacuoles) in a general process known as **endocytosis**. Three major types of endocytosis are recognized, as summarized in Table 2–2 and Figure 2–6.

1. **Phagocytosis** ("cell eating") is the ingestion of particles such as bacteria or dead cell remnants. Certain blood-derived cells, such as macrophages and neutrophils, are specialized for this activity. When a bacterium becomes bound to the surface of a neutrophil, it becomes surrounded by extensions of plasmalemma and cytoplasm which project from the cell in a process dependent on cytoskeletal changes. Fusion of the membranous folds encloses the bacterium in an intracellular vacuole called a **phagosome**, which then merges with a lysosome for degradation of its contents as discussed later in this chapter.

2. **Pinocytosis** ("cell drinking") involves smaller invaginations of the cell membrane which fuse and entrap extracellular fluid and its dissolved contents. The resulting **pinocytotic vesicles** (~80 nm in diameter) then pinch off inwardly from the cell surface and either fuse with lysosomes or move to the opposite cell surface where they fuse with the membrane and release their contents outside the cell. The latter process, called **transcytosis**, accomplishes bulk transfer of dissolved substances across the cell.

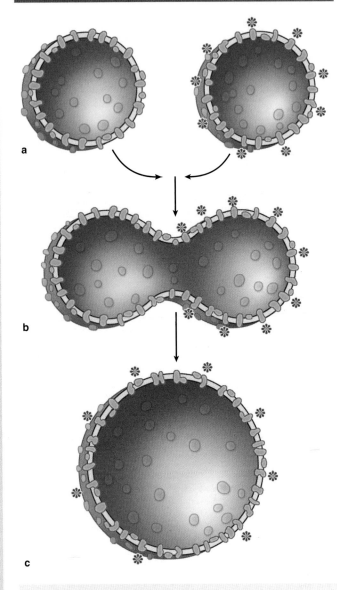

(a) Two types of cells were grown in tissue cultures, one with fluorescently labeled transmembrane proteins in the plasmalemma (right) and one without.

(b) Cells of each type were fused together experimentally into hybrid cells.

(c) Minutes after the fusion of the cell membranes, the fluorescent proteins of the labeled cell spread to the entire surface of the hybrid cells. Such experiments provide important data supporting the fluid mosaic model. However, many membrane proteins show more restricted lateral movements, being anchored in place by links to the cytoskeleton.

3. **Receptor-mediated endocytosis:** Receptors for many substances, such as low-density lipoproteins and protein hormones, are integral membrane proteins at the cell surface.

High-affinity binding of such **ligands** to their receptors causes these proteins to aggregate in special membrane regions that then invaginate and pinch off internally as vesicles.

The formation and fate of vesicles in receptor-mediated endocytosis also often depend on specific peripheral proteins on the cytoplasmic side of the membrane (Figure 2–7). The occupied cell-surface receptors associate with these cytoplasmic proteins and begin to invaginate as **coated pits**. The electron-dense coating on the cytoplasmic surface of such pits contains several polypeptides, the major one being **clathrin**. Clathrin molecules interact like the struts of a geodesic dome, forming that region of cell membrane into a cage-like invagination that soon pinches off into the cytoplasm as a **coated vesicle** (Figure 2–7b) with the receptor-bound ligands inside. Another type of receptor-mediated endocytosis prominent in very thin cells produces invaginations called **caveolae** (L. *caveolae*, little caves) that involve a family of integral membrane proteins called caveolins associated with diverse peripheral proteins called cavins.

In all these endocytotic processes the vesicles or vacuoles produced quickly enter and fuse with the **endosomal compartment**, a dynamic collection of membranous tubules and vacuoles in the peripheral cytoplasm (Figure 2–7). Phagosomes and pinocytotic vesicles typically fuse with lysosomes within the endosomal compartment for digestion of their contents, while molecules entering by receptor-mediated endocytosis may be directed down other pathways. The membranes of many late endosomes have ATP-driven H^+ pumps that acidify their interior, activating the hydrolytic enzymes of lysosomes, and in other endosomes causing ligands to uncouple from their receptors, after which the two molecules are sorted into separate endosomes. Receptors are often sorted into recycling endosomes and returned to the cell surface for reuse. Low-density lipoprotein receptors, for example, undergo repeated rounds of recycling. Other endosomes may release their entire contents at a separate domain of the cell membrane (transcytosis), which occurs in many epithelial cells.

Clathrin molecules separate from coated vesicles and recycle back to the cell membrane for the formation of new coated pits. Vesicle trafficking through the endosomal compartment includes direction by peripheral membrane G-proteins called **Rab proteins**, small GTPases that bind guanine nucleotides and associated proteins.

Movement of large molecules from inside to outside the cell usually involves vesicular transport in the process of **exocytosis**. In exocytosis, a cytoplasmic vesicle containing the molecules to be secreted fuses with the plasma membrane, resulting in the release of its contents into the extracellular space without compromising the integrity of the plasma membrane (see "Transcytosis" in Figure 2–7a). Exocytosis is triggered in many cells by a transient increase in cytosolic Ca^{2+}. Membrane fusion during exocytosis is highly regulated, with selective interactions between several specific membrane proteins.

FIGURE **2–5**   Major mechanisms by which molecules cross membranes.

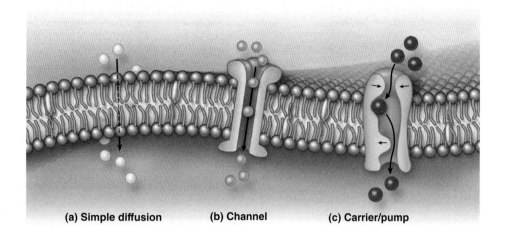

(a) Simple diffusion   **(b) Channel**   **(c) Carrier/pump**

Lipophilic and some small, uncharged molecules can cross membranes by **simple diffusion (a).**

Most ions cross membranes in multipass proteins called **channels (b)** whose structures include transmembrane ion-specific pores. Many other larger, water-soluble molecules require binding to sites on selective **carrier proteins (c)**, which then change their conformations and release the molecule to the other side of the membrane.

Diffusion, channels, and most carrier proteins translocate substances across membranes using only kinetic energy. In contrast, **pumps** are carrier proteins for active transport of ions or other solutes and require energy derived from ATP.

Exocytosis of macromolecules made by cells occurs via either of two pathways:

- **Constitutive secretion** is used for products that are released from cells continuously, as soon as synthesis is complete, such as collagen subunits for the ECM.
- **Regulated secretion** occurs in response to signals coming to the cells, such as the release of digestive enzymes from pancreatic cells in response to specific stimuli. Regulated exocytosis of stored products from epithelial cells usually occurs specifically at the apical domains of cells, constituting a major mechanism of glandular secretion (see Chapter 4).

Portions of the cell membrane become part of the endocytotic vesicles or vacuoles during endocytosis; during exocytosis membrane returns to the cell surface, a process referred to as **membrane trafficking** (see Figure 2–7a). Trafficking of membrane components occurs continuously in most cells and is not only crucial for maintaining the cell size but also for physiologically important processes such as reducing blood lipid levels.

In many cells subpopulations of vacuoles and tubules within the endosomal compartment accumulate small vesicles *within* their lumens by further invaginations of their limiting membranes, becoming **multivesicular bodies**. Multivesicular bodies may merge with lysosomes for selective degradation of their content, or they may also fuse with the plasma membrane and release their intraluminal vesicles outside the cell as **exosomes**. These small (50-150 nm diameter) released vesicles can fuse with other cells, transferring their contents and membranes in another form of cell-to-cell communication.

Signal Reception & Transduction

Cells in a multicellular organism communicate with one another to regulate tissue and organ development, to control their growth and division, and to coordinate their functions. Adjacent cells often form communicating **gap junctions** that couple the two cells and allow exchange of ions and small molecules (see Chapter 4).

Cells also use about two dozen families of **receptors** to detect and respond to various extracellular molecules and physical stimuli. Each cell type in the body contains a distinctive set of cell surface and cytoplasmic receptor proteins that enable it to respond to a complementary set of signaling molecules in a specific, programmed way. Cells bearing receptors for a specific ligand are the **target cells** for that molecule. The routes signal molecules take from source to target cells provide one way to categorize signaling processes:

- In **endocrine signaling**, the signal molecules (here called **hormones**) move in the blood from their sources to target cells throughout the body.
- In **paracrine signaling**, the chemical ligand diffuses in extracellular fluid but is rapidly metabolized, limiting its effect only local to target cells near its source.
- In **synaptic signaling**, a specialized type of paracrine interaction, neurotransmitters act on adjacent cells through special contact areas called **synapses** (see Chapter 9).

TABLE **2–2**	Mechanisms of transport across the plasma membrane.	
Process	**Type of Movement**	**Example**
PASSIVE PROCESSES	Movement of substances down a concentration gradient due to the kinetic energy of the substance; no expenditure of cellular energy is required; continues until equilibrium is reached (if unopposed)	
Simple diffusion	Unassisted net movement of small, nonpolar substances down their concentration gradient across a selectively permeable membrane	Exchange of oxygen and carbon dioxide between blood and body tissues
Facilitated diffusion	Movement of ions and small, polar molecules down their concentration gradient; assisted across a selectively permeable membrane by a transport protein	
Channel-mediated	Movement of ion down its concentration gradient through a protein channel	Na^+ moves through Na^+ channel into cell
Carrier-mediated	Movement of small, polar molecule down its concentration gradient by a carrier protein	Transport of glucose into cells by glucose carrier
Osmosis	Diffusion of water across a selectively permeable membrane; direction is determined by relative solute concentrations; continues until equilibrium is reached	Solutes in blood in systemic capillaries "pulls" fluid from interstitial space back into the blood
ACTIVE PROCESSES	Movement of substances requires expenditure of cellular energy	
Active transport	Transport of ions or small molecules across the membrane against a concentration gradient by transmembrane protein pumps	
Primary	Movement of substance up its concentration gradient; powered directly by ATP	Ca^{2+} pumps transport Ca^{2+} out of the cell Na^+/K^+ pump moves Na^+ out of the cell and K^+ into the cell
Secondary	Movement of a substance up its concentration gradient is powered by harnessing the movement of a second substance (eg, Na^+) down its concentration gradient	
Symport	Movement of substance up its concentration gradient in the same direction as Na^+	Na^+/glucose transport
Antiport	Movement of substance up its concentration gradient in the opposite direction from Na^+	Na^+/H^+ transport
Vesicular transport	Vesicle formed or lost as material is brought into a cell or released from a cell	
Exocytosis	Bulk movement of substance out of the cell by fusion of secretory vesicles with the plasma membrane	Release of neurotransmitter by nerve cells
Endocytosis	Bulk movement of substances into the cell by vesicles forming at the plasma membrane	
Phagocytosis	Type of endocytosis in which vesicles are formed as particulate materials external to the cell are engulfed by pseudopodia	White blood cell engulfing a bacterium
Pinocytosis	Type of endocytosis in which vesicles are formed as interstitial fluid is taken up by the cell	Formation of small vesicles in capillary wall to move substances
Receptor-mediated endocytosis	Type of endocytosis in which plasma membrane receptors first bind specific substances; receptor and bound substance then taken up by the cell	Uptake of cholesterol into cells

FIGURE 2–6 Three major forms of endocytosis.

a Phagocytosis

c Receptor-mediated endocytosis

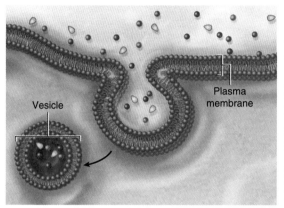

b Pinocytosis

There are three general types of endocytosis:

(a) Phagocytosis involves the extension from the cell of surface folds or pseudopodia which engulf particles such as bacteria, and then internalize this material into a cytoplasmic vacuole or **phagosome**.

(b) In **pinocytosis** the cell membrane forms similar folds or invaginates (dimples inward) to create a pit containing a drop of extracellular fluid. The pit pinches off inside the cell when the cell membrane fuses and forms a pinocytotic vesicle containing the fluid.

(c) Receptor-mediated endocytosis includes membrane proteins called **receptors** that bind specific molecules (ligands). When many such receptors are bound by their ligands, they aggregate in one membrane region, which then invaginates and pinches off to create a vesicle or **endosome** containing both the receptors and the bound ligands.

- In **autocrine signaling**, signals bind receptors on the same cells that produced the signal molecule.
- In **juxtacrine signaling**, important in early embryonic tissue interactions, the signaling molecules are cell membrane-bound proteins, which bind surface receptors of the target cell when the two cells make direct physical contact.

Receptors for hydrophilic signaling molecules, including polypeptide hormones and neurotransmitters, are usually transmembrane proteins in the plasmalemma of target cells. Figure 2–8 shows three important functional classes of such receptors:

- **Channel-linked receptors** open associated channels upon ligand binding to promote transfer of molecules or ions across the membrane.
- **Enzymatic receptors** are usually protein kinases in which ligand binding induces activation and phosphorylation of other proteins.
- **G-protein–coupled receptors** upon ligand binding stimulate associated G-proteins to bind the guanine nucleotide GTP and be released to activate other cytoplasmic proteins.

›› MEDICAL APPLICATION

Certain diseases are caused by defective receptors. For example, **pseudohypoparathyroidism** and one type of **dwarfism** involve nonfunctioning parathyroid and growth hormone receptors, respectively. In these two conditions, the glands produce the respective hormones, but the target cells cannot respond because they lack normal receptors.

Ligands binding such receptors in a cell membrane represent first messengers, beginning a process of **signal transduction** by activating a series of intermediary enzymes downstream to produce changes in the cytoplasm, the nucleus, or both. Channel-mediated ion influx or activation of kinases can activate various cytoplasmic proteins, amplifying the signal. Activated G-proteins target ion channels or other membrane-bound effectors that also propagate the signal further into the cell (Figure 2–8). One such effector protein is the enzyme adenyl cyclase which generates the second messenger molecule, cyclic adenosine monophosphate (cAMP). Other second messengers include 1,2-diacylglycerol (DAG) and inositol 1,4,5-triphosphate (IP_3). Production of ionic changes or second messengers amplifies the first signal and triggers a

FIGURE **2–7**   Receptor-mediated endocytosis involves regulated membrane trafficking.

Major steps during and after endocytosis are indicated diagrammatically in part **a**. Ligands bind with high affinity to specific surface receptors, which then associate with specific cytoplasmic proteins, including clathrin and adaptor proteins, and aggregate in membrane regions to form **coated pits**. Clathrin facilitates invagination of the pits, and another peripheral membrane protein, **dynamin**, forms constricting loops around the developing neck of the pit, causing the invagination to pinch off as a **coated vesicle**. The clathrin lattice of coated pits **(CP)** and vesicles **(CV)** is shown ultrastructurally in part **b**.

Internalized vesicles lose their clathrin coats, which are recycled, and fuse with other endosomes that comprise the **endosomal compartment**. Ligands may have different fates within the endosomal compartment:

- Receptors and ligands may move to late endosomes and then to lysosomes for degradation.
- Ligands may separate from their receptors, with the empty receptors sequestered into recycling endosomes and returned to the cell surface for reuse.
- Other endosomal vesicles containing ligands may move to and fuse with another cell surface, where the ligands are released again outside the cell in the process of transcytosis.

(Figure 2–7b, reproduced with permission from Dr John Heuser, Department of Cell Biology and Physiology, Washington University School of Medicine, St. Louis, MO.)

cascade of enzymatic activity, usually including kinases, leading to changes in gene expression or cell behavior. Second messengers may diffuse through the cytoplasm or be retained locally by scaffold proteins for more focused amplification of activity.

Low-molecular-weight *hydrophobic* signaling molecules, such as steroids and thyroid hormones, bind reversibly to carrier proteins in the blood plasma for transport through the body.

Such hormones are lipophilic and pass by diffusion through cell membranes, binding to specific cytoplasmic receptor proteins in target cells. With many steroid hormones, receptor binding activates that receptor, enabling the complex to move into the nucleus and bind with high affinity to specific DNA sequences. Typically, this increases the level of transcription of those genes. Each steroid hormone specifically binds a different member of a family of homologous receptor proteins.

FIGURE 2–8 Major types of membrane receptors.

a **Channel-linked receptors**

b **Enzymatic receptors**

c **G-protein–coupled receptors**

Protein and most small ligands are hydrophilic molecules that bind transmembrane protein receptors to initiate changes in the target cell.

(a) Channel-linked receptors bind ligands such as neurotransmitters and open to allow influx of specific ions.

(b) Enzymatic receptors are usually protein kinases that are activated to phosphorylate (and usually activate) other proteins upon ligand binding.

(c) G-protein–coupled receptors bind ligand, changing the conformation of its G-protein subunit, allowing it to bind GTP, and activating and releasing this protein to in turn activate other proteins such as ion channels and adenyl cyclase.

❯ CYTOPLASMIC ORGANELLES

Inside the cell membrane, the fluid cytoplasm (or cytosol) bathes metabolically active structures called **organelles**, which may be membranous (such as mitochondria) or nonmembranous protein complexes (such as ribosomes and proteasomes). Most organelles assume their locations in the cytoplasm by movements along the polymers of the **cytoskeleton**, which also determines a cell's shape and motility.

Cytosol also contains hundreds of enzymes, such as those of the glycolytic pathway, which produce building blocks for larger molecules and break down small molecules to liberate energy.

Oxygen, CO_2, electrolytic ions, low-molecular-weight substrates, metabolites, and waste products all diffuse through cytoplasm, either freely or bound to proteins, entering or leaving organelles where they are used or produced.

Ribosomes

Ribosomes are macromolecular machines, about 20×30 nm in size, which assemble polypeptides from amino acids on molecules of transfer RNA (tRNA) in a sequence specified by mRNA. A functional ribosome has two differently sized subunits bound to a strand of mRNA. The core of the small ribosomal subunit is a highly folded ribosomal RNA (rRNA) chain associated with more than 30 unique proteins; the core of the large subunit has three other rRNA molecules and nearly 50 other basic proteins.

The rRNA molecules in the ribosomal subunits not only provide structural support but also position the tRNA molecules bearing amino acids in the correct "reading frame" and catalyze the formation of the peptide bonds. The more peripheral proteins of the ribosome seem to function primarily to stabilize the catalytic RNA core.

These ribosomal proteins are themselves synthesized in cytoplasmic ribosomes but then move to the nucleus where they associate with newly synthesized rRNA. The ribosomal subunits thus formed then move from the nucleus to the cytoplasm for use and reuse in translation of any mRNA strand.

During protein synthesis multiple ribosomes typically bind the same strand of mRNA to form larger complexes, called **polyribosomes** or **polysomes** (Figure 2–9). In stained preparations of cells polyribosomes are intensely basophilic because the phosphate groups in their RNA molecules make these constituents polyanionic. Thus, cytoplasmic regions that stain intensely with hematoxylin and basic dyes, such as methylene and toluidine blue, indicate sites of active protein synthesis.

Proper folding of new proteins occurs with protein chaperones. Denatured proteins or those that cannot be refolded properly become conjugated to the protein ubiquitin which targets

them for breakdown by proteasomes (discussed later). As indicated in Figure 2–9, proteins synthesized for use within the cytosol (eg, glycolytic enzymes) or for import into the nucleus and certain other organelles emerge from polyribosomes existing as isolated cytoplasmic clusters. Polyribosomes attached to membranes of the endoplasmic reticulum translate mRNAs coding for membrane proteins of that structure, the Golgi apparatus, and the cell membrane; enzymes for storage in lysosomes; and proteins to undergo exocytosis from secretory vesicles.

Endoplasmic Reticulum

The cytoplasm of most cells contains this convoluted membranous network called the **endoplasmic reticulum (ER)**. As shown in Figure 2–10, the network (or reticulum) extends from the surface of the nucleus throughout the cytoplasm and encloses a series of intercommunicating channels called **cisternae** (L. *cisternae*, reservoirs). With a membrane surface up to 30 times that of the plasma membrane, the ER is a major site for vital cellular activities, including biosynthesis of proteins and lipids. Polyribosomes attached to the membrane in different regions of ER allow two types of ER to be distinguished.

Rough Endoplasmic Reticulum

Rough endoplasmic reticulum (RER) is prominent in cells specialized for protein secretion, such as pancreatic acinar

---

FIGURE 2–9 Polyribosomes: free or bound to the endoplasmic reticulum.

Free polyribosomes (not attached to the endoplasmic reticulum, or ER) synthesize cytosolic and cytoskeletal proteins and proteins for import into the nucleus, mitochondria, and peroxisomes.

Proteins that are to be incorporated into membranes, stored in lysosomes, or eventually secreted from the cell are made on polysomes attached to the membranes of ER. The proteins produced by these ribosomes become segregated during translation into the interior of the ER's membrane cisternae.

In both pathways, misfolded proteins are conjugated to ubiquitin and targeted for proteasomal degradation.

FIGURE **2–10** Rough and smooth endoplasmic reticulum.

Nucleus

Cisternae

Ribosomes

a

Ribosomes   Rough ER   Smooth ER

b

c

Functions of Endoplasmic Reticulum
I. **Synthesis:** Provides a place for chemical reactions
a. Smooth ER is the site of lipid synthesis and carbohydrate metabolism
b. Rough ER synthesizes proteins for secretion, incorporation into the plasma, membrane, and as enzymes within lysosomes
2. **Transport:** Moves molecules through cisternal space from one part of the cell to another, sequestered away from the cytoplasm
3. **Storage:** Stores newly synthesized molecules
4. **Detoxification:** Smooth ER detoxifies both drugs and alcohol

(a) The **endoplasmic reticulum** is an anastomosing network of intercommunicating channels or **cisternae** formed by a continuous membrane, with some regions that bear polysomes appearing rough and other regions appearing smooth. While RER is the site for synthesis of most membrane-bound proteins, three diverse activities are associated with smooth ER: (1) lipid biosynthesis, (2) detoxification of potentially harmful compounds, and (3) sequestration of Ca++ ions. Specific cell types with well-developed SER are usually specialized for one of these functions.

(b) By TEM cisternae of RER appear separated, but they form a continuous channel or compartment in the cytoplasm. The

interconnected membranous cisternae of RER are flattened, while those of SER are frequently tubular. (×14,000)

(c) Here, with fluorescence microscopy and immunocytochemistry of intact epithelial cells in culture, the lacelike ER (yellow/green) is seen to be continuous with the nuclear envelope and most abundant in the surrounding area, but present throughout the cytoplasm. ER was visualized with a fluorescently tagged antibody against an enzyme specific to that organelle. Cell nuclei stain bright blue with DAPI (4′,6-diamidino-2-phenylindole) and microtubules red with a fluorescent antibody against tubulin.

(Figure 2–10c Reproduced with permission from The Human Protein Atlas project.)

cells (making digestive enzymes), fibroblasts (collagen), and plasma cells (immunoglobulins). The RER consists of saclike as well as parallel stacks of flattened cisternae (Figure 2–10), each limited by membranes that are continuous with the outer membrane of the cell's nucleus. Polyribosomes on the cytosolic surface of the RER confer basophilic staining properties on this organelle.

As mentioned above the major function of RER is production of membrane-associated proteins, proteins of membranous organelles, and proteins destined for exocytosis. Production here includes the initial (core) glycosylation of glycoproteins, certain other posttranslational modifications

of newly formed polypeptides, and the assembly of multichain proteins. These activities involve resident enzymes of the RER and protein complexes that function as chaperones guiding the folding of nascent proteins, inhibiting aggregation, and generally monitoring protein quality within the ER.

Protein synthesis begins on polyribosomes in the cytosol. The 5′ ends of mRNAs for proteins destined for the RER encode an N-terminal **signal sequence** of 15-40 amino acids that includes a series of six or more hydrophobic residues. As shown in Figure 2–11, the newly translated signal sequence is bound by a protein complex called the **signal-recognition**

FIGURE **2–11** Movement of polypeptides into the RER.

The newly translated amino terminus of a protein to be incorporated into membranes or sequestered into vesicles contains 15-40 amino acids that include a specific sequence of hydrophobic residues comprising the **signal sequence** or signal peptide. This sequence is bound by a signal-recognition particle (SRP), which then recognizes and binds a receptor on the ER. Another receptor in the ER membrane binds a structural protein of the large

ribosomal subunit, more firmly attaching the ribosome to the ER. The hydrophobic signal peptide moves through a protein pore (translocon) in the ER membrane, and the SRP is freed for reuse. The signal peptide is removed from the growing protein by a peptidase and translocation of the growing polypeptide continues until it is completely segregated into the ER cisterna.

particle (SRP), which inhibits further polypeptide elongation. The SRP–ribosome–nascent peptide complex binds to SRP receptors on the ER membrane. SRP then releases the signal sequence, allowing translation to continue with the nascent polypeptide chain transferred to a **translocator complex** (also called a translocon) through the ER membrane (Figure 2–11). Inside the lumen of the RER, the signal sequence undergoes removal by the enzyme, signal peptidase. With the ribosome docked at the ER surface, translation continues with the growing polypeptide pushing itself while chaperones and other proteins serve to "pull" the nascent polypeptide through the translocator complex. Upon release from the ribosome, posttranslational modifications and proper folding of the polypeptide continue.

RER has a highly regulated system to prevent forwarding of nonfunctional proteins to the channel for secretion or to other organelles. New proteins unable to be folded or assembled properly by chaperones undergo ER-associated degradation (ERAD), in which these unsalvageable proteins are translocated back into the cytosol, conjugated to ubiquitin, and then degraded by proteasomes.

As mentioned, proteins synthesized in the RER can have various destinations: intracellular storage (eg, in lysosomes), provisional storage in cytoplasmic vesicles prior to exocytosis (eg, in most pancreatic cell granules), and as integral membrane proteins. Diagrams in Figure 2–12 show four cell types with distinct differences in the destinations of their major

protein products and how these differences determine the cell's histologic features.

>> **MEDICAL APPLICATION**

Quality control during protein production in the RER and properly functioning ERAD to dispose of defective proteins are extremely important and several inherited diseases result from malfunctions in this system. For example, in some forms of osteogenesis imperfecta bone cells synthesize and secrete defective procollagen molecules that cannot assemble properly and produce very weak bone tissue.

Smooth Endoplasmic Reticulum

Regions of ER that lack bound polyribosomes make up the **smooth endoplasmic reticulum (SER)**, which is continuous with RER but frequently less abundant (Figure 2–10). Lacking polyribosomes, SER is not basophilic and best visualized by TEM. Unlike the cisternae of RER, SER cisternae are more tubular or saclike, with interconnected channels of various shapes and sizes rather than stacks of flattened cisternae.

SER has three main functions, which vary in importance in different cell types.

■ Enzymes in the SER perform *synthesis of phospholipids and steroids*, major constituents of cellular membranes. These lipids then move from the SER to other

FIGURE **2–12**   Protein localization and cell morphology.

(a) Erythroblast

(b) Eosinophilic leukocyte

(c) Plasma cell

(d) Pancreatic acinar cell

The ultrastructure and general histologic appearance of a cell are determined by the nature of the most prominent proteins the cell is making.

(a) Cells that make few or no proteins for secretion have scant RER, with essentially all polyribosomes free in the cytoplasm.

(b) Cells that synthesize, segregate, and store various proteins in specific secretory granules or vesicles always have RER, a Golgi apparatus, and a supply of granules containing the proteins ready to be secreted.

(c) Cells with extensive RER and a well-developed Golgi apparatus show few secretory granules because the proteins undergo exocytosis immediately after Golgi processing is complete. Many cells, especially those of epithelia, are *polarized*, meaning that the distribution of RER and secretory vesicles is different in various regions or poles of the cell.

(d) Epithelial cells specialized for secretion have distinct polarity, with RER abundant at their basal ends and mature secretory granules at the apical poles undergoing exocytosis into an enclosed extracellular compartment, the lumen of a gland.

membranes by lateral diffusion, by phospholipid transfer proteins, or by vesicles that detach from the SER for movement along the cytoskeleton and fusion with other membranous organelles. In cells that secrete steroid hormones (eg, cells of the adrenal cortex), SER occupies a substantial portion of the cytoplasm.

■ Other SER enzymes, including those of the cytochrome P450 family, allow *detoxification of potentially harmful exogenous molecules* such as alcohol, barbiturates, and other drugs. In liver cells these enzymes also process endogenous molecules such as the components of bile.

■ SER vesicles are also responsible for *sequestration and controlled release of Ca²⁺*, which is part of the rapid response of cells to various stimuli. This function is well developed in striated muscle cells, where the SER has a key role in the contraction process and assumes a specialized form called the **sarcoplasmic reticulum** (see Chapter 10).

❯❯ MEDICAL APPLICATION

Jaundice denotes a yellowish discoloration of the skin and is caused by accumulation in extracellular fluid of bilirubin and other pigmented compounds, which are normally metabolized by SER enzymes in cells of the liver and excreted as bile. A frequent cause of jaundice in newborn infants is an underdeveloped state of SER in liver cells, with failure of bilirubin to be converted to a form that can be readily excreted.

Golgi Apparatus

The dynamic organelle called the **Golgi apparatus**, or Golgi complex, completes posttranslational modifications of proteins produced in the RER, while packaging and addressing these proteins to their proper destinations. The organelle, named for histologist Camillo Golgi who discovered it in 1898, consists of many smooth membranous saccules, some vesicular, others tubular or flattened, all containing enzymes and new proteins being processed. In most cells, small Golgi complexes assume locations near the nucleus (Figure 2–13).

As shown in Figure 2–13, the Golgi apparatus has two distinct functional sides or faces, formed by the complex system of cytoplasmic tubules and vesicles. New proteins exit the ER in small, membrane-enclosed **transport vesicles** moved along cytoskeletal polymers by motor proteins. The transport vesicles merge with the Golgi-receiving region, or *cis face*. On the opposite side of the Golgi network, at its shipping or *trans face*, larger saccules or vacuoles accumulate, condense, and generate other vesicles that carry completed protein products to organelles away from the Golgi (Figures 2–13 and 2–14).

Formation of transport vesicles and secretory vesicles involves assembly of protein coat complexes, which also regulate vesicular traffic to and through the Golgi apparatus. Forward movement of vesicles in the *cis* Golgi network involves the coat protein complex **COP-II**, which also sorts and concentrates proteins exiting the RER, while retrograde and other poorly understood movements in that region involve **COP-I**. These coat protein complexes, along with other membrane

FIGURE **2–13** Golgi apparatus.

The **Golgi apparatus** is a highly plastic, morphologically complex system of membrane vesicles and cisternae in which proteins and other molecules made in the RER undergo further modification and sorting into specific vesicles destined for distinct roles in the cell.

(a) TEM of the Golgi apparatus provided early evidence about how this organelle functions. Near the cell nucleus (**N**) are small portions of electron-dense **RER** cisternae, adjacent to which is the face of the *cis Golgi network* (**CGN**), or the receiving face of the Golgi apparatus, the first of several wide, flattened Golgi cisternae. This adjoins a stack of characteristically flattened and curved medial Golgi cisternae. Cytological and molecular data indicate that transport vesicles (**TV**) move proteins serially into and through these cisternae until at the *trans Golgi network* (**TGN**), the Golgi's shipping region, such vesicles condense to form larger secretory vesicles (**SV**) or other vacuoles that emerge to carry their content of modified proteins elsewhere in the cell. Formation, fusion, and movement of transport vesicles through the Golgi apparatus occur under the control of specific membrane proteins. (×30,000).

(b) Morphological aspects of the Golgi apparatus are revealed more clearly by SEM, which shows a three-dimensional image of the Golgi membrane compartments, with numerous transport vesicles and the *trans* side facing the lower right. Cells may have multiple Golgi apparatuses, each with the general organization shown here and typically situated near the cell nucleus. (×35,000)

(c) The Golgi apparatus can be clearly localized in fluorescent microscopy of intact cultured cells processed by immunocytochemistry with a fluorescent antibody against a Golgi-specific protein (Golgi reassembly-stacking protein 1), which shows complexes of Golgi vesicles (green), near cell nuclei (blue, DAPI-stained), against a background of microtubules stained red with a fluorescent antibody against tubulin. This perinuclear location of Golgi complexes and their proximity to RER are characteristic of this organelle. Because of the abundance of lipids in its many membranes, the Golgi apparatus is difficult to visualize in typical paraffin-embedded, H&E-stained sections. In developing white blood cells with active Golgi complexes, the organelle can sometimes appear as a faint unstained juxtanuclear region (sometimes called a "Golgi ghost") surrounded by basophilic cytoplasm.

(Figure 2–13c reproduced with permission from The Human Protein Atlas project.)

FIGURE **2–14** Summary of functions within the Golgi apparatus.

Rough ER

Polyribosome

RER

Transporting vesicle from RER to Golgi

cis Golgi

medial Golgi cisternae

Transporting vesicles

trans Golgi

Lysosome

Secretory granule

Exocytosis

Membrane proteins

In the RER
- New proteins are translocated into ER cisternae
- Preassembled mannose-rich *oligosaccharides* are added to specific asparagine residues (N-linked)
- Proteins are folded, guided by *chaperones*, with strict quality control
- *Disulfide bonds* are formed between specific cysteine residues

In the *cis* Golgi network (CGN),
- Vesicle movement from RER and forward through the CGN is promoted by the coat protein COP-II
- Similarly, COP-I controls retrograde vesicle movements
- *Mannose-6-phosphate* is added to future lysosomal enzymes
- N-linked oligosaccharides are trimmed and other sugars added

Vesicles move to the medial Golgi cisternae where
- *New glycosylation* occurs on –OH groups of some lipids and serine and threonine residues (O-linked)
- N-linked oligosaccharides on proteins are modified further
- Glycoproteins and glycolipids are *sorted* into specific vesicles

In the *trans* Golgi network
- Sialic acid is added as the terminal sugar to certain oligosaccharides
- *Sulfation* of tyrosine residues and some sugars occurs
- Specific vesicles with different destinations are separated and sorted

The main molecular processes are listed at the right, with the major compartments where they occur. In the *trans* Golgi network, the proteins and glycoproteins combine with specific receptors that guide them to the next stages toward their destinations.

proteins, receptors and promoters of membrane fusion organize the vesicles and tubular network of the Golgi apparatus. The dynamic activity of these various proteins, the mechanisms of which remain an active area of research, directs new proteins toward different Golgi regions and gives rise to lysosomes or secretory vesicles for exocytosis.

As indicated in Figure 2–14, sequentially located Golgi saccules contain different enzymes at the various *cis*, *medial*, and *trans* levels. These enzymes promote glycosylation, sulfation, phosphorylation, and limited proteolysis of the transported proteins. Following these activities the Golgi apparatus initiates packaging, concentration, and storage of secretory products.

Secretory Granules

Originating as condensing vesicles in the Golgi apparatus, **secretory granules** predominate in cells that store a product until its release by exocytosis, often signaled by a metabolic, hormonal, or neural message (regulated secretion). These membrane-bound granules contain a densely concentrated form of the secretory product (Figure 2–15). The contents of some secretory granules may be up to 200 times more concentrated than those in the cisternae of the RER. The term "**zymogen granules**" refers to the secretory granules containing digestive enzymes in cells of the gastrointestinal tract and its associated glands.

FIGURE **2–15** Secretory granules.

TEM of one area of a pancreatic acinar cell shows numerous mature, electron-dense **secretory granules (S)** in association with condensing vacuoles **(C)** of the Golgi apparatus **(G)**. Such granules form as the contents of the Golgi vacuoles become more condensed. In H&E-stained sections, secretory granules are often shown as intensely eosinophilic structures, which in polarized epithelial cells are concentrated at the apical region prior to exocytosis. (×18,900)

Lysosomes

Lysosomes are sites of intracellular digestion and turnover of cellular components. Lysosomes (Gr. *lysis*, solution, + *soma*, body) are membrane-limited vesicles that contain about 40 different hydrolytic enzymes and are particularly abundant in cells with great phagocytic activity (eg, macrophages, neutrophils). Although the nature and activity of lysosomal enzymes vary depending on the cell type, the most common are acid hydrolases such as proteases, nucleases, phosphatase, phospholipases, sulfatases, and β-glucuronidase. As this list shows, lysosomal enzymes can break down most macromolecules.

Lysosomes are usually spherical, range in diameter from 0.05 to 0.5 μm, and present a uniformly granular, electron-dense appearance in the TEM (Figure 2–16). In macrophages and neutrophils, lysosomes are slightly larger and visible with the light microscope, especially after histochemical staining.

The membrane surrounding each lysosome shields cytoplasmic components from the degradative enzymes. Moreover, since these enzymes have optimal activity at an acidic pH (~5.0), leaked lysosomal enzymes are inactive at the cytosolic pH (~7.2) and harmless to the cell.

After synthesis in the RER lysosomal hydrolases move to the Golgi apparatus, where the enzymes are modified and packaged in vacuoles that form lysosomes. Addition of mannose-6-phosphate (M6P) by a phosphotransferase in the *cis* Golgi occurs only on the N-linked oligosaccharides of hydrolases destined for lysosomes. Membrane receptors for M6P-containing proteins in the *trans* Golgi network bind these proteins and divert them from the secretory pathway for segregation into developing lysosomes.

Digestion of material taken from outside the cell by endocytosis occurs when the membrane of the phagosome or pinocytotic vesicle fuses with a lysosome. This mixes the endocytosed material with the lysosomal enzymes and activates proton pumps in the lysosomal membrane that acidify the contents, allowing digestion. The composite activated

FIGURE **2–16** Lysosomes.

Lysosomes are spherical membrane-enclosed vesicles that function as sites of intracellular digestion and are particularly numerous in cells active after the various types of endocytosis. Lysosomes are not well shown on H&E-stained cells but can be visualized by light microscopy after staining with toluidine blue.

(a) Cells in a kidney tubule show numerous purple lysosomes **(L)** in the cytoplasmic area between the basally located nuclei **(N)** and apical ends of the cells at the center of the tubule. Using endocytosis, these cells actively take up small proteins in the lumen of the tubule, degrade the proteins in lysosomes, and then release the resulting amino acids for reuse. (×300) 35

(b) The wide distribution of small lysosomes (green) within intact cultured epithelial cells is shown by immunocytochemistry with

an antibody against a granulin precursor specific for these organelles. Microtubules (red) occur through the full extent of cytoplasm, especially around the cells' nuclei (blue).

(c) In the TEM lysosomes **(L)** have a characteristic very electron-dense appearance and are shown here near groups of Golgi cisternae **(G)**. The less electron-dense lysosomes represent heterolysosomes in which digestion of the contents is under way. The cell is a macrophage with fine cytoplasmic extensions (arrows). (×15,000)

(Figure 2–16b, reproduced with permission from The Human Protein Atlas project.)

organelles, now termed secondary or **heterolysosomes**, have a more heterogeneous appearance in the TEM because of the wide variety of materials they may be digesting (Figure 2–16c).

During the digestion of macromolecules, released nutrients diffuse into the cytosol through the lysosomal membrane. Indigestible material remains within a small vacuolar remnant

called a **residual body** (Figure 2–17). In certain long-lived cells (eg, neurons, heart muscle), residual bodies can accumulate over time as granules of **lipofuscin**.

Besides degrading exogenous macromolecules lysosomes also function in a process called **autophagy**, which eliminates excess organelles or large aggregates of nonfunctional

FIGURE **2–17** Lysosomal functions.

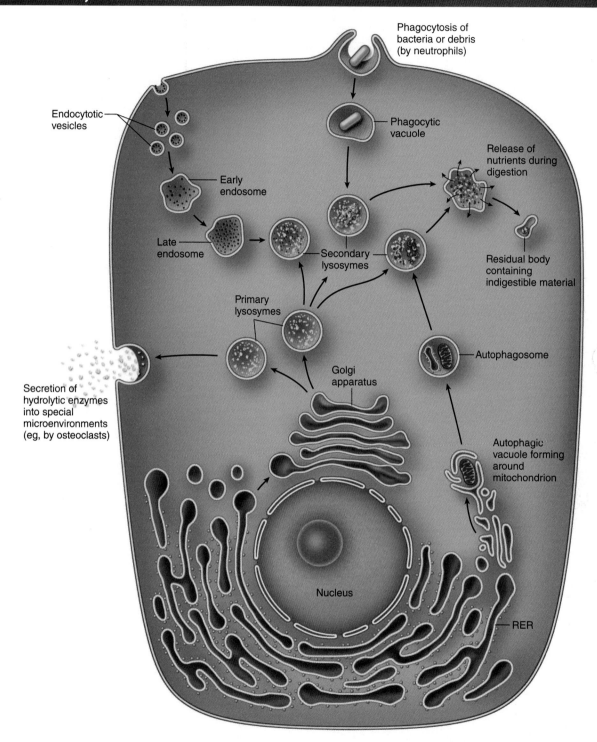

Synthesis of lysosomal enzymes occurs in the RER, with packaging in the Golgi apparatus. Endocytosis produces vesicles that fuse with **endosomes** before merging with **lysosomes**. Phagocytic vacuoles (or phagosomes) fuse with primary lysosomes to become **secondary lysosomes** (or heterolysosomes), in which ingested material is degraded. **Autophagosomes**, such as those depicted here with a mitochondrion in the process of digestion, are formed after nonfunctional or surplus organelles become enclosed with membrane, and the resulting structure fuses with a lysosome. The products of lysosomal digestion are recycled to the cytoplasm, but indigestible molecules remain in a membrane-enclosed **residual body**, which may accumulate in long-lived cells as lipofuscin. In certain cells, such as osteoclasts, the lysosomal enzymes are secreted into a restricted extracellular compartment.

FIGURE **2–18** Autophagy.

RB

Autophagy is a process in which the cell uses lysosomes to dispose of excess or nonfunctioning organelles or membranes. Membrane that appears to emerge from the SER encloses the organelles destined for destruction, forming an autophagosome that then fuses with a lysosome for digestion of the contents. In this TEM, the two autophagosomes at the **upper left** contain portions of RER more electron dense than the neighboring normal RER and one near the **center** contains what may be mitochondrial membranes plus RER. Also shown is a vesicle with features of a residual body **(RB)**. (×30,000)

macromolecules in cytoplasm (Figures 2–17 and 2–18). During autophagy a lipid bilayer membrane forms around and isolates the cytoplasmic portion to be removed, producing an **autophagosome** (Gr. *autos,* self, + *phagein,* to eat, + *soma*),

which then fuses with a lysosome for digestion of the enclosed material. Cell starvation or nutrient stress enhances autophagic activity. Amino acids, nucleotides, and other digestion products released from autophagosomes serve as sources of energy or in new synthetic reactions.

❯❯ MEDICAL APPLICATION

Diseases categorized as *lysosomal storage disorders* stem from defects in one or more of the digestive enzymes present in lysosomes, usually due to a mutation leading to a deficiency of one of the enzymes, or defects due to faulty posttranslational processing. In cells that must digest the substrate of the missing or defective enzyme following autophagy, the lysosomes cannot function properly. Such cells accumulate large secondary lysosomes or residual bodies filled with the indigestible macromolecule. The accumulation of these vacuoles may eventually interfere with normal cell or tissue function, producing symptoms of the disease. A few lysosomal storage diseases are listed in Table 2–3, with the enzyme involved for each and the tissue affected.

Proteasomes

Proteasomes are abundant, membrane-free cytoplasmic and nuclear protein complexes, each approximately the size of the small ribosomal subunits. They function to degrade denatured or otherwise nonfunctional polypeptides. Proteasomes also remove proteins no longer needed by the cell and provide an important mechanism for restricting the activity of a specific protein to a certain window of time. Whereas lysosomes digest organelles or membranes by autophagy, proteasomes deal primarily with free proteins as individual macromolecules.

As shown diagrammatically in Figure 2–9, the proteasome is a cylindrical structure made of four stacked rings, each composed of seven proteins including proteases. At each end of the cylinder is a regulatory particle that contains ATPase and recognizes proteins with attached molecules of **ubiquitin**, an abundant cytosolic 76-amino acid protein found in all cells. Proteasomal chaperones recognize misfolded or denatured proteins, or short-lived proteins with oxidized amino acids and target them for destruction by other enzyme complexes which conjugate ubiquitin to lysine residues of the protein, forming a polyubiquitin chain. Ubiquitinated proteins are recognized

TABLE **2–3**	Examples of lysosomal storage diseases caused by defective lysosomal enzymes.	
Disease	**Faulty Enzyme**	**Main Organs Affected**
Hurler syndrome (MPS I)	α-L-Iduronidase	Skeleton and nervous system
McArdle syndrome	Muscle phosphorylase	Skeletal muscles
Tay–Sachs	GM_2-gangliosidase	Nervous system
Gaucher	Glucocerebrosidase	Liver and spleen
I-cell disease	Phosphotransferase for M6P formation	Skeleton and nervous system

by the regulatory particles of proteasomes, unfolded by the ATPase, and then translocated into the core of the cylindrical structure for degradation by endopeptidases, releasing the ubiquitins for reuse. Peptides produced in proteasomes may undergo further breakdown to amino acids or may have other specialized destinations, such as the antigen-presenting complexes of cells activating an immune response.

❯❯ MEDICAL APPLICATION

Failure of proteasomes or other aspects of a cell's protein quality control can allow large aggregates of protein to accumulate in affected cells. Such aggregates may adsorb other macromolecules to them and damage or kill cells. Aggregates released from dead cells can accumulate in the ECM of the tissue. In the brain, this can interfere directly with cell function and lead to neurodegeneration. **Alzheimer disease** and **Huntington disease** are two neurologic disorders caused initially by such protein aggregates.

Mitochondria

Mitochondria (Gr. *mitos*, thread, + *chondros*, granule) are membrane-enclosed organelles with arrays of enzymes specialized for aerobic respiration and production of **adenosine triphosphate (ATP)**, with high-energy phosphate bonds, which supplies energy for most cellular activities. Cytoplasmic enzymes convert glucose anaerobically to pyruvate, releasing a small amount of energy by glycolysis. Importation of pyruvate into mitochondria and oxidizing it to CO_2 and H_2O allows the capture of additional energy. Mitochondrial enzymes yield 15 times more ATP than that produced by glycolysis alone. A small part of the energy released in mitochondria escapes bondage in ATP and dissipates as heat helping to maintain body temperature.

Mitochondria are usually elongated structures with diameters of 0.5-1 μm and lengths up to 10 times greater. They are highly plastic, rapidly changing shape, fusing with one another and dividing, while being moved through the cytoplasm along microtubules. The number of mitochondria corresponds to a cell's energy requirement: cells with a high-energy metabolism (eg, cardiac muscle, cells of some kidney tubules) have abundant mitochondria, whereas cells with a low metabolic rate have few mitochondria. Similarly, mitochondria of differentiated cells localize preferentially in cytoplasmic regions where energy utilization is more intense.

❯❯ MEDICAL APPLICATION

Myoclonic epilepsy with ragged-red fibers (MERRF) is a rare disease occurring in individuals in whom cells of specific tissues, notably regions of skeletal muscle, inherit mitochondrial DNA with a mutated gene for lysine-tRNA, leading to defective synthesis of respiratory chain proteins that can produce structural abnormality in muscle fibers and other cells.

Mitochondria are often sufficiently large to be visible with the light microscope as discrete eosinophilic organelles (Figure 2–19). With the TEM each mitochondrion is seen to have two separated and quite different membranes that together create two compartments: the innermost **matrix** and a narrow **intermembrane space** (Figure 2–20a). Both mitochondrial membranes contain a higher density of protein molecules than other membranes in the cell and have reduced fluidity. The **outer membrane** is sievelike, containing many transmembrane proteins called **porins** that form channels through which small molecules such as pyruvate and other metabolites readily pass from the cytoplasm to the intermembrane space.

The **inner membrane** has many long folds called **cristae**, which project into the matrix and greatly increase the membrane's surface area (Figure 2–20). The number of cristae in mitochondria also corresponds to the energy needs of the cell. The lipid bilayer of the inner membrane contains unusual phospholipids and is highly impermeable to ions (Figure 2–20). Integral proteins include various transport proteins that make the inner membrane selectively permeable to the small molecules required by enzymes in the matrix. Mitochondrial matrix enzymes include those that oxidize pyruvate and fatty acids to form acetyl coenzyme A (CoA) and those of the citric acid cycle that oxidize acetyl CoA, releasing CO_2 as waste and small energy-rich molecules that provide electrons for transport along the **electron-transport chain** (or respiratory chain). Enzymes and other components of this chain occur in the inner membrane and allow oxidative phosphorylation, which produces most of the ATP in animal cells.

Formation of ATP by oxidative phosphorylation enzymes occurs by a **chemiosmotic process**. Membrane proteins guide the small electron carrier molecules through tightly packed enzyme complexes so that the electrons move sequentially along the chain. Electron transfer is coupled with oriented proton uptake and release, with protons accumulating in the intermembrane space (Figure 2–20) and producing an **electrochemical gradient** across the inner membrane. Membrane-associated proteins of the **ATP synthase** system form large (10 nm), multisubunit, globular complexes on stalk-like structures projecting from the matrix side of the inner membrane (Figure 2–20). This enzyme complex contains a channel through which protons flow down the electrochemical gradient, passing through the membrane back into the matrix. Passage of protons through this channel causes rotation of specific polypeptides in the globular ATP synthase complex, converting the energy of proton flow into the mechanical energy of protein movement. Mechanical energy is stored in the new phosphate bond of ATP by other subunit polypeptides binding adenosine diphosphate (ADP) and inorganic phosphate (Figure 2–20). A steady torrent of protons along the gradient allows each of these remarkable synthase complexes to produce more than 100 molecules of ATP per second.

Another role for mitochondria occurs at times of cell stress when the protein cytochrome c dislodges from the inner membrane's electron-transport chain and leaves the organelle.

FIGURE **2–19** Mitochondria in the light microscope.

(a) In certain sectioned cells stained with H&E, mitochondria appear throughout the cytoplasm as small eosinophilic structures. The mitochondria usually appear round or slightly elongated and are more abundant in cytoplasmic regions with higher energy demands, such as near the cell membrane in cells undergoing much active transport. The central nuclei are also clearly seen in these cells.

(b) The distribution and morphology of mitochondria (yellow/green) is shown here with intact cultured epithelial cells.

Mitochondria are most abundant near cell nuclei (blue), reflecting the greater need for ATP in the synthetic activities within that region. Such preparations also show that mitochondrial shape can be quite plastic and variable. The length of these organelles, while usually only a few times their diameters, can be greatly elongated as seen here. Such mitochondria tend to be oriented along microtubules (not stained here).

(Figure 2–19b, reproduced with permission from The Human Protein Atlas project.)

In the cytoplasm this protein activates sets of enzymes that degrade all cellular components in a regulated process called **apoptosis** which results in rapid cell death (see Chapter 3).

New mitochondria originate by growth and division (fission) of preexisting mitochondria. During cell division, each daughter cell typically receives half the mitochondria in the parent cell.

Unlike most organelles, mitochondria are partly autonomous of nuclear genes and activities. The mitochondrial matrix contains a small circular chromosome of DNA, ribosomes, mRNA, and tRNA, all with similarities to the corresponding bacterial components. Protein synthesis occurs in mitochondria but because of the reduced amount of mitochondrial DNA produces only a small subset of mitochondrial proteins locally. Most such proteins are encoded by nuclear DNA and synthesized on free polyribosomes of the cytosol with short terminal amino acid sequences that serve as signals for their uptake across the mitochondrial membranes. The observation that mitochondria have certain bacterial characteristics led to the understanding that mitochondria evolved from an ancestral aerobic prokaryote that lived symbiotically within an ancestral eukaryotic host cell.

Peroxisomes

Peroxisomes are spherical organelles enclosed by a single membrane and named for their enzymes which produce and degrade hydrogen peroxide, H_2O_2 (Figure 2–21). **Oxidases** located here oxidize substrates by removing hydrogen atoms that bind molecular oxygen (O_2), producing H_2O_2. Peroxidases such as **catalase** immediately break down H_2O_2, which can potentially damage cells. These enzymes also inactivate various potentially toxic molecules, including certain prescription drugs, particularly in the large and abundant peroxisomes of liver and kidney cells.

Other diverse enzymes in peroxisomes complement certain functions of the SER and mitochondria in the metabolism of lipids and other molecules. Thus, β-oxidation of long-chain fatty acids (18 carbons and longer) preferentially utilizes peroxisomal enzymes differing from their mitochondrial counterparts.

FIGURE **2–20** Mitochondrial structure and ATP formation (Legend Opposite).

(a) The two mitochondrial membranes and the innermost matrix can be seen in the TEM and small diagram. The **outer membrane** is smooth and the **inner membrane** has many sharp folds called **cristae** that increase its surface area greatly. The **matrix** is a gel with a high concentration of enzymes.

(b) Metabolites such as pyruvate and fatty acids enter mitochondria via membrane porins and are converted to acetyl CoA by matrix enzymes of the **citric acid cycle** (or Krebs cycle), yielding some ATP and NADH (nicotinamide adenine dinucleotide), a major source of electrons for the **electron-transport chain**. The movement of electrons through the protein complexes of the inner membrane's electron-transport system is accompanied by

the directed movement of protons (H^+) from the matrix into the intermembranous space, producing an electrochemical gradient across the membrane. Other membrane-associated proteins make up the **ATP synthase** systems, each of which forms a globular complex on a stalk-like structure projecting from the matrix side of the inner membrane. A channel in this enzyme complex allows proton flow down the electrochemical gradient and across the membrane back into the matrix. The flow of protons causes rapid spinning of specific polypeptides in the globular ATP synthase complex, converting the energy of proton flow into mechanical energy, which other subunit proteins store in the new phosphate bond of ATP.

Certain reactions leading to the formation of bile acids and cholesterol also occur in peroxisomes.

Peroxisomes form in two ways: budding of precursor vesicles from the ER or growth and division of preexisting

peroxisomes. Peroxisomal proteins emerge from free polyribosomes and have targeting sequences of amino acids at either terminus recognized by receptors located in the peroxisomal membrane for import into the organelle.

FIGURE **2–21** Peroxisomes.

Peroxisomes are small spherical, membranous organelles, containing enzymes that use O_2 to remove hydrogen atoms from fatty acids, in a reaction that produces hydrogen peroxide (H_2O_2) that must be broken down to water and O_2 by another enzyme, **catalase.**

(a) By TEM peroxisomes **(P)** display matrices of moderate electron density. The aggregated electron-dense particles here represent glycogen (G). (×30,000)

(b) Peroxisomes **(P)** in most species characteristically contain central, more electron-dense crystalloid aggregates of constituent enzymes, as shown here. (×60,000)

(c) The small size, abundance, and widespread cellular distribution of peroxisomes (green) is shown in cultured osteosarcoma cells processed for immunocytochemistry with a fluorescent antibody against a protein specific to this organelle. Cell nuclei appear bright blue with DAPI staining.

(Figure 2–21c reproduced with permission from The Human Protein Atlas project.)

⟩ THE CYTOSKELETON

The cytoplasmic **cytoskeleton** is a complex array of (1) microtubules, (2) microfilaments (also called actin filaments), and (3) intermediate filaments. These protein polymers determine the shapes of cells, play key roles in the movements of organelles and cytoplasmic vesicles, as well as allowing movements of entire cells. Table 2–4 summarizes important properties, functions, and locations of the cytoskeletal components.

TABLE **2–4**	Properties of cytoskeletal components (microtubules, microfilaments, and intermediate filaments).

General Function of Cytoskeleton

1. **Structural:** Provides structural support to cells; stabilizes junctions between cells
2. **Movement:** Assists with cytosol streaming and cell motility; helps move organelles and materials throughout cell; helps move chromosomes during cell division

	Microtubules	Microfilaments	Intermediate Filaments
Subunit	Heterodimers of αβ-tubulin	G–actin monomers	Antiparallel tetramers of two rodlike dimers
Overall structure	Hollow tube with a wall of 13 parallel protofilaments	Two intertwined filaments of F-actin	Cable of four intertwined protofibrils, each consisting of bundled tetramers associated end-to-end
Diameter	25 nm	5–7 nm	8–10 nm
Monomeric proteins	α and β tubulin (54 kDa)	Globular G-actin (42 kDa)	Various α-helical rodlike proteins (~55 kDa, Table 2–5)
Polarity	+ and – ends	+ and – ends	No apparent polarity
Relative stability	Dynamic in cytoplasm; stable in axonemes	Dynamic	Stable
General locations	Radiating through cytoplasm from concentration at centrosomes; axonemes	Concentrated beneath cell membrane; in cell extensions like microvilli	Arrayed throughout cytoplasm; at desmosomes; inside nuclear envelope
Key functions	Maintain cell's shape and polarity; provide tracks for organelle and chromosome movement; move cilia and flagella	Contract and move cells; change cell shape; cytokinesis; cytoplasmic transport and streaming	Strengthen cell and tissue structure; maintain cell shape; maintain nuclear shape (lamins)

Microtubules

Within the cytoplasm of all eukaryotic cells are fine tubular structures known as **microtubules** (Table 2–4; Figure 2–22), most of which are highly dynamic in length. Microtubules

FIGURE 2–22 Microtubules and actin filaments in cytoplasm.

(a) Microtubules (MT) and actin microfilaments (MF) can both be clearly distinguished in this TEM of fibroblast cytoplasm, which provides a good comparison of the relative diameters of these two cytoskeletal components. (×60,000)

(b) Arrays of microfilaments and microtubules are easily demonstrated by immunocytochemistry using antibodies against their subunit proteins, as in this cultured cell. Actin filaments (red) are most concentrated at the cell periphery, forming prominent circumferential bundles from which finer filaments project into cellular extensions and push against the cell membrane. Actin filaments form a dynamic network important for cell shape changes such as those during cell division, locomotion, and formation of cellular processes, folds, pseudopodia, lamellipodia, microvilli, etc., which serve to change a cell's surface area or give direction to a cell's crawling movements.

Microtubules (green/yellow) are oriented in arrays that generally extend from the centrosome area near the nucleus into the most peripheral extensions. Besides serving to stabilize cell shape, microtubules form the tracks for kinesin-based transport of vesicles and organelles into the cell periphery and dynein-based transport toward the cell nucleus.

(Figure 2–22b, reproduced with permission from Dr Albert Tousson, University of Alabama—Birmingham High Resolution Imaging Facility, Birmingham.)

also form key elements of larger, more stable arrays termed **axonemes** in the cytoplasmic extensions called cilia (discussed in Chapter 4) and flagella. Each microtubule is hollow, with an outer diameter of 25 nm and a 5-nm-thick wall, a structure that confers significant rigidity to help maintain cell shape. Microtubules vary in length but can become many micrometers long. Two or more microtubules often become linked side-by-side by protein arms or bridges, which are particularly important in the axonemes of cilia and flagella.

As indicated in Table 2–4 the protein subunit of a microtubule is a heterodimer of **α and β tubulin**, each with a molecular mass of about 50 kDa. Under appropriate conditions, the tubulin heterodimers polymerize to form the microtubules, which have a slightly spiral organization. The tubulin subunits align lengthwise as protofilaments, with 13 parallel protofilaments forming the circumference of each microtubule wall.

Polymerization of tubulins occurs within **microtubule-organizing centers (MTOCs)**, which contain short assemblies of tubulin that function as nucleating sites for further polymerization. Microtubules are polarized structures, with growth (polymerization) occurring more rapidly at the (+) end (Figure 2–23). Microtubules show **dynamic instability**, with continuous cycles of polymerization and depolymerization at steady-state conditions, which depend on concentrations of tubulin, Ca^{2+}, Mg^{2+}, and the presence of various **microtubule-associated proteins (MAPs)**. Energy for assembly comes from GTP bound to incoming tubulin subunits. Individual microtubules shorten as depolymerization exceeds growth. Microtubule stability varies with the cellular location and function; microtubules of cilia are very stable, while those of the mitotic spindle are short-lived.

The dominant MTOC in most cells is the **centrosome**, which develops around two cylindrical **centrioles**, each about 0.2 μm in diameter and 0.3-0.5 μm in length. Each centriole consists of nine highly organized microtubule triplets (Figure 2–24). With their long axes at right angles, the paired centrioles organize nearby tubulin complexes and other proteins as a pericentriolar matrix found close to the nucleus of nondividing cells. Before cell division, more specifically during the period of DNA replication, the centrosome duplicates itself to form two centrosomes, each with a pair of centrioles. During mitosis the new centrosomes move to opposite poles of the cell and become organizing centers for the microtubules of the mitotic spindle.

Microtubules also form part of the system for intracellular transport of membranous vesicles, macromolecular complexes, and organelles. Well-studied examples include axoplasmic transport in neurons, melanin transport in pigment cells, chromosome movements by the mitotic spindle, and vesicle movements among different cell compartments. In each of these examples, movement ceases if microtubules are disrupted. Transport occurs along the outer microtubule surface and requires proteins called **motor proteins**, which use ATP in moving the larger structures. **Kinesins** carry material away from the MTOC near the nucleus toward the plus end of microtubules (anterograde transport); **cytoplasmic dyneins**

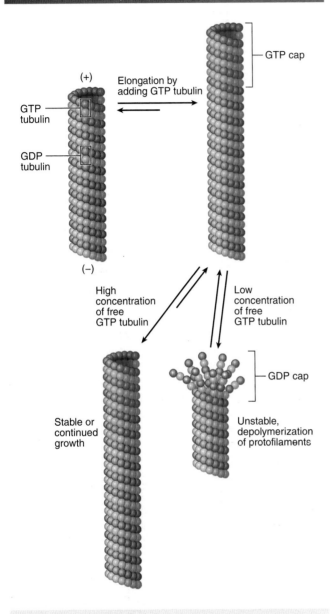

At stable tubulin concentrations some microtubules grow while others shrink, each existing in a condition called dynamic instability. In cytoplasmic areas where the tubulin concentration is high, tubulin GTP polymerizes at a microtubule's (+) end faster than the incorporated GTP can be hydrolyzed. The resulting "GTP cap" stabilizes that end of the microtubule and promotes further rapid growth. As free tubulin concentrations decrease, the rate of growth also decreases, thereby allowing GTP hydrolysis to catch up. The resulting "GDP cap" at the microtubule end is unstable and favors rapid depolymerization (termed "catastrophe"). This increases the local concentration of free, monomeric tubulin that "rescues" the microtubule before it completely disappears and produces another short period of microtubule elongation.

Dynamic instability allows the growing ends of microtubules to explore the cytoplasm and become stabilized when they contact stabilizing structures, such as kinetochores on chromosomes early in mitosis (see Chapter 3).

carry material along microtubules in the opposite direction (retrograde transport), toward the nucleus. Important roles for this system include extending the ER from the nuclear envelope to the plasmalemma and moving vesicles to and through the Golgi apparatus.

>> **MEDICAL APPLICATION**

Several inhibitory compounds used by cell biologists to study details of microtubule dynamics are also widely used in cancer chemotherapy to block activity of the mitotic spindle in rapidly growing neoplastic cells. Such drugs include vinblastine, vincristine, and paclitaxel, all of which were originally discovered as plant derivatives.

Microfilaments (Actin Filaments)

Microfilaments are composed of **actin** subunits and allow motility and most contractile activity in cells, using reversible assembly of the actin filaments as well as interactions between these filaments and associated **myosin** family proteins. Actin filaments are thin (5-7 nm diameter), polarized polymers, shorter and more flexible than microtubules (Figure 2–22). They are composed of globular G-actin monomers that assemble in the presence of K^+ and Mg^{2+} into a double-stranded helix of filamentous F-actin (Table 2–4). G-actin is generally added to preexisting filaments, but new filaments can arise from a pool of G-actin by the action of nucleating proteins, such as formin. Another nucleating factor, a complex of polypeptides called Arp2/3, also binds to the side of preexisting actin filaments and induces a new F-actin branch, a process that can lead to formation of a microfilament network.

Like microtubules, actin filaments are highly dynamic. Monomers polymerize rapidly at the (+) or barbed end, with ATP hydrolysis at each addition; at the same time monomers dissociate at the (−) or pointed end. This leads to migration of subunits through the polymer, a rapid process called *treadmilling* (Figure 2–25). In cells both the assembly and disassembly of subunits from F-actin are promoted by other proteins, such as *profilin* and *cofilin*, respectively.

Actin is very abundant in all cells and becomes concentrated in networks of actin filaments and as free G-actin subunits near the cell membrane, a cytoplasmic region often called the **cell cortex**. Arp2/3 activity produces an important branched network of microfilaments in this region. Microfilament-rich cellular extensions, including surface folds or ruffles, are important for endocytosis, and microfilaments of the cortex underlie endosomal trafficking. Cell movements on firm substrates involve sheetlike protrusions, or lamellipodia, in which the concentrated actin filaments are continuous with deeper parallel F-actin bundles called **stress fibers** (Figure 2–13c).

Actin-binding proteins, such as formin and others just mentioned, change the dynamic physical properties of microfilaments, particularly their lengths and interactions with other structures, and this determines the viscosity and other mechanical properties of the local cytoplasm. Cross-linking

FIGURE **2–24** Centrosome.

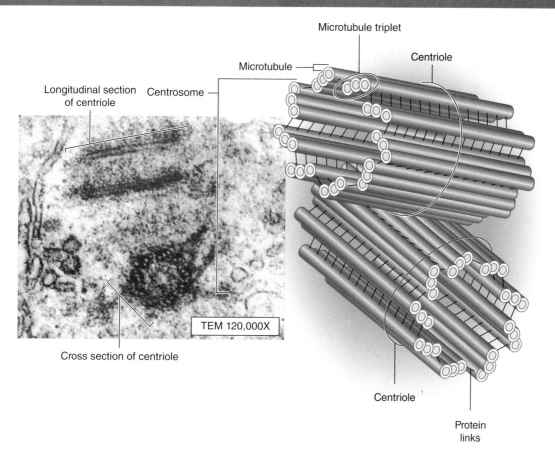

The **centrosome** is the microtubule-organizing center for the mitotic spindle and consists of paired centrioles. The TEM reveals that the two centrioles in a centrosome exist at right angles to each other in a dense matrix of free tubulin subunits and other proteins. Each centriole consists of **nine microtubular triplets**. In a poorly understood process, the centrosome duplicates itself and the pair divides equally during a cell's interphase, each half having a duplicated centriole pair. At the onset of mitosis, the two daughter centrosomes move to opposite sides of the nucleus and become the two poles of the mitotic spindle of microtubules attaching to chromosomes.

(Micrograph reproduced with permission from Dr Gwen V. Childs, University of Arkansas for Medical Sciences, Department of Neurobiology and Developmental Sciences.)

within networks of F-actin increases cytoplasmic viscosity, while severing (and capping) the filaments tends to decrease viscosity. The lengths and other physical properties of actin filaments depend on activities of various other actin-binding proteins, including those indicated in Figure 2–26.

Just as the molecular motors kinesin and dynein move structures along microtubules, various **myosin motors** use ATP to transport cargo along F-actin. Movement is usually toward the barbed (+) ends of actin filaments; unconventional myosin VI moves cargo in the other direction. Interactions between F-actin and myosins form the basis for various cell movements:

- Transport of organelles, vesicles, and granules in the process of *cytoplasmic streaming*
- Contractile rings of microfilaments with myosin II constricting to produce two cells by *cytokinesis* during mitosis

- Membrane-associated molecules of myosin I whose movements along microfilaments produce the cell surface changes during *endocytosis*.

Stabilized arrays of actin filaments integrated with arrays of thicker (16 nm) myosin filaments permit very forceful contractions in specialized cells such as those of muscle (see Chapter 10).

Intermediate Filaments

The third class of cytoskeletal components includes filaments intermediate in size between the other two, with a diameter averaging 10 nm (Table 2–4). Unlike microtubules and actin filaments, these **intermediate filaments** are stable, confer increased mechanical stability to cell structure, and consist of different protein subunits in different cell types. More than a dozen proteins, ranging in size from 40 to 230 kDa, serve as

FIGURE **2–25** Actin filament treadmilling.

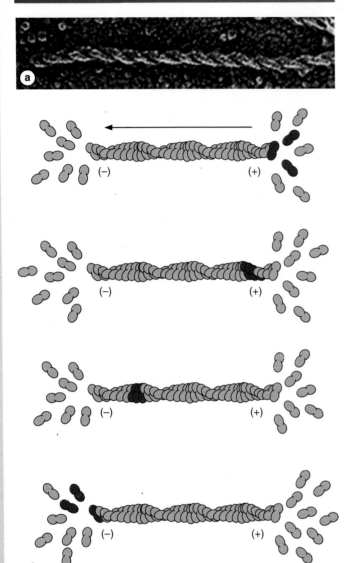

b

FIGURE **2–26** Roles of major actin-binding proteins in regulating the organization of microfilaments.

(a) Actin filaments or microfilaments are helical two-stranded polymers assembled from **globular actin subunits**.

(b) Assembly of actin filaments (F-actin) is polarized, with G-actin subunits added to the plus (+) end and removed at the minus (−) end. Even actin filaments of a constant length are highly dynamic structures, balancing G-actin assembly and disassembly at the opposite ends, with a net movement or flow along the polymer known as **treadmilling**.

(Figure 2–25a, reproduced with permission from John Heuser, Washington University School of Medicine, St. Louis, MO.)

Many proteins regulate the assembly of microfilaments and the interactions of these filaments with one another. By altering microfilament length and cross-linking, such proteins influence physical properties of the local cytoplasm.

subunits of various intermediate filaments and can be localized by immunohistochemistry in various cells. As indicated in Table 2–4 nearly all these subunits are coiled, rodlike dimers that form antiparallel tetramers, which self-assemble into large cable-like bundles or protofibrils stabilized by further lateral interactions. Table 2–5 lists six classes of intermediate

filament proteins forming rodlike subunits, their sizes, and cell distributions.

Important intermediate filament proteins include the following:

■ **Keratins** (Gr. *keras*, horn) or **cytokeratins** are a diverse family of acidic and basic isoforms that compose heterodimer subunits of intermediate filaments in all epithelial cells (see Chapter 4). Over 30 related genes encode keratin subunits, which produce filaments with different chemical and immunologic properties for various functions. Intermediate filaments of keratins form large bundles or tonofibrils that attach to certain junctions between epithelial cells (Figure 2–27). In skin epidermal cells, cytokeratins accumulate during differentiation in the process of *keratinization,* producing an outer layer of nonliving cells that reduces dehydration.

TABLE **2–5**	Major classes and representatives of intermediate filament proteins, their sizes and locations.		
Class	**Protein**	**Size (kDa)**	**Cell Distribution**
I	Acidic cytokeratin	40–65	Epithelial cells
II	Basic cytokeratin	51–68	Epithelial cells
III	Desmin	53	Muscle cells
	Synemin	190	Muscle cells
	GFAP	50	Astrocytes (less in other glial cells)
	Peripherin	57	Neurons
	Vimentin	54	Mesenchymal cells
IV	NF-L	68	Neurons
	NF-M	110	Neurons
	NF-H	130	Neurons
	α-Internexin	55	Embryonic neurons
V	Lamins	62–72	Nuclei of all cells
VI	Nestin	230	Neural stem cells

FIGURE **2–27** Intermediate filaments of keratin.

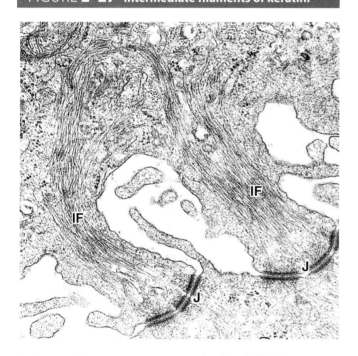

Intermediate filaments (IF) display an average diameter of 8-10 nm, between that of actin filaments and microtubules, and serve to provide mechanical strength or stability to cells. A large and important class of intermediate filaments is composed of **keratin** subunits, which are prominent in epithelial cells. Bundles of keratin filaments called **tonofibrils** associate with certain classes of intercellular junctions **(J)** common in epithelial cells and are easily seen with the TEM, as shown here in two extensions in an epidermal cell bound to a neighboring cell. (×60,000)

Keratinization of skin made terrestrial life possible during vertebrate evolution. Keratinization also provides some protection from minor abrasions and produces various hard protective structures of skin, such as nails (as well as feathers, beaks, horns, and the scales of reptiles).

▪ **Vimentin** is the most common class III intermediate filament protein and occurs in most cells derived from embryonic mesenchyme. Important vimentin-like proteins include **desmin** found in most muscle cells and **glial fibrillar acidic protein (GFAP)** found especially in astrocytes, supporting cells of central nervous system tissue. Figure 1–12a shows desmin filaments of a cultured cell stained immunocytochemically.

▪ **Neurofilament** proteins of three distinct sizes make heterodimers that form the subunits of the major intermediate filaments of neurons.

▪ **Lamins** make up a family of seven isoforms present in the cell nucleus, where they form a structural framework called the **nuclear lamina** just inside the nuclear envelope (see Chapter 3).

›› MEDICAL APPLICATION

The presence of a specific type of intermediate filament in tumors can often reveal the cellular origin of the tumor, information important for diagnosis and treatment of the cancer. Identification of intermediate filament proteins by means of immunocytochemical methods is a routine procedure. One example is the use of GFAP to identify **astrocytomas**, the most common type of brain tumor.

FIGURE **2–28** Cellular inclusions.

Inclusions are cytoplasmic structures or deposits filled with stored macromolecules and are not present in all cells.

(a) Lipid droplets are abundant in cells of the adrenal cortex and appear with the TEM as small spherical structures with homogenous matrices **(L)**. Mitochondria are also seen here. As aggregates of hydrophobic lipid molecules, these inclusions are enclosed by a single monolayer of phospholipids with various peripheral proteins, including enzymes for lipid metabolism. In routine processing of tissue for paraffin sections, fat droplets are generally removed, leaving empty spaces in the cells. The most common fat cells have cytoplasm filled with one large lipid droplet. (×19,000)

(b) TEM of a liver cell cytoplasm shows numerous individual or clustered electron-dense particles representing **glycogen granules**, although these granules lack membrane. Glycogen granules usually form characteristic aggregates such as those shown. Glycogen is a ready source of energy, and such granules are often abundant in cells with high metabolic activity. (×30,000)

(c) Pigment deposits (PD) occur in many cell types and may contain various complex substances, such as **lipofuscin** or melanin. Lipofuscin granules represent an accumulating by-product of lysosomal digestion in long-lived cells, but melanin granules serve to protect cell nuclei from damage to DNA caused by light. Many cells contain pigmented deposits of **hemosiderin granules** containing the protein ferritin, which forms a storage complex for iron. Hemosiderin granules are very electron dense, but with the light microscope, they appear brownish and resemble lipofuscin. The liver cells shown have large cytoplasmic regions filled with pigment deposits, which probably represent iron-containing hemosiderin. (×400; Giemsa)

❯ INCLUSIONS

Cytoplasmic **inclusions** contain accumulated metabolites or other substances, but unlike organelles have little or no metabolic activity themselves. Most inclusions are transitory structures not enclosed by membrane. Figure 2–28 shows features of important and commonly seen inclusions, which include the following:

- **Lipid droplets**, accumulations of lipid-filling adipocytes (fat cells) and present in various other cells.
- **Glycogen granules**, aggregates of the carbohydrate polymer storing glucose, visible as irregular clumps of periodic acid–Schiff (PAS)-positive or electron-dense material in several cell types, notably liver cells.
- Pigmented deposits of naturally colored material, including **melanin**, dark brown granules which in skin serve to protect cells from ultraviolet radiation; **lipofuscin**, a pale brown granule found in many cells, especially in stable nondividing cells (eg, neurons, cardiac muscle), containing a complex mix of material partly derived from

residual bodies after lysosomal digestion; and **hemosiderin**, a dense brown aggregate of denatured ferritin proteins with many atoms of bound iron, prominent in phagocytic cells of the liver and spleen, where it results from phagocytosis of red blood cells.

❯❯ MEDICAL APPLICATION

A condition termed **hemosiderosis**, in which the iron-containing inclusion **hemosiderin** occurs in cells of organs throughout the body, may be seen with increased uptake of dietary iron, impaired iron utilization, or with excessive lysis of red blood cells. Hemosiderosis itself does not damage cell or organ function. However, extreme accumulations of iron in cellular hemosiderin can lead to disorders, such as hemochromatosis and iron overload syndrome, in which tissues of the liver and other organs are damaged.

Table 2–6 presents a summary of the major structural and functional features of all cytoplasmic components.

TABLE **2-6**   Summary of cellular structural components.

Component	Structure	Major Function	Appearance
Plasma membrane	Phospholipid bilayer containing cholesterol and proteins (integral and peripheral) and some carbohydrates (externally); forms a selectively permeable boundary of the cell	Acts as a physical barrier to enclose cell contents; regulates material movement into and out of the cell; establishes and maintains an electrical charge difference across the plasma membrane; functions in cell communication	
Cilia	Short, numerous membrane extensions supported by microtubules, which occur on exposed membrane surfaces of some cells	Move substances (eg, mucus and dissolved materials) over the cell surface	
Flagellum	Long, singular membrane extension supported by microtubules; present on sperm cells	Propels sperm	
Microvilli	Numerous thin membrane folds projecting from the free cell surface; supported by microfilaments	Increase membrane surface area for greater absorption	
Nucleus	Large structure enclosed within a double membrane; contains chromatin, nucleolus, and nucleoplasm	Houses the DNA that serves as the genetic material for directing protein synthesis	
Nuclear envelope	Double membrane boundary between cytoplasm and nuclear contents; continuous with rough endoplasmic reticulum	Separates nucleus from cytoplasm	
Nuclear pores	Openings through the nuclear envelope	Allow passage of materials between the cytoplasm and nucleoplasm, including ribonucleic acid (RNA), protein, ions, and small water-soluble molecules	
Nucleolus	Large, prominent structure within the nucleus	Functions in synthesis of ribosomes	
Cytoplasm	Contents of cells between the plasma membrane and nuclear envelope	Responsible for many cellular processes	
Cytosol	Viscous fluid medium with dissolved solutes (eg, ions, proteins, carbohydrates, lipids)	Provides support for organelles; serves as the viscous fluid medium through which diffusion occurs	
Organelles	Membrane-bound and nonmembrane-bound structures	Carry out specific metabolic activities of the cell	
Rough endoplasmic reticulum (rough ER)	Extensive interconnected membrane network that varies in shape (eg, cisternae, tubules); ribosomes attached on cytoplasmic surface	Modifies, transports, and stores proteins produced by attached ribosomes; these proteins are secreted, become components of the plasma membrane, or serve as enzymes of lysosomes	
Smooth endoplasmic reticulum (smooth ER)	Extensive interconnected membrane network lacking ribosomes	Synthesizes, transports, and stores lipids (eg, steroids); metabolizes carbohydrates; detoxifies drugs, alcohol, and poisons; forms vesicles and peroxisomes	

(Continued)

TABLE **2–6**	Summary of cellular structural components. (Continued)		
Component	**Structure**	**Major Function**	**Appearance**
Golgi apparatus	Series of several elongated, flattened saclike membranous structures	Modifies, packages, and sorts materials that arrive from the ER in transport vesicles; forms secretory vesicles and lysosomes	
Vesicles	Spherical-shaped membrane-bound sacs; contain various types of materials to be transported through the cell	Transport cellular material	
Lysosomes	Spherical-shaped membrane-bound organelles formed from the Golgi apparatus; contain digestive enzymes	Digest microbes or materials (eg, ingested by the cell, worn-out cellular components, or the entire cell)	
Peroxisomes	Smaller, spherical-shaped membrane-bound organelles formed from the ER or through fission; contain oxidative enzymes	Detoxify specific harmful substances either produced by the cell or taken into the cell; engage in beta oxidation of fatty acids to acetyl CoA	
Mitochondria	Double membrane-bound organelles containing a circular strand of DNA (genes for producing mitochondrial proteins)	Synthesize most ATP during aerobic cellular respiration by digestion of fuel molecules (eg, glucose) in the presence of oxygen	
Ribosomes	Organelles composed of both protein and ribosomal RNA (rRNA) that are organized into both a large and small subunit; may be bound to a membrane or free in cytosol	Engage in protein synthesis: Bound ribosomes produce proteins that are secreted, incorporated into plasma membrane, and within lysosomes; free ribosomes produce proteins used within the cell	Bound ribosomes Free ribosomes
Cytoskeleton	Organized network of protein filaments and hollow tubules, including microfilaments, intermediate filaments, and microtubules	Maintains intracellular structural support and organization of cells; participates in cell division; facilitates movement	Cytoskeleton Intermediate filament Microfilament Microtubule
Microfilaments	Actin protein monomers organized into two thin, intertwined protein filaments (actin filaments)	Maintain cell shape; support microvilli; separate two cells during cytokinesis (a process of cell division); facilitate change in cell shape; participate in muscle contraction	
Intermediate filaments	Various protein components	Provide structural support; stabilize junctions between cells	
Microtubules	Hollow cylinders composed of tubulin protein	Maintain cell shape and rigidity; organize and move organelles; support cilia and flagella; participate in vesicular transport; separate chromosomes during the process of cell division	
Centrosome	Amorphous region adjacent to nucleus; contains a pair of centrioles	Organizes microtubules; participates in mitotic spindle formation during cell division	Centriole Centrosome
Proteasomes	Large, barrel-shaped protein complexes located in both the cytosol and nucleus	Degrade and digest damaged or unneeded proteins; ensure quality of exported proteins	
Inclusions	Aggregates of specific types of molecules (eg, melanin protein, glycogen, or lipid)	Serve as temporary storage for these molecules	Variable appearance

The Cytoplasm SUMMARY OF KEY POINTS

- **Cell differentiation** is the process by which cells of an embryo become specialized structurally to augment specific cytoplasmic activities for functions at the level of tissues and organs.
- **Organelles** are metabolically active structures or complexes, with or without membranes, in the cytoplasm of eukaryotic cells.

Plasma Membrane

- The **plasma membrane (cell membrane** or **plasmalemma)** is the lipid bilayer with embedded proteins that surrounds a cell and is seen only with the TEM.
- The **lipid bilayer** forms from amphipathic **phospholipids, stabilized** by **cholesterol**, and contains many **embedded (integral) proteins** and many **peripheral proteins** on its cytoplasmic surface.
- Membrane proteins move laterally within the lipid bilayer, with less movement in areas referred to as **lipid rafts**, which have higher concentrations of cholesterol and saturated fatty acids.
- Integral membrane proteins include **receptors** for external ligands, **channels** for passive or active movement of molecules across the membrane, and **pumps** for active membrane transport.
- **Endocytosis** is cellular uptake of macromolecules or fluid by plasma membrane engulfment or invagination, followed by the "pinching off" of a filled membranous vesicle in the cytoplasm.
- Major types of endocytosis include **phagocytosis** (uptake of particulate material), **pinocytosis** (uptake of dissolved substances), and **receptor-mediated endocytosis** (uptake of specific molecules bound to integral membrane receptor proteins).
- **Exocytosis** is a type of cellular secretion in which cytoplasmic membrane vesicles fuse with the plasma membrane and release their contents to the extracellular space.
- All types of **cell signaling** use membrane receptor proteins often linked to enzymes such as kinases or adenylyl cyclase whose activities initiate intracellular signaling pathways.

Ribosomes

- The two **ribosomal subunits**, each a complex of rRNA and many proteins, attach to mRNA and translate that message into protein.
- Multiple ribosomes on the same mRNA make up a **polyribosome (polysome)**, and an abundance of these produces basophilic cytoplasm after H&E staining.

Endoplasmic Reticulum

- The ER is a convoluted network of membrane enclosing continuous spaces called **cisternae** and extending from the nucleus to the plasma membrane.
- **Rough ER** has a **granular, basophilic cytoplasmic surface** due to the presence of polysomes making most membrane proteins, proteins in certain other organelles, or for exocytosis; RER is always well developed in cells actively secreting proteins.
- Proteins to be processed through the RER contain initial **signal peptides** that bind receptors in the ER membrane, localizing them to that organelle.
- After **translocation** across the membrane into the cisterna, the proteins undergo **posttranslational modification and folding** in a process monitored by RER molecular chaperones and enzymes.
- **Smooth ER (SER)** lacks ribosomes but includes enzymes for **lipid and glycogen metabolism**, for **detoxification reactions**, and for temporary **Ca²⁺ sequestration**.

Golgi Apparatus

- The **Golgi apparatus** is a dynamic organelle consisting of stacked membranous cisternae in which proteins made in RER are **processed** further and **packaged** for secretion or other roles.
- Proteins in **transport vesicles** enter the cis or receiving face of the Golgi, move through medical cisternae of the Golgi network for enzymatic modifications, and are released in other vesicles at the trans face.

- Vesicle movement through the Golgi apparatus occurs under the control of specific **coat protein complexes,** such as COPII and COPI.
- Important protein modifications in the Golgi apparatus include **sulfation** and **glycosylation** reactions.
- Modified proteins leave the Golgi apparatus after packaging in vesicles with coat proteins that direct movement to lysosomes, the plasma membrane, or secretion by exocytosis.

Lysosomes

- **Primary lysosomes** emerge from the Golgi apparatus containing inactive acid hydrolases specific for degrading a wide variety of cellular macromolecules.
- **Secondary lysosomes** are more heterogeneous, having fused with vesicles produced by endocytosis that contain material to be digested by the hydrolytic enzymes.
- During **autophagy**, lysosomes digest unneeded or nonfunctional organelles after these become surrounded by membrane that then fuses with a lysosome.
- Products of digestion in secondary lysosomes are released to the cytoplasm for reuse; final condensed vesicles containing any indigestible molecules are called **residual bodies**.

Proteasomes

- Proteasomes are small cytoplasmic protein complexes that degrade improperly folded proteins tagged with the polypeptide **ubiquitin**.

Mitochondria

- **Mitochondria** are the major sites of **ATP synthesis** and are abundant in cells or cytoplasmic regions where large amounts of energy are expended.
- Mitochondria are usually **elongated organelles** and form by fission of preexisting mitochondria.
- Mitochondria have two membranes: a **porous outer membrane** encloses the intermembrane space and an **inner membrane with many folds (cristae)** encloses a gel-like matrix.
- The **mitochondrial matrix** contains enzymes for β-oxidation of fatty acids and the citric acid (Krebs) cycle.
- The inner membrane includes enzyme assemblies of the **electron-transport system and ATP synthase**.
- Mitochondria of stressed cells may release **cytochrome c** from the inner membrane, triggering a regulated series of events culminating in cell death (**apoptosis**).

Peroxisomes

- Peroxisomes are small spherical organelles containing enzymes for various metabolic reactions, notably **for oxidation and detoxification**, and **catalase** that breaks down the H₂O₂ resulting from those reactions.

Cytoskeleton

- The cytoskeleton contains three types of polymers: (1) **microtubules** 25 nm in diameter; (2) actin filaments or **microfilaments** (5–7 nm); and (3) **intermediate filaments** (8–10 nm).
- Microtubules are semirigid tubular structures with walls composed of **polymerized tubulin** heterodimers; their structure is often very dynamic, with steady addition and dissociation of tubulin.
- Microtubules are important in **maintaining cell shape** and as **tracks for transport** of vesicles and organelles by the **motor proteins kinesin** and **dynein**.
- Microfilaments are short, flexible, highly dynamic filaments of **actin subunits**, in which changes in length and interactions with binding proteins regulate cytoplasmic viscosity and movement.
- **Myosins** are **motor proteins** that bind and move along actin filaments, carrying vesicles or producing cytoplasmic movement.
- Movements of cytoplasm produced by actin filaments and myosins are important for endocytosis, cell cleavage after mitosis, and cell locomotion on substrates.

- **Intermediate filaments** are the most stable cytoskeletal component, conferring strong mechanical stability to cells.
- Intermediate filaments are composed of various protein subunits in different cells; these include **vimentin**, nuclear **lamins**, **neurofilament proteins**, and **keratins**, which are especially important in epithelial cells.

Inclusions

- Unlike organelles, **inclusions** are not metabolically active and are primarily storage sites, such as **lipid droplets**, **glycogen granules**, **pigment granules**, and **residual bodies** (also called **lipofuscin**).

The Cytoplasm ASSESS YOUR KNOWLEDGE

1. In TEM preparations of cells, the cell membrane often appears as a trilaminar structure having two parallel dark-staining components on either side of an unstained middle layer. This central poorly stained region of the membrane is primarily responsible for which of the following functions?
   a. Creation of a barrier to water-soluble molecules
   b. Binding by cellular receptions to specific ligands
   c. Catalyzing membrane-associated activities
   d. Transport of ions
   e. Connections to the cytoskeleton

2. Chaperonins are cytoplasmic proteins most likely to be found in which of the following organelles?
   a. Lysosomes
   b. Golgi complexes
   c. Rough endoplasmic reticulum
   d. Smooth endoplasmic reticulum
   e. Mitochondria

3. Which of the following best defines the term "exocytosis"?
   a. The discharge of ions or small molecules from a cell by protein pumps in the cell membrane
   b. The uptake of material at one domain of a cell's surface and its discharge from the opposite side of the cell
   c. The process by which proteins move from one cytoplasmic compartment to another
   d. The discharge of proteins in cytoplasmic vesicles from a cell following fusion of the vesicles with the plasmalemma
   e. Diffusion of lipid-soluble molecules from a cell across the cell membrane

4. Cytoplasm often stains poorly because its lipid content is removed by the organic solvents used in the clearing step in routine histological preparations. This problem is most likely to occur with cytoplasmic regions rich in which of the following organelles?
   a. Free polysomes
   b. Mitochondria
   c. Lysosomes
   d. Smooth endoplasmic reticulum
   e. Rough endoplasmic reticulum

5. Polarity in microtubules is important in determining which of the following?
   a. The strength of vinblastine binding to microtubules
   b. The velocity of transport along microtubules with myosin motors
   c. The overall dynamic instability of the microtubules
   d. The linkage of microtubules to intermediate filaments
   e. The direction of vesicular transport along microtubules

6. Which of the following proteins is/are most likely to have initially contained a "signal peptide" that bound a "signal-recognition particle" during its translation?
   a. An enzyme of the respiratory chain
   b. Lamins
   c. Proteins in secretory granules
   d. F-actin
   e. Proteins in the large ribosomal subunit

7. Vesicles of a Golgi apparatus that are destined to become part of other organelles most likely have which of the following on their membranes?
   a. Channel proteins
   b. Clathrin
   c. COP II
   d. Actin
   e. GTP

8. About 3 years ago, a 39-year-old construction worker became increasingly uncoordinated. His wife describes bouts of depression and apathy beginning about a decade ago. Laboratory tests are normal. MRI and CT reveal striatal and caudate atrophy with "boxcar ventricles." His mini-mental status examination score is 24/30. The cranial nerve examination shows dysarthria, saccadic extraocular eye movements, and a hyperactive gag reflex. There is increased tone in all extremities. Polymerase chain reaction reveals one normal band with 20 CAG (trinucleotide) repeats and the other with 49 CAG repeats. Modulation of respiration and mitochondrial membrane potential and bioenergetic failure are associated with the abnormal gene in this disease. Which of the following mechanisms used to establish the mitochondrial electrochemical gradient may be altered in this disease?
   a. The action of ATP synthase
   b. Transfer of electrons from NADH to O_2 in the intermembrane space
   c. Pumping of protons into the mitochondrial matrix by respiratory chain activity
   d. Proton-translocating activity in the inner membrane
   e. Transport of ATP out of the matrix compartment by a specific transporter

9. A 56-year-old man has been taking atorvastatin because of a poor lipid profile and a family history of cardiovascular disease. The statin family of drugs enhances endocytosis of low-density lipoprotein (LDL) from the blood. Endocytosis of LDL differs from phagocytosis of bacterial cells in which of the following ways?
   a. Use of membrane-enclosed vesicles in the uptake process
   b. Coupling with the lysosomal system
   c. Dependence on acidification
   d. Use of clathrin-coated pits
   e. Use of hydrolases

10. A 14-year-old boy is diagnosed with epidermolysis bullosa simplex (EBS). His skin blisters easily with rubbing or scratching. Blisters occur primarily on his hands and feet and heal without leaving scars. Genetic analysis shows mutations in the *KRT5* and *KRT14* genes, which code keratin 5 and keratin 14. What is the primary function of those proteins?
    a. Generate movement
    b. Provide mechanical stability
    c. Carry out nucleation of microtubules
    d. Stabilize microtubules against disassembly
    e. Transport organelles within the cell

Answers: 1a, 2c, 3d, 4d, 5e, 6c, 7c, 8d, 9d, 10b

3 The Nucleus

ontaining the code for all of a cell's enzymes and other proteins, the **nucleus** is the command center of the cell. The nucleus also holds the molecular machinery to replicate the DNA and to synthesize and process all types of RNA. Between cell divisions pore complexes in the membrane enclosing the nucleus regulate macromolecular transfer between the nuclear and cytoplasmic compartments. Mature RNA molecules pass into the cytoplasm for their roles in protein synthesis, while proteins needed for nuclear activities are imported there from the cytoplasm. Restricting protein synthesis to the cytoplasm helps ensure that newly made RNA molecules do not become involved in translation before processing is completed.

❯ COMPONENTS OF THE NUCLEUS

The nucleus usually appears as a large rounded or oval structure, often near the cell's center (Figure 3–1). Typically, the largest structure within a cell, it consists of a **nuclear envelope** enclosing the **chromatin**, the mass of DNA, and its associated proteins, with one or more specialized chromatin regions called **nucleoli**. In specific tissues, the size and shape of cell nuclei normally tend to be uniform.

Nuclear Envelope

The **nuclear envelope** forms a selectively permeable barrier between the nuclear and cytoplasmic compartments. Electron microscopy reveals that the envelope has two concentric membranes separated by a narrow (30–50 nm) **perinuclear space** (Figures 3–2 and 3–3). This space and the outer nuclear membrane are continuous with the extensive cytoplasmic network of the rough endoplasmic reticulum (RER). Closely associated with the inner nuclear membrane is a highly organized meshwork of proteins called the **nuclear lamina** (Figure 3–4),

which stabilizes the nuclear envelope. Major components of this layer comprise the class of intermediate filament proteins called **lamins** that bind to membrane proteins and associate with chromatin in nondividing cells.

The inner and outer nuclear membranes are bridged at **nuclear pore complexes** (Figures 3–2 through 3–6). Each nuclear pore complex's core proteins, called **nucleoporins**, display eightfold symmetry around a lumen. Ions and small solutes pass through the lumen by simple diffusion, but nucleoporins regulate the movement of macromolecules between nucleus and cytoplasm. A growing cell has 3000–4000 such pores, each providing passage for up to 1000 macromolecules per second, with individual channels permitting molecular transfer in both directions simultaneously. Macromolecules shipped out of the nucleus include ribosomal subunits and other RNAs associated with proteins, while inbound traffic consists of chromatin proteins, ribosomal proteins, transcription factors, and enzymes. Using mechanisms similar to that by which specific proteins are recognized and translocated across the RER membrane, proteins of complexes destined for the cytoplasm have specific nuclear export sequences and proteins to be imported have nuclear localization sequences. The latter bind specifically to transport proteins (**importins**) that in turn interact with proteins of the pore complexes for transfer across the nuclear envelope. Energy for the transport is derived from guanosine 5′-triphosphate (GTP), with specific GTPases helping provide directionality to the transfer.

Chromatin

Chromatin consists of DNA and all the associated proteins involved in the organization and function of DNA. In humans, each cell's chromatin (except that of eggs and sperm) is divided among 46 **chromosomes** (23 pairs). After DNA replication but before cell division, each chromosome consists of two

FIGURE **3–1** Nuclei of large, active cells.

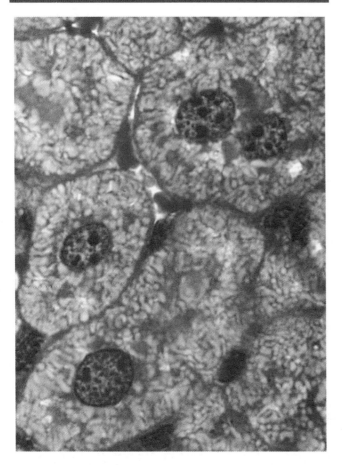

Liver cells have large, central nuclei. One or more highly basophilic nucleoli are visible within each nucleus, indicating intense protein synthesis by these cells. Most of the chromatin is light staining or euchromatic, with small areas of more darkly stained heterochromatin scattered throughout the nucleus and just inside the nuclear envelope. This superficial heterochromatin allows the boundary of the organelle to be seen more easily by light microscopy. One cell here has two nuclei, which is fairly common in the liver. (×500; Pararosaniline–toluidine blue)

identical chromatin units called **chromatids** held together by complexes of cohesin proteins.

DNA of each human cell is approximately 2 meters long, with 3.2 billion base pairs (bp), and therefore must be extensively packaged within the nucleus. This occurs initially by the DNA associating with sets of small basic proteins called **histones**. The structural unit of DNA and histones, called a **nucleosome** (Figures 3–7 and 3–8), has a core of eight histones (two copies each of histones H2A, H2B, H3, and H4), around which is wrapped about 150 bp of DNA. Each nucleosome also has a larger histone (H1) associated with both the wrapped DNA and the surface of the core. In the EM the series of nucleosomes on DNA resembles a 10-nm wide "string of

beads" with 50–80 bp of linker DNA separating each bead. Nucleosomes are structurally dynamic; modification and rearrangement of the histones allows temporary unwrapping of the DNA and arrival of enzymes and other proteins required for replication and gene transcription.

DNA wrapped around nucleosomes spirals further for greater compaction within the nucleus and for regulation of gene activity. The 10-nm filament of nucleosomes and DNA undergoes helical folding to yield a fiber with a diameter of 30 nm (Figure 3–8). The 30-nm chromatin fiber then self-interacts to form loops hundreds or thousands of kilobases long. Such loops have multiple nonstructural functions, mediating specific interactions with gene regulatory elements to control transcription in a precise spatial and temporal manner. These fibers with their loops then fold further into chromatin domains which associate with each other to create chromatin compartments. Large protein complexes maintain these compartments structurally and compact them further during cell division, producing visibly discrete chromosomes (Figure 3–8).

Microscopically two categories of chromatin can be distinguished in nuclei of most nondividing cells (Figure 3–3). **Euchromatin** is visible as finely dispersed granular material in the electron microscope and as lightly stained basophilic areas in the light microscope. **Heterochromatin** (Gr. *heteros*, other + *chroma*, color) appears as coarse, electron-dense material in the electron microscope and as intensely basophilic clumps in the light microscope.

DNA in the more open structure of euchromatin includes most genes, although not all genes are transcribed in all cells. Heterochromatin is always more compact than euchromatin, shows little or no transcriptional activity, and includes at least two types of genomic material called constitutive and facultative heterochromatin. *Constitutive heterochromatin* is generally similar in all cell types and contains mainly repetitive, gene-poor DNA sequences, including the large chromosomal regions called **centromeres** and **telomeres**, located near the middle (most often) and at the ends of chromosomes, respectively. *Facultative heterochromatin* contains other regions of DNA with gene transcription variably inactivated in different cells by epigenetic mechanisms, undergoing reversible transitions from compact, transcriptionally silent states to more open, transcriptionally active conformations.

The ratio of heterochromatin to euchromatin seen with nuclear staining can provide a rough indicator of a cell's metabolic and biosynthetic activity (Figure 3–3). Euchromatin predominates in active cells such as large neurons, while heterochromatin prevails in cells with little synthetic activity such as circulating lymphocytes. Facultative heterochromatin also occurs in the small, dense "sex chromatin" or **Barr body**, one of the two large X chromosomes present in human females but not males. The Barr body remains tightly coiled, while the other X chromosome is euchromatic and transcriptionally active. Cells of males have one X chromosome and one Y chromosome; like the other chromosomes, the single X chromosome here remains largely euchromatic.

FIGURE 3–2 Relationship of nuclear envelope to the rough ER (RER).

Nucleus

Nuclear pores

Nuclear envelope

Nucleolus

Chromatin

Ribosome

Rough endoplasmic reticulum

Functions of the Nucleus

1. **Cellular regulation:** Houses genetic material, which directs all cellular activities and regulates cellular structure
2. **Production:** Produces ribosomal subunits in nucleolus and exports them into cytoplasm for assembly into ribosomes

Three-dimensional representation of a cell nucleus shows a single large nucleolus and the distribution of the nuclear pores in the nuclear envelope. The outer membrane of the nuclear envelope is continuous with the RER. (TEM ×20,000)

>> **MEDICAL APPLICATION**

Barr bodies or gender chromatin permit gender to be determined microscopically in patients whose external sex organs do not permit that determination, as in hermaphroditism and pseudohermaphroditism. Sex chromatin analysis also helps reveal other anomalies involving the sex chromosomes, such as the presence of XXY chromosomes (Klinefelter syndrome), which causes testicular abnormalities and azoospermia (absence of sperm).

Although heterochromatin tends to be scattered or concentrated near the nuclear lamina, routine microscopy provides little evidence for spatial organization of chromatin. Recent in situ hybridization studies of nuclei in cultured human fibroblasts have used differently labeled fluorescent probes for sequences on each individual chromosome to reveal that these structures occupy discrete **chromosomal territories** within dispersed chromatin (Figure 3–9). Such studies show further that chromosomal domains with few genes form a layer beneath the nuclear envelope, while domains with many active genes occur deeper in the nucleus.

The X and Y sex chromosomes contain genes determining whether an individual will develop as a female or a male. In addition to the pair of sex chromosomes, cells contain 22 pairs of autosomes. Each pair contains one chromosome originally derived from the mother and one from the father. The members of each chromosomal pair are called **homologous**

because, although from different parents, they contain forms (alleles) of the same genes. Cells of most tissues (somatic cells) are considered **diploid** because they contain these chromosome pairs and two sex chromosomes: XX in females, XY in males. Geneticists refer to diploid cells as $2n$, where n is the number of unique chromosomes in a species, 23 in humans. Sperm cells and mature oocytes (germ cells) are **haploid**, with half the diploid number of chromosomes, each pair having been separated during meiosis (described later in the chapter).

Microscopic analysis of chromosomes usually begins with cultured cells arrested in mitotic metaphase by colchicine or other compounds that disrupt microtubules. After processing and nuclear staining the condensed chromosomes of one nucleus are photographed by light microscopy and rearranged digitally to produce a **karyotype**, facilitating analysis of the stained chromosomes (Figure 3–10).

>> **MEDICAL APPLICATION**

Karyotyping is important for many prenatal diagnoses, in which chromosomal analysis of cultured cells from the fetus or amnion can detect certain genetic anomalies. As with karyotypes of adults, missing or extra chromosomes and chromosomal deletions or translocations are readily seen. New methods of chromosomal staining and molecular techniques, such as fluorescence in situ hybridization (FISH), are continuously being developed and used for cytogenetic diagnosis.

FIGURE **3–3** Ultrastructure of a nucleus.

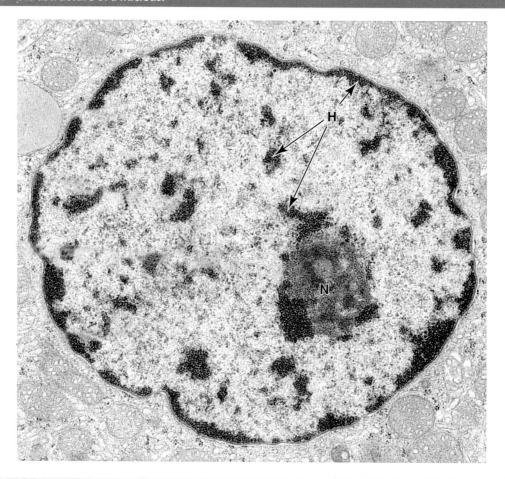

Regions of euchromatin and heterochromatin display variable electron densities with the transmission electron microscope (TEM). An active nucleus typically has much diffuse, light-staining euchromatin and smaller subdomains of electron-dense heterochromatin (**H**), with many of these associated at the periphery associated with the nuclear lamina. The more heterogeneous electron-dense subdomain is the nucleolus (**N**), the site of rRNA synthesis, and ribosomal subunit assembly. (×25,000)

Nucleolus

The **nucleolus** is a nonmembranous, compact, and highly basophilic subdomain of nuclei in cells actively engaged in protein synthesis (Figures 3–1 through 3–3). Here the intense basophilia indicates not heterochromatin but rather the presence of concentrated ribosomal RNA (rRNA) undergoing transcription, processing, and assembly into ribosomal subunits. Chromosomal regions with the genes for rRNA organize to form one or more nucleoli in cells requiring intense ribosome production for protein synthesis during growth or secretion. Ultrastructural analysis of an active nucleolus reveals fibrillar and granular subregions with different staining characteristics that reflect stages of rRNA maturation, as described in Figure 3–11. Molecules of rRNA are processed in the nucleolus and very quickly associate with the ribosomal proteins imported from the cytoplasm via nuclear pores.

The newly organized small and large ribosomal subunits then undergo export back to the cytoplasm through those same nuclear pores.

❯❯ MEDICAL APPLICATION

Tissues with either stable or rapidly renewing cell populations can include cells that become transformed to grow at a higher rate and in an uncoordinated manner. Such **neoplastic proliferation** typically follows damage to the DNA of proto-oncogenes and failure of the cells to be eliminated. Neoplastic growth can be either benign (with slow growth and no invasiveness to neighboring organs) or malignant (with rapid growth and great capacity to invade other organs). **Cancer** is the common term for all malignant tumors.

FIGURE **3–4** The nuclear envelope, nuclear lamina, and nuclear pore complexes.

Perinuclear space · Rough ER · Nuclear pore complex · Inner and outer nuclear membrane · Nuclear lamina · Chromatin

NL · NPC · NL

(a) Bound to the inner membrane of the nuclear envelope is the **nuclear lamina**, a meshwork assembled from lamins (class V intermediate filament proteins). The 100-nm wide **nuclear pore complexes** (NPC) each contain approximately 34 nucleoporin proteins forming a symmetric core of inner and outer rings which stabilize the extreme curvature of the nuclear envelope's inner and outer membranes where they abut the pore. Proteins in the cytoplasm that are destined for the nucleus bind to importin proteins, which in turn bind filamentous polypeptides that extend from the NPC outer ring and facilitate import into the nucleus. On the inside of the NPC, a basket-like assembly of other nucleoporins interacts with the transcriptional machinery in chromatin and facilitates export of newly made messenger ribonucleoprotein particles into the cytoplasm. Nuclear pores simultaneously transport macromolecules in both directions, utilizing energy derived locally from GTP, and unlike most cell membrane channels or transporters do not open and close while regulating transport.

(b) Scanning EM of the inner nuclear membrane (nucleoplasmic face) showing portions of the nuclear lamina (**NL**) meshwork with many embedded nuclear pore complexes (**NPC**). The preparation is from an actively growing amphibian oocyte. Nuclei of these very large cells can be isolated manually, facilitating ultrastructural studies of the nuclear envelope. (×100,000)

(Reproduced with permission from Dr M.W. Goldberg, Department of Biological and Biomedical Sciences, Durham University, UK.)

FIGURE **3–5** Nuclear pores.

C · N

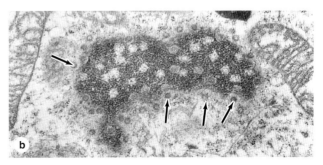

(a) A TEM section through the nuclear envelope between nucleus (**N**) and cytoplasm (**C**) shows its two-membrane structure. The electron-dense nuclear pore complexes bridging the nuclear envelope can also be seen (arrows). Electron-dense heterochromatin is adjacent to the envelope, except at the nuclear pores.

(b) A tangential section through a nuclear envelope shows the nuclear pore complexes (arrows) and the electron-lucent patches in the peripheral heterochromatin, which represent the areas just inside pores. (×80,000)

FIGURE 3–6 **Cryofracture of nuclear envelope showing nuclear pores.**

An electron micrograph obtained by freeze-fractured cell shows the two layers of the nuclear envelope and nuclear pores. The fracture plane occurs partly *between* the two nuclear envelope membranes (left) but mostly just *inside* the envelope with the chromatin removed. The size and distribution of the nuclear pore complexes are clearly seen. (×60,000)

❱❱ MEDICAL APPLICATION

Certain mutations in the gene coding for lamin A are associated with a subtype of the disorder progeria, which causes premature aging. In this and other rare "laminopathies," the nuclear envelope is abnormal, but how this is linked to the disorder is unclear. Laminopathies affect some tissues much more than others, although the lamins involved are in all the body's cells.

❱ THE CELL CYCLE

Before differentiation most cells undergo repeated cycles of macromolecular synthesis (growth) and division (mitosis). The regular sequence of events that produce new cells comprises the **cell cycle**. Improved knowledge about controls on each phase of the cell cycle and about quality control during DNA replication has led to understanding the causes of many types of cancer, in which cells proliferate without those restrictions.

The cell cycle has four distinct phases: **mitosis** and periods termed G_1 (the time gap between mitosis and the beginning of DNA replication), **S** (the period of DNA synthesis), and G_2 (the gap between DNA duplication and the next mitosis). Figure 3–12 illustrates the approximate durations of these phases in rapidly dividing human cells. The G_1 phase, usually the longest and most variable part of the cycle, involves active RNA and protein synthesis, including proteins controlling progress through the cell cycle. Also in G_1, the cell volume, reduced by half during mitosis, returns to its previous size. The S phase includes DNA replication, histone synthesis, and the beginning of centrosome duplication. In the relatively short G_2 phase, proteins required for mitosis accumulate. As new postmitotic cells specialize and differentiate, cell cycle activities may be temporarily or permanently suspended, with the cells sometimes referred to as being in the G_0 phase. Some differentiated cells renew cycling under certain conditions, such as those of the liver following partial hepatectomy; others, including most muscle and nerve cells, are *terminally differentiated*.

Cycling begins in postmitotic G_0 cells with protein signals from the extracellular environment called **mitogens** or **growth factors** binding to cell surface receptors and triggering a cascade of kinase signaling in the cells. The cells are then maintained at the *restriction point* at the G_1/S "boundary" until sufficient nutrients and enzymes required for DNA synthesis have accumulated, and when all is ready DNA replication (S phase) begins.

As shown in Figure 3–13, entry or progression through other phases of the cycle occurs with monitoring at other

FIGURE **3–7** Components of a nucleosome.

Core of 8 histone molecules: H2A, H2B, H3, and H4

H1 histone

Central DNA

Link DNA

6 nm

10 nm

Nucleosomes are structures that produces the initial organization of free double-stranded DNA into chromatin. Each nucleosome has an octameric core complex made up of four types of **histones**, two copies each of H2A, H2B, H3, and H4. Around this core is wound DNA approximately 150 bp in length. One H1 histone is located outside the DNA on the surface of each nucleosome. DNA associated with nucleosomes in vivo thus resembles a long string of beads. Nucleosomes are very dynamic structures, with H1 loosening and DNA unwrapping at least once every second to allow other proteins, including transcription factors and enzymes, access to the DNA.

specific *checkpoints*, where certain conditions must be met before the cell continues cycling. A family of cytoplasmic proteins called **cyclins** regulates cycling overall. With different cyclins present during different cell cycle phases, each activates one or more specific **cyclin-dependent kinases (CDKs)**. Each activated CDK then phosphorylates specific proteins, including enzymes, transcription factors for specific sets of genes, and cytoskeletal subunits, triggering the activities that characterize the next phase of the cycle. With completion of each successive set of activities, the cyclin controlling that cell cycle phase is ubiquitinated and removed rapidly by proteasomes and a new cyclin that promotes activities for the next phase takes over. In this way, diverse cellular activities occur in coordination with specific phases of the cell cycle. Table 3–1 summarizes the major cyclins, CDKs, and their important target proteins.

❯❯ MEDICAL APPLICATION

Many mitogenic growth factors for research are produced commercially from microorganisms or cells with recombinant DNA, and some have important medical uses. Important examples include analogs of granulocyte colony-stimulating factor (G-CSF), which stimulates neutrophil production in immunocompromised patients, and erythropoietin, which can stimulate red blood cell formation in patients with anemia.

FIGURE **3–8** From DNA to chromatin.

DNA — 2 nm

Nucleosomes (DNA and core histones) — 10 nm

Packed nucleosomes in 30-nm chromatin fiber — 30 nm

Extended loops of transcriptionally active chromatin, tethered to protein scaffold — 300 nm

Heterochromatin

Condensed heterochromatin and dispersed euchromatin

Euchromatin — 700 nm

Entire chromosome at metaphase

Centromere

1400 nm

Chromatids

Several orders of DNA folding occur in chromatin and during chromatin condensation. The top drawing shows the 2-nm DNA double helix, followed by its association with histones to form 10-nm filaments of **nucleosomes** connected by DNA ("beads on a string"). The string of nucleosomes then self-assembles as a more compact 30-nm diameter **chromatin fiber**. DNA in many regions of these fibers self-interacts, forming large loops tethered at their ends to scaffold-like complexes of transcriptional repressor proteins. These and other gene regulatory proteins contribute to precise spatial and temporal control of gene expression within the loops. The entire length of a 30-nm fiber then folds further into variably condensed, topologically associated chromatin domains maintained structurally by protein complexes. Domains with loops and active gene transcription comprise **euchromatin** and fill most of the nucleus in synthetically active cells. **Heterochromatin**, with many fewer loops and little gene activity, remains more highly condensed, largely at the nuclear periphery. The bottom drawing shows a metaphase chromosome, with maximum packing of DNA mediated by other large complexes of proteins during cell division to form visibly discrete chromosomes. The **chromosome** consists of two **chromatids** held together at a constriction called the **centromere**.

FIGURE **3–9** Chromosome territories of a human fibroblast nucleus.

Fluorescence in situ hybridization (FISH) can be used with a combination of labeled probes, each specific for sequences on different chromosomes. A nucleus of a cultured human fibroblast was processed by 24-color FISH, photographed by confocal microscopy in appropriate channels, and the results superimposed to form an RGB (red-green-blue) image **(a)** of the 24 differently labeled chromosome types (1–22, X, and Y). Individual chromosome territories in the image were identified and false-colored after classification by software developed for such analyses **(b)**.

(Reproduced with permission from Dr Thomas Cremer, Department of Biology II, Anthropology and Human Genetics, Ludwig Maximilian University, Munich, Germany.)

FIGURE **3–10** Human karyotype.

Karyotypes provide light microscopic information regarding the number and morphology of chromosomes in an organism. Such preparations are made by staining and photographing the chromosomes of a cultured cell arrested with colchicine during mitosis, when chromosomes are maximally condensed. From the image individual chromosomes are typically placed together in pairs. With certain stains, each chromosome has a particular pattern of banding that facilitates its identification and shows the relationship of the banding pattern to genetic anomalies. Hybridization with fluorescent probes specific for each chromosome (FISH) followed by karyotyping yields an image like that shown here. Note that the 22 pairs of autosomes, as well as the X and Y chromosomes, differ in size, morphology, and location of the centromere.

repair of the damage before the cell enters S phase, so that the damaged DNA does not reproduce gene defects during replication. If the problem encountered at any checkpoint cannot be corrected quickly while cycling is halted, proteins encoded by tumor suppressor genes are activated and that cell's activity is redirected toward cell suicide or apoptosis.

❯❯ MEDICAL APPLICATION

Many genes coding for proteins important in the control of cell proliferation and differentiation are often called **proto-oncogenes**; changes in the structure or expression of these can convert them to **oncogenes** causing uncontrolled cell growth and a potential for cancer. Altered proto-oncogenes are associated with many types of tumors and hematologic cancers. Proto-oncogenes can encode almost any protein involved in the control of mitotic activity, including various specific growth factors, the receptors for growth factors, and various kinases and other proteins involved in intracellular signaling of growth factors.

Progression through the cell cycle stops with adverse conditions such as inadequate nutrition (nutrient stress), inappropriate cellular microenvironments, or DNA damage. Nuclear DNA is monitored very closely, and damage here can arrest the cell cycle not only at the G_1 **restriction point** but also during S or at a checkpoint in G_2 (Figure 3–13). G_1 arrest may permit

FIGURE **3–11** Regions within a nucleolus.

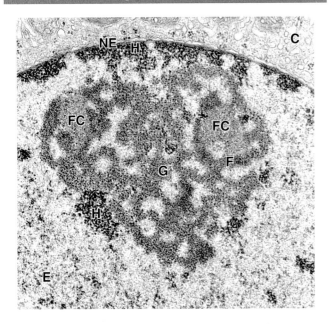

TEM of a nucleolus reveals morphologically distinct regions, which correspond loosely to major subcompartments for ribosomal subunit synthesis. Variably light-staining areas comprise the fibrillar centers (**FC**) containing clustered "nucleolar organizer" rRNA genes undergoing transcription. Surrounding these centers are areas of a dense fibrillar component (**F**) in which the new rRNA transcripts accumulate and undergo processing. Other areas display a more distinctly granular component (**G**) with large and small ribosomal subunits being assembled from mature rRNAs and ribosomal proteins imported from the cytoplasm. Areas of heterochromatin (**H**) are also typically found near the nucleolus besides being scattered in the euchromatin (**E**) and adjacent to the nuclear envelop (**NE**) which separates chromatin from cytoplasm (**C**). (×35,000)

›› MEDICAL APPLICATION

Retinoblastoma is a type of cancer occurring in the eyes, usually in young children. One form of the disease is inherited or familial. Research on the genetic basis of this disease led to the discovery of Rb, a gene coding for a key protein active at the G_1 restriction point that blocks cell cycle progression until a mitogenic stimulus arrives. A kinase activated by a growth factor receptor phosphorylates the Rb protein, causing it to release the E2F transcription factor. This factor then activates genes needed for DNA replication.

DNA changes (mutations) resulting from damage are not always detected and corrected (or eliminated). If such a change occurs in a gene important for cell cycle activities, such as genes for certain growth factors, their receptors or signaling kinases, normal controls on the cell cycle may be affected and growth may occur in a less-regulated manner usually detected by the tumor suppressor proteins such as p53.

Failure to detect unregulated cell cycling can lead to additional defects and the cellular changes found in the various types of cancer. Mutations in the gene for the key tumor suppressor p53 itself characterize many forms of human cancer, thus reducing the ability to eliminate cells with damaged DNA and facilitating proliferation of cells with new genetic defects.

› MITOSIS

During the period of cell division, or **mitosis** (Gr. *mitos*, a thread), the only cell cycle phase distinguishable by routine light microscopy, a parent cell divides and each of the two daughter cells receives a chromosomal set identical to that of the parent cell. The chromosomes duplicated during the preceding S phase are distributed to the daughter cells. The long period between mitoses (the G_1, S, and G_2 phases) constitutes the so-called **interphase**, while the events of mitosis itself occur in four rapid, major stages (Figure 3–12). Important details of each mitotic phase, shown in Figure 3–14, are summarized here. During the relatively long **prophase**, several changes occur:

- The nucleolus disappears, and the replicated chromatin (DNA and associated proteins) condenses into discrete threadlike chromosomes, each consisting of duplicate sister chromatids joined at the centromere.
- The two centrosomes with their now-duplicated centrioles separate and migrate to opposite poles of the cell and organize the microtubules of the **mitotic spindle**.
- Late in prophase, lamins and inner nuclear membrane are phosphorylated, causing the nuclear lamina and nuclear pore complexes to disassemble and disperse in cytoplasmic membrane vesicles.

During **metaphase**, chromosomes condense further and large protein complexes called **kinetochores** (Gr. *kinetos*, moving), located at the centromere DNA region of each chromosome, attach to the mitotic spindle (Figure 3–15). The cell assumes a spherical shape and microtubules move the chromosomes into alignment at the equatorial plate.

In **anaphase**, sister chromatids (now called chromosomes themselves) separate and move toward opposite spindle poles by a combination of microtubule motor proteins and dynamic changes in the lengths of the microtubules as the spindle poles move farther apart.

At **telophase**, the following occur:

- The two sets of chromosomes are at the spindle poles and begin reverting to their uncondensed state.
- Microtubules of the spindle depolymerize, and the nuclear envelope begins to reassemble around each set of daughter chromosomes.
- A belt-like contractile ring of actin filaments associated with myosins develops in the cortical cytoplasm at the cell's equator. During **cytokinesis** at the end of telophase constriction of this ring produces a cleavage furrow that progressively divides the cytoplasm and its organelles into two daughter cells, each with one nucleus.

FIGURE **3–12** The cell cycle.

The ability to recognize cells microscopically during both mitosis and DNA replication (by autoradiography after administering radiolabeled thymidine) led to the concept of the cell "cycle" with the phases occurring as shown here. In rapidly dividing cells, **G₁** is a period in which cells accumulate the enzymes and nucleotides required for DNA replication, **S** is the period devoted primarily to DNA replication, **G₂** is a usually short period of preparation for

mitosis, and **M** includes all phases of mitosis itself. In rapidly growing human tissues, the cell cycle varies from 24 to 36 hours. The length of G₁ depends on many factors and is usually the longest and most variable period; the length of S is largely a function of the genome size. G₂ and mitosis together normally last only 2–3 hours. Differentiating cells in growing tissues may have very long G₁ periods and such cells are often said to be in the **G₀** phase of the cell cycle.

FIGURE **3–13** Controls at cell cycle checkpoints.

Each phase of the cell cycle has one or more checkpoints where the quality of specific cell activities is checked. Progression to the next phase of the cycle does not occur until all activities of the preceding phase are completed satisfactorily. Three important checkpoints are shown here, including:

- The *start or restriction checkpoint* just before the start of S
- The *G₂/M checkpoint* that ensures that DNA replication is complete

- The metaphase *spindle checkpoint* that ensures that all chromosomes will be segregated

Overall progression in the cycle is regulated by proteins called **cyclins** and **cyclin-dependent kinases (CDKs)** that phosphorylate/activate enzymes and other proteins needed for phase-specific functions. Major cyclins, their CDKs, and important protein targets are summarized in Table 3–1.

TABLE **3–1**	Major cyclin and cyclin-dependent kinase complexes regulating the human cell cycle and important target proteins.	
Cycle Phase or Checkpoint	**Active Cyclin-CDK Complex**	**Examples of Target Proteins**
Early G_1	Cyclin D-CDK4 or 6	Phosphorylates Rb protein, releasing E2F, a transcription factor that activates genes for many G_1 activities and for cyclin A
Late G_1/entry of S	Cyclin E-CDK2	Further activation E2F-mediated gene transcription; protein p53; other kinases
Progression through S	Cyclin A-CDK2	DNA polymerase and other proteins for DNA replication
G_2/entry of M	Cyclin A-CDK1	Specific phosphatases and cyclin B
Progression through M	Cyclin B-CDK1	Nuclear lamins; histone H1; chromatin- and centrosome-associated proteins

Most tissues undergo cell turnover with slow cell division and cell death. Nerve tissue and cardiac muscle are exceptions because their differentiated cells cannot undergo mitosis. As discussed in later chapters, a capacity for mitosis within a tissue, either by differentiated cells or by a reserve of stem cells, largely determines the tissue's potential for regeneration. Rapid cell turnover characterizes the epithelium lining the digestive tract and uterus or covering the skin. Mitotic cells are usually difficult to identify conclusively in sections of adult organs but may often be detected in rapidly growing tissues by their condensed chromatin (Figure 3–16).

FIGURE **3–14** Phases of mitosis.

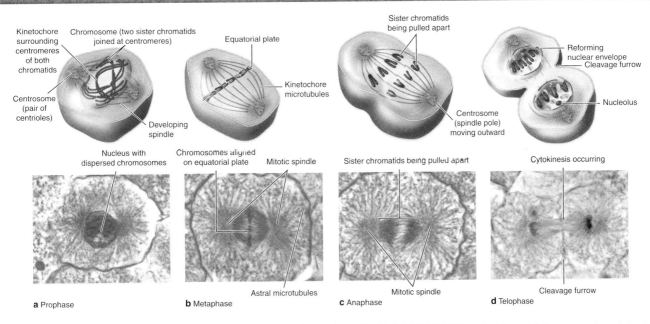

Kinetochore surrounding centromeres of both chromatids — Chromosome (two sister chromatids joined at centromeres) — Centrosome (pair of centrioles) — Developing spindle — Nucleus with dispersed chromosomes

Equatorial plate — Kinetochore microtubules — Chromosomes aligned on equatorial plate — Mitotic spindle — Astral microtubules

Sister chromatids being pulled apart — Centrosome (spindle pole) moving outward — Sister chromatids being pulled apart — Mitotic spindle

Reforming nuclear envelope — Cleavage furrow — Nucleolus — Cytokinesis occurring — Cleavage furrow

a Prophase **b** Metaphase **c** Anaphase **d** Telophase

The chromosomal changes that occur during mitosis are easily and commonly studied in the large cells of very early embryos of fish after sectioning, such as the mitotic cells shown here.

(a) During the relatively long **prophase**, the **centrosomes** move to opposite poles, the nuclear envelope disappears by fragmentation, and the chromosomes condense and become visible. Having undergone DNA replication, each chromosome consists of two chromatids joined at their centromere regions by **kinetochore** protein complexes.

(b) At the short **metaphase**, the chromosomes have become aligned at the **equatorial plate** as a result of their attachments to the dynamic microtubules of the **mitotic spindle** organized by the centrosomes. The spindle consists of **kinetochore microtubules**, polar microtubules which interdigitate near the equatorial plate, and shorter astral microtubules anchoring the spindle to the cell membrane.

(c) During **anaphase**, the kinetochores separate and the chromatids (now called chromosomes themselves) are pulled on their microtubules toward each centrosome.

(d) In **telophase**, the cell pinches itself in two by contraction of the F-actin bundle in the cell cortex, after which the chromosomes decondense, transcription resumes, nucleoli reappear, and the nuclear lamina and nuclear envelope reassemble. (All ×500; H&E)

FIGURE **3–15** Mitotic spindle and metaphase chromosomes.

TEM of a sectioned metaphase cell shows several features of the mitotic apparatus, including the very electron-dense chromosomes bound at kinetochores (arrows) to the microtubules of the spindle. The microtubules converge on the centrosomes (**C**), each containing a pair of centrioles. The flattened membrane vesicles near the mitotic spindle may represent fragments of the nuclear envelope, which begin to reassemble during late telophase. (×19,000)

(*Reproduced with permission from Richard McIntosh, Department of Molecular, Cellular and Developmental Biology, University of Colorado, Boulder.*)

FIGURE **3–16** Mitotic cells in adult tissues.

Dividing cells in recognizable stages of mitosis are rarely observed in adult tissues because they are rare and the cells are small, with variable shapes and orientations. However, *mitotic figures*, nuclei with clumped, darkly stained chromatin, can sometimes be identified, as shown here in various rapidly renewing tissues.

(a) In the lining of the small intestine, many mitotic *transit amplifying cells* can be found in the area above the most basal region of the intestinal crypts. Condensed chromosomes of cells in late anaphase and prophase phase can be distinguished here.

(b) Metaphase cell in a gland of proliferating uterine endometrium.

(c) Telophase cell in the esophagus lining.

(d) Metaphase in the basal layer of epidermis. (×400; H&E)

STEM CELLS & TISSUE RENEWAL

Throughout an individual's lifetime, many tissues and organs contain a small population of undifferentiated **stem cells** whose cycling serves to renew the differentiated cells of tissues as needed. Many stem cells divide infrequently and asymmetrically; that is, one daughter cell remains as a stem cell, while the other becomes committed to a path that leads to differentiation (Figure 3–17). Stem cells of many tissues occur in specific locations or niches where the microenvironment helps maintain their uniquely undifferentiated properties, often remaining rare and inconspicuous by routine histologic methods.

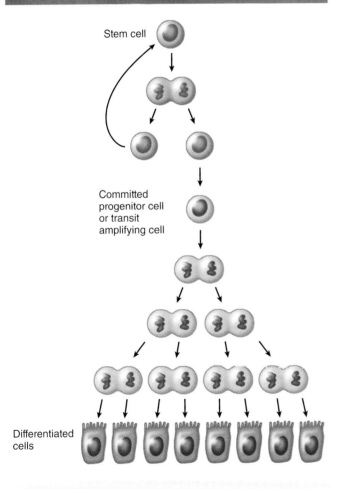

Stem cell

Committed progenitor cell or transit amplifying cell

Differentiated cells

In rapidly growing adult tissues and perhaps in other tissues, there are slowly dividing populations of **stem cells**. Stem cells divide asymmetrically, producing one cell that remains as a stem cell and another that becomes committed to a differentiative pathway but divides a few more times at a more rapid rate. Such cells have been termed **progenitor cells**, or "transit amplifying cells," each of which eventually stops dividing and becomes fully differentiated.

Stem cells are best studied in tissues with *rapidly renewing cell populations*, including blood cells, skin cells, and cells lining the digestive tract. Most mitotic cells here do not represent stem cells, but rather the more rapidly dividing progeny of the cells committed to differentiation (Figure 3–17). These are commonly called **progenitor cells** or transit amplifying cells because they are in transit along the path from the stem cell niche to a differentiated state, while still amplifying by mitosis the number of new cells available for the differentiated tissue. Cells formed by progenitor cells may become terminally differentiated, meaning that renewed cycling cannot occur and the specialized cells exist for only a short time.

In tissues with *stable cell populations*, such as most connective tissues, smooth muscle, and the cells lining blood vessels, stem cells are not readily apparent, and differentiated cells appear to undergo slow and episodic division to maintain tissue integrity.

MEIOSIS

A specialized process involving *two* unique and closely associated cell divisions, **meiosis** occurs only in the cells that will form sperm and egg cells. Chapters 21 and 22 fully cover differentiation of these two "germ cells" or **gametes**, but chromosomal aspects of meiosis are described here for comparison with the events of mitosis (Figure 3–18).

Two key features characterize meiosis. (1) Early in the process, the homologous chromosomes of each pair (one from the mother, one from the father) come together in an activity termed **synapsis**. During synapsis double-stranded breaks and repairs occur in the DNA, some of which result in reciprocal DNA exchanges called **crossovers** between the aligned homologous chromosomes. This produces new combinations of genes in the chromosomes so that few if any chromosomes in the germ cells are exactly like those in the mother and father. (2) The cells produced are **haploid**, having just one chromosome from each pair present in the body's somatic cells. The union of haploid eggs and sperm at fertilization forms a new diploid cell (the zygote) that can develop into a new individual.

As shown in Figure 3–18, the important events of meiosis unfold as follows:

- A cell approaching the first meiotic division has just completed a typical S phase and replicated its DNA; each chromosome contains the two identical DNA molecules called *sister chromatids* bound by cohesin proteins.
- During a greatly elongated prophase of the first meiotic division (prophase I), the partially condensed chromatin of homologous chromosomes begins to come together and physically associate along their lengths during synapsis. Because each of the paired chromosomes has two chromatids, geneticists refer to synaptic chromosomes as *tetrads* to emphasize that four copies of each genetic

FIGURE 3–18 Mitosis and meiosis.

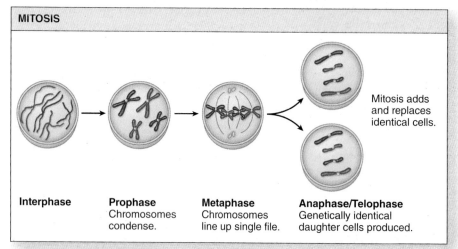

MITOSIS

Interphase

Prophase
Chromosomes
condense.

Metaphase
Chromosomes
line up single file.

Anaphase/Telophase
Genetically identical
daughter cells produced.

Mitosis adds
and replaces
identical cells.

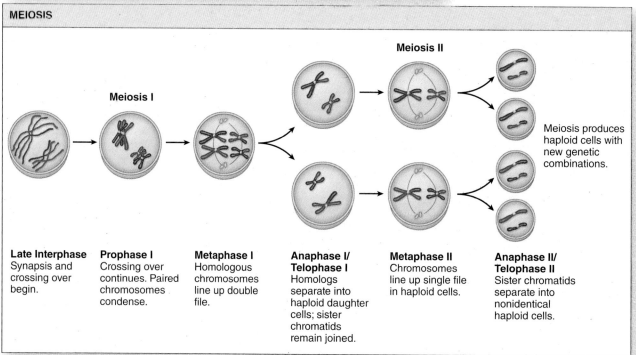

MEIOSIS

Meiosis I

Meiosis II

Late Interphase
Synapsis and
crossing over
begin.

Prophase I
Crossing over
continues. Paired
chromosomes
condense.

Metaphase I
Homologous
chromosomes
line up double
file.

**Anaphase I/
Telophase I**
Homologs
separate into
haploid daughter
cells; sister
chromatids
remain joined.

Metaphase II
Chromosomes
line up single file
in haploid cells.

**Anaphase II/
Telophase II**
Sister chromatids
separate into
nonidentical
haploid cells.

Meiosis produces
haploid cells with
new genetic
combinations.

Mitosis and meiosis share many aspects of chromatin condensation and separation but differ in key ways. Mitosis produces *two diploid cells* that are the same genetically. In meiosis, the two homologous maternal and paternal chromosomes physically align in **synapsis**, and regions are exchanged during *crossing over* or genetic recombination. This is followed by **two meiotic divisions** with no intervening S phase, producing *four haploid cells*.

sequence are present. During synapsis recombination or crossing over occurs among the four chromatids, which mixes up the genes inherited from each parent and yields a new and different set of genes to be passed on to the next generation. In human, spermatogenesis prophase I normally lasts for 3 weeks; oocytes arrest in this meiotic phase from the time of their formation in the fetal ovary through the woman's reproductive maturity, that is, for about 12 years to nearly five decades.

▪ With completion of synapsis and crossing over the chromosomes become fully condensed and undergo metaphase, anaphase, and telophase as the cell divides.

This first meiotic division separates the homologous chromosomes that paired up during synapsis; each of the separated chromosomes still contains two chromatids held together by cohesins at the centromeric DNA.

■ Each of the two new cells now divides again, much more rapidly and without an intervening S phase. In this second meiotic division, cohesin proteins are lost and the chromatids separate to opposite poles as individual chromosomes. In each new cell, a nuclear envelope forms around this new haploid set of chromosomes.

In summary, meiosis and mitosis share many aspects of chromatin condensation and separation (Figure 3–18), but differ in key ways:

■ Mitosis culminates in cell division producing *two diploid cells.* Meiosis involves two cell divisions and produces *four haploid cells.*

■ During meiotic crossing over, new combinations of genes arise, with every haploid cell genetically unique. Lacking synapsis and the opportunity for DNA recombination, mitosis yields two cells that are the same genetically.

❯❯ MEDICAL APPLICATION

In humans, chromosome 21 is a very small chromosome and the one most likely to be "overlooked" at the metaphase/anaphase checkpoint. Failure of these homologous chromosomes to separate (nondisjunction) in the first meiotic division also occurs with greater frequency in older oocytes (or sperm progenitor cells). A gamete retaining this chromosome pair forms a viable zygote after fertilization, but the developing **trisomy 21** individual has morphologic and cognitive impairments associated with Down syndrome.

❯ APOPTOSIS

Less evident, but no less important than cell proliferation for body functions, is the process of cell suicide called **apoptosis** (Gr. *apo*, off + *ptosis*, a falling), a rapid and highly regulated cellular activity that shrinks and eliminates defective and unneeded cells (Figure 3–19). Apoptosis results in small membrane-enclosed *apoptotic bodies,* which quickly undergo phagocytosis by neighboring cells or cells specialized for debris removal. Apoptotic cells do not rupture or release their contents, unlike cells that die after an injury and undergo *necrosis,* a difference important for neighboring cells. Necrotic release of cellular components triggers local inflammatory reactions and immigration of leukocytes, a potentially hazardous tissue response avoided by apoptosis

FIGURE **3–19** Apoptotic cells.

Apoptotic cells in adult tissues are rare because the process is completed very rapidly. Moreover, with their highly condensed chromatin in pyknotic nuclei and rounded shape, cells early in apoptosis may superficially resemble some mitotic cells. Shown here are apoptotic cells (**A**) in the epithelium covering an intestinal villus (**a**), in a corpus luteum beginning to undergo involution (**b**), in the epithelium of a uterine endometrial gland at the onset of menstruation (**c**), and in the liver (**d**). (×400; H&E)

following arrested cycling in defective cells or as part of normal organ development.

❯❯ MEDICAL APPLICATION

Cancer cells often deactivate the genes that control the apoptotic process, thus preventing cell elimination and allowing their progression toward a more malignant state. The Bcl-2 family of proteins that controls the onset of apoptosis was first identified by a genetic mutation in a specific B-cell lymphoma, which provided the name for the original protein.

The **Bcl-2 family** of cytoplasmic proteins initiates apoptosis, regulating release of suicide-promoting factors from mitochondria. Triggered by either irreversible internal damage or external signals, specific Bcl-2 proteins induce a process with the following features:

- **Loss of mitochondrial function and caspase activation:** Activated Bcl-2 proteins in the outer mitochondrial membrane compromise membrane integrity, stopping normal activity and releasing cytochrome c into the cytoplasm where it activates proteolytic enzymes called **caspases**. The initial caspases activate a cascade of other caspases, resulting in protein degradation throughout the cell.

- **Fragmentation of DNA:** Caspase-activated **DNase** cleaves DNA between nucleosomes into small fragments. (The new ends produced in the fragmented DNA allow apoptotic cells to be stained histochemically using an appropriate enzyme that adds labeled nucleotides at these sites.)

- **Shrinkage of nuclear and cell volumes:** Destruction of the cytoskeleton and chromatin causes the cell to shrink quickly, producing small structures with dense, darkly stained **pyknotic nuclei** that may be identifiable with the light microscope (Figure 3–19).

- **Cell membrane changes:** The plasma membrane of the shrinking cell undergoes dramatic shape changes, such as "blebbing," as membrane proteins disappear and lipid mobility increases.

- **Phagocytic removal:** Membrane-bound remnants of cytoplasm and nucleus separate as small **apoptotic bodies** (Figure 3–20). Newly exposed phospholipids on these bodies induce their phagocytosis by neighboring cells or white blood cells.

❯❯ MEDICAL APPLICATION

Nuclei of cells in malignant tumors are often enlarged, abnormally shaped, and extremely dark staining, with abnormal nucleoli, in comparison with nuclei of normal cells. Such changes are useful to pathologists looking for evidence of cancer during microscopic examinations of biopsies.

A few examples of apoptosis emphasize its significance. In the ovary, apoptosis provides for both the monthly loss of luteal cells and the removal of excess oocytes and their follicles. First discovered as "programmed cell death" in embryos, apoptosis helps shape developing organs or body regions, such as the free spaces between embryonic fingers and toes. Apoptosis of excess nerve cells plays an important role in the final development of the central nervous system.

Triggered by p53 and other tumor suppressor proteins, apoptosis eliminates cells in which damage caused by free radicals, radiation, or nutrient starvation blocks survival. In all these examples, apoptosis occurs very rapidly, in less time than required for mitosis, and the affected cells are removed without a trace.

FIGURE 3–20 Late apoptosis—apoptotic bodies.

TEM of a cell in late apoptosis shows radical changes in cell shape, with membrane blebbing and the formation of many membrane-bound cytoplasmic regions. These apoptotic bodies may separate from one another but remain enclosed by plasma membrane so that no contents are released into the extracellular space. The membrane changes are recognized by neighboring cells, and macrophages and apoptotic bodies are very rapidly phagocytosed. (×10,000)

The Nucleus SUMMARY OF KEY POINTS

Nuclear Envelope

- Cytoplasm is separated from nucleoplasm by the **nuclear envelope**, a double set of membranes with a narrow perinuclear space; the outer membrane binds ribosomes and is continuous with the RER.
- The nuclear envelope is penetrated by **nuclear pore complexes**, large assemblies of nucleoporins with eightfold symmetry through which proteins and protein–RNA complexes move in both directions.
- The nuclear envelope is supported internally by a meshwork, the nuclear lamina, composed of intermediate filament subunits called **lamins**.

Chromatin

- Chromatin is the combination of DNA and its associated proteins.
- Chromatin with DNA that is active in transcription stains lightly and is called **euchromatin**; inactive chromatin stains more darkly and is called **heterochromatin**.
- The DNA molecule initially wraps around complexes of basic proteins called **histones** to form **nucleosomes**, producing a structure resembling beads on a string.
- Additional levels of chromatin fiber condensation are less well understood and involve nonhistone proteins, including scaffolds of large protein complexes.
- The extra X chromosome in cells of female mammals forms facultative heterochromatin and can be seen as the Barr body.

Nucleolus

- The **nucleolus** is a very basophilic or electron-dense area of chromatin localized where **rRNA transcription and ribosomal subunits assembly** occur.
- By TEM, an active nucleolus is seen to have **fibrous and granular parts** where rRNA forms and ribosomal subunits are assembled, respectively.

The Cell Cycle

- The **cell cycle** is the sequence of events that controls cell growth and division.
- The G_1 phase, the longest part of the cycle, begins immediately after mitosis and includes all preparations for DNA replication.
- The period of DNA (and histone) synthesis is the **S phase**.
- In a short G_2 **phase** the cell prepares for division during **mitosis (M)**.
- Cell cycling is controlled by the sequential appearance of key cytoplasmic proteins, the **cyclins**, which bind **CDKs**.
- CDKs phosphorylate and activate the enzymes and transcription factors whose functions characterize each phase of the cell cycle.
- Progress through the cell cycle stages is monitored at checkpoints, including the G_1 **restriction point**; only when each phase's activities are completed are the cyclins changed to trigger those of the next phase.

Mitosis

- Stages of mitotic cell divisions include **prophase**, when chromosomes condense, the nuclear envelope disassembles, and the microtubular spindle forms; **metaphase**, when chromosomes are aligned; **anaphase**, when they begin to separate toward the two centrosomes; and **telophase**, when nuclear envelope re-forms around the separated chromosomes.
- Telophase ends with **cytokinesis** or cell cleavage into two daughter cells by a contractile ring of actin filaments and myosin.

Stem Cells & Tissue Renewal

- **Stem cells** occur in all tissues with rapid cell turnover; they divide slowly in an **asymmetric** manner, with one daughter cell remaining a stem cell and one becoming committed toward differentiation.
- Cells committed to differentiate (**transit amplifying or progenitor cells**) typically divide more rapidly than stem cells before slowing or stopping division to differentiate.

Meiosis

- **Meiosis** is the process by which two successive cell divisions produce cells called **gametes** containing half the number of chromosomes found in somatic cells.
- Prophase of the first meiotic division is a unique, extended period in which homologous chromosomes pair and undergo genetic recombination during the process called **synapsis**.
- Synaptic pairs separate toward two daughter cells at the first meiotic division.
- The second meiotic division occurs with no intervening S phase and separates the sister chromatids into two final cells that are **haploid**.

Apoptosis

- **Apoptosis** is the process by which redundant or defective cells are rapidly eliminated in a manner that does not provoke a local inflammatory reaction in the tissue.
- Apoptosis involves a cascade of events controlled by the **Bcl-2 family of proteins** regulating the release of death-promoting factors from mitochondria.
- Cytochrome c from mitochondria activates cytoplasmic proteases called **caspases**, which degrade proteins of the cytosol, cytoskeleton, and cell membrane.
- **Endonucleases** are activated, which degrade all nuclear DNA.
- Cell and nuclear volumes shrink rapidly, and the cell membrane changes produce extensive blebbing of the cell surface.
- Late in apoptosis, the cell breaks into many small **apoptotic bodies** that undergo **phagocytosis** by neighboring cells.
- Apoptosis occurs rapidly, with little or no release of proteins that would trigger inflammation, unlike the **death of injured cells by necrosis** that typically induces local inflammation.

The Nucleus   ASSESS YOUR KNOWLEDGE

1. Which of the following facilitates breakdown of the nuclear envelope during the onset of mitosis?

   a. Disassembly of nucleosomes in the associated constitutive heterochromatin
   b. Increased export of material by the nuclear pore complexes into the perinuclear space
   c. Phosphorylation of lamin subunits by a CDK
   d. Activities triggered at a restriction point late in G_1
   e. The activity of proteasomes

2. Binding of histone H1 proteins to importins is important for which of the following?

   a. Transport through the nuclear pore complexes
   b. Properly directed vesicular transport through the Golgi apparatus
   c. Transport from the granular part of the nucleolus
   d. Further binding to the "linker DNA" and proper assembly of nucleosomes
   e. Phosphorylation of cyclins

3. Which of the following is a region of chromatin that is well-developed in large neurons active in protein synthesis?

   a. Heterochromatin
   b. The nucleolus
   c. The Nissl substance (neuronal RER)
   d. The Barr body
   e. The nucleosome

4. Which of the following is found during meiosis but not mitosis?

   a. Chromatids
   b. Polar microtubules
   c. Metaphase
   d. Synapsis
   e. Cytokinesis

5. Transitions in the cell cycle from one phase to the next are regulated by protein kinases whose activity depends on what other proteins?

   a. Tumor suppressors
   b. Cyclins
   c. Actins
   d. Lamins
   e. Importins

6. Mitotic figures visible in a tissue section from the lining of the small intestine are most likely to belong to which of the following categories?

   a. Terminally differentiated cells
   b. Partially differentiated cells
   c. Blood cells
   d. Stem cells
   e. Progenitor cells

7. Key differences between apoptotic and necrotic cell death include which of the following?

   a. Apoptotic cells do not release factors that induce inflammation.
   b. Necrosis does not trigger inflammation.
   c. Apoptosis does not utilize intracellular proteases.
   d. Apoptosis usually follows lethal physical damage to a cell.
   e. Necrosis is involved in formation of some organs during embryonic development.

8. A 29-year-old woman presents with a 101°F fever, pericardial effusions and Libman–Sachs endocarditis, arthralgia, and facial rash across the malar region ("butterfly rash") that is accentuated by sun exposure. Laboratory tests show creatine 1.7 mg/dL (normal 0.5–1.1 mg/dL), high titers of antinuclear autoantibodies (ANA), Smith antigen, and antinucleosome antibodies in the blood. Which one of the following is most likely to be directly affected by the disruption of nucleosomes in this patient?

   a. Packaging of genetic material in a condensed form
   b. Transcribing DNA
   c. Forming pores for bidirectional nuclear-cytoplasmic transport
   d. Forming the nuclear lamina
   e. Holding together adjacent chromatids

9. A 32-year-old man and his 30-year-old wife are referred for a reproductive endocrinologist infertility (REI) consult after 2 years of "trying to get pregnant." He is diagnosed with oligozoospermia. Ejaculated mature sperm are collected and undergo genetic analysis. Using gene linkage analysis, his REI specialist determines that he has aberrations in spermatogenic meiotic recombination, including both diminished frequency and suboptimal location, resulting in high frequency of aneuploid sperm. In explaining the diagnosis, she explains meiosis and recombination attributing the problem to a specific phase of the meiosis. Which part of meiosis is most closely associated with recombination?

   a. Metaphase I
   b. Anaphase I/Telophase I
   c. Prophase I
   d. Prophase II
   e. Anaphase II/Telophase II

10. A newborn boy is diagnosed with Apert syndrome. He has craniosynostosis, hypoplasia of the middle part of the face with retrusion of the eyes, and syndactyly that includes fusion of the skin, connective tissue, and muscle of the first, middle, and ring fingers with moderate fusion of those digits. There is very limited joint mobility past the first joint. Which one of the following is most likely *decreased* in cells of the interdigital regions of the developing hand of this newborn child?

   a. Random DNA degradation
   b. Inflammation
   c. Cell swelling
   d. Bcl-2
   e. DNA degradation by endonucleases

4 Epithelial Tissue

During embryonic development animal cells differentiate and become integrated into **four basic tissue types:** epithelial, connective, muscular, and nervous tissues, each an assemblage of similarly specialized cells united in performing specific functions. The basic tissues, each containing extracellular matrix (ECM) as well as cells, associate with one another in the variable proportions and morphologies characteristic of each organ. Table 4–1 summarizes the main features of the basic tissue types.

Characteristically, connective tissue contains cells producing very abundant ECM, muscle tissue has elongated cells specialized for contraction and movement, and nervous tissue includes cells with long, fine processes specialized to receive, generate, and transmit nerve impulses. Most organs can be divided into the **parenchyma**, which is composed of the cells responsible for the organ's specialized functions, and the **stroma**, the cells of which play a supporting role in the organ. Except in the brain and spinal cord, the stroma always consists of connective tissue.

Epithelial tissues are composed of closely aggregated polyhedral cells adhering strongly to one another and to a thin layer of ECM, forming cellular sheets that line the cavities of organs and cover the body surface. Epithelia (Gr. *epi*, upon + *thele*, nipple) line all external and internal surfaces of the body and all substances that enter or leave an organ must cross this type of tissue.

The principal functions of epithelial tissues include the following:

- **Covering, lining, and protecting surfaces** (eg, epidermis)
- **Absorption** (eg, the intestinal lining)
- **Secretion** (eg, parenchymal cells of glands)

Specific cells of certain epithelia may be contractile (myoepithelial cells) or specialized sensory cells, such as those of taste buds or the olfactory epithelium.

› CHARACTERISTIC FEATURES OF EPITHELIAL CELLS

The shapes and dimensions of epithelial cells vary greatly, ranging from tall **columnar** to **cuboidal** to low **squamous** cells. The cells' major functions generally dictate their size and morphology. Epithelial cell nuclei differ in shape and may be

TABLE 4–1	Main characteristics of the four basic types of tissues.		
Tissue	**Cells**	**Extracellular Matrix**	**Main Functions**
Epithelial	Aggregated polyhedral cells	Small amount	Lining of surface or body cavities; glandular secretion
Connective	Several types of fixed and wandering cells	Abundant amount	Support and protection of tissues/organs
Muscle	Elongated contractile cells	Moderate amount	Strong contraction; body movements
Nervous	Elongated cells with extremely fine processes	Very small amount	Transmission of nerve impulses

elliptic (oval), spherical, or flattened, with nuclear shape corresponding roughly to cell shape. Columnar cells generally have elongated nuclei, squamous cells have flattened nuclei, and cuboidal or pyramidal cells have more spherical nuclei (Figure 4–1).

The shape and density of the stained nuclei in epithelia help indicate cell shape and density since the lipid-rich membranes of epithelial cells frequently remain indistinguishable by routine light microscopy. The nuclei also allow one to determine the number of cell layers in an epithelium, a primary morphologic criterion for classifying epithelia.

Most epithelia adjoin a layer of connective tissue containing blood vessels from which the epithelial cells receive nutrients and O₂. Even thick epithelia do not themselves normally contain blood vessels. The connective tissue layer that underlies the epithelia lining the organs of the digestive, respiratory, and urinary systems is called the **lamina propria**. The area of contact between the two tissues may be increased by small evaginations called **papillae** (L. *papula*, nipple) projecting from the connective tissue into the epithelium. Papillae occur most frequently in epithelial tissues subject to friction, such as the covering of the skin or tongue.

Epithelial cells show **polarity**, with organelles and membrane proteins distributed unevenly within the cell. The region of the cell contacting the ECM and connective tissue comprises the **basal pole** and the opposite end, usually facing a space, the **apical pole**, with the two poles differing significantly in both structure and function. Regions of cuboidal or columnar cells that adjoin neighboring cells encompass the cells' **lateral surfaces**; cell membranes here often have numerous folds which increase the area and functional capacity of that surface.

Basement Membranes

The basal surface of all epithelia rests on a thin extracellular, felt-like sheet of macromolecules referred to as the **basement membrane** (Figure 4–1), a semipermeable filter for substances reaching epithelial cells from below. Glycoproteins and other components in this structure can often be stained and visualized with the light microscope (Figure 4–2).

With the transmission electron microscope (TEM) two parts of the basement membrane may be resolved. Nearest the epithelial cells is the **basal lamina**, a thin, electron-dense, sheetlike layer of fine fibrils, and beneath this layer is a more diffuse and fibrous **reticular lamina** (Figure 4–3a). The terms "basement membrane" and "basal lamina" are sometimes used interchangeably, but "basal lamina" usually denotes the fine extracellular layer visualized ultrastructurally and "basement membrane" the entire structure beneath the epithelial cells visible by light microscopy.

FIGURE **4–1** Epithelia and adjacent connective tissue.

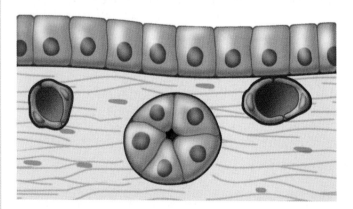

Cuboidal or pyramidal cells of epithelia generally have spherical nuclei, while nuclei of squamous epithelial cells are flattened. An extracellular **basement membrane** (red) always lies at the interface of epithelial cells and connective tissue. Nutrients for epithelial cells must diffuse across the basement membrane. Nerve fibers normally penetrate this structure, but small blood capillaries (being epithelial themselves) normally never enter epithelia.

FIGURE **4–2** Basement membranes.

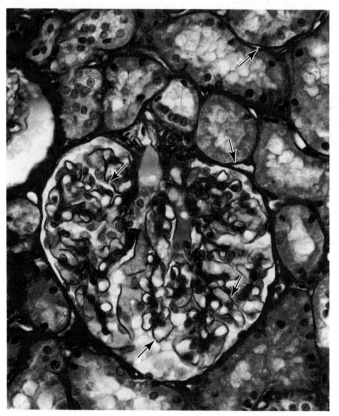

This section of kidney shows the well-stained basement membranes (arrows) of epithelia forming structures within the large, round renal glomerulus and its surrounding tubules. In kidney glomeruli, the basement membrane, besides having a supporting function, has a highly developed role as a filter that is key to renal function. (×100; Picrosirius-hematoxylin [PSH])

FIGURE **4–3** Basal and reticular laminae of basement membranes.

(a) The ultrastructural components of the basement membrane are revealed by TEM. The dense **basal lamina (BL)**, 20-100 nm thick, may appear with thin clear zones on each side and is anchored to a thicker, more diffuse **reticular lamina (RL)** containing collagen III fibers. **Hemidesmosomes (H)** bind the basal surface of the epithelial cell (**C**) to the basal lamina. (×54,000)

(b) Laminin, a major glycoprotein within basal laminae, is shown here by immunohistochemistry and identifies the basement membranes of the stratified epithelium (**E**) and the simple epithelium lining a small blood vessel (**V**). Laminin also occurs in the **external laminae** surrounding nerves (**N**) and muscle (**M**) fibers, seen here in cross-section. (×200)

The macromolecules of the basal lamina are secreted from the basal poles of the epithelial cells and form a sheetlike array. Chapter 5 describes all ECM components more fully, but those specific to basal laminae characteristically include the following:

- **Type IV collagen:** Monomers of type IV collagen self-assemble into a two-dimensional network of evenly spaced subunits resembling the mesh of a window screen.
- **Laminins:** These are large glycoproteins that attach to transmembrane **integrin** proteins in the basal cell membrane and project through the mesh formed by the type IV collagen.
- **Nidogen** and **perlecan:** Respectively a short, rodlike protein and a proteoglycan, both cross-link laminins to the type IV collagen network, helping to provide the basal lamina's three-dimensional structure, to bind the epithelium to that structure, and to determine its porosity and the size of molecules able to filter through it.

Basal laminae often called *external laminae* but with similar composition also exist as thin sleeves surrounding muscle cells, nerves (Figure 4–3b), and fat-storing cells, where they serve as semipermeable barriers regulating macromolecular exchange between the enclosed cells and connective tissue.

The more diffuse meshwork of the reticular lamina contains **type III collagen** and adheres to the basal lamina through

anchoring fibrils of **type VII collagen**, with both these collagens produced by cells of the connective tissue (Figure 4–3).

Besides acting as filters, functions of basement membranes include helping to provide structural support for epithelial cells and attach epithelia to underlying connective tissue. Basal lamina components help organize integrins and other proteins in the plasma membrane of epithelial cells, maintaining cell polarity and helping to localize endocytosis, signal transduction, and other activities. Basement membrane proteins also mediate many cell-to-cell interactions involving epithelia and mark routes for certain cell migrations along epithelia. Finally, the basement membrane also serves as a scaffold that allows rapid epithelial repair and regeneration.

Intercellular Adhesion & Other Junctions

Several membrane-associated structures make up junctions providing adhesion and communication between cells. Some such junctions occur in other tissues, but all are particularly numerous and prominent in epithelia. Epithelial cells adhere strongly to neighboring cells and basal laminae, particularly in epithelia subject to friction or other mechanical forces.

As shown in Figure 4–4 and summarized in Table 4–2, lateral surfaces of epithelial cells have complexes of several specialized intercellular junctions with different functions:

- **Tight** or **occluding junctions** form a seal between adjacent cells.

FIGURE **4–4** Junctional complexes of epithelial cells.

Microvilli

Tight junction
(occluding junction)

Adherens junction
(anchoring junction)

Desmosome
(anchoring junction)

Intermediate
filament

Gap junction
(communicating junction)

Hemidesmosome
(anchoring junction)

Basal lamina

Most cuboidal or columnar epithelial cells have intercellular junctional complexes with the different types of junctions shown schematically here. At the apical end, **tight junctions** (zonulae occludens) and **adherent junctions** (zonulae adherens) are typically close together and each forms a continuous band around the cell. Multiple ridges of the tight junction prevent passive flow of material between the cells but are not very strong; the adhering junctions immediately below them serve to stabilize and strengthen the circular occluding bands and help hold the cells together.

Both **desmosomes** and **gap junctions** are spot-like, not circular, structures between two cells. Bound to intermediate filaments inside the cells, desmosomes form very strong attachment points that supplement the zonula adherens and play a major role to maintain the integrity of an epithelium. Gap junctions, each a patch of many **connexons** in the adjacent cell membranes, have little strength but serve as intercellular channels for flow of molecules. All these junctional types are also found in certain other cell types besides epithelia. **Hemidesmosomes** bind epithelial cells to the underlying basal lamina.

TABLE **4–2**	Epithelial cell junctions, their major structural features and functions, and medical significance.				
Junction	Tight Junction (Zonula Occludens)	Adherens Junction (Zonula Adherens)	Desmosome (Macula Adherens)	Hemidesmosome	Gap Junction (Nexus)
Major transmembrane link proteins	Occludins, claudins, ZO proteins	E-cadherin, catenin complexes	Cadherin family proteins (desmogleins, desmocollin)	Integrins	Connexin
Cytoskeletal components	Actin filaments	Actin filaments	Intermediate filaments (keratins)	Intermediate filaments	None
Major functions	Seals adjacent cells to one another, controlling passage of molecules between them; separates apical and basolateral membrane domains	Provides points linking the cytoskeletons of adjacent cells; strengthens and stabilizes nearby tight junctions	Provides points of strong intermediate filament coupling between adjacent cells, strengthening the tissue	Anchors cytoskeleton to the basal lamina	Allows direct transfer of small molecules and ions from one cell to another
Medical significance	Defects in occludins may compromise the fetal blood–brain barrier, leading to severe neurologic disorders	Loss of E-cadherin in epithelial cell tumors (carcinomas) promotes tumor invasion and the shift to malignancy	Autoimmunity against desmoglein I leads to dyshesive skin disorders characterized by reduced cohesion of epidermal cells	Mutations in the integrin-β4 gene are linked to some types of epidermolysis bullosa, a skin blistering disorder	Mutations in various connexin genes have been linked to certain types of deafness and peripheral neuropathy

- **Adherent** or **anchoring junctions** create sites of strong cell adhesion.
- **Gap junctions** act as channels for communication between adjacent cells.

In many epithelia, these junctions develop in a definite order at the apical end of the cells. **Tight junctions**, the most apical of the set, are also called *zonulae occludens*, with the term "zonula" indicating that the junction forms a band completely encircling each cell. In TEM the adjacent membranes at these junctions appear fused or very tightly apposed (Figure 4–5). The seal between the two cell membranes results from tight interactions between the transmembrane proteins: **claudin** and **occludin**. Tight junctions appear clearly after cryofracture of epithelia (Figure 4–6), where they resemble a band of branching strands in the membrane around each cell's apical end. The intercellular seal of tight junctions ensures that molecules crossing an epithelium in either direction do so by going *through* the cells (a transcellular path) rather than *between* them (the paracellular pathway). Epithelia with one or very few fused sealing strands (eg, proximal renal tubule) are more permeable to water and solutes than epithelia with many fused strands (eg, the lining of the urinary bladder).

Epithelial tight junctions also serve a related purpose: these continuous zones within cell membranes serve as fences restricting movements of fluid membrane lipids and proteins at the apical cell pole into the lateral and basal surfaces, and vice versa. The tight junctions thus maintain two distinct membrane domains (apical and basolateral) with different sets of components, which allows these two sides of the epithelium to display different receptors and other proteins and to function differently. Apical cell membranes of epithelia make up part of the luminal compartment of a tissue or an organ, while the basolateral domains comprise part of a basal compartment that also encompasses the underlying connective tissue.

›› MEDICAL APPLICATION

Proteins of **tight junctions** provide the targets for certain common bacteria of medical importance. The enterotoxin secreted by *Clostridium perfringens*, which causes "food poisoning," binds claudin molecules of intestinal cells, prevents insertion of these proteins during maintenance of tight junctions, and causes loss of tissue fluid into the intestinal lumen via the paracellular pathway.

Similarly, *Helicobacter pylori*, an important factor in the etiology of **gastric ulcers**, binds the extracellular domains of tight-junction proteins in cells of the stomach and inserts a protein into these cells, which targets ZO-1 and disrupts signaling from the junction.

The second junction type, the **adherens junction** or zonula adherens (Figures 4–4 and 4–5), also encircles the epithelial cell, usually immediately below the tight junction. As an adherent junction, this type firmly anchors a cell to its

FIGURE **4–5** Epithelial cell junctional complex.

Ultrastructural view of the apical region near microvilli (**MV**) of two epithelial cells, revealing a junctional complex with a tight junction (**TJ**) or zonula occludens, an adherent junction (**AJ**) or zonula adherens, and a desmosome (**D**) associated with intermediate filaments (**IF**). The functions and major protein components of these junction types are summarized in Table 4–2. (×195,000)

FIGURE **4–6** View of a tight junction after cryofracture.

Just below the apical microvilli (**MV**) of this epithelial cell, a cryofracture plane splitting fused cell membranes reveals the fused strands of transmembrane proteins forming the tight junction (**TJ**, or zonula occludens). (×100,000)

❯❯ MEDICAL APPLICATION

Various **blistering (bullous) diseases**, such as pemphigus vulgaris, involving the epidermis or stratified squamous epithelia of the oral mucosa, are due to abnormal desmosome function caused by autoimmune reactions against specific desmogleins that reduce cell-to-cell adhesion. Similar disorders arise with genetic mutations for various junctional proteins.

neighbors. Cell adhesion here depends on **cadherins**, transmembrane glycoproteins of each cell that bind each other in the presence of Ca^{2+}. At their cytoplasmic ends, cadherins bind **catenins** that link to actin filaments with actin-binding proteins. The actin filaments linked to the adherens junctions form part of the "terminal web," a cytoskeletal feature at the apical pole in many epithelial cells. Together, the tight and adherent junctions encircling the apical ends of epithelial cells function like the plastic bands that hold a six-pack of canned drinks together.

Another anchoring junction is the **desmosome** (Gr., *desmos*, binding and *soma*, body) or *macula adherens* (L. *macula*, spot), a term indicating that this junction resembles a single "spot-weld" and does not form a belt around the cell. Desmosomes consist of disc-shaped structures in the lateral surface of one cell that match with identical structures of adjacent cells (Figures 4–4 and 4–5). Desmosomes contain larger members of the cadherin family called desmogleins and desmocollins. The cytoplasmic ends of these clustered transmembrane proteins bind plakoglobins, catenin-like proteins that link to larger proteins called desmoplakins in an electron-dense plaque. Desmoplakins in turn bind intermediate filament proteins rather than actins. Epithelial desmosomes attach to cable-like intermediate filaments of cytokeratin, sometimes referred to as tonofilaments. These intermediate filaments bound to desmosomes provide firm cellular adhesion and considerable tensile strength throughout the epithelium.

Gap junctions, shown in Figure 4–7, mediate intercellular communication rather than adhesion or occlusion between cells. Abundant in many epithelia, gap junctions also occur with functional importance in nearly all mammalian tissues. Cryofracture preparations show that gap junctions consist of aggregated transmembrane protein complexes that form circular patches in the plasma membrane (Figure 4–7b).

The transmembrane gap junction proteins, **connexins**, form hexameric complexes called **connexons**, each of which has a central hydrophilic pore about 1.5 nm in diameter. When two cells attach, connexins in the adjacent cell membranes move laterally and align to produce connexons between the two cells (Figures 4–4 and 4–7a), with each such "junction" having dozens or hundreds of aligned connexon pairs. Gap junctions permit intercellular exchange of molecules with small (<1.5 nm) diameters. Some molecules mediating signal transduction, such as cyclic nucleotides and ions, move rapidly through gap junctions, allowing cells in many tissues to act in a coordinated manner rather than as independent units. For example, in heart and visceral muscles, gap junctions help produce rhythmic contractions.

FIGURE **4–7** Gap junctions.

Cell A   Cell B

(a) A diagram of a gap junction shows the structural elements that allow the exchange of nutrients and signal molecules between cells without loss of material into the intercellular space. The communicating channels are formed by pairs of abutting particles (**connexons**), which are in turn each composed of six protein subunits (connexins) that span the lipid bilayer of each cell membrane. The channel formed by paired connexons (arrow) is about 1.5 nm in diameter, limiting the size of transmitted molecules.

(b) A cryofracture preparation of a gap junction, showing the patch of aggregated transmembrane protein complexes, the connexons. (×150,000)

(c) A section perpendicular to a gap junction between two cells shows that their cell membranes are very closely apposed, separated only by a 2-nm-wide electron-dense space. Individual connexons are not resolved in sections prepared for TEM. (×150,000)

On the basal epithelial surface, cells (Figure 4–4) attach to the basal lamina by anchoring junctions called **hemidesmosomes** (Gr. *hemi*, half + *desmos* + *soma*), best seen by TEM (Figure 4–3). These adhesive structures resemble a half-desmosome ultrastructurally, but unlike desmosomes the clustered transmembrane proteins that indirectly link to cytokeratin intermediate filaments are integrins rather than cadherins. The integrins of hemidesmosomes bind primarily to laminin molecules in the basal lamina.

The **focal adhesion**, or focal contact, represents another basal anchoring junction found in cells moving during epithelial repair or reorganization. Although resembling hemidesmosomes superficially, focal adhesions are smaller, more numerous, and consist of integrins linked indirectly to bundled actin filaments, not intermediate filaments. Importantly, integrins of focal adhesions also bind via paxillin to **focal adhesion kinase**, a signaling protein which upon integrin binding to laminin or other specific ECM proteins initiates a cascade of intracellular protein phosphorylation affecting cell adhesion, mobility, and gene expression. Focal adhesions also occur in migrating nonepithelial cells such as fibroblasts.

❯ SPECIALIZATIONS OF THE APICAL CELL SURFACE

The apical ends of many columnar and cuboidal epithelial cells have specialized structures projecting from the cells. These function either to increase the apical surface area for better absorption or to move substances along the epithelial surface.

Microvilli

Many cells have cytoplasmic projections best seen with the electron microscope. Such extensions usually reflect the movements and activity of actin filaments and may be both temporary and variable in their length, shape, and number. However, in epithelia specialized for absorption the apical cell surfaces often become filled with an array of projecting **microvilli** (L. *villus*, tuft), usually of uniform length. In cells such as those lining the small intestine, densely packed microvilli constitute the **brush** or **striated border** projecting into the lumen (Figure 4–8). With the average microvillus about 1 μm long and 0.1 μm wide and with hundreds or thousands present on the end of each absorptive cell, the total apical surface area

FIGURE **4–8** Microvilli.

- Formin and other proteins for F-actin capping

- Fimbrin, villin (cross-linking F-actin)

- Myosin I (anchoring F-actin to membrane)

- Actin filaments (microfilaments)

Myosin II

d   Intermediate filaments (keratins)

Absorptive cells lining the small intestine demonstrate the highly uniform microvilli of a striated or brush border particularly well.

(a) A pseudo-colored TEM of one such cell shows many parallel microvilli and their connections to the terminal web (**TW**) in the underlying cytoplasm. (×6500)

(b) SEM of a sectioned epithelial cell shows both the internal and surface structure of individual microvilli and the association with actin filaments and intermediate filaments of the terminal web (**TW**). (×7000)

(c) TEM of microvilli sectioned longitudinally and transversely (inset) reveals the microfilament arrays that form the core of these projections. The terminal web (**TW**) of the cytoskeleton is also seen. The glycocalyx (**G**) extending from glycoproteins and glycolipids of the microvilli plasmalemma contains certain enzymes for late stages of macromolecule digestion. (×15,000)

(d) The diagram shows a few microfilaments in a microvillus, with various actin-binding proteins important for F-actin assembly, capping, cross-linking, and movement. Like

microfilaments in other regions of the cytoskeleton, those of microvilli are highly dynamic with treadmilling and various myosin-based interactions. Myosin motors import various microvilli components along the actin filaments.

(Figure 4–8b, reproduced with permission from Dr John Heuser, Washington University School of Medicine, St. Louis, MO.)

increases by 20- or 30-fold with a brush border. The thick gly-cocalyx covering microvilli of the intestinal cells' brush border includes membrane-bound proteins and enzymes for diges-tion of certain macromolecules.

Each microvillus contains bundled actin filaments capped and bound to the surrounding plasma membrane by actin-binding proteins (Figure 4–8d). Although microvilli are rela-tively stable, the microfilament arrays remain dynamic and undergo various myosin-based movements, which help main-tain optimal conditions for absorption via numerous channels, receptors, and other proteins in the plasmalemma. The actin filaments insert into the **terminal web** of cortical microfila-ments at the base of the microvilli.

>> MEDICAL APPLICATION

Celiac disease, also called **gluten-sensitive enteropathy** or **sprue**, is a disorder of the small intestine in which one of the first pathologic changes is loss of the microvilli brush border of the absorptive cells. This is caused by an immune reaction against the wheat protein gluten during its digestion, which produces diffuse enteritis (intestinal inflammation), changes to the epithelial cells leading to malabsorption, and eventu-ally to pathologic changes in the intestinal wall. The mal-absorption problems and structural changes are reversible when gluten is removed from the diet.

Stereocilia

Stereocilia are a much less common type of apical process, best seen on the absorptive epithelial cells lining the male reproductive system (Figure 4–9). Like microvilli, stereocilia increase the cells' surface area, facilitating absorption. More specialized stereocilia with a motion-detecting function occur as important components of inner ear sensory cells.

Stereocilia resemble microvilli in containing arrays of microfilaments and actin-binding proteins, with similar diam-eters, and with similar connections to the cell's terminal web. However, stereocilia typically have much greater length and less motility than microvilli, and may show branching distally.

Cilia

Cilia are long, highly motile apical structures, larger than microvilli, and contain internal arrays of microtubules not microfilaments (Figure 4–10). In addition to cilia on epithelial cells, most (if not all) other cell types have at least one short projection called a *primary cilium*, not specialized for motil-ity but enriched with receptors and signal transduction com-plexes for detection of light, odors, motion, and flow of liquid past the cells.

Numerous motile cilia occur apically on cuboidal or columnar cells of many epithelia. Cilia have lengths of 5-10 μm and diameters of 0.2 μm, much longer and two times wider than typical microvilli. As shown in Figure 4–11, each cilium has a core structure consisting of nine outer or peripheral microtubule doublets (in which a few tubulin protofilaments

FIGURE **4–9** Stereocilia.

At the apical ends of the tall epithelial cells lining organs such as the epididymis (shown here) are numerous very long ste-reocilia, which increase the surface area available for absorp-tion. Stereocilia are much longer than microvilli and often have distal branching. (×400; H&E)

are shared) arrayed around a central pair of singlet micro-tubules. This **9 + 2 assembly** of microtubules makes up an **axoneme** (Gr. *axon*, axis + *nema*, thread). As with other microtubules, kinesin and cytoplasmic dynein motors move along the outer microtubules transporting macromolecular complexes into and out of cilia, respectively. Occurring at an average velocity of 3 μm/sec, such intraciliary transport of axonemal components as well as membrane-associated and even transmembrane proteins is fundamentally important for ciliary growth and maintenance.

Microtubules of axonemes have continuity with those of **basal bodies**, cytoplasmic structures just below the cell membrane (Figures 4–10 and 4–11). Basal bodies' composi-tion resembles somewhat that of centrioles, with triplets of microtubules and dynamic tubulin protofilaments forming rootlets anchoring the entire structure to the cytoskeleton.

Cilia exhibit rapid beating patterns that move a current of fluid and suspended matter in one direction along the epi-thelium. Ciliary motion occurs through successive changes in the conformation of the axoneme, in which various accessory proteins make each cilium relatively stiff, but elastic. Complexes with **axonemal dynein** bound to one microtubule in each doublet extend as "arms" toward a microtubule of the next dou-blet. With energy from ATP dynein-powered sliding of adjacent doublets relative to each other bends the axoneme and a rapid, repetitive series of these sliding movements produces the beat-ing motion of the cilium. The long flagellum that extends from each fully differentiated sperm cell has an axonemal structure like that of a cilium and moves with a similar mechanism.

FIGURE **4–10** Cilia.

Epithelial cells lining the respiratory tract have many very well-developed cilia.

(a) By light microscopy cilia (**C**) on the columnar cells appear as a wave of long projections, interrupted by nonciliated, mucus-secreting goblet cells (**G**). (×400; Toluidine blue)

(b) SEM of the apical surfaces of this epithelium shows the density of the cilia (**C**) and the scattered goblet cells (**G**). (×600)

(c) TEM of cilia (**C**) sectioned longitudinally reveals central and peripheral microtubules (arrowheads) of the axonemes, with cross-sections (inset) clearly showing the 9 + 2 array of the microtubule doublets. At the base of each cilium is a basal body (**B**) anchoring the axoneme to the apical cytoplasm. Much shorter microvilli (**MV**) can be seen between the cilia. (×59,000; Inset: ×80,000)

›› MEDICAL APPLICATION

Several mutations have been described in the proteins of the cilia and flagella. These cause **immotile cilia syndrome** (Kartagener syndrome), whose symptoms include chronic respiratory infections due to the lack of the cleansing action of cilia in the respiratory tract and immotile spermatozoa, causing male infertility.

› TYPES OF EPITHELIA

Epithelia include two main types or groups: **covering (lining) epithelia** and **secretory (glandular) epithelia**. This represents an arbitrary functional division; in some lining epithelia all the cells also secrete (eg, the lining of the stomach) and others have glandular cells distributed among the lining cells (eg, mucous cells in the small intestine or trachea).

Covering or Lining Epithelia

Cells of covering epithelia become organized into one or more layers that cover the surface or line the cavities of an organ. As summarized in Table 4–3, such epithelia are classified according to the number of cell layers and the cell morphology in the outer layer. **Simple epithelia** consist of only one cell layer and **stratified epithelia** have two or more layers.

Based on cell shape, simple epithelia are further classified as **squamous** (thin, flat cells), **cuboidal** (cell width and thickness roughly similar), or **columnar** (cells taller than they are wide). Figures 4–12 through 4–14 show examples of these epithelial types.

For most stratified epithelia (Figure 4–15) classification utilizes the shape of the superficial cells in the outer layer(s): again **squamous**, **cuboidal**, or **columnar**.

The very thin surface cells of stratified squamous epithelia can be "keratinized" (packed with keratin filaments) or "non-keratinized" (with relatively sparse keratin). **Stratified squamous keratinized epithelium** is found mainly in the skin epidermis, where it helps prevent dehydration from underlying tissue (Figure 4–15a). Its cells form many layers, with the less differentiated cuboidal cells near the basement membrane. These cells have many desmosomes and become more irregular in shape, and then flatten as they accumulate keratin in the process of **keratinization** and are moved progressively toward the skin surface, where they become thin, metabolically inactive packets (squames) of keratin lacking nuclei.

C H A P T E R

FIGURE **4–11** Ciliary axoneme.

Microtubule protofilament

Dynein "arms"

Radial spoke to central microtubule

Nexin-link protein to next doublet

Distal tips of cilia contain dynamic pools of tubulin, other ciliary precursor proteins, and motor proteins

Pair of dynein arms

Central microtubules

Microtubule doublet

Inner sheath

Nexin cross-links between doublets

b

Transport of proteins upward through cilia involves kinesin II motors moving along microtubules of peripheral doublets

Plasma membrane

Transport of proteins back to base of cilium involves cytoplasmic dynein motors moving along microtubules of peripheral doublets

Basal body

Microtubule triplet

Rootlet

a

(a) A diagram of a ciliary **axoneme** consisting of **two central microtubules** surrounded by **nine peripheral (outer) microtubular doublets** associated with other proteins. In the doublets tubule A is complete, with 13 protofilaments, whereas tubule B shares three of A's protofilaments. Elastic but relatively stiff, axoneme structure also involves nexins linking the outer doublets, protein complexes sheathing the central pair of microtubules, and other protein assemblies radiating like spokes from microtubule A toward the central pair.

The axoneme is continuous with a **basal body** located in the apical cytoplasm. Basal bodies are structurally somewhat like centrioles, consisting of nine relatively short **microtubular triplets** linked together in a pinwheel-like arrangement. Dynamic pools of tubulin and other proteins exist around basal bodies and at the distal tips of axonemes, with proteins transported distally along outer tubules

by **kinesin** (anterograde transport) and proximally along the same tubules (retrograde transport) by **cytoplasmic dynein** motors. Such transport, involving both axonemal components and membrane proteins, is crucial for ciliary growth and maintenance.

(b) Ciliary movement involves a rapid series of changes in the shape of the axoneme. Along the length of each doublet, a series of paired "arms" with **axonemal dynein** is bound to microtubule A, with each pair extended toward microtubule B of the next doublet. When activated by ATP, the dynein arms briefly bind the neighboring microtubule, and the doublets slide past each other slightly. The sliding motion is restricted by nexin cross-links between the doublets, causing the axoneme to bend. A rapid succession of this movement along the axoneme produces ciliary motion.

TABLE **4–3**	Common types of covering epithelia.		
Major Feature	**Cell Form**	**Examples of Distribution**	**Main Function**
Simple (one layer of cells)	Squamous	Lining of vessels (endothelium); Serous lining of cavities: pericardium, pleura, peritoneum (mesothelium)	Facilitates the movement of the viscera (mesothelium), active transport by pinocytosis (mesothelium and endothelium), secretion of biologically active molecules (mesothelium)
	Cuboidal	Covering the ovary, thyroid	Covering, secretion
	Columnar	Lining of intestine, gallbladder	Protection, lubrication, absorption, secretion
Stratified (two or more layers of cells)	Squamous keratinized (dry)	Epidermis	Protection; prevents water loss
	Squamous nonkeratinized (moist)	Mouth, esophagus, larynx, vagina, anal canal	Protection, secretion; prevents water loss
	Cuboidal	Sweat glands, developing ovarian follicles	Protection, secretion
	Transitional	Bladder, ureters, renal calyces	Protection, distensibility
	Columnar	Conjunctiva	Protection
Pseudostratified (layers of cells with nuclei at different levels; not all cells reach surface but all adhere to basal lamina)		Lining of trachea, bronchi, nasal cavity	Protection, secretion; cilia-mediated transport of particles trapped in mucus out of the air passages

As discussed with skin, this surface layer of cells helps protect against water loss across this epithelium. **Stratified squamous nonkeratinized epithelium** (Figures 4–15b and c) lines moist internal cavities (eg, mouth, esophagus, and vagina) where water loss is not a problem. Here the flattened cells of the surface layer retain their nuclei and most metabolic functions.

Stratified cuboidal and **stratified columnar epithelia** are both relatively rare. Stratified cuboidal epithelium appears in

FIGURE **4–12** Simple squamous epithelium.

This is a single layer of thin cells, in which the **cell nuclei** (arrows) are the thickest and most visible structures. Simple epithelia are typically specialized as lining of vessels and cavities, where they regulate passage of substances into the underlying tissue. The thin cells often exhibit transcytosis. Examples shown here are those lining the thin renal loops of Henle **(a)**, covering the outer wall of the intestine **(b)**, and lining the inner surface of the cornea **(c)**. The simple squamous epithelium lining the vasculature or the cornea is also called **endothelium**, while that lining large body cavities is called **mesothelium** and secretes a lubricant film called **serous fluid**. (a, c ×400; b ×600; H&E)

FIGURE **4–13** Simple cuboidal epithelium.

Cells here are roughly as tall as they are wide. Their greater thickness allows cytoplasm to be rich in mitochondria and other organelles for a high level of active transport across the epithelium and other functions. Examples shown here are from a renal collecting tubule **(a)**, a large thyroid follicle **(b)**, and the thick mesothelium covering an ovary **(c)**. (All ×400; H&E)

FIGURE **4–14** Simple columnar epithelium.

Cells here are always taller than they are wide, with apical cilia or microvilli, and are often specialized for absorption. Complexes of tight and adherent junctions, sometimes called "terminal bars" in light microscopic images, are present at the apical ends of cells. The examples shown here are from a renal collecting duct **(a)**, the oviduct lining, with both secretory and ciliated cells **(b)**, and the lining of the gallbladder **(c)**. (All ×400; H&E)

>> **MEDICAL APPLICATION**

In individuals with chronic vitamin A deficiency, epithelial tissues of the type found in the bronchi and urinary bladder may gradually be replaced by stratified squamous epithelium.

the excretory ducts of salivary and sweat glands (Figure 4–15d). Stratified columnar epithelium occurs in the conjunctiva lining the eyelids, where it is both protective and mucus-secreting.

Unique **transitional epithelium** or **urothelium** lines much of the urinary tract, extending from the kidneys to the proximal part of the urethra, and characterized by a superficial layer of large, dome-like cells sometimes called **umbrella cells** (Figure 4–16). As discussed further with the urinary system, these cells become specialized to protect underlying tissues from the hypertonic and potentially cytotoxic effects of urine. Importantly, unique morphological features of the cells allow *distension* of transitional epithelium as the urinary bladder fills.

A final morphological type of epithelium is called **pseudostratified columnar epithelium** (Figure 4–17). Here tall, irregular cells all remain attached to the basement membrane, but not all cells extend to the apical epithelial surface and the cell nuclei occur at different levels, giving the cells a stratified appearance. A good example of pseudostratified columnar epithelium is that lining the trachea, where the cells are also heavily ciliated.

FIGURE **4–15** Stratified epithelium.

Epithelium

Basement
membrane

Lamina propria

Stratified squamous epithelia usually have protective functions: protection against easy invasion of underlying tissue by microorganisms and protection against water loss. These functions are particularly important in the epidermis **(a)** in which differentiating cells become **keratinized**, that is, filled with keratin and other substances, eventually lose their nuclei and organelles, and form superficial layers of flattened squames that impede water loss. Keratinized cells are sloughed off and replaced by new cells from more basal layers, which are discussed fully with the skin in Chapter 18.

Nonkeratinized stratified squamous epithelia occur in many organs, such as the esophageal lining **(b)** or outer covering of the cornea **(c)**. Here cells accumulate much less keratin and retain their nuclei but still provide protection against microorganisms.

Stratified cuboidal or columnar epithelia are rare but occur in excretory ducts of certain glands, such as sweat glands **(d)** where the double layer of cells allows additional functions. All ×400; (b) PT, (a, c, and d) H&E.

❯❯ MEDICAL APPLICATION

In **chronic bronchitis**, common among habitual smokers, the number of goblet cells in the lining of airways in the lungs often increases greatly. This leads to excessive mucus production in areas where there are too few ciliated cells for its rapid removal and contributes to obstruction of the airways. The ciliated pseudostratified epithelium lining the bronchi of smokers can also be transformed into stratified squamous epithelium by metaplasia.

Secretory Epithelia & Glands

Epithelial cells that function mainly to produce and secrete various macromolecules may occur in epithelia with other major functions or comprise specialized organs called **glands**. Secretory cells may synthesize, store, and release proteins (eg, in the pancreas), lipids (eg, adrenal, sebaceous glands), or complexes of carbohydrates and proteins (eg, salivary glands). Epithelia of mammary glands secrete all three substances. The cells of some glands (eg, sweat glands) have little synthetic activity and secrete mostly water and electrolytes (ions) transferred from the blood.

Scattered secretory cells, sometimes called unicellular glands, are common in simple cuboidal, simple columnar, and pseudostratified epithelia. An important, easily seen example are the **goblet cells** abundant in the lining of the small intestine (Figure 4–18) and respiratory tract (Figure 4–17), which secrete lubricating mucus that aids the function of these organs.

FIGURE **4–16** Transitional epithelium or urothelium.

Urothelium is stratified and lines much of the urinary tract. The superficial cells are rounded or dome-shaped and have specialized membrane features enabling them to withstand the hypertonic effects of urine and protect underlying cells from this toxic solution. Cells of this epithelium are also able to adjust their relationships with one another and undergo a transition in their appearance as the urinary bladder fills and the wall is distended. These unique features of transitional epithelium are discussed more extensively in Chapter 19. (×400; H&E)

FIGURE **4–17** Pseudostratified epithelium.

Cells of pseudostratified epithelia appear to be in several layers, but their basal ends all rest on the basement membrane. The pseudostratified columnar epithelium of the upper respiratory tract shown here contains many ciliated cells, as well as other cells with their nuclei at different levels. (×400; H&E)

Glands develop from covering epithelia in the fetus by cell proliferation and growth into the underlying connective tissue, followed by further differentiation (Figure 4–19). **Exocrine glands** remain connected with the surface epithelium, the connection forming the tubular ducts lined with epithelium that deliver the secreted material where it is used. **Endocrine glands** lose the connection to their original epithelium and therefore lack ducts. Thin-walled blood vessels (capillaries) adjacent to endocrine cells absorb their secreted hormone products for transport in blood to target cells throughout the body.

As shown in Figure 4–20, epithelia of exocrine glands become organized as a continuous system of many small **secretory portions** and **ducts** that transport the secretion out of the gland. A connective tissue stroma supports the secretory units in both exocrine and endocrine glands. In larger glands, denser layers of connective tissue also surround the larger ducts, form partitions or *septa* separating the gland into lobules, each containing secretory units connected to a small part of the duct system, and enclose the entire gland as its *capsule* (Figure 4–20).

The structures of their secretory portions and ducts allow exocrine glands to be classified as shown schematically in Table 4–4. Although the three-dimensional morphology is often not prominent in histologic sections, the key points are summarized as follows:

- Glands can be **simple** (ducts not branched) or **compound** (ducts with two or more branches).
- Secretory portions can be **tubular** (either short, or long and **coiled)** or **acinar** (rounded and saclike); either type of secretory unit may be **branched**, even if the duct is not branched.
- **Compound** glands can have branching ducts as well as multiple tubular, acinar, or tubuloacinar secretory portions.

Three basic mechanisms for releasing the product are commonly used by cells specialized for secretion (Figure 4–21), and cells engaged in each type of secretion can be distinguished histologically:

FIGURE **4–18**   Goblet cells: unicellular glands.

The simple columnar epithelium lining the small intestine shows many isolated goblet cells secreting mucus into the lumen.

(a) With a stain for the oligosaccharide components of mucin glycoproteins, the cytoplasmic secretory granules of two goblet cells and secreted mucus are stained purple. (×600; PAS-PT)

(b) As shown ultrastructurally, goblet cells always have basal nuclei surrounded by RER (**R**), a large Golgi complex (**G**), and abundant apical cytoplasm filled with large secretory granules (**SG**). After exocytosis mucin components are hydrated and become mucus. A brush border of microvilli (**M**) is seen on neighboring columnar cells. (×17,000)

1. **Merocrine secretion:** This is the most common method of protein or glycoprotein secretion and involves typical exocytosis from membrane-bound vesicles or secretory granules.

2. **Holocrine secretion:** Here cells accumulate product continuously as they enlarge and undergo terminal differentiation, culminating in complete cell disruption that releases the product and cell debris into the gland's lumen. This is best seen in the sebaceous glands producing lipid-rich material in skin (Figure 4–22).

3. **Apocrine secretion:** Here product accumulates at the cells' apical ends, portions of which are then pinched off to release the product surrounded by a small amount of cytoplasm and cell membrane. Unlike the small membrane-enclosed vesicles called exosomes (see Chapter 2), these secretory products generally occur in large vesicles, do not generally involve formation within multivesicular bodies, and are released into ducts. Epithelial cells of mammary glands use merocrine secretion to add proteins to milk, but their release of lipid droplets represents the best-studied example of apocrine secretion (Figure 4–23).

›› MEDICAL APPLICATION

The holocrine sebaceous glands represent the primary structure involved in the common form of **acne**, acne vulgaris. Excessive holocrine secretion of sebum and keratin triggered by the surge of the steroid hormone testosterone that occurs in both genders at puberty frequently leads to blocked ducts within the gland. Activity of the normal commensal skin bacterium *Propionibacterium acnes* within the blocked duct commonly produces localized inflammation.

Exocrine glands with merocrine secretion can be further categorized as either **serous** or **mucous** according to the nature of their secretory products, which give distinct staining properties to the cells. Serous cells synthesize abundant proteins that are mostly not glycosylated, such as digestive enzymes. Such cells have well-developed RER and Golgi complexes and are filled apically with secretory granules in different stages of maturation (Figure 4–24). Serous cells, therefore, stain intensely with basophilic or acidophilic stains. Serous cells make up the acini of the pancreas and parotid salivary glands.

Mucous cells, such as goblet cells, also have RER and Golgi complexes and apical regions filled with secretory granules, but here these contain heavily glycosylated proteins called **mucins**. Following exocytosis mucins quickly become hydrated and form a viscous, apical layer of **mucus** on the epithelium. Most hydrophilic mucins usually get washed out of cells during routine histological preparations, causing the secretory granules to stain poorly with eosin (Figure 4–25). Sufficient oligosaccharides remain in developing mucinogen granules, however, to allow staining of mucous cells by the periodic acid-Schiff (PAS) method (Figure 4–18a).

Mixed **seromucous glands** have both serous acini and mucous tubules with clustered serous cells and occur in some salivary glands (see Figure 16–5). The product of such glands is a mixture of digestive enzymes and watery mucus.

In addition to secretory cells, epithelia of many exocrine glands (eg, sweat, lachrymal, salivary, and mammary glands) contain contractile **myoepithelial cells** at the basal ends of the secretory cells (Figure 4–26). Long processes of these cells embrace an acinus like an octopus might embrace a rounded boulder. Bound to the basal lamina by hemidesmosomes and

FIGURE **4–19** Formation of glands from covering epithelia.

During fetal development, epithelial cells proliferate and penetrate the underlying connective tissue. These cells may—or may not—maintain a connection with the surface epithelium. The connection is maintained to form a duct in exocrine glands; it is lost as endocrine glands develop without ducts. Exocrine glands secrete substances to specific organs via duct systems. Endocrine glands produce hormones and are always rich in capillaries. Hormones are released outside the cells and picked up by these blood vessels for distribution throughout the body, where specific target cells are identified by receptors for the hormones. Endocrine glands can have secretory cells arranged as irregular cords (left) or as rounded follicles (right) with lumens for temporary storage of the secretory product.

connected to the other epithelial cells by both gap junctions and desmosomes, myoepithelial cells are rich in actin filaments and myosins. Strong contractions in these cells serve to help propel secretory products from acini into the duct system.

Endocrine glands lack myoepithelial cells and become specialized either for protein or steroid **hormone** synthesis, with cytoplasmic staining characteristic of RER or SER, respectively. The proteins are released by exocytosis and the lipophilic steroids by diffusion through the cell membrane for uptake by binding proteins outside the cell. As mentioned

previously, endocrine signaling involves hormone transport in the blood to target cells throughout the body, often within other endocrine glands. The receptors may also appear on cells very close to the hormone-secreting cell or on the secreting cell itself, signaling which is termed paracrine or autocrine, respectively.

Important but inconspicuous endocrine or paracrine cells also occur singly or in small groups in epithelia of the digestive, respiratory, and other organ systems. Hormone secretion also happens from some cells specialized for other functions, such

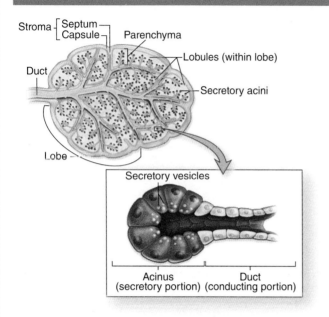

FIGURE **4–20** General structure of exocrine glands.

Exocrine glands have ducts that lead to another organ or the body surface. Inside the gland, the duct runs through the connective tissue of septa and branches repeatedly, until its smallest branches end in the secretory portions of the gland.

as certain cardiac muscle cells or fat cells. The pancreas contains both endocrine and exocrine cells. Liver cells exert both functions in the same cells, secreting bile components into a duct system and releasing other products to the bloodstream.

❯ TRANSPORT ACROSS EPITHELIA

Many cells can actively transport certain ions against concentration and electrical potential gradients. An important example involves the extrusion of Na$^+$ from cells by the transmembrane protein Na$^+$/K$^+$-ATPase, also called the Na$^+$/K$^+$ pump, which allows cells to maintain the required low intracellular sodium concentration (5-15 mmol/L vs ~140 mmol/L in extracellular fluid).

Some epithelial cells specialize in the transfer of ions (by ion pumps) and water (via the membrane channels called aquaporins) in either direction across the epithelium, the process known as **transcellular transport** (Figure 4–27). Apical tight junctions prevent paracellular diffusion or backflow *between* the cells.

Epithelia of kidney tubules, with major roles in maintaining the body's overall balance of salts and water, exemplify key

sites for such ion and water transport. Cells of the proximal renal tubules become specialized structurally for transcellular transport. The apical surface at the tubule lumen allows free entry to Na$^+$, while the basolateral cell membranes have sodium pumps for the active extrusion of Na$^+$ into the interstitial fluid surrounding the tubules. Maintenance of osmotic and electrical balances occurs by the passive transfer of chloride ions (Cl$^-$) and water into the cell. These cells have elaborately folded basal membranes, with abundant mitochondria within the folds to supply ATP for Na$^+$/K$^+$ pumps (Figure 4–28). Regulated transfer of ions and water by various epithelial cells along the renal tubules helps maintain the ionic balance within the body and allows excretion of excess water and salts in the urine.

All cells can also internalize extracellular molecules and fluid using endocytosis and formation of cytoplasmic, membrane-bound vesicles. This process actively occurs in the simple squamous epithelial cells lining blood and lymphatic capillaries (endothelia) or body cavities (mesothelia). These thin cells have few organelles other than the abundant pinocytotic vesicles, which cross the thin cells in both directions and release their contents on the opposite side by exocytosis. This process of **transcytosis** also occurs between the apical and basolateral membrane domains in cells of simple cuboidal and columnar epithelia and underlies many physiologic processes.

❯ RENEWAL OF EPITHELIAL CELLS

Epithelial tissues are relatively labile structures whose cells undergo continuous renewal by mitotic activity and stem cell populations. The rate of renewal varies widely: fast in tissues such as the intestinal epithelium, turning over every week, or very slow, as in the large glands. In stratified epithelial tissues, stem cells and mitosis occur only within the basal layer in contact with the basal lamina. In some functionally complex epithelia, stem cells occur only in restricted niches some distance from the transit amplifying cells and differentiating cells. For example, the epithelium lining the small intestine derives completely from stem cells found in the simple glands between the intestinal villi. In the epidermis many stem cells localize at a characteristic position along the wall of hair follicles.

> ❯❯ **MEDICAL APPLICATION**

Both benign and malignant tumors can arise from most types of epithelial cells. Malignant tumors of epithelial origin are called **carcinomas** (Gr. *Karkinos*, cancer + *oma*, tumor). Malignant tumors derived from glandular epithelial tissue are called **adenocarcinomas** (Gr. *Adenos*, gland + *karkinos*). Adenocarcinomas are by far the most common tumors in adults after age 45.

TABLE **4–4**	Structural classes of exocrine glands, features of each class, and examples.

SIMPLE Glands (Ducts Do Not Branch)

Class	Simple Tubular	Branched Tubular	Coiled Tubular	Acinar (or Alveolar)	Branched Acinar
Features	Elongated secretory portion; duct usually short or absent	Several long secretory parts joining to drain into 1 duct	Secretory portion is very long and coiled	Rounded, saclike secretory portion	Multiple saclike secretory parts entering the same duct
Examples	Mucous glands of colon; intestinal glands or crypts (of Lieberkühn)	Glands in the uterus and stomach	Sweat glands	Small mucous glands along the urethra	Sebaceous glands of the skin

COMPOUND Glands (Ducts from Several Secretory Units Converge into Larger Ducts)

Class	Tubular	Acinar (Alveolar)	Tubuloacinar
Features	Several elongated coiled secretory units and their ducts converge to form larger ducts	Several saclike secretory units with small ducts converge at a larger duct	Ducts of both tubular and acinar secretory units converge at larger ducts
Examples	Submucosal mucous glands (of Brunner) in the duodenum	Exocrine pancreas	Salivary glands

Epithelia typically undergo rapid repair and replacement of apoptotic or damaged cells. In some large glands, most notably the liver, mitotic activity normally occurs at a slow rate but is stimulated greatly following major damage to the organ. When a portion of liver tissue is removed surgically or lost by the acute effects of toxic substances, cells of undamaged regions quickly begin active proliferation, regenerating a new mass of functional liver tissue.

›› MEDICAL APPLICATION

Some epithelial cells are prone to abnormal growth or dysplasia, which can progress to precancerous growth called **neoplasia**. Early neoplastic growth is often reversible and does not always result in cancer.

Under certain abnormal conditions, one type of epithelial tissue may undergo transformation into another type in another reversible process called **metaplasia**. In heavy cigarette smokers, the ciliated pseudostratified epithelium lining the bronchi can be transformed into stratified squamous epithelium.

FIGURE **4–21** Mechanisms of exocrine gland secretion.

Secretory contents

Secretory vesicle

Nucleus

Secretory vesicles releasing their contents via exocytosis

(a) **Merocrine gland**

Disintegrating cells with contents becoming the secretion

Cells dividing

(b) **Holocrine gland**

Secretions

Nucleus of secretory cell

Pinching off of apical portion of secretory cell

(c) **Apocrine gland**

Three basic types of secretion are used by cells of exocrine glands, depending on what substance is being secreted.

(a) Merocrine secretion releases products, usually containing proteins, by means of exocytosis at the apical end of the secretory cells. Most exocrine glands are merocrine.

(b) Holocrine secretion is produced by the disintegration of the secretory cells themselves as they complete their terminal differentiation, which involves becoming filled with product. Sebaceous glands of hair follicles are the best examples of holocrine glands.

(c) Apocrine secretion involves loss of membrane-enclosed apical cytoplasm, usually containing one or more lipid droplets. Apocrine secretion, along with merocrine secretion, is seen in mammary glands.

Epithelial Tissue SUMMARY OF KEY POINTS

- An **epithelium** is a tissue in which cells are bound tightly together structurally and functionally to form a sheetlike or tubular structure with little extracellular material between the cells.
- Cells in epithelia each have an **apical side** facing the sheet's free surface and a **basal side** facing a basement membrane and underlying connective tissue.
- Epithelia are often specialized for absorption or **transcytosis**, pinocytosis of material at the apical side and exocytosis at the basolateral side (or vice versa).
- Cells of most epithelia exhibit **continuous renewal**, with the locations of stem cells and rates of cell turnover variable in various specialized epithelia.

Basement Membrane

- The **basement membrane** of all epithelia is a thin extracellular layer of specialized proteins, usually having two parts: a basal lamina and a more fibrous reticular lamina.
- The **basal lamina** is a thin meshwork of type IV collagen and laminin produced by the epithelial cells.
- The **reticular lamina** contains type III collagen and anchoring fibrils of VII collagen, all secreted by cells of the immediately adjacent connective tissue.

- Together, these components **attach** epithelia to connective tissue, regulate (**filter**) substances passing from connective tissue into epithelia, provide a guide or **scaffold** during tissue regeneration after injury, and **compartmentalize** epithelial cells from other tissues.

Intercellular Junctions

- Intercellular junctions are well developed in epithelia and consist of three major types, with different functions.
- **Tight or occluding junctions** are formed by interacting transmembrane proteins such as **claudin** and **occludin**; linear arrangements of these linked proteins surround the apical ends of the cells and **prevent paracellular passage** of substances (between the cells.)
- **Adherent or anchoring junctions**, formed by interacting proteins of the **cadherin** family, are points of strong **attachment** holding together cells of the epithelium.
- Adherent junctions may form **zonula adherens** that encircle epithelial cells just below their tight junctions and attach indirectly to **actin filaments**, or scattered, spot-like attachment sites called **desmosomes** or **maculae adherens**, which attach to **keratin intermediate filaments**.

FIGURE **4–22** Holocrine secretion in a sebaceous gland.

In **holocrine secretion**, best seen in the sebaceous gland adjacent to hair follicles, entire cells fill with a lipid-rich product as they differentiate. Mature (terminally differentiated) cells separate and completely disintegrate, releasing the lipid that serves to protect and lubricate adjacent skin and hair. Sebaceous glands lack myoepithelial cells; cell proliferation inside a dense, inelastic connective tissue capsule continuously forces product into the duct. (×200; H&E)

FIGURE **4–23** Apocrine secretion in the mammary gland.

The secretory portions of a mammary gland demonstrate **apocrine secretion**, characterized by extrusion of the secretion product along with a bit of apical cytoplasm enclosed within a small amount of plasma membrane, which is quickly lost after separation from the secretory cell (**arrows**). The released portion of cell contains lipid droplet(s), the major product of apocrine secretion. Merocrine secretion also occurs from the same and other cells of the mammary gland. (×400; PSH)

- **Hemidesmosomes** composed of transmembrane **integrins** attach cells to proteins of the basal lamina.
- **Gap or communicating junctions** are points of cell contact where both plasma membranes have numerous hexameric complexes of transmembrane **connexons**, each forming a channel allowing passage of small molecules from one cell to the other.

Apical Structures of Epithelial Cells

- **Microvilli** are small membrane projections with cores of **actin filaments** that generally function to increase epithelial cells' apical surface area for **absorption**.
- **Stereocilia** are long microvilli with specialized mechanosensory function in cells of the inner ear and for absorption in tissues of the male reproductive tract.
- **Cilia** are larger projecting structures with a well-organized core of **microtubules** (in a 9 + 2 arrangement called the **axoneme**) in which restricted, dynein-based sliding of microtubules causes ciliary movement that propels material along an epithelial surface.

Morphological Types of Epithelia

- An epithelium in which the basement membrane underlies one cell layer is **simple**; the cells of different simple epithelia range widely in height, from very thin or **squamous**, to roughly **cuboidal**, to very tall or **columnar**.
- Epithelia with two or more layers of cells are **stratified** and almost all such epithelia are stratified squamous, in which the outer cell layers are thin and flattened.
- Cells of stratified squamous epithelia move gradually from the basal to the surface layers, changing shape and becoming filled with **keratin** intermediate filaments.
- Stratified squamous epithelia such as the epidermis cover the body surface, **protecting** underlying tissues from excess water loss (dehydration) and microbial invasion.
- **Pseudostratified epithelia** are thick and appear to have several cell layers; all cells attach to the basal lamina but not all extend to the free epithelial surface.

FIGURE 4–24 Serous cells.

The small **serous acini** of the exocrine pancreas each have 5-10 cells facing a very small central lumen. Each acinar cell is roughly pyramidal, with its apex at the lumen. **(a)** As seen by light microscopy, the apical ends are very eosinophilic due to the abundant secretory granules present there. The cells' basal ends contain the nuclei and an abundance of RER, making this area basophilic.

A small duct (**D**) is seen, but lumens of acini are too small to be readily visible. The enclosed area is comparable to that shown in part **b**. (×300; H&E) **(b)** A portion of one acinar cell is shown ultrastructurally, indicating the abundant RER (**R**), a Golgi complex (**G**), apical secretory granules (**SG**), and the small acinar lumen (**L**). (×13,000)

- **Transitional epithelium or urothelium**, found only in the lining of the urinary system, is stratified, with large, rounded surface cells protective against urine.

Epithelial Secretion/Glands

- The major function in many epithelial cells is synthesis and secretion of specialized products; organs composed primarily of such epithelia are called **glands**.
- **Exocrine glands** have epithelial ducts carrying secretions to specific sites; the ducts of **simple glands** are unbranched and those of **compound glands** are branched.
- The secretory portions of exocrine glands may form round, saclike **acini** (also called **alveoli**) or elongated **tubules**; both types of secretory units may themselves branch.

- **Endocrine glands** lack ducts; secreted substances are hormones carried throughout the body by the interstitial fluid and blood, with specificity produced by the hormone receptors of target cells.
- Glands have three basic secretory mechanisms: **merocrine**, which uses exocytosis; **holocrine**, in which terminally differentiated cells filled with lipid products are released; and **apocrine**, in which apical, product-filled areas of cells are extruded.
- Exocrine glands producing mucus, or similar individual cells called **goblet cells**, are called **mucous glands**; oligosaccharide components of mucus stain poorly with routine dyes but stain well with PAS stain.
- Exocrine glands producing largely enzymes (proteins) are called **serous glands** and stain darkly with H&E due to the cells' content of RER and secretory granules.

FIGURE **4–25** Mucous cells.

Mucous cells of salivary glands are typically larger than serous cells, with flattened basal nuclei. Most of the cytoplasm is filled with secretory granules containing mucinogen like that of goblet cells. The RER and Golgi complexes of mucous cells produce heavily glycosylated glycoproteins with water-binding properties. The lumens (arrows) of mucous tubules are larger than those of serous acini. Much connective tissue surrounds the mucous tubules and ducts (**D**). (×200; PT)

FIGURE **4–26** Myoepithelial cells.

(a) The TEM shows two salivary gland cells containing secretory granules, with an associated **myoepithelial cell** (**M**). (×20,000)

(b) A myoepithelial cell immunostained brown with antibodies against actin shows its association with cells of an acinus stained by H&E. Contraction of the myoepithelial cell compresses the acinus and aids in the expulsion of secretory products into the duct. (×200)

Epithelial Tissue ASSESS YOUR KNOWLEDGE

1. Functions of the basement membrane include which of the following?
   a. Contractility
   b. Molecular filtering
   c. Active ion transport
   d. Excitability
   e. Modification of secreted proteins

2. Using immunohistochemistry, a population of cells is shown to be positive for the protein connexin. From this, we can infer that the cells are connected by what type of junction?
   a. Tight (occluding) junctions
   b. Zonula adherens
   c. Gap junctions
   d. Hemidesmosomes
   e. Desmosomes (macula adherens)

3. An individual genetically unable to synthesize normal occludin is likely to have epithelia with defective regulation in which of the following?
   a. Material crossing the epithelium between the cells (paracellular movement)
   b. Communication between the cells
   c. Attachment to the basement membrane
   d. Strong attachment to neighboring cells
   e. Movement of membrane proteins in the apical domains of cells

4. An intermediate filament protein found in cytoplasm of most epithelial cells is which of the following?
   a. Actin
   b. Vimentin
   c. Laminin
   d. Myosin
   e. Keratin

FIGURE 4–27 Ion and water absorption and secretion.

Ion and water transport across epithelia can occur in either direction, depending on the organ involved.

(a) Absorption is the process of transport from an organ or duct's lumen to capillaries near the epithelial basement membrane and involves movement from the apical to the basolateral cell membrane domains. Absorption occurs, for example, in the epithelium of the gallbladder and intestine where it serves to concentrate bile or obtain water and ions from digested material.

(b) Secretion involves transport in the other direction from the capillaries into a lumen, as in many glands and the choroid plexus. Secretion by epithelial cells removes water from the neighboring interstitial fluid or plasma and releases it as part of the specialized aqueous fluids in such organs.

No matter whether an epithelium is involved in absorption or secretion, apical occluding junctions are necessary to maintain tight separation of the apical and basolateral compartments of either side of the epithelium.

5. Which of the following cellular features is used in naming types of epithelia?
    a. Shape of cells in the basal layer
    b. Number of cell layers
    c. Presence of a basal lamina
    d. Size of the nuclei
    e. Nature of the cell junctions that are present

6. The release of lipid droplets from cells is which type of secretion?
    a. Merocrine
    b. Serous
    c. Apocrine
    d. Mucous
    e. Holocrine

7. Exocrine glands in which the acini all produce a secretion of heavily glycosylated, hydrophilic proteins are an example of which type of gland?
    a. Serous gland
    b. Mixed gland
    c. Mucous gland
    d. Tubuloacinar gland
    e. Simple gland

8. With a 5-year history of chronic respiratory infections, a 23-year-old, non-smoking man is referred to an otolaryngologist. A bronchial biopsy indicates altered structures in the epithelial cells. Which of the following, if altered to reduce function, is most likely involved in this patient's condition?
    a. Hemidesmosomes
    b. Cilia
    c. Basolateral cell membrane folds
    d. Microvilli
    e. Tight junctions

FIGURE **4–28** Features of absorptive cells.

A diagram and TEM photo showing the major ultrastructural features of a typical epithelial cell highly specialized for absorption, cells of proximal convoluted tubule of the kidney. The apical cell surface has a brush border consisting of uniform microvilli (**MV**) that increase the area of that surface to facilitate all types of membrane transport.

Vesicles formed during pinocytosis may fuse with lysosomes as shown in (**a**) or mediate transcytosis by secreting their contents at the basolateral cell membrane. The basal cell surface is also enlarged, here by invaginations of the cell membrane, which are associated with mitochondria (**M**) providing ATP for active transport. Basolateral membrane infoldings from neighboring cells (the more heavily stippled structures) also with mitochondria interdigitate with those of this cell. Various ions entering through the apical membranes of renal epithelial cells undergo active transport out of the cells across the basolateral membrane.

Immediately below the basal lamina shown in (**b**) is a capillary (**C**) that removes water and other substances absorbed across the epithelium. Junctional complexes between individual cells separate the apical and basolateral compartments on either side of the epithelium. Epithelial cells also show lateral membrane interdigitations with neighboring cells. (×9600)

9. An 11-month-old girl is referred to a pediatric gastroenterology clinic due to a history of generalized weakness, slow growth, and refractory diarrhea. For the past month, she has been hospitalized regularly to receive parenteral nutrition. Examination of the epithelium lining her small intestine confirms that the failure to absorb nutrients is most likely due to a significant decrease in which of the following?

a. Microvilli
b. Gap junctions
c. Cilia
d. Cell layers
e. Basement membrane thickness

10. A 42-year-old woman of Mediterranean descent presents with multiple oral blisters and a few cutaneous blisters on her back and buttocks. The superficial bullae are fragile, some have unroofed to form ulcerated lesions, and there is a positive Nikolsky sign. Blood tests reveal antibodies to a subfamily of cadherins and immunohistochemical staining of a biopsy from the oral mucosa shows distribution of the antigen throughout the epithelium. In what structures is the defect that is causing this patient's condition?

a. Desmosomes
b. Tight junctions
c. Hemidesmosomes
d. Gap junctions
e. Reticular lamina

5 Connective Tissue

onnective tissue provides a matrix supporting and physically connecting other tissues and cells to form the organs of the body. The interstitial fluid of connective tissue gives metabolic support to cells, serving as the direct medium for diffusion of nutrients and waste products.

Unlike the other tissue types (epithelium, muscle, and nerve) which consist mainly of cells, connective tissues always include very large amounts of **extracellular matrix (ECM)**. Extracellular matrices contain different combinations of long **protein fibers** (collagen and elastic fibers) and **ground substance**, a complex of anionic hydrophilic proteoglycans, glycosaminoglycans (GAGs), and multiadhesive glycoproteins (laminin, fibronectin, and others). As described briefly in Chapter 4 with the basal lamina, such glycoproteins help stabilize the ECM by binding to other matrix components and to integrins in cell membranes. Water within ground substance allows the exchange of nutrients and metabolic wastes between cells and the blood supply.

The variety of connective tissue types in the body reflects differences in composition and amount of the cells, fibers, and ground substance, which together are responsible for the remarkable structural, functional, and pathologic diversity of connective tissue.

All connective tissues originate from embryonic **mesenchyme**, a tissue developing mainly from the middle layer of the embryo, the mesoderm. Mesenchyme consists largely of viscous ground substance with few collagen fibers (Figure 5–1). **Mesenchymal cells** have large nuclei with fine chromatin and prominent nucleoli. Often described as "spindle-shaped," with their scant cytoplasm extended as two or more thin cytoplasmic processes, mesenchymal cells appear undifferentiated and evenly scattered through the ECM. Mesodermal cells migrate from their site of origin in the embryo, surrounding and penetrating developing organs. In addition to producing all types of connective tissue proper and the specialized connective tissues, bone and cartilage, the embryonic mesenchyme includes stem cells for other tissues, such as blood, the vascular endothelium, and muscle. This chapter describes the features of soft, supportive connective tissue proper.

›› MEDICAL APPLICATION

Some cells in mesenchyme are **multipotent stem cells** potentially useful in **regenerative medicine** after grafting to replace damaged tissue in certain patients. Mesenchyme-like cells remain present in some adult connective tissues, including that of tooth pulp and some adipose tissue, and are being investigated as possible sources of stem cells for therapeutic repair and organ regeneration.

› CELLS OF CONNECTIVE TISSUE

Fibroblasts are the key cells in connective tissue proper (Figure 5–2 and Table 5–1). Fibroblasts originate locally from mesenchymal cells and become permanent residents of connective tissue. Other cells found here, such as **macrophages**, **plasma cells**, and **mast cells**, originate from hematopoietic stem cells in bone marrow, circulate in the blood, and then move into connective tissue where they function. These and other white blood cells (leukocytes) reside transiently in most connective tissues, where they perform various functions for a short period as needed and then die by apoptosis.

FIGURE **5-1** Embryonic mesenchyme.

Mesenchyme consists of a population of undifferentiated cells, generally elongated but with many shapes, having large euchromatic nuclei and prominent nucleoli indicating high levels of synthetic activity. These **mesenchymal cells** are surrounded by an ECM they produced consisting largely of a simple ground substance rich in hyaluronan (hyaluronic acid), but with very little collagen. (×200; Mallory trichrome)

Fibroblasts

Fibroblasts (Figure 5–3), the most common cells in connective tissue proper, produce and maintain most of the tissue's extracellular components. Fibroblasts synthesize and secrete collagen (the most abundant protein of the body) and elastin, which both form large fibers, as well as the GAGs, proteoglycans, and multiadhesive glycoproteins comprising the ground substance. As described later, most of the secreted ECM components undergo further modification outside the cell before assembling as a matrix.

Distinct levels of fibroblast activity can be observed histologically (Figure 5–3b) because cells with intense synthetic activity differ morphologically from the quiescent fibroblasts dispersed within matrix they have already synthesized. Some histologists reserve the term "fibroblast" to denote the active cell and use "fibrocyte" to denote the quiescent cell. The active fibroblast has more abundant and irregularly branched cytoplasm, containing much rough endoplasmic reticulum (RER) and a well-developed Golgi apparatus, with a large, ovoid, euchromatic nucleus and a prominent nucleolus. The quiescent cell is smaller than the active fibroblast, with fewer cytoplasmic extensions, much less RER, and a darker, more heterochromatic nucleus.

Fibroblasts respond to many families of proteins called **growth factors** which influence cell growth and differentiation. In adults, connective tissue fibroblasts rarely undergo division. However, stimulated by locally released growth factors, cell cycling and mitotic activity resume when the tissue requires additional fibroblasts, for example, to repair a damaged organ. Fibroblasts involved in wound healing, sometimes called **myofibroblasts**, have a well-developed contractile function, being enriched with a form of actin also found in smooth muscle cells.

›› MEDICAL APPLICATION

The regenerative capacity of connective tissue is clearly observed in organs damaged by ischemia, inflammation, or traumatic injury. Spaces left after such injuries, especially in tissues whose cells divide poorly or not at all (eg, cardiac muscle), become filled by connective tissue, forming dense irregular **scar tissue**. The healing of surgical incisions and other wounds depends on the reparative capacity of connective tissue, particularly on activity and growth of fibroblasts.

In some rapidly closing wounds, a cell called the myofibroblast, with features of both fibroblasts and smooth muscle cells, is also observed. These cells have most of the morphologic characteristics of fibroblasts but contain increased amounts of actin microfilaments and myosin and behave much like smooth muscle cells. Their activity is important for the phase of tissue repair called **wound contraction**.

Adipocytes

Adipocytes (L. *adeps*, fat + Gr. *kytos*, cell), or fat cells, occur in the connective tissue of many organs. These large, mesenchymally derived cells become specialized to store lipid as neutral fats or less commonly, to produce heat. Tissue with a large population of adipocytes, called adipose connective tissue, serves to cushion and insulate the skin and other organs. Adipose tissue has major metabolic significance with considerable medical importance and is discussed separately in Chapter 6.

Macrophages & the Mononuclear Phagocyte System

Macrophages have highly developed phagocytic ability and specialize in turnover of protein fibers and removal of apoptotic cells, tissue debris, or other particulate material, being especially abundant at sites of inflammation. Size and shape vary considerably, corresponding to their state of functional activity. A typical macrophage measures between 10 and 30 μm in diameter and has an eccentrically located, oval or kidney-shaped nucleus. Macrophages exist in the connective tissue of most organs and are sometimes referred to by pathologists as "histiocytes."

FIGURE 5–2 Cellular and extracellular components of connective tissue.

Blood vessel

Ground substance

Extracellular matrix

Protein fibers

Elastic fiber
Collagen fiber
Reticular fiber

Resident cells

Mesenchymal cell
Macrophage
Adipocyte
Fibroblast

Connective tissue consists of **fibroblasts** and other cells and an **ECM** with various protein fibers, all of which are surrounded by watery **ground substance**. In all types of connective tissue the extracellular volume exceeds that of the cells.

TABLE 5–1	Functions of cells in connective tissue proper.
Cell Type	**Major Product or Activity**
Fibroblasts (fibrocytes)	Extracellular fibers and ground substance
Plasma cells	Antibodies
Lymphocytes (several types)	Various immune/defense functions
Eosinophilic leukocytes	Modulate allergic/vasoactive reactions and defense against parasites
Neutrophilic leukocytes	Phagocytosis of bacteria
Macrophages	Phagocytosis of ECM components and debris; antigen processing and presentation to immune cells; secretion of growth factors, cytokines, and other agents
Mast cells and basophilic leukocytes	Pharmacologically active molecules (eg, histamine)
Adipocytes	Storage of neutral fats

❯❯ MEDICAL APPLICATION

Besides their function in turnover of ECM fibers, macrophages comprise a key component of an organism's innate immune defense system, removing cell debris, neoplastic cells, bacteria, and other invaders. Macrophages also function as important antigen-presenting cells required for the activation and specification of lymphocytes.

When stimulated (by injection of foreign substances or by infection) macrophages change their morphologic characteristics and properties, becoming **activated macrophages**. In addition to showing an increase in their capacity for phagocytosis and intracellular digestion, activated macrophages exhibit enhanced metabolic and lysosomal enzyme activity. Macrophages are also secretory cells producing an array of substances, including various enzymes for ECM breakdown and various growth factors or cytokines that help regulate immune cells and reparative functions.

With adequate stimulation macrophages may increase in size and fuse to form **multinuclear giant cells**, usually found only in pathologic conditions.

FIGURE **5–3** Fibroblasts.

(a) Fibroblasts typically have large active nuclei and eosinophilic cytoplasm that tapers off in both directions along the axis of the nucleus, a morphology often referred to as "spindle-shaped." Nuclei (**arrows**) are clearly seen, but the eosinophilic cytoplasmic processes resemble the collagen bundles (**C**) that fill the ECM and are difficult to distinguish in H&E-stained sections.

(b) Both active and quiescent fibroblasts may sometimes be distinguished, as in this section of dermis. Active fibroblasts have large, euchromatic nuclei and basophilic cytoplasm, while inactive fibroblasts (or **fibrocytes**) are smaller with more heterochromatic nuclei (**arrows**). The round, very basophilic round cells are in leukocytes. (Both ×400; H&E)

In the TEM macrophages display characteristic irregular surfaces with pleats, protrusions, and indentations, features related to their active pinocytotic and phagocytic activities (Figure 5–4). They generally have well-developed Golgi complexes and many lysosomes.

Macrophages derive from precursor cells called **monocytes** circulating in the blood (see Chapter 12). Monocytes cross the epithelial wall of small vessels called venules to enter connective tissue, where they mature, and acquire the morphologic features of macrophages. Monocytes formed in the yolk sac during early development circulate and become residents in developing organs throughout the embryo, comprising a group of related cells called the **mononuclear phagocyte system**. Many of these macrophage-like cells with prominent functions in various organs have specialized names (Table 5–2). These are typically long-lived cells, surviving with relative inactivity in tissues for months or years. During inflammation and tissue repair which follow organ damage, macrophages become activated and play very important roles. Under such conditions, these cells increase in number, mainly in the connective tissue stroma, both by proliferation and by recruiting additional monocytes formed in the bone marrow (see Chapter 13).

The transformation from monocytes to macrophages in connective tissue involves increase in cell size, increased protein synthesis, and increase in the number of Golgi complexes and lysosomes. In addition to debris removal, macrophages secrete growth factors important for tissue repair and function in the uptake, processing, and presentation of antigens for lymphocyte activation, a role discussed later with the immune system.

Mast Cells

Mast cells are oval or irregularly shaped cells of connective tissue, between 7 and 20 μm in diameter, filled with basophilic secretory granules that often obscure the central nucleus (Figure 5–5). These electron-dense granules vary in size, ranging from 0.3 to 2.0 μm in diameter. Because of the high content of acidic radicals in their sulfated GAGs, mast cell granules display **metachromasia**, which means that they can change the color of some basic dyes (eg, toluidine blue) from blue to purple or red. Common fixatives preserve the granules poorly so mast cells may be difficult to identify in routinely prepared slides.

Mast cells function in the localized release of many bioactive substances important in the local inflammatory response,

FIGURE 5–4 Macrophage ultrastructure.

Characteristic features of macrophages seen in this TEM of one such cell include the prominent nucleus (**N**) and the nucleolus (**Nu**) and the numerous secondary lysosomes (**L**). The arrows indicate phagocytic vacuoles near the protrusions and indentations of the cell surface. (×10,000)

innate immunity, and tissue repair. A partial list of molecules released from these cells' secretory granules includes the following:

- **Heparin**, a sulfated GAG that acts locally as an anticoagulant

- **Histamine**, which promotes increased vascular permeability and smooth muscle contraction
- **Serine proteases**, which activate various mediators of inflammation
- **Eosinophil** and **neutrophil chemotactic factors**, which attract those leukocytes

TABLE 5–2   Distribution and main functions of the cells of the mononuclear phagocyte system.

Cell Type	Major Location	Main Function
Monocyte	Blood	Precursor of macrophages
Macrophage	Connective tissue, lymphoid organs, lungs, bone marrow, pleural and peritoneal cavities	Production of cytokines, chemotactic factors, and several other molecules that participate in inflammation (defense), antigen processing, and presentation
Kupffer cell	Liver (perisinusoidal)	Same as macrophages
Microglial cell	Central nervous system	Same as macrophages
Langerhans cell	Epidermis of skin	Antigen processing and presentation
Dendritic cell	Lymph nodes, spleen	Antigen processing and presentation
Osteoclast (from fusion of several macrophages)	Bone	Localized digestion of bone matrix
Multinuclear giant cell (several fused macrophages)	In connective tissue under various pathological conditions	Segregation and digestion of foreign bodies

FIGURE **5–5** Mast cells.

Mast cells are components of loose connective tissues, often located near small blood vessels (**BV**).

(a) They are typically oval shaped and have cytoplasm filled with strongly basophilic granules. (×400; PT)

(b) Ultrastructurally mast cells show little else around the nucleus (**N**) besides these cytoplasmic granules (**G**), except for occasional mitochondria (**M**). The granule staining in the TEM is heterogeneous and variable in mast cells from different tissues; at higher magnifications some granules may show a characteristic scroll-like substructure (inset) that contains preformed mediators such as histamine and proteoglycans. The ECM near this mast cell includes elastic fibers (**E**) and bundles of collagen fibers (**C**).

- **Cytokines**, polypeptides directing activities of leukocytes and other cells of the immune system
- **Phospholipid** precursors, which get converted to prostaglandins, leukotrienes, and other important lipid mediators of the inflammatory response.

Occurring in connective tissue of many organs, mast cells become especially numerous near small blood vessels in skin and mesenteries (*perivascular* mast cells) and in the tissue that lines digestive and respiratory tracts (*mucosal* mast cells); the granule content of the two populations differs somewhat. These major locations indicate that mast cells develop strategically to function as sentinels detecting invasion by microorganisms.

Release of certain chemical mediators stored in mast cells promotes the allergic reactions known as **immediate hypersensitivity reactions** which occur within a few minutes after the appearance of an antigen in an individual previously sensitized to that antigen. Among many examples of immediate hypersensitivity reaction, anaphylactic shock represents a dramatic, potentially fatal condition. Anaphylaxis consists of the following sequential events (Figure 5–6). The first exposure to an antigen (allergen), such as bee venom, causes antibody-producing cells to produce an immunoglobulin of the IgE class that binds avidly to receptors on the surface of mast cells. Upon a second exposure to the antigen, it reacts with the IgE on the mast cells, triggering rapid release of histamine, leukotrienes, chemokines, and heparin from the mast cell granules that can produce the sudden onset of the allergic reaction. Degranulation of mast cells also occurs because of the action of the complement molecules that participate in the immunologic reactions described in Chapter 14.

Like macrophages, mast cells originate from progenitor cells in the bone marrow, which circulate in the blood, cross the wall of venules, and enter connective tissues, where they mature. Although mast cells resemble basophilic leukocytes in many respects, they appear to have a different lineage at least in humans.

Plasma Cells

Derived from lymphocytes, **plasma cells** produce and secrete antibodies. These relatively large, ovoid cells have basophilic cytoplasm rich in RER and a large Golgi apparatus near the nucleus that may appear pale in routine histologic preparations (Figure 5–7).

The nucleus of the plasma cell is generally spherical but eccentrically placed. Many of these nuclei contain compact, peripheral regions of heterochromatin alternating with lighter areas of euchromatin. At least a few plasma cells occur in most common connective tissues, with average life spans of only 10–20 days.

FIGURE 5–6 Mast cell secretion.

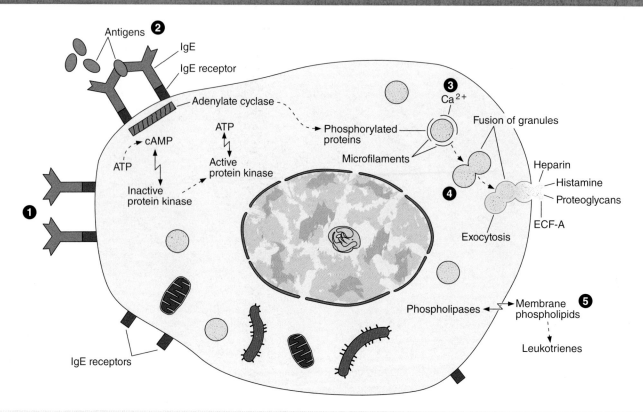

Mast cell secretion is triggered by reexposure to certain antigens and allergens. Molecules of IgE antibody produced in an initial response to an allergen such as pollen or bee venom are bound to surface receptors for IgE (**1**), of which 300,000 are present per mast cell.

When a second exposure to the allergen occurs, IgE molecules bind this antigen and a few IgE receptors very rapidly become cross-linked (**2**). This activates adenylate cyclase, leading to phosphorylation of specific proteins (**3**), entry of Ca^{2+}, and rapid exocytosis of some granules (**4**). In addition, phospholipases act on specific membrane phospholipids, leading to production and release of leukotrienes (**5**).

The components released from granules, as well as the leukotrienes, are immediately active in the local microenvironment and promote a variety of controlled local reactions that together normally comprise part of the inflammatory process called the **immediate hypersensitivity reaction**. "ECF-A" refers to the eosinophil chemotactic factor of anaphylaxis.

›› MEDICAL APPLICATION

Plasma cells derive from B lymphocytes and mature for the synthesis of immunoglobulin antibodies. Each antibody is specific for the one antigen that stimulated the clone of B cells and reacts only with that antigen or molecules resembling it (see Chapter 14). The results of the antibody–antigen reaction are variable, but they usually neutralize harmful effects caused by antigens. An antigen that is a toxin (eg, tetanus, diphtheria) may lose its capacity to do harm when it is bound by a specific antibody. Bound antigen–antibody complexes are quickly removed from tissues by phagocytosis.

Leukocytes

Other white blood cells, or **leukocytes**, besides macrophages and plasma cells normally comprise a population of wandering cells in connective tissue. Derived from circulating blood cells, they leave blood by migrating between the endothelial cells of venules to enter connective tissue. This process increases greatly during inflammation, a vascular and cellular defensive response to injury or foreign substances, including pathogenic bacteria or irritating chemical substances.

Inflammation begins with the local release of chemical mediators from various cells, the ECM and blood plasma proteins. These substances act on local blood vessels, mast cells, macrophages, and other cells to induce events characteristic of

FIGURE **5–7** Plasma cells.

Variable numbers of antibody-secreting plasma cells occur in the connective tissue of many organs.

(a) Plasma cells are large, ovoid cells, with basophilic cytoplasm. The round nuclei frequently show peripheral clumps of heterochromatin, giving the structure a "clock-face" appearance. (×640; H&E)

(b) Plasma cells become more abundant in infected tissues, as in the inflamed lamina propria shown here. A large pale **Golgi apparatus** (arrows) at a juxtanuclear site in each cell is actively involved in the terminal glycosylation of the antibodies (glycoproteins). Plasma cells leave their sites of origin in lymphoid tissues, move to connective tissue, and produce antibodies that mediate immunity. (×400; PT)

inflammation, for example, increased blood flow and vascular permeability, entry and migration of leukocytes, and activation of macrophages for phagocytosis.

Most leukocytes function in connective tissue only for a few hours or days and then undergo apoptosis. However, as discussed with the immune system, some lymphocytes and phagocytic antigen-presenting cells normally leave the interstitial fluid of connective tissue, enter blood or lymph, and move to selected lymphoid organs.

❯❯ MEDICAL APPLICATION

Increased vascular permeability is caused by the action of vasoactive substances such as histamine released from mast cells during **inflammation**. Classically, the major signs of inflamed tissues include "redness and swelling with heat and pain" (*rubor et tumor cum calore et dolore*). Increased blood flow and vascular permeability produce local tissue **swelling (edema)**, with increased redness and warmth. **Pain** is due mainly to the action of the chemical mediators on local sensory nerve endings. All these activities help protect and repair the inflamed tissue. **Chemotaxis** (Gr. *chemeia*, alchemy + *taxis*, orderly arrangement), the phenomenon by which specific cell types are attracted by specific molecules, draws much larger numbers of leukocytes into inflamed tissues.

❯ FIBERS

The fibrous components of connective tissue form as elongated structures produced as their protein subunits polymerize after secretion from fibroblasts (Figure 5–2). The three main types of fibers include **collagen**, **reticular**, and **elastic fibers**. Proteins of the collagen family make up subunits for collagen and reticular fibers, while elastic fibers are composed mainly of the protein **elastin**. These fibers occur unequally among the different types of connective tissue, with the predominant fiber type conferring most specific tissue properties.

Collagen

Collagens constitute a family of proteins selected during evolution for their ability to form various extracellular fibers, sheets, and networks, all extremely strong and resistant to normal shearing and tearing forces. A key element of all connective tissues, collagen also forms the basis of epithelial basement membranes and the external laminae of muscle and nerve cells.

Collagen is the most abundant protein in the human body, representing 30% of its dry weight. A major activity of fibroblasts, collagen secretion also occurs in several other cell types which make collagen subunits distinguishable by their molecular compositions, morphologic characteristics, distribution, functions, and pathologies. A family of 28 collagens exists in vertebrates, named with Roman numerals in the order of their identification. These exist as three major functional groups, as listed in Table 5–3, with each collagen type categorized according to the structures formed by their interacting subunits:

- **Fibrillar collagens**, notably **collagen types I, II**, and **III**, have polypeptide subunits that aggregate to form large fibrils clearly visible in the electron or light microscope (Figure 5–8). Collagen type I, the most abundant and widely distributed collagen, forms large, eosinophilic bundles usually called **collagen fibers**. These often densely fill the connective tissue, forming structures such as tendons, organ capsules, and dermis.
- **Network or sheet-forming collagens** such as **type IV collagen** have subunits produced by epithelial cells and represent major structural proteins of external laminae and all epithelial basal laminae.
- **Linking/anchoring collagens** occur as short collagens linking fibrillar collagens to one another (forming larger fibers) and to other components of the ECM. **Type VII collagen** binds type IV collagen and anchors the basal lamina to the underlying reticular lamina in basement membranes (see Figure 4–3).

Collagen synthesis occurs in many cell types but is a specialty of fibroblasts. To start the process, **procollagen α chains** assemble in the cell's RER. Different α chains of variable lengths and sequences arise by transcription of related collagen genes. In the ER, three α chains are selected, aligned, and stabilized by disulfide bonds at their carboxyl terminals, and folded as a **triple helix**, another defining feature of collagens.

TABLE 5–3	Collagen types.				
Type	**α-Chain Composition**	**Structure**	**Optical Microscopy**	**Major Location**	**Main Function**
Fibril-Forming Collagens					
I	$[\alpha1\,(I)]_2[\alpha2\,(I)]$	300-nm molecule, 67-nm-banded fibrils	Thick, highly picrosirius birefringent, fibers	Skin, tendon, bone, dentin	Resistance to tension
II	$[\alpha1\,(II)]_3$	300-nm molecule, 67-nm-banded fibrils	Loose aggregates of fibrils, birefringent	Cartilage, vitreous body	Resistance to pressure
III	$[\alpha1\,(III)]_3$	67-nm-banded fibrils	Thin, weakly birefringent, argyrophilic (silver-binding) fibers	Skin, muscle, blood vessels, frequently together with type I	Structural maintenance in expansible organs
V	$[\alpha1\,(V)]_3$	390-nm molecule, N-terminal globular domain	Frequently forms fiber together with type I	Fetal tissues, skin, bone, placenta, most interstitial tissues	Participates in type I collagen function
XI	$[\alpha1\,(XI)]\,[\alpha2\,(XI)]$ $[\alpha3\,(XI)]$	300-nm molecule	Small fibers	Cartilage	Participates in type II collagen function
Network-Forming Collagens					
IV	$[\alpha1\,(IV)]_2\,[\alpha2\,(IV)]$	Two-dimensional cross-linked network	Detected by immunocytochemistry	All basal and external laminae	Support of epithelial cells; filtration
X	$[\alpha1(X)]_3$	Hexagonal lattices	Detected by immunocytochemistry	Hypertrophic cartilage involved in endochondral bone formation	Increases density of the matrix
Linking/Anchoring Collagens					
VII	$[\alpha1\,(VII)]_3$	450 nm, globular domain at each end	Detected by immunocytochemistry	Epithelial basement membranes	Anchors basal laminae to underlying reticular lamina
IX	$[\alpha1\,(IX)]\,[\alpha2\,(IX)]$ $[\alpha3\,(IX)]$	200-nm molecule	Detected by immunocytochemistry	Cartilage, vitreous body	Binds various proteoglycans; associated with type II collagen
XII	$[\alpha1\,(XII)]_3$	Large N-terminal domain	Detected by immunocytochemistry	Placenta, skin, tendons	Interacts with type I collagen
XIV	$[\alpha1\,(XIV)]_3$	Large N-terminal domain; cross-shaped molecule	Detected by immunocytochemistry	Placenta, bone	Binds type I collagen fibrils, with types V and XII, strengthening fiber formation

FIGURE **5–8** Type I collagen.

Subunits of type I collagen, the most abundant collagen, assemble to form extremely strong fibrils, which are then bundled together further by other collagens into much larger structures called **collagen fibers**.

(a) TEM shows fibrils cut longitudinally and transversely. In longitudinal sections, fibrils display alternating dark and light bands; in cross section, the cut ends of individual collagen molecules appear as dots. Ground substance completely surrounds the fibrils. (×100,000)

(b) The large bundles of type I collagen fibrils (**C**) appear as acidophilic collagen fibers in connective tissues, where they may fill the extracellular space. Subunits for these fibers were secreted by the fibroblasts (**arrows**) associated with them. (×400; H&E)

The triple helix undergoes exocytosis and cleavage to a rod-like **procollagen molecule** (Figure 5–9), the basic subunit from which the fibers or sheets assemble. These subunits may be homotrimeric, with all three chains identical, or heterotrimeric, with two or all three chains having different sequences. Different combinations of procollagen α chains produce the various collagen types with different structures and functional properties.

›› MEDICAL APPLICATION

Keloids, localized swellings caused by abnormally large amounts of collagen forming in skin scars, occur most often in individuals of African descent and often represent a troublesome clinical problem to manage. Not only can they be disfiguring, but excision is almost always followed by recurrence.

FIGURE **5–9** The collagen subunit.

8.6 nm

In the most abundant form of collagen, type I, each **procollagen** molecule or subunit has two α₁- and one α₂-peptide chains, each with a molecular mass of approximately 100 kDa, intertwined in a right-handed helix and held together by hydrogen bonds and hydrophobic interactions. The length of each molecule (sometimes called tropocollagen) is 300 nm, and its width is 1.5 nm. Each complete turn of the helix spans a distance of 8.6 nm.

Many steps make up the pathway from procollagen synthesis, through post-translational processing and secretion, to the final assembly of collagen in the ECM. Most thoroughly studied for type I collagen, which accounts for 90% of all the body's collagen, the most important parts of this process are summarized in Figure 5–10 and described briefly here:

1. The procollagen α chains assemble on polyribosomes of the RER and translocate into its cisternae. These chains typically have long central domains rich in proline and lysine, with every third amino acid glycine.

2. **Hydroxylase** enzymes in the RER cisternae add hydroxyl (-OH) groups to some prolines and lysines in reactions requiring O_2, Fe^{2+}, and ascorbic acid (vitamin C) as cofactors.

3. Glycosylation of some hydroxylysine residues also occurs to different degrees in various collagen types.

4. Both the amino- and carboxyl-terminal sequences of α chains lack the Gly-X-Y repeats and assume globular structures. In the RER the C-terminal regions of three selected α chains (α1, α2) become stabilized by cysteine disulfide bonds, which align the three polypeptides and facilitate their central domains folding as the triple helix. With its globular terminal sequences intact, the trimeric procollagen molecule undergoes transport through the Golgi apparatus, packaging in vesicles, and secretion.

5. Outside the cell, specific proteases called **procollagen peptidases** remove the terminal globular peptides, converting the procollagen molecules to collagen molecules. These now self-assemble in an entropy-driven process to form polymeric collagen fibrils, usually in specialized niches near the cell surface.

6. Certain proteoglycans and other collagens (eg, types V and XII) associate with the new collagen fibrils, stabilize these assemblies, and promote the formation of larger fibers from the fibrils.

7. Fibrillar structure is reinforced and disassembly prevented by the formation of covalent cross-links between the collagen molecules, a process catalyzed by **lysyl oxidase**.

The other fibrillar and sheetlike collagens form in processes like that described for collagen type I and are stabilized by linking or anchoring collagens. Because of the many steps in collagen biosynthesis, many points occur at which the process can be interrupted or changed by defective enzymes or by disease processes (Table 5–4).

Type I collagen fibrils have diameters ranging from 20 to 90 nm and can be several micrometers in length. Adjacent rodlike collagen subunits of the fibrils are staggered by 67 nm, with small gaps (lacunar regions) between their ends (Figure 5–11). This structure produces a characteristic feature of type I collagen visible by EM: transverse striations with a regular periodicity (Figure 5–11). Type I collagen fibrils assemble further to form large, extremely strong collagen fibers that may be further bundled by linking collagens and proteoglycans. Collagen type II (present in cartilage) occurs as more delicate fibrils but does not form fibers or bundles. Sheet-forming collagen type IV subunits assemble as a latticelike network in epithelial basal laminae.

When they fill the ECM (eg, in tendons or the sclera of the eye), bundles of collagen appear white. The highly regular orientation of subunits makes collagen fibers birefringent with polarizing microscopy (see Figure 1–7). In routine light microscopy, collagen fibers are acidophilic, staining pink with eosin, blue with Mallory trichrome stain, and red with Sirius red. Because collagen bundles are long and tortuous, their length and diameter appear more readily in spread preparations rather than sections, as shown in Figure 1–7a. A very small mesentery is frequently used for this purpose; when spread on a slide, this structure is sufficiently thin to let the light pass through and can be stained and examined directly under the microscope.

Collagen turnover and renewal in normal connective tissue generally occurs as a very slow but ongoing process. In some musculoskeletal organs, such as tendons and ligaments, collagen is very stable, whereas other tissues, like the periodontal ligament surrounding teeth, have high collagen turnover rates. To be renewed, the collagen must first be degraded. Degradation begins with specific enzymes called **collagenases**, members of an enzyme class called **matrix metalloproteinases (MMPs)**, which clip collagen fibrils or sheets in ways that render them susceptible to further degradation by nonspecific proteases. Various MMPs are secreted by macrophages and play an important role in remodeling the ECM during tissue repair.

›› MEDICAL APPLICATION

Normal collagen function depends on the expression of many different genes and adequate execution of several posttranslational events. It is not surprising; therefore, many pathologic conditions are directly attributable to insufficient or abnormal collagen synthesis. A few such genetic disorders or conditions are listed in Table 5–4.

Reticular Fibers

Found in delicate connective tissue of many organs, notably in the immune system, **reticular fibers** consist mainly of collagen type III, which forms an extensive network (reticulum) of thin (diameter 0.5–2 μm) fibers for the support of many different cells. Reticular fibers stain poorly in hematoxylin and eosin (H&E) preparations but characteristically appear black after impregnation with silver salts (Figure 5–12) and are thus termed **argyrophilic** (Gr. *Argyros*, silver). Reticular fibers also stain with periodic acid–Schiff (PAS), which, like argyrophilia, involves the high content of sugar chains bound to type III collagen α chains. Reticular fibers contain up to 10% carbohydrate as opposed to 1% in most other collagen fibers.

FIGURE 5–10 Collagen synthesis.

Intracellular environment

Nucleus

Formation of mRNA for each type of α chain.

RER

Synthesis of procollagen α chains with propeptides at both ends. Clipping of signal peptide.

Hydroxylation of specific prolyl and lysyl residues in the endoplasmic reticulum. Vitamin C dependent.

Attachment of soluble galactosyl and glucosyl sugars to specific hydroxylysyl residues.

Assembly of procollagen molecules (triple helix).

Nonhelical propeptides.

Transfer vesicles

Transport of soluble procollagen to Golgi complex.

Golgi

Centrioles

Packaging of soluble procollagen in secretory vesicles.

Secretory vesicles

Secretory vesicles assisted by microtubules and microfilaments transport soluble procollagen molecules to cell surface.

Extracellular environment

Procollagen peptidases   Procollagen peptidases

Collagen molecules

Microtubule arrays

Exocytosis of procollagen molecules to extracellular space. Procollagen peptidases cleave most of the nonhelical terminal peptides, transforming procollagen into insoluble collagen molecules, which aggregate to form collagen fibrils.

Fibrillar structure is reinforced by the formation of covalent cross-links between collagen molecules catalyzed by the enzyme lysyl oxidase.

Hydroxylation and glycosylation of procollagen α chains and their assembly into triple helices occur in the RER, and further assembly into fibrils occurs in the ECM after secretion of procollagen. Because there are many slightly different genes for procollagen α chains and collagen production depends on several posttranslational events involving several other enzymes, many diseases involving defective collagen synthesis have been described.

TABLE **5–4**	Examples of clinical disorders resulting from defects in collagen synthesis.	
Disorder	**Defect**	**Symptoms**
Ehlers–Danlos type IV	Faulty transcription or translation of collagen type III	Aortic and/or intestinal rupture
Ehlers–Danlos type VI	Faulty lysine hydroxylation	Increased skin elasticity, rupture of eyeball
Ehlers–Danlos type VII	Decrease in procollagen peptidase activity	Increased articular mobility, frequent luxation
Scurvy	Lack of vitamin C, a required cofactor for prolyl hydroxylase	Ulceration of gums, hemorrhages
Osteogenesis imperfecta	Change of 1 nucleotide in genes for collagen type I	Spontaneous fractures, cardiac insufficiency

FIGURE **5–11** **Assembly of type I collagen.**

Shown here are the relationships among type I collagen molecules, fibrils, fibers, and bundles.

1. Rodlike triple-helix collagen molecules, each 300 nm long, self-assemble in a highly organized, lengthwise arrangement of overlapping regions.

2. The regular, overlapping arrangement of subunits continues as large collagen fibrils are assembled.

3. This structure causes fibrils to have characteristic cross striations with alternating dark and light bands when observed in the EM.

4. Fibrils assemble further and are linked together in larger collagen fibers visible by light microscopy.

5. Type I fibers often form into still larger aggregates bundled and linked together by other collagens.

The photo shows an SEM view of type I collagen fibrils closely aggregated as part of a collagen fiber. Striations are visible on the surface of the fibrils.

FIGURE **5–12** Reticular fibers.

In these silver-stained sections of adrenal cortex **(a)** and lymph node **(b)**, networks of delicate, black **reticular fibers** are prominent. These fibers serve as a supportive stroma in most lymphoid and hematopoietic organs and many endocrine glands. The fibers consist of type III collagen that is heavily glycosylated, producing the black argyrophilia, an affinity for stains containing silver salts. Type III collagen is also known as **reticulin**. Cell nuclei also appear dark, but cytoplasm is unstained. (×100) Fibroblasts specialized for reticular fiber production in hematopoietic and lymphoid organs are often called reticular cells.

Reticular fibers produced by fibroblasts occur in the reticular lamina of basement membranes and typically also surround adipocytes, smooth muscle and nerve fibers, and small blood vessels. Delicate reticular networks serve as the supportive stroma for the parenchymal secretory cells and rich microvasculature of the liver and endocrine glands. Abundant reticular fibers also characterize the stroma of hemopoietic tissue (bone marrow), the spleen, and lymph nodes where they support rapidly changing populations of proliferating cells and phagocytic cells.

Elastic Fibers

Also thinner than type I collagen fibers, **elastic fibers** form sparse networks interspersed with collagen bundles in many organs, particularly those subject to regular stretching or bending. As the name implies, elastic fibers have rubberlike properties that allow tissue containing these fibers, such as the stroma of the lungs, to be stretched or distended and return to their original shape. In the wall of large blood vessels, especially arteries, elastin also occurs as fenestrated sheets called **elastic lamellae**. Elastic fibers and lamellae are not strongly acidophilic and stain poorly with H&E; they are stained more darkly than collagen with other stains such as orcein and aldehyde fuchsin (Figure 5–13).

Elastic fibers (and lamellae) are a composite of **fibrillin** (350 kDa), which forms a network of **microfibrils**, embedded in a larger mass of cross-linked **elastin** (60 kDa). Both proteins emerge by secretion from fibroblasts (and smooth muscle cells in vascular walls) and give rise to elastic fibers in a stepwise manner as shown in Figure 5–14. Initially, microfibrils with diameters of 10 nm develop from fibrillin and various glycoproteins. The microfibrils act as scaffolding upon which elastin is then deposited. Elastin accumulates around the microfibrils, eventually making up most of the elastic fiber, and conferring the rubberlike property.

The elastic properties of these fibers and lamellae result from the structure of the elastin subunits and the unique cross-links holding them together. Elastin molecules have many lysine-rich regions interspersed with hydrophobic

FIGURE **5–13**   Elastic fibers.

Elastic fibers or lamellae (sheets) add resiliency to connective tissue. Such fibers may be difficult to discern in H&E-stained tissue, but elastin has a distinct, darker-staining appearance with other staining procedures.

(a) The length, diameter, distribution, and density of dark **elastic fibers** are easily seen in this spread preparation of nonstretched connective tissue in a mesentery. (×200; Hematoxylin and orcein)

(b) In sectioned tissue at higher magnification, **elastic fibers** can be seen among the acidophilic collagen bundles of dermis. (×400; Aldehyde fuchsin)

(c) Elastic lamellae in the wall of the aorta are more darkly stained, incomplete sheets of elastin between the layers of eosinophilic smooth muscle. (×80; H&E)

FIGURE **5–14**   Formation of elastic fibers.

Stages in the formation of elastic fibers can be seen by TEM.

(a) Initially, a developing fiber consists of many 10-nm-diameter **microfibrils** composed of **fibrillin** subunits secreted by fibroblasts and smooth muscle cells.

(b) Elastin is deposited on the scaffold of microfibrils, forming growing, amorphous composite structures. The elastin molecules are also secreted by the fibroblasts and quickly become covalently cross-linked into larger assemblies.

(c) Elastin accumulates and ultimately occupies most of the electron-dense center of the single elastic fiber shown here. Fibrillin microfibrils typically remain visible at the fiber surface. Collagen fibrils, seen in cross section, are also present surrounding the elastic fiber. (All ×50,000)

FIGURE **5–15** Molecular basis of elastic fiber elasticity.

Relaxed

Cross-link Stretched Single elastin molecule

The diagram shows a small piece of an elastic fiber, in two conformations. Elastin polypeptides, the major components of elastic fibers, have multiple random-coil domains that straighten or stretch under force, and then relax. Most of the cross-links between elastin subunits consist of the covalent, cyclic structure **desmosine**, each of which involves four converted lysines in two elastin molecules. This unusual type of protein cross-link holds the aggregate together with little steric hindrance to elastin movements. These properties give the entire network its elastic quality.

domains rich in lysine and proline that are thought to form extensible, random-coil conformations (like natural rubber). During deposition on the fibrillin microfibrils, lysyl oxidase converts the lysines' amino groups to aldehydes and four oxidized lysines on neighboring elastin molecules then condense covalently as a **desmosine** ring, cross-linking the polypeptides. Bound firmly by many desmosine rings, but maintaining the rubberlike properties of their hydrophobic domains, elastic fibers stretch reversibly when force is applied (Figure 5–15). Elastin resists digestion by most proteases, but is hydrolyzed by pancreatic **elastase**.

❯❯ MEDICAL APPLICATION

Fibrillins comprise a family of proteins involved in making the scaffolding necessary for the deposition of elastin. Mutations in the fibrillin genes result in **Marfan syndrome**, a disease characterized by a lack of resistance in tissues rich in elastic fibers. Because the walls of large arteries are rich in elastic components and because the blood pressure is high in the aorta, patients with this disease often experience aortic swellings called **aneurysms**, which are life-threatening conditions.

❯ GROUND SUBSTANCE

The ground substance of the ECM is a highly hydrated (with much bound water), transparent, complex mixture of three major kinds of macromolecules: **glycosaminoglycans (GAGs)**, **proteoglycans**, and **multiadhesive glycoproteins**. Filling the space between cells and fibers in connective tissue, ground substance allows diffusion of small molecules and, due to its viscosity, acts as both a lubricant and a barrier to the penetration of invaders. Physical properties of ground substance also profoundly influence various cellular activities. When adequately fixed for histologic analysis, its components aggregate as fine, poorly resolved material that appears in TEM preparations as electron-dense filaments or granules (Figure 5–16a).

GAGs (also called mucopolysaccharides) are long polymers of repeating disaccharide units, usually a hexosamine and uronic acid. The hexosamine can be glucosamine or galactosamine, and the uronic acid can be glucuronate or iduronate. The largest and most ubiquitous GAG, **hyaluronan** (also called hyaluronate or hyaluronic acid), has molecular weight from hundreds to thousands of kDa, and assembles as a very long polymer of the glucosamine-glucuronate disaccharide. Uniquely among GAGs, hyaluronan synthesis occurs directly into the ECM by an enzyme complex, **hyaluronan synthase**, located in the cell membrane of many cells. Hyaluronan forms a viscous, pericellular network binding a considerable amount of water and giving it an important role in both allowing molecular diffusion through connective tissue and lubricating various organs and joints.

All other GAGs are much smaller (5–40 kDa), sulfated, bound to proteins (as parts of proteoglycans), and synthesized in Golgi complexes. The four major GAGs found in proteoglycans are **dermatan sulfate**, **chondroitin sulfates**, **keratan sulfate**, and **heparan sulfate**, all of which have different disaccharide units modified further with carboxyl and sulfate groups and different tissue distributions (Table 5–5). The high negative charges in GAGs produce extended conformations and cause them to sequester cations as well as water. These features provide GAGs with space-filling, cushioning, and lubricant functions.

A **proteoglycan** consists of a core protein with various numbers and combinations of sulfated GAGs covalently attached. Like glycoproteins, they assemble on RER, mature in the Golgi apparatus, where the GAG side chains are added, and undergo secretion from cells by exocytosis. As an important difference from glycoproteins, proteoglycans have attached GAGs that often comprise a greater mass than the protein core. As shown in Figure 5–16b, after secretion proteoglycans become bound to hyaluronan polymers by link proteins and their GAG side chains associate further with collagen fibers and other ECM components.

The great diversity found in proteoglycans owes in part to enzymatic differences in the Golgi complexes. A region of ECM may contain several different core proteins, each with one or many sulfated GAGs of different lengths and

FIGURE 5–16 Ground substance of the ECM.

(a) TEM of connective tissue ECM reveals **ground substance** as areas containing only fine granular material among the collagen (**C**) fibers, elastic (**E**) fibers, and fibroblast processes (**F**). (×100,000)

(b) As shown here schematically, connective tissue ground substance contains a vast complex of **proteoglycans** linked to very long **hyaluronan** molecules. Each proteoglycan monomer has a **core protein** with a few or many side chains of the sulfated GAGs listed in Table 5–5. Synthesized in the RER and Golgi apparatus like glycoproteins, proteoglycan monomers are distinguished by often

being more heavily glycosylated and by the addition and sulfation of GAGs, which vary significantly among proteoglycans in their number, length, and the degree to which the sugar polymers are modified. **Aggrecan**, the most abundant and important proteoglycan in the articular cartilage of joints (see Chapter 8), is a very large macromolecule with a 250-kDa core protein approximately 400 nm long with roughly 100 chondroitin sulfate side chains, each 20 kDa, and 30–60 keratan sulfate side chains, each 5–15 kDa.

composition. As mentioned with epithelia, **perlecan** occurs as the key proteoglycan in all basal laminae. One of the best-studied proteoglycans, **aggrecan,** is very large, having a 250-kDa core protein heavily bound with chondroitin and keratan sulfate chains. A link protein joins aggrecan to hyaluronan (Figure 5–16b). Abundant in cartilage, aggrecan–hyaluronan complexes fill the space between collagen fibers and cells and contribute greatly to the physical properties of this tissue. Other proteoglycans include decorin, with very few GAG side

chains that bind the surface of type I collagen fibrils, and syndecan, with an integral membrane core protein providing an additional attachment of ECM to cell membranes.

Embryonic mesenchyme (Figure 5–1) is very rich in hyaluronan and water, producing the characteristic wide spacing of cells and a matrix ideal for cell migrations and growth. In both developing and mature connective tissues, core proteins and GAGs (especially heparan sulfate) of many proteoglycans bind and sequester various growth factors and

TABLE **5–5**	Composition and distribution of glycosaminoglycans in connective tissue and their interactions with collagen fibers.				
	Repeating Disaccharides				
Glycosaminoglycan	**Hexuronic Acid**	**Hexosamine**	**Distribution**	**Electrostatic Interaction with Collagen**	
Hyaluronic acid	D-glucuronic acid	D-glucosamine	Umbilical cord, synovial fluid, vitreous humor, cartilage		
Chondroitin 4-sulfate	D-glucuronic acid	D-galactosamine	Cartilage, bone, cornea, skin, notochord, aorta	High levels of interaction, mainly with collagen type II	
Chondroitin 6-sulfate	D-glucuronic acid	D-galactosamine	Cartilage, umbilical cord, skin, aorta (media)	High levels of interaction, mainly with collagen type II	
Dermatan sulfate	L-iduronic acid or D-glucuronic acid	D-galactosamine	Skin, tendon, aorta (adventitia)	Low levels of interaction, mainly with collagen type I	
Heparan sulfate	D-glucuronic acid or L-iduronic acid	D-galactosamine	Aorta, lung, liver, basal laminae	Intermediate levels of interaction, mainly with collagen types III and IV	
Keratan sulfate	D-galactose	D-glucosamine	Cartilage, nucleus pulposus, annulus fibrosus	None	

other signaling proteins. Degradation of such proteoglycans during the early phase of tissue repair releases these stored growth factors, which then help stimulate new cell growth and ECM synthesis.

❯❯ MEDICAL APPLICATION

The degradation of proteoglycans is carried out by several cell types and depends in part on the presence of several lysosomal enzymes. Several disorders have been described, including a deficiency in certain lysosomal enzymes that degrade specific GAGs, with the subsequent accumulation of these macromolecules in tissues. The lack of specific hydrolases in the lysosomes has been found to be the cause of several disorders, including the **Hurler**, **Hunter**, **Sanfilippo**, and **Morquio syndromes**.

Because of their high viscosity, hyaluronan and proteoglycans tend to form a barrier against bacterial penetration of tissues. Bacteria that produce hyaluronidase, an enzyme that hydrolyzes hyaluronan and disassembles proteoglycans complexes, reduce the viscosity of the connective tissue ground substance and have greater invasive power.

Making up the third major class of ground substance macromolecules, **multiadhesive glycoproteins** all have multiple binding sites for cell surface integrins and for other matrix macromolecules. Adhesive glycoproteins consist of large molecules with branched oligosaccharide chains and allow adhesion of cells to their substrate. One example, the large (200–400 kDa) trimeric glycoprotein **laminin**, possesses binding sites for integrins, type IV collagen, and specific proteoglycans, thus providing adhesion for epithelial and other cells. As described in the previous chapter, all basal and external laminae contain much laminin, the adhesive glycoprotein essential for the assembly and maintenance of these structures.

Another such glycoprotein, **fibronectin** (L. *fibra*, fiber + *nexus*, interconnection), a 235–270-kDa dimer synthesized largely by fibroblasts, has binding sites for collagens and certain GAGs, and forms insoluble fibrillar networks throughout connective tissue (Figure 5–17). The fibronectin substrate provides specific binding sites for integrins, an interaction important for both cellular adhesion and migration through the ECM.

Integrins, as briefly described in Chapter 2, represent integral membrane proteins that act as matrix receptors for specific sequences on laminin, fibronectin, some collagens, and certain other ECM proteins. Integrins bind their ECM ligands with relatively low affinity, allowing cells to explore their environment without losing attachment to it or becoming glued to it. All integrins are heterodimers with two transmembrane polypeptides: the α and β chains. Great diversity in the subsets of integrin α and β chains which cells express allows cells to have different specific ECM ligands.

Integrin–microfilament complexes become clustered on fibroblasts and other mesenchymal cells, forming structures called **focal adhesions** demonstrable by TEM or immunocytochemistry. As mentioned in Chapter 4, this type of adhesive junction typically forms at the ends of actin filaments bundled by α-actinin as cytoplasmic stress fibers, and focal adhesion kinases provide a mechanism by which pulling forces or other physical properties of the ECM can change various cellular activities.

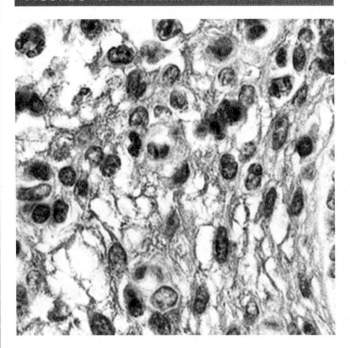

FIGURE **5–17** Fibronectin localization.

Like laminin of basement membranes, **fibronectin** is a multi-adhesive glycoprotein, with binding sites for ECM components and for integrins at cell surfaces and has important roles in cell migration and the maintenance of tissue structure. As shown here by immunohistochemistry, fibronectin forms a fine network throughout the ECM of connective tissue. (×400)

Water in the ground substance of connective tissue, also known as **interstitial fluid**, has an ion composition like that of blood plasma. Interstitial fluid also contains plasma proteins of low molecular weight that pass through the thin walls of the smallest blood vessels, the capillaries. Although plasma proteins constitute only a small proportion of connective tissue proteins, it is estimated that as much as one-third of the body's plasma proteins normally occur in the interstitial fluid of connective tissue because of its large volume and wide distribution.

>> **MEDICAL APPLICATION**

Edema is the excessive accumulation of interstitial fluid in connective tissue. This water comes from the blood, passing through the capillary walls that become more permeable during inflammation and normally produces at least slight swelling.

Capillaries in connective tissue also bring the various nutrients required by cells and carry away their metabolic waste products to the detoxifying and excretory organs, the liver and kidneys. Interstitial fluid provides the solvent for all these substances.

As shown in Figure 5–18, two main forces act on the water in capillaries:

- the **hydrostatic pressure** of the blood caused by the pumping action of the heart, which forces water out across the capillary wall and
- the colloid **osmotic pressure** produced by plasma proteins such as albumin, which draws water back into the capillaries.

The colloid osmotic pressure exerted by the blood proteins which cannot pass through the capillary walls tends to pull back into the capillary the water forced out by hydrostatic pressure (Figure 5–18). (Because the ions and low-molecular-weight compounds that pass easily through the capillary walls have similar concentrations inside and outside these blood vessels, the osmotic pressures they exert remain approximately equal on either side of the capillaries and cancel each other.)

The quantity of water drawn back into capillaries is often less than that which was forced out. This excess fluid does not normally accumulate in connective tissue but drains continuously into lymphatic capillaries that eventually return it to the blood. Discussed later with the lymphoid system, lymphatic capillaries originate in connective tissue as delicate endothelial tubes (Figure 5–18).

› TYPES OF CONNECTIVE TISSUE

Different combinations and densities of the cells, fibers, and other ECM components produce graded variations in histological structure within connective tissue. Descriptive names or classifications used for the various types of connective tissue typically denote either a structural characteristic or a major component. Table 5–6 gives a classification commonly used for the main types of connective tissue. Adipose tissue, an important specialized connective tissue, and two other supporting tissues, cartilage and bone, are covered in Chapters 6, 7, and 8, respectively.

Connective Tissue Proper

Connective tissue proper grades broadly as either "loose" or "dense," terms that refer to the amount of collagen present (Figure 5–19). **Loose connective tissue** occurs widely, forming a layer beneath the epithelial lining of many organs and filling internal spaces of muscle and nerve (Figure 5–19).

Also called **areolar tissue**, loose connective tissue typically contains cells, fibers, and ground substance in roughly equal parts. Fibroblasts predominate among the cells, but the other types of connective tissue cells also normally occur, along with nerves and small blood vessels.

FIGURE **5–18** Movement of fluid in connective tissue.

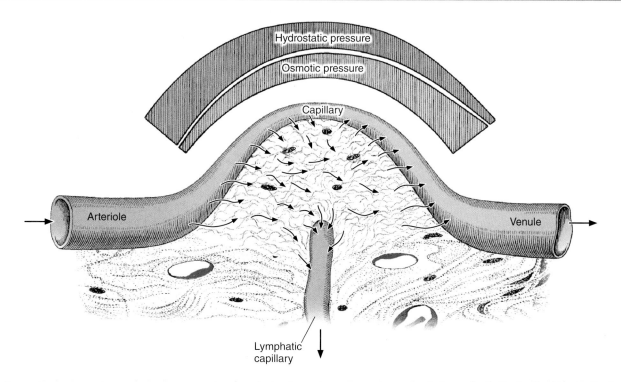

Water normally passes through capillary walls into the ECM of surrounding connective tissues primarily at the arterial end of a capillary because the **hydrostatic pressure** is greater than the colloid **osmotic pressure**. However, hydrostatic pressure decreases toward the venous end of the capillary, as indicated at the top of the figure. The fall in hydrostatic pressure parallels a rise in osmotic pressure of the capillary blood because the plasma protein concentration increases as water is pushed out across the capillary wall.

As a result of the increased protein concentration and decreased hydrostatic pressure, osmotic pressure at the venous end is greater than hydrostatic pressure, and water is drawn back into the capillary. In this way plasma and interstitial fluid constantly mix, nutrients in blood circulate to cells in connective tissue, and cellular wastes are removed.

Not all water that leaves capillaries by hydrostatic pressure is drawn back in by osmotic pressure. This excess tissue fluid is normally drained by the lymphatic capillaries, open-ended vessels that arise in connective tissue and enter the one-way lymphatic system that eventually delivers the fluid (now called **lymph**) back to the bloodstream via the thoracic and right lymphatic ducts, as described in Chapter 11.

Collagen fibers outnumber other types, but elastic and reticular fibers are also present. With at least a moderate amount of ground substance, loose connective tissue has a delicate consistency, providing flexibility but not much resistance to stress.

Dense connective tissue has similar components as loose connective tissue, but with fewer cells, almost all fibroblasts, and a clear predominance of bundled type I collagen fibers over ground substance. The abundance of collagen here protects organs and strengthens them structurally. In **dense irregular connective tissue**, bundles of collagen fibers appear randomly interwoven, with no definite orientation. The tough three-dimensional collagen network provides considerable resistance to stress from all directions. Examples of dense irregular connective tissue include the deep dermis layer of skin and the capsules surrounding most organs. Dense irregular and loose connective tissues often develop in proximity, with the two types grading into each other and making distinctions between them somewhat arbitrary (Figure 5–19).

Dense regular connective tissue consists mostly of type I collagen bundles and fibroblasts aligned in parallel for great resistance to prolonged or repeated stresses from the same direction (Figure 5–20).

The best examples of dense regular connective tissue are the very strong and flexible **tendons** (Figure 5–20), cords connecting muscles to bones; **aponeuroses**, essentially sheet-like tendons; and **ligaments**, bands or sheets holding together components of the skeletal system. Consisting almost entirely of densely packed parallel collagen fibers separated by very little ground substance and having very few blood vessels, these inextensible structures appear white in the fresh state.

TABLE 5–6	Classification of connective or supporting tissues.		
	General Organization	Major Functions	Examples
Connective Tissue Proper			
Loose (areolar) connective tissue	Much ground substance; many cells and little collagen, randomly distributed	Supports microvasculature, nerves, and immune defense cells	Lamina propria beneath epithelial lining of digestive tract
Dense irregular connective tissue	Little ground substance; few cells (mostly fibroblasts); much collagen in randomly arranged fibers	Protects and supports organs; resists tearing	Dermis of skin, organ capsules, submucosa layer of digestive tract
Dense regular connective tissue	Almost completely filled with parallel bundles of collagen; few fibroblasts, aligned with collagen	Provide strong connections within musculoskeletal system; strong resistance to force	Ligaments, tendons, aponeuroses, corneal stroma
Embryonic Connective Tissues			
Mesenchyme	Sparse, undifferentiated cells, uniformly distributed in matrix with sparse collagen fibers	Contains stem/progenitor cells for all adult connective tissue cells	Mesodermal layer of early embryo
Mucoid (mucous) connective tissue	Random fibroblasts and collagen fibers in viscous matrix	Supports and cushions large blood vessels	Matrix of the fetal umbilical cord
Specialized Connective Tissues			
Reticular connective tissue (see Chapter 14)	Delicate network of reticulin/collagen III with attached fibroblasts (reticular cells)	Supports blood-forming cells, many secretory cells, and lymphocytes in most lymphoid organs	Bone marrow, liver, pancreas, adrenal glands, all lymphoid organs except the thymus
Adipose Tissue (see Chapter 6)			
Cartilage (see Chapter 7)			
Bone (see Chapter 8)			
Blood (see Chapter 12)			

Fibrocytes with elongated nuclei lie parallel to the collagen fibers in dense regular connective tissue, with cytoplasmic folds enveloping portions of the collagen bundles, as shown by TEM in Figure 5–20b. H&E-stained preparations typically fail to demonstrate this sparse cytoplasm in such "**tendinocytes**" because it shows acidophilia like that of the collagen. In aponeuroses, the parallel bundles of collagen exist as multiple layers alternating at 90° angles to one another. Some ligaments, such as the elastic ligaments along the vertebral column, contain many parallel bundles of elastic fibers in addition to collagen.

On their outer surface tendons and ligaments have a layer of dense irregular connective tissue continuous with the outermost layers of the adjacent muscles and bones. Collagen bundles vary in size in different tendons and ligaments, but all dense regular connective tissue structures remain poorly vascularized, allowing only slow repair of damage in this tissue. Ligaments and tendons will be discussed again in Chapters 8 and 10, respectively, with bone, joints, and muscle.

❯❯ MEDICAL APPLICATION

Overuse of tendon–muscle units can result in **tendonitis**, characterized by inflammation of the tendons and their attachments to muscle. Common locations are the elbow, the Achilles tendon of the heel, and the shoulder rotator cuff. The swelling and pain produced by the localized inflammation restricts the affected area's normal range of motion and can be relieved by injections of anti-inflammatory agents such as cortisone. Fibroblasts eventually repair damaged collagen bundles of the area.

Reticular Tissue

Reticular tissue, characterized by abundant fibers of type III collagen (Figure 5–12), forms a delicate network supporting various types of cells. Also known as **reticulin**, type III collagen is produced by modified fibroblasts also often called **reticular cells**, which remain associated with and partially cover the collagen fibers (Figure 5–21). The loose disposition

FIGURE **5–19** Loose connective tissue and dense irregular connective tissue.

Examples of these connective tissue types shown here indicate the close association that often occurs between these two types.

(a) Loose connective tissue (**L**) of a gland contains faintly stained ground substance with fine fibers of collagen and frequently forms a thin layer near epithelia, while dense irregular connective tissue (**D**) forms a thicker layer and is invariably much richer in larger bundles of collagen. Scattered leukocytes can be seen in both connective tissues, along with the large irregular spaces of lymphatic vessels (left). (×100; H&E)

(b) Trichrome staining of a section from skin demonstrates the blue staining of collagen with this method and its relative density

in loose (**L**) and dense irregular (**D**) connective tissue. (×100; Mallory trichrome)

(c) Another example of dense irregular connective tissue, showing the randomly arranged large collagen bundles. The arrangement of collagen strengthens the tissues and resists tearing from all directions. (×150; H&E)

(d) Dense irregular connective tissue (**D**) forms a thick, protective capsule around many organs such as the testis shown here. Here the capsule is covered by a simple squamous epithelium of serous mesothelial cells (**S**), which produce a hyaluronate-rich lubricant around such organs. (×150; H&E)

FIGURE **5–20** Dense regular connective tissue.

(a) Micrograph shows a longitudinal section of dense regular connective tissue in a tendon. Long, parallel bundles of collagen fibers fill the spaces between the elongated nuclei of fibrocytes. (×100; H&E stain)

(b) The electron micrograph shows one **fibrocyte** in a cross section of tendon, revealing that the sparse cytoplasm of the fibrocytes is divided into numerous thin cytoplasmic processes extending among adjacent collagen fibers. (×25,000)

FIGURE **5–21** Reticular tissue.

(a) The diagram shows only the fibers and attached **reticular cells** (free, transient cells are not represented). **Reticular fibers** of type III collagen, or reticulin, are produced and enveloped by the reticular cells, forming an elaborate network through which interstitial fluid or lymph and wandering cells from blood pass continuously.

(b) The micrograph shows a silver-stained section of lymph node in which reticular fibers are seen as irregular black lines. Reticular cells are also heavily stained and dark. Most of the smaller, more lightly stained cells are lymphocytes passing through the lymph node. (×200; Silver) of glycosylated reticular fibers provides a framework with specialized microenvironments for cells in hemopoietic tissue and some lymphoid organs (bone marrow, lymph nodes, and spleen). The resulting cell-lined system creates a meshwork for the passage of leukocytes and lymph. Macrophages and dendritic cells (also in the mononuclear phagocyte family) are also dispersed within these reticular tissues to monitor cells formed there or passing through removing debris.

Mucoid Tissue

Mucoid (or mucous) connective tissue represents the principal component of the fetal umbilical cord, where it is referred to as **Wharton's jelly**. With abundant ground substance composed chiefly of hyaluronan, mucoid tissue is gelatinous, with sparse collagen fibers and scattered fibroblasts (Figure 5–22). This population of fibroblastic cells includes many mesenchymal stem cells, items of much research interest for their potential in regenerative medicine. Mucoid connective tissue shows some similarities to tissue found in the vitreous chambers of eyes and pulp cavities of young teeth.

FIGURE **5–22** **Mucoid tissue.**

A section of umbilical cord shows large fibroblasts surrounded by a large amount of very loose ECM containing mainly ground substances very rich in hyaluronan, with wisps of collagen. Histologically mucoid (or mucous) connective tissue resembles embryonic mesenchyme in many respects and is rarely found in adult organs. (×200; H&E)

Connective Tissue SUMMARY OF KEY POINTS

- Connective tissue is specialized to physically **support** and **connect** other tissues and maintain the water required for metabolite diffusion to and from cells.
- Connective tissues all consist primarily of **extracellular** material rather than cells.
- Within most organs connective tissue proper forms the supportive **stroma**, which supports the organ's unique functional components or **parenchyma**.
- The **ECM** of connective tissue proper usually consists of both large protein **fibers** and nonfibrous areas of unstained **ground substance** rich in various GAGs and water.
- All adult connective tissues are derived from an embryonic form of connective tissue called **mesenchyme**, which contains uniformly undifferentiated cells scattered in a gel-like matrix.

Cells of Connective Tissue

- **Fibroblasts** (fibrocytes), the major cells of connective tissue proper, are elongated, irregularly shaped cells with oval nuclei that synthesize and secrete most components of the ECM.
- **Adipocytes** (fat cells) are very large cells specialized for storage of triglycerides; they predominate in a specialized form of connective tissue called **adipose tissue**.
- **Macrophages** are short-lived cells that differentiate in connective tissue from precursor cells called **monocytes** circulating in the blood; they function in ECM turnover, phagocytosis of dead cells and debris, and antigen presentation to lymphocytes.
- **Mast cells** also originate from blood cell precursors and are filled with granules for the release of various vasoactive agents and other substances during inflammatory and allergic reactions.
- **Plasma cells** are short-lived cells that differentiate from B lymphocytes and are specialized for the abundant secretion of specific antibodies (immunoglobulins).

- Besides macrophages and plasma cells, other **leukocytes** normally wander through all types of connective tissue proper, providing surveillance against bacterial invaders and stimulating tissue repair.

Fibers of Connective Tissue

- The most important and abundant fibers of connective tissue are composed of the protein **collagen**, of which there are some 20 related types.
- Synthesis of collagen by fibroblasts and certain other cells involves posttranslational modifications in the RER, notably **hydroxylation** of the numerous prolines and lysines, and formation of helical trimeric subunits of **procollagen**.
- Upon exocytosis, the nonhelical ends of the procollagen subunits are removed, forming trimeric **collagen molecules** that aggregate and become covalently bound together in large **collagen fibrils**.
- The highly regular assembly of collagens in the fibrils produces a characteristic pattern of **crossbanding** visible ultrastructurally along the fibrils of some collagen types.
- Fibrils of type I collagen are bundled together by other forms of nonfibrillar, linking collagens to produce large **collagen bundles**.
- Collagen fibrils are degraded by collagenase enzymes classified as **MMPs**, produced primarily by macrophages.
- Type III collagen produces a network of delicate **reticular fibers**, which stain very dark with silver stains and are abundant in immune and lymphoid tissues.
- **Elastic fibers**, or sheets called **elastic lamellae**, are composed of the proteins **elastin** and **fibrillin**, which exist in a stretchable conformation that provides elastic properties to connective tissues rich in this material.

Ground Substance

- **Ground substance** is the watery, largely unstained extracellular material that is more abundant than fibers in some types of connective tissue proper.
- Ground substance is rich in **hydrated GAGs, proteoglycans**, and **multiadhesive glycoproteins**.
- The major types of GAGs are **hyaluronan** (hyaluronic acid), which is a very long polymer of the disaccharide glucosamine-glucuronate, and various shorter chains of **sulfated GAGs** composed of other disaccharide polymers.
- Sulfated GAGs such as **chondroitin sulfate** and **keratan sulfate** have various sizes and compositions, but they are all bound to the core proteins of **proteoglycans** and are produced in the Golgi apparatus before secretion.
- Proteoglycans attach to polymers of HA via **linker proteins** to form huge complexes in ground substance that bind water and other substances, including certain polypeptide growth factors that help regulate fibroblast proliferation.
- **Multiadhesive glycoproteins** such as fibronectin and laminin have binding sites for collagens and for integrin proteins in cell membranes, thus allowing temporary attachments between cells and the ECM required for cell migration and positioning.

Types of Connective Tissue

- **Connective tissue proper** is usually classified as loose or dense according to the amount of collagen and ground substance present.
- **Loose connective tissue** (or **areolar tissue**) has relatively more ground substance than collagen, and it typically surrounds small blood vessels and occupies areas adjacent to other types of epithelia.
- **Dense irregular connective tissue** is filled primarily with randomly distributed bundles of type I collagen, with some elastic fibers, providing resistance to tearing from all directions as well as some elasticity.
- **Dense regular connective tissue**, prominent in tendons and ligaments, features bundles of essentially parallel type I collagen, providing great strength (but little stretch) in binding together components of the musculoskeletal system.
- **Reticular tissue** consists of delicate networks of type III collagen and is most abundant in certain lymphoid organs where the fibers form attachment sites for lymphocytes and other immune cells.
- **Mucoid tissue** is a gel-like connective tissue with few cells found most abundantly around blood vessels in the umbilical cord.

Connective Tissue ASSESS YOUR KNOWLEDGE

1. Which of the following connective tissue components is located in the ECM but not in the ground substance?
   a. Collagen bundles
   b. Fibronectin
   c. GAGs
   d. Hyaluronan
   e. Proteoglycans

2. What cells numerous in loose connective tissue are filled with secretory granules and stain with metachromasia?
   a. Macrophages
   b. Mast cells
   c. Fibrocytes
   d. Active fibroblasts
   e. Leukocytes

3. What is the first step of collagen production that occurs after the protein undergoes exocytosis?
   a. Cross-linking of collagen fibrils with a short-linking collagen
   b. Removal of the terminal nonhelical domains by peptidases
   c. Hydroxylation of lysine and proline
   d. Assembly of subunits to form a larger structure
   e. Disulfide bond formation

4. What is an important part of the role played by macrophages during maintenance and renewal of strong extracellular fibers in connective tissue?
   a. Storage for a major energy source needed for ECM maintenance
   b. Production of specific collagen subunits
   c. A sentinel function against invaders entering the ECM
   d. Secretion of MMPs
   e. Presentation of antigens important for assembly of collagen bundles

5. Sulfated GAGs are important constituents of what extracellular structures?
   a. Hyaluronan
   b. Elastic fibers
   c. Type I collagen
   d. Proteoglycans
   e. Multiadhesive glycoproteins

6. Which of the following contains binding sites for integrins and is an important part of the ECM in both loose connective tissue and dense irregular connective tissue?
   a. Aggrecan
   b. Fibronectin
   c. Perlecan
   d. Fibrillin
   e. Most types of collagen

7. Dense regular connective tissue typically involves which of the following features?
   a. Contains mostly synthetically active fibroblasts
   b. Contains much ground substance
   c. Contains a similar cell population as areolar connective tissue
   d. Predominant tissue type in the stroma of most organs
   e. Predominantly located in tendons and ligaments

8. Research scientists at a small biotech firm are investigating new methods of controlling the growth and metastasis of malignant cells in patients diagnosed with breast cancer. They have developed a novel peptide-based drug, potentially deliverable therapeutically, that disrupts the tumor cells' ability to adhere to the ECM, which in turn triggers apoptosis. Which of the following is the most likely target of such drugs?
   a. Cadherins
   b. Adhesins
   c. Integrins
   d. Glycolipids of the cell membrane
   e. Fibrillin

9. A 36-year-old man is referred by his family physician to the pulmonary clinic. He complains of shortness of breath following physical activity and decreased capacity for exercise. He says that strenuous exercise including yard work is impossible without sitting down and resting every few minutes. After taking several deep breaths during the physical examination, he begins to wheeze. He is not a smoker and works in an office not exposed to dust, fumes, or other irritants. He appears slightly jaundiced. Serum alpha-1-antitrypsin (AAT) concentration analysis is below normal and is followed up with AAT phenotype and DNA testing that indicates one copy of S and one of Z mutations with 40% abnormal AAT production. Urinalysis shows elevated levels of desmosine and isodesmosine. These excreted compounds normally contribute to efficient lung function by which of the following mechanisms?

   a. Posttranslational modification of fibrillin
   b. Cross-linking elastin
   c. Activating elastase
   d. Activating AAT
   e. Binding type IV collagen to elastin

10. A 33-year-old homeless woman has been living in an abandoned building and eating dried meat and bread from the dumpster behind a delicatessen. She smokes cigarettes "bummed" from others. She presents at a free clinic with bleeding under the skin, particularly around hair follicles, and bruises on her arms and legs. She is irritable, clinically depressed, and fatigued with general muscle weakness. Her gums are bleeding, swollen, purple, and spongy, with several loose teeth. She has an infected toe, which may be broken. She is afebrile, a glucose finger-stick is normal, and the urine dipstick shows no sugar, protein, or ketones. You suspect a vitamin deficiency. What might be the underlying mechanism for this patient's symptoms?

   a. Decreased degradation of collagen
   b. Stimulation of prolyl hydroxylase
   c. Formation of unstable collagen helices
   d. Excessive callus formation in healing fractures
   e. Organ fibrosis

6 Adipose Tissue

Areolar connective tissue in which fat-storing cells or **adipocytes** predominate comprises **adipose tissue**. Typically found in isolation or small groups within loose or dense irregular connective tissue, adipocytes are large cells aggregated as adipose tissue or "fat" in many organs and body regions. Adipose tissue normally represents 15%–20% of the body weight in men, somewhat more in women. Besides serving as storage depots for neutral fats, chiefly triglycerides (long-chain fatty acyl esters of glycerol), adipocytes function as key regulators of the body's overall energy metabolism. With a growing epidemic of obesity and its associated health problems, including diabetes and heart disease, adipocytes and adipose tissue now constitute a major area of medical research.

Two properties of triglyceride lipids explain their selection as the preferred form of nutrient storage. Insoluble in water, lipids can become concentrated with no adverse osmotic effects on cells. Also, the caloric density of triglycerides (9.3 kcal/g) is twice that of proteins or carbohydrates, including glycogen, making these simple lipids the most efficient means of storing calories. Adipocytes specialize in concentrating triglycerides as lipid droplet(s), with other cells normally accumulating relatively little lipid.

Adipocytes are metabolically active cells, responding to both nervous and hormonal stimuli. They release hormones and various other important substances. Adipose tissue represents a widespread endocrine organ at the center of nutritional homeostasis. With its unique physical properties, tissue rich in fat conducts heat poorly and provides thermal insulation for the body. Adipose tissue also fills spaces between other tissues, helping to keep some organs in place. Subcutaneous layers of adipose tissue help shape the body surface, and cushion regions subject to repeated mechanical stress such as the palms, heels, and toe pads.

There are two major types of adipose tissue with different locations, structures, colors, and functions. **White adipose tissue**, the more common type specialized for fat storage, consists of cells each containing one large cytoplasmic droplet of whitish-yellow fat. **Brown adipose tissue** contains cells with multiple lipid droplets interspersed among abundant mitochondria, which helps give this tissue a darker appearance. Brown adipocytes release heat and function to warm the blood. Both types of adipose tissue have a rich blood supply, and adipocytes, unlike other cells of connective tissue proper, are individually surrounded by a thin external lamina containing type IV collagen.

❯ WHITE ADIPOSE TISSUE

Specialized for relatively long-term energy storage, adipocytes of white adipose tissue become spherical when isolated but are polyhedral when closely packed in situ. When completely developed, a white adipocyte is very large, between 50 and 150 μm in diameter, and contains a single huge droplet of lipid filling almost the entire cell. Having a single large droplet of triglycerides, white adipocytes are also called **unilocular** (Figure 6–1). Sometimes described as having a signet-ring appearance, an adipocyte's single lipid droplet displaces most cytoplasm and flattens the nucleus against the cell membrane (Figure 6–1d). Because lipid undergoes removal from cells by xylene or other solvents used in routine histological techniques, unilocular adipocytes often appear empty in standard light microscopy. This membrane and the thin rim of cytoplasm that remains after such loss of the stored lipid frequently shrinks, collapses, or ruptures, distorting cell and tissue structure.

❯❯ MEDICAL APPLICATION

Unilocular adipocytes can generate relatively common benign tumors called **lipomas**, although malignant adipose tumors (**liposarcomas**) occur infrequently. Fetal lipomas of brown fat are sometimes called **hibernomas**.

FIGURE **6–1** White adipose tissue.

White or unilocular adipose tissue is commonly seen in sections of many human organs.

(a) Large white adipocytes (**A**) are seen in the connective tissue associated with small blood vessels. The fat cells are empty because lipid was dissolved away in slide preparation. Nuclei at the cell membranes are visible in some of the fat cells. (×100; H&E)

(b) Large (empty) adipocytes predominate in this typical white adipose tissue, which shows only a small portion of microvasculature. In a single histologic section, nuclei of most very large adipocytes are not included. (×100; H&E)

(c) Tissue was fixed here with osmium tetroxide, which preserves lipid (**L**) and stains it black. Many adipocytes in this slide retain at least part of their large lipid droplets. (×440; Osmium tetroxide)

(d) In this specimen from a young mammal the smaller adipocytes marked with asterisks are not unilocular, having many lipid droplets of various sizes. Such cells in white fat represent those in which differentiation is incomplete as well as a small subpopulation of beige cells with brown fat-forming potential. The eccentric nuclei of the unilocular cells are indicated by arrowheads. (×200; PT)

Most cytoplasmic organelles in a white adipocyte localize near the peripheral nucleus, including mitochondria, a small Golgi apparatus, a few cisternae of RER, and free polyribosomes. The thin, submembranous layer of cytoplasm surrounding the lipid droplet contains cisternae of smooth ER (SER) and pinocytotic vesicles. Transmission electron microscopy (TEM) reveals a great abundance of caveolae in the cell membranes of most adipocytes, especially immature cells, and numerous minute lipid droplets in addition to the large droplet. In this cell type caveolae play important roles in lipid trafficking and formation of the large triglyceride storage droplet.

As shown in Figure 6–1, partitions of connective tissue containing a vascular bed and a nerve network subdivide white fat into incomplete lobules. Fibroblasts, macrophages, and other cells typically comprise about half the total cell number in white adipose tissue. Reticular fibers form a fine interwoven network supporting individual fat cells and binding them together. The microvasculature between adipocytes may not always be apparent in tissue sections.

The distribution of white adipose tissue changes significantly through childhood and adult life, partly regulated by sex hormones controlling adipose deposition in the breasts and thighs. The color of freshly dissected white adipose tissue depends on the diet, varying from white to yellow with increasing amounts of carotenoid dissolved in the lipid.

Storage & Mobilization of Lipids

White adipocytes can store triglycerides derived from three sources:

- Dietary fats brought to the cells via the circulation as **chylomicrons**,
- Lipids synthesized in the liver and transported in blood with **very low-density lipoproteins (VLDLs)**, and
- Free fatty acids and glycerol synthesized by the adipocytes.

Chylomicrons (Gr. *chylos*, juice + *micros*, small) represent particles of variable size, up to 1200 nm in diameter, formed from ingested lipids in epithelial cells lining the small intestine and transported in the blood and lymph. They consist of a core containing mainly triglycerides, surrounded by a stabilizing monolayer of phospholipids, cholesterol, and several apolipoproteins.

VLDLs appear as much smaller complexes (30–80 nm, providing a greater surface-to-volume ratio) of similar lipid and protein composition to chylomicrons, but undergo synthesis and release in liver cells. Clinical tests for circulating levels of lipoproteins routinely measure blood lipids after fasting to allow depletion of chylomicrons. Varying levels of apoproteins and triglycerides in the complexes allow their categorization according to density, from VLDL to high-density lipoprotein (HDL).

In adipose tissue both chylomicrons and VLDLs become hydrolyzed at the luminal surfaces of blood capillaries by **lipoprotein lipase**, an enzyme synthesized by the adipocytes and transferred to the capillary cell membrane (Figure 6-2). Free fatty acids then enter the adipocytes by both active transport and diffusion. Within the adipocytes the fatty acids combine with glycerol phosphate, supplied by glucose metabolism, to again form triglycerides, which then get deposited in the growing lipid droplet. **Insulin** stimulates glucose uptake by adipocytes and accelerates its conversion into triglycerides, and the production of lipoprotein lipase.

Upon adipocyte stimulation by nerves or various hormones, stored lipids become mobilized and cells release fatty acids and glycerol. **Norepinephrine** released in the adrenal gland and by postganglionic sympathetic nerves in adipose tissue activates a **hormone-sensitive lipase** that breaks down triglycerides at the surface of the stored lipid droplets (Figure 6-2). Growth hormone (GH) from the pituitary gland also stimulates this lipase activity. The free fatty acids diffuse across the membranes of the adipocyte and the capillary endothelium and bind the protein albumin in blood for transport throughout the body. The more water-soluble glycerol remains free in blood for uptake in the liver. Insulin inhibits the hormone-sensitive lipase, reducing fatty acid release, and stimulates enzymes for lipid synthesis. Besides insulin and GH, other peptide hormones also cooperate in regulating lipid synthesis and mobilization in adipocytes.

Hormonal activity of white adipocytes themselves includes production of the 16-kDa polypeptide hormone **leptin** (Gr. *leptos*, thin), a "satiety factor" with target cells in the hypothalamus, other brain regions, and peripheral organs, which helps regulate the appetite under normal conditions and participates in regulating the formation of new adipose tissue.

FIGURE 6–2 Lipid storage and mobilization from adipocytes.

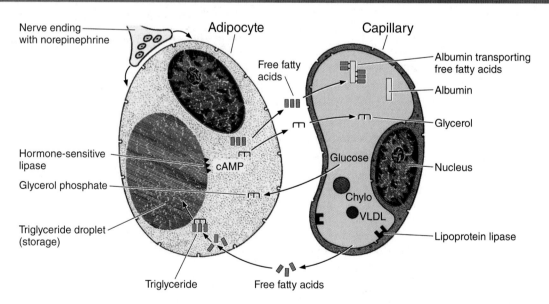

Triglycerides are transported by blood and lymph from the intestine and liver in lipoprotein complexes known as **chylomicrons (Chylo)** and **VLDLs**. In the capillary endothelial cells of adipose tissue, these complexes are partly broken down by **lipoprotein lipase**, releasing free fatty acids and glycerol. The free fatty acids diffuse from the capillary into the adipocyte, where they are reesterified to glycerol phosphate, forming triglycerides that are stored in the lipid droplet until needed.

Norepinephrine from nerve endings stimulates the cyclic AMP (cAMP) system, which activates **hormone-sensitive lipase** to hydrolyze the stored triglycerides to free fatty acids and glycerol. These substances diffuse into the capillary, where the fatty acids bind albumin for transport throughout the body for use as an energy source.

Abundant caveolae in the adipocyte plasmalemma are rich in cholesterol and other lipids and appear to mediate endocytosis of fatty acids necessary for growth of the lipid storage droplet.

Although white adipose tissue associated with different organs appears histologically similar, differences in gene expression have been noted between visceral deposits (in the abdomen) and subcutaneous deposits of white fat. Such differences may have importance for medical risks of obesity; it is well established that increased visceral adipose tissue raises the risk of diabetes and cardiovascular disease, whereas increased subcutaneous fat does not. The release of visceral fat products directly to the portal circulation of the liver may also influence the medical relevance of this form of obesity.

In response to body needs, lipids undergo mobilization rather uniformly from white adipocytes in all parts of the body, although adipose tissue in the palms, soles, and fat pads behind the eyes resists even long periods of starvation. During starvation, adipocytes can lose nearly all their fat and become polyhedral or spindle-shaped cells with only very small lipid droplets.

Histogenesis of White Adipose Tissue

Like other connective tissue, skeletal and muscle cells, adipocytes develop from mesenchymal stem cells. Adipose development first produces **preadipocytes**, which look rather like larger fibroblasts with cytoplasmic lipid droplets (Figure 6–3). Initially, the droplets of white adipocytes are separate from one another but they soon fuse to form the single large droplet (Figure 6–1).

As shown in Figure 6–3, white adipocytes develop together with a smaller population of cells termed beige adipocytes, which remain within white adipose tissue and have histological and metabolic features generally intermediate between white and brown adipocytes. With adaptation to cold temperatures beige adipocytes change reversibly, forming many more small lipid droplets, adopting a gene expression profile more like that of brown fat and begin to release heat as described below.

FIGURE **6–3** Development of white and brown fat cells.

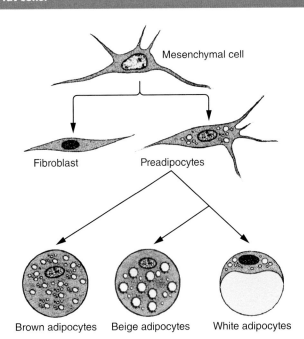

Mesenchymal cell

Fibroblast   Preadipocytes

Brown adipocytes   Beige adipocytes   White adipocytes

Mesenchymal stem cells differentiate as progenitor cells for all types of connective tissue, including **preadipocytes**. These are initially of at least two types. Preadipocytes developing within the lateral mesoderm of the embryo produce large number of **white adipocytes** (forming white adipose tissue) and a smaller number of so-called "beige" adipocytes with cytological features and gene expression patterns of both white and brown adipocytes. White adipocytes are unilocular, with one large lipid droplet occupying most of the cytoplasm. The white adipocyte is usually much larger than that shown here in relation to the other cell types.

Brown adipocytes differentiate from another population of preadipocytes located in paraxial embryonic mesoderm and remain multilocular (having many small lipid droplets) with numerous mitochondria (not shown here). Mitochondrial metabolism of lipid in brown adipocytes releases heat rather than ATP. Cells functioning as brown adipocytes can also develop from beige adipocytes during adaptation to cold temperatures.

At birth humans have stores of white adipose tissue, which begin to accumulate by the 14th week of gestation. Both visceral and subcutaneous fat becomes well developed after this time. Proliferation of progenitor cells diminishes by late gestation, and adipose tissue increases mainly by the filling of existing adipocytes until around age 10, followed by a period of new fat cell differentiation that lasts through adolescence. New adipocyte formation occurs around small blood vessels, where undifferentiated mesenchymal cells are most abundant.

Excessive adipose tissue accumulation, or obesity, occurs when nutritional intake exceeds energy expenditure, an increasingly common condition in modern, sedentary lifestyles. Although adipocytes can differentiate from mesenchymal stem cells throughout life, adult-onset obesity mainly involves increasing the size of existing adipocytes (hypertrophy). Childhood obesity, in contrast, often involves increases in both adipocyte size and numbers due to the differentiation of more preadipocytes from mesenchymal cells (hyperplasia). Weight loss after dietary changes results from reductions in adipocyte volume, but not their overall number.

❯ BROWN ADIPOSE TISSUE

Brown adipose tissue constitutes 2%–5% of the newborn body weight, located mainly in the back, neck, and shoulders, but becomes greatly reduced during childhood and adolescence. In adults, it occurs only in scattered areas, especially around the kidneys, adrenal glands, aorta, and mediastinum. Brown adipocytes contain many small lipid inclusions and are therefore called **multilocular** (Figure 6–3). The color of **brown fat** is due to both the very abundant mitochondria (containing cytochrome pigment) scattered among the lipid droplets of the fat cells and the large number of blood capillaries in this tissue. The small lipid droplets, abundant mitochondria, and rich vasculature all help mediate this tissue's principal function of **heat production** and warming the blood.

Cells of brown fat are polygonal and generally smaller than white adipocytes; their smaller lipid droplets allow the nucleus to be more centrally located (Figure 6–4). Brown adipocytes often localize closely around large capillaries, and the tissue becomes subdivided by connective tissue partitions into lobules that are better delineated than the lobules of white

FIGURE **6–4** Brown adipose tissue.

(a) Brown adipose tissue with closely packed cells is shown here around a small blood vessel (**BV**), with adjacent white adipose tissue at the top of the photo. Brown adipocytes are slightly smaller and characteristically contain many small lipid droplets and central spherical nuclei. If the lipid has been dissolved from the cells, as shown here, the many mitochondria among the lipid spaces are retained and can be easily discerned. (×200; PT)

(b) A diagram of a single brown, **multilocular adipocyte** showing the central nucleus, many small lipid droplets (yellow), and very numerous mitochondria. Also shown is a sympathetic nerve ending that releases norepinephrine to stimulate mitochondrial production of heat, the principal function of brown adipose tissue.

adipose tissue. Cells of this tissue receive direct sympathetic innervation which regulates their metabolic activity.

Function of Brown Adipocytes

The main function of these multilocular adipose cells is heat production by nonshivering **thermogenesis**. The physiology of brown fat is best understood from studies of the tissue in hibernating species. In animals ending their hibernation period, and in newborn humans, nerve impulses liberate norepinephrine into brown adipose tissue. As in white fat, this neurotransmitter activates the hormone-sensitive lipase of adipocytes, promoting hydrolysis of triglycerides to fatty acids and glycerol. However, unlike the process in white fat, liberated fatty acids of multilocular adipocytes are not released but are quickly metabolized, with a consequent increase in O_2 consumption and heat production. This raises the temperature within the tissue and warms the locally circulating blood, which then distributes the heat throughout the body.

Heat production in brown adipocytes greatly exceeds that of other cells because their inner mitochondrial membranes have greatly upregulated levels of the transmembrane protein **uncoupling protein-1 (UCP1)** or **thermogenin**. In the presence of free fatty acids, UCP1 permits the flow of protons from the intermembranous space to the matrix without passing through ATP synthetase complexes. Instead of producing ATP, the energy associated with this proton flow dissipates as heat.

Histogenesis of Brown Adipose Tissue

Brown adipose tissue also develops from mesenchyme but involves preadipocytes in a different embryonic location (paraxial) from those producing white adipose tissue. Brown adipocytes also emerge earlier than white fat during fetal development. In humans the amount of brown fat is maximal relative to body weight at birth, when thermogenesis is most needed, and partially disappears by involution and apoptosis during childhood. Lean adults have greater amounts and more active brown fat than other people.

The number of brown adipocytes increases during cold adaptation, usually appearing as clusters of multilocular cells in white adipose tissue. As indicated earlier, this increase involves the reversible shift of beige cells to functional brown adipocytes, but may also include proliferation and differentiation of new adipocytes from preexisting progenitor cells. Besides stimulating thermogenic activity, autonomic nerves also promote brown adipocyte differentiation and prevent apoptosis in mature brown fat cells.

Adipose Tissue SUMMARY OF KEY POINTS

- The defining cells of adipose tissue (fat), **adipocytes**, are very large cells derived from mesenchyme and specialized for energy storage in lipid droplet(s) with **triglycerides**.
- Adipocytes store lipids from three sources: from dietary fats packaged as **chylomicrons** in the intestine; from triglycerides produced in the liver and circulating as **VLDLs**; and from fatty acids synthesized locally.
- Lipids are mobilized from adipocytes by **hormone-sensitive lipase** activated by **norepinephrine** released from the adrenal gland and various peptide hormones.
- Cells of adipose tissue are supported by reticular fibers, with connective tissue septa dividing the tissue into lobules of various sizes.
- There are two types of adipose tissue: **white fat** and **brown fat**.

White Adipose Tissue

- **White adipose tissue** is found in many organs throughout the body, typically forming about 20% of the body weight in adults.
- Adipocytes of white fat are typically very **large cells**, ranging in diameter from 50 to 150 μm.

- These cells each contain primarily **one large lipid droplet** (they are **unilocular**), causing the nucleus and remaining cytoplasm to be pushed against the plasmalemma.
- Fatty acids are released from white adipocytes by **lipase** activity when nutrients are needed and carried throughout the body on plasma proteins such as albumin.
- **Leptin** is a polypeptide hormone with target cells in the hypothalamus that is released from white adipocytes and helps regulate eating behavior.

Brown Adipose Tissue

- **Brown fat** comprises up to 5% of the newborn body weight but smaller amounts in adults.
- Adipocytes of this tissue are typically smaller than those of white fat and contain primarily **many small lipid droplets** (they are **multilocular**) in cytoplasm containing many mitochondria and a central nucleus.
- Fatty acids released in adipocytes of brown fat are metabolized in mitochondria of these cells for **thermogenesis** rather than ATP synthesis, using **uncoupling protein-1**.

Adipose Tissue ASSESS YOUR KNOWLEDGE

1. White adipocytes are derived developmentally from what precursor cells?

   a. Monocytes
   b. Fibroblasts
   c. Mesenchymal cells
   d. Brown adipocytes
   e. Mast cells

2. What are the relatively large particles formed in the intestinal epithelial cells and rich in ingested lipids?

   a. Fatty acids
   b. Chylomicrons
   c. Glycerols
   d. Very low-density lipoproteins
   e. Adipocytes

3. What substance, released from the adrenal gland and some autonomic neurons, increases lipolytic activity in white adipocytes?

   a. Leptin
   b. Insulin
   c. Norepinephrine
   d. Glycogen
   e. Triglyceride

4. What is the most important form of lipid storage in both white and brown adipocytes?

   a. Free fatty acids
   b. Cholesterol
   c. Chylomicrons
   d. Glycerol
   e. Triglycerides

5. Important target cells of leptin are found in which organ?

   a. Small intestine
   b. White adipose tissue
   c. Large intestine
   d. Hypothalamus
   e. Brown adipose tissue

6. The hormone-sensitive lipase in the cells of adipose tissue acts primarily on what substrate?

   a. Glucose
   b. Free fatty acids
   c. Glycerol
   d. Triglycerides
   e. Very low-density lipoproteins

7. Applied to adipocytes, the term "multilocular" refers to which of the following?

   a. The large number of small cytoplasmic lipid droplets
   b. The proliferation of the cells in an obese individual
   c. The large number of mitochondria in the cells
   d. The high density of nerves supplying the tissue
   e. The type of mesenchymal cells also present

8. Fully differentiated white adipocytes are large cells, typically having diameters of approximately what size?

   a. 5 μm
   b. 10 μm
   c. 100 μm
   d. 500 μm
   e. 1000 μm

9. Ten days after birth, a full-term newborn boy develops firm, erythematous nodules, and plaques over his trunk, arms, buttocks, thighs, and cheeks. His mother's pregnancy was complicated by placenta previa, and his airway was cleared of aspirated meconium immediately after birth. A biopsy of subcutaneous tissue shows necrosis within the brown adipose tissue. What metabolic activity is liable to be affected in this patient?

   a. Export of fatty acids from fat
   b. Thermal insulation
   c. Oxidation of fatty acids for thermogenesis
   d. Activation of the adenylate cyclase system
   e. Initiation of shivering

10. A 44-year-old woman of African ancestry visits her family physician for a physical examination at the urging of her husband. She has no current complaints and is taking no medications. She is allergic to erythromycin. She works as a software developer and lives with her 52-year-old husband and 12-year-old daughter. She is a nonsmoker and drinks an occasional glass of wine when she and her husband go out to dinner. She is involved in no regular exercise. Her mother is 66 and suffers from type 2 diabetes, hyperlipidemia, and hypertension and had a myocardial infarction last year. The patient's father died of a stroke last year at the age of 72. On examination, the patient's blood pressure is 155/100 mm Hg, pulse 84 beats/min, weight 215 lb (increased from 180 lb 3 years ago), and height 5 ft 7 in. In this patient, during the period of weight gain, which one of the following responses would be most likely in her white fat?

    a. Increased synthesis of growth hormone
    b. Decreased synthesis of leptin
    c. Increased release of chylomicrons to the blood
    d. Decreased conversion of beige adipocytes to unilocular white adipocytes
    e. Increased incorporation of fatty acids into triglycerides

CHAPTER **7** Cartilage

Cartilage, a tough and durable form of supporting connective tissue, characteristically displayss an **extracellular matrix** (ECM) with very high concentrations of GAGs and proteoglycans, all interacting with collagen and elastic fibers. Structural features of its matrix make cartilage ideal for a variety of mechanical and protective roles within the adult skeleton and elsewhere (Figure 7–1).

Cartilage ECM has a firm yet flexible consistency that allows the tissue to bear mechanical stresses without permanent distortion. In the respiratory tract, ears and nose, cartilage forms the framework supporting softer tissues. Because of its resiliency and smooth, lubricated surface, cartilage provides cushioning and sliding regions within skeletal joints and facilitates bone movements. As described in Chapter 8, cartilage also guides development and growth of long bones, both before and after birth.

Cartilage consists of cells called **chondrocytes** (Gr. *chondros*, cartilage + *kytos*, cell) and **chondroblasts** embedded in the ECM which, unlike connective tissue proper, contains no other cell types. Chondroblasts undergo mitosis and secrete ECM components, maturing as *nondividing* chondrocytes which also produce the ECM and maintain it longterm. As cartilage develops the cells occupy matrix cavities called **lacunae**.

The physical properties of cartilage depend on electrostatic bonds between **type II collagen** fibrils, **hyaluronan**, and the sulfated GAGs on densely packed **proteoglycans**. Its semirigid consistency relates to the water binding the negatively charged hyaluronan and GAG chains that extend from proteoglycan core proteins, all components enclosed within a complex meshwork of thin type II collagen fibrils. The high content of bound water allows cartilage to serve as a shock absorber, an important functional role.

All types of cartilage lack vascular supplies with chondrocytes receiving nutrients and oxygen by diffusion from capillaries in surrounding connective tissue (the perichondrium). In some skeletal elements, large blood vessels do traverse cartilage to supply other tissues, but these vessels release few nutrients to the chondrocytes. As expected of cells in an avascular tissue, chondrocytes exhibit low metabolic activity. Cartilage also lacks nerves.

The **perichondrium** (Figure 7–2), a sheath of dense connective tissue surrounding most cartilaginous structures, forms an interface between the cartilage and tissues supported by the cartilage. The perichondrium harbors the blood supply serving the cartilage and a small neural component. Articular cartilage, which covers the ends of bones in movable joints and erodes during arthritic degeneration, lacks perichondrium but its chondrocytes receive sufficient oxygen and nutrients from the synovial fluid.

As shown in Figure 7–1, variations in the composition of the matrix characterize three main types of cartilage: hyaline cartilage, elastic cartilage, and fibrocartilage. Table 7–1 summarizes the notable features of each.

> **›› MEDICAL APPLICATION**
>
> Many genetic conditions in humans or mice that cause defective cartilage, joint deformities, or short limbs are due to recessive mutations in genes for collagen type II, the aggrecan core protein, the sulfate transporter, and other proteins required for normal chondrocyte function.

› HYALINE CARTILAGE

Hyaline (Gr. *hyalos*, glass) cartilage, the most common of the three types, appears homogeneous and semitransparent in the fresh state. In adults hyaline cartilage can be found in the articular surfaces of movable joints, in the walls of larger respiratory passages (nose, larynx, trachea, bronchi), in the ventral ends of ribs, where they articulate with the sternum, and in the epiphyseal plates of long bones, where it makes possible longitudinal bone growth (Figure 7–1). In the embryo, hyaline cartilage forms the temporary skeleton later gradually replaced by bone.

FIGURE 7–1 Distribution of cartilage in adults.

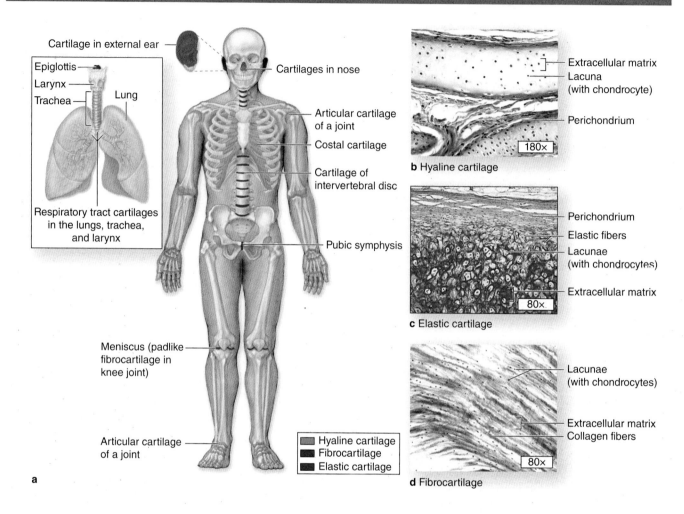

Cartilage in external ear

Epiglottis
Larynx
Trachea
Lung

Respiratory tract cartilages
in the lungs, trachea,
and larynx

Cartilages in nose

Articular cartilage
of a joint

Costal cartilage

Cartilage of
intervertebral disc

Pubic symphysis

Meniscus (padlike
fibrocartilage in
knee joint)

Articular cartilage
of a joint

Hyaline cartilage
Fibrocartilage
Elastic cartilage

a

b Hyaline cartilage

Extracellular matrix
Lacuna
(with chondrocyte)

Perichondrium

180×

c Elastic cartilage

Perichondrium
Elastic fibers
Lacunae
(with chondrocytes)

Extracellular matrix

80×

d Fibrocartilage

Lacunae
(with chondrocytes)

Extracellular matrix
Collagen fibers

80×

(a) There are three types of adult cartilage associated with areas of the skeleton, particularly in joints and where pliable support is useful, as in the ribs, ears and nose. Cartilage support of other tissues throughout the respiratory tract is also prominent.

The photomicrographs show the key features of **(b) hyaline cartilage**, **(c) elastic cartilage** and **(d) fibrocartilage**. Dense connective tissue of perichondrium appears here with hyaline and elastic cartilage.

≫ MEDICAL APPLICATION

Osteoarthritis, a chronic condition that commonly occurs during aging, involves the gradual loss or changed physical properties of the hyaline cartilage that lines the articular ends of bones in joints. Joints that are weight-bearing (knees, hips) or heavily used (wrist, fingers) are most prone to cartilage degeneration. Fragments released by wear-and-tear to the articular cartilage trigger secretion of matrix metalloproteinases and other factors from macrophages in adjacent tissues, which exacerbate damage and cause pain and inflammation within the joint.

Matrix

Collagen makes up 40% of hyaline cartilage's dry weight, with all of it embedded in the firm, hydrated gel of proteoglycans and structural glycoproteins. In routine histology preparations, the proteoglycans confer variable basophilia on this matrix, making the thin collagen fibrils barely discernible. **Type II collagen** predominates in hyaline cartilage, with lesser amounts of minor collagens also present.

Aggrecan (core protein 250 kDa), with approximately 150 GAG side chains of chondroitin sulfate and keratan sulfate, makes up the most abundant proteoglycan of hyaline cartilage. Hundreds of these proteoglycans bind noncovalently by link proteins to long polymers of hyaluronan, as shown schematically in Figure 7–2a and discussed in Chapter 5. These proteoglycan complexes adhere further to the surface of type II collagen fibrils (Figure 7–2a). Water bound to GAGs in the proteoglycans constitutes up to 60%–80% of the weight of fresh hyaline cartilage.

The structural multiadhesive glycoprotein **chondronectin** represents another key component of cartilage matrix.

FIGURE **7–2** The structure of cartilage matrix and cells.

a

b

(a) A schematic representation of the most abundant molecules in cartilage matrix shows the interaction between type II collagen fibrils and proteoglycans linked to hyaluronan. Link proteins noncovalently bind the protein core of proteoglycans to the linear hyaluronan molecules. The chondroitin sulfate side chains of the proteoglycan electrostatically bind to the collagen fibrils, forming a cross-linked matrix. The circled area is enlarged in the lower part of the figure. Physical properties of these matrix components produce a highly hydrated, pliable material with great strength. Water represents approximately 75% of the wet weight of hyaline cartilage.

(b) A diagram of the transitional area between the perichondrium and the cartilage matrix. Fibroblast-like progenitor cells in the perichondrium give rise to larger chondroblasts, which divide and differentiate as chondrocytes. These functional cells produce matrix components and exist in lacunae surrounded by the matrix. The ECM immediately around each lacuna, called the **territorial matrix**, contains mostly proteoglycans and sparse collagen; that more distant from lacunae, the **interterritorial matrix**, contains more collagen and may be less basophilic.

TABLE **7–1** | Important features of the major cartilage types.

	Hyaline Cartilage	Elastic Cartilage	Fibrocartilage
Main features of the extracellular matrix	Homogeneous, with type II collagen and aggrecan	Type II collagen, aggrecan, and darker elastic fibers	Type II collagen and large areas of dense connective tissue with type I collagen
Major cells	Chondrocytes, chondroblasts	Chondrocytes, chondroblasts	Chondrocytes, fibroblasts
Typical arrangement of chondrocytes	Isolated or in small isogenous groups	Usually in small isogenous groups	Isolated or in isogenous groups arranged axially
Presence of perichondrium	Yes (except at epiphyses and articular cartilage)	Yes	No
Main locations or examples	Many components of upper respiratory tract; articular ends and epiphyseal plates of long bones; fetal skeleton	External ear, external acoustic meatus, auditory tube; epiglottis and certain other laryngeal cartilages	Intervertebral discs, pubic symphysis, meniscus, and certain other joints; insertions of tendons
Main functions	Provides smooth, low-friction surfaces in joints; structural support for respiratory tract	Provides flexible shape and support of soft tissues	Provides cushioning, tensile strength, and resistance to tearing and compression

Like fibronectin in other connective tissues, chondronectin binds specifically to GAGs, collagen and integrins, mediating transient adherence of chondrocytes to the ECM.

Staining variations within the matrix reflect local differences in its molecular composition. Immediately surrounding each chondrocyte, the ECM is richer in GAGs than collagen, often causing these areas of **territorial matrix** to stain more darkly than the intervening areas of interterritorial matrix (Figures 7–2b and 7–3).

Cartilage Cells

Cells occupy only a small volume of hyaline cartilage. At the periphery of the cartilage, young chondrocytes and **chondroblasts** have an elliptic shape, with the long axes parallel to the surface (Figure 7–3). Deeper in the cartilage they become rounded and often appear in small groups of cells called **isogenous aggregates**, originating from a single chondroblast by mitotic divisions. As these chondrocytes become more active in secreting collagens and other ECM components, the new matrix separates the cells which then occupy separate lacunae.

Cartilage cells and matrix may shrink slightly during routine histologic preparation, resulting in both the irregular shape of the chondrocytes and their retraction from the matrix. In living tissue, chondrocytes fill their lacunae completely.

Because of the cartilage matrix avascularity, chondrocytes respire under low-oxygen tension. Hyaline cartilage cells metabolize glucose by anaerobic glycolysis primarily. Nutrients from the blood diffuse to all the chondrocytes from the cartilage surface, with movement of water and solutes in the cartilage matrix promoted by intermittent tissue compression and decompression during body movements. The limits of such diffusion define the maximum thickness of hyaline cartilage, which usually exists as small, thin plates.

❯❯ MEDICAL APPLICATION

In contrast to other forms of cartilage and most other tissues, hyaline cartilage is susceptible to partial or isolated regions of **calcification** during aging, especially in the costal cartilage adjacent to the ribs. Calcification of the hyaline matrix, accompanied by degenerative changes in the chondrocytes, is a common part of the aging process and in many respects resembles endochondral ossification by which bone is formed.

FIGURE 7–3 Hyaline cartilage.

(a) The upper part of the photo shows the perichondrium (**P**), an example of dense connective tissue consisting of type I collagen primarily. Among the fibroblastic cells of the perichondrium are indistinguishable mesenchymal stem cells. There is a gradual transition and differentiation of cells from the perichondrium to the cartilage, with elongated fibroblast-like cells becoming larger and more rounded as chondroblasts and chondrocytes (**C**). These become localized within lacunae surrounded by the matrix (**M**) which these cells secreted. (×200; H&E)

(b) The thin region of hyaline cartilage shown here has perichondrium (**P**) on both sides and shows larger lacunae containing isogenous groups of chondrocytes (**C**) within the matrix (**M**). Such groups of two, four or more cells arise by mitosis of chondroblasts; the cells will separate into individual lacunae as they begin to secrete matrix. Territorial matrix immediately around the chondrocytes displays more intense basophilia than interterritorial matrix farther from the cells, indicating its greater density of sulfated GAGs. (×160; H&E)

Several hormones and growth factors accelerate blast synthesis of sulfated GAGs and secretion of proteoglycans, with the pituitary-derived protein called growth hormone or **somatotropin** serving as a major regulator of hyaline cartilage growth. This hormone acts indirectly, promoting the endocrine release from the liver of insulin-like growth factors, or somatomedins, which directly stimulate the cells of hyaline cartilage.

> **>> MEDICAL APPLICATION**
>
> Cells of cartilage can give rise to either benign (**chondroma**) or slow-growing, malignant (**chondrosarcoma**) tumors in which cells produce normal matrix components. Chondrosarcomas seldom metastasize and are generally removed surgically.

Perichondrium

Except in the articular cartilage of joints, all hyaline cartilage has a covering layer of dense connective tissue, the **perichondrium**, essential for the growth and maintenance of the cartilage (Figures 7–2b and 7–3). The outer region of the perichondrium consists primarily of collagen type I fibers and fibroblasts, but an inner layer adjoining the cartilage matrix also contains mesenchymal stem cells that provide a source for new chondroblasts that divide and differentiate into chondrocytes.

❯ ELASTIC CARTILAGE

Elastic cartilage has features essentially like those of hyaline cartilage except that in addition to the meshwork of collagen type II fibrils it contains an abundant network of elastic fibers (Figures 7–4 and 7–1c), which give fresh elastic cartilage a yellowish color. With appropriate staining the elastic fibers usually appear as dark bundles distributed unevenly through the matrix.

More flexible than hyaline cartilage, elastic cartilage occurs in the external ear, the walls of the external auditory

FIGURE 7–4 Elastic cartilage.

The chondrocytes (**C**) and overall organization of elastic cartilage resemble those of hyaline cartilage, but the matrix (**M**) also contains elastic fibers that can be seen as darker components with proper staining. The abundant elastic fibers provide greater flexibility to this type of cartilage. The section in part **b** includes perichondrium (**P**) that is also like that of hyaline cartilage. **(a)** ×160; Hematoxylin and orcein. **(b)** ×180; Weigert resorcin and van Gieson.

canals, the auditory (Eustachian) tubes, the epiglottis, and the upper respiratory tract. Elastic cartilage in these locations includes a perichondrium like that of most hyaline cartilage. Throughout elastic cartilage the cells resemble those of hyaline cartilage both physiologically and structurally.

› FIBROCARTILAGE

Fibrocartilage takes various forms in different structures but appears as a mixture of hyaline cartilage and dense connective tissue (Figures 7–5 and 7–1d). It develops in intervertebral discs, in attachments of certain ligaments, and in the pubic symphysis—all places where it serves as very tough, yet cushioning support tissue for bone.

Cells of fibrocartilage occur singly and often in aligned isogenous aggregates, producing a sparse ECM of type II collagen and other matrix components. Areas with chondrocytes and hyaline matrix become separated by other regions with fibroblasts and dense bundles of type I collagen, which confer extra tensile strength to this tissue (Figure 7–5). The relative scarcity of proteoglycans overall makes fibrocartilage matrix more acidophilic than that of hyaline or elastic cartilage. Fibrocartilage lacks a distinct surrounding perichondrium.

Intervertebral discs of the spinal column consist primarily of fibrocartilage and act as lubricated cushions and shock absorbers, held in place by ligaments and preventing damage to adjacent vertebrae from abrasive forces or impacts. Intervertebral discs are discussed further with joints in Chapter 8.

Again, Table 7–1 summarizes the important features of the three major types of cartilage.

› CARTILAGE FORMATION, GROWTH, & REPAIR

All cartilage develops from embryonic mesenchyme in the process of **chondrogenesis** (Figure 7–6). The first indications of cell differentiation appear as the rounding of mesenchymal cells, which retract their extensions, multiply rapidly and become more densely packed together. As mentioned, the terms "chondroblasts" and "chondrocytes," respectively, generally refer to the cartilage cells during and after the period of rapid proliferation. At both stages, the cells have basophilic cytoplasm rich in RER for collagen synthesis (Figure 7–7). ECM production first encloses the cells in their lacunae and then gradually separates chondroblasts from one another. During embryonic development cartilage differentiation takes place primarily from the center outward. Therefore, the more central cells have the characteristics of chondrocytes, whereas the peripheral cells are typical chondroblasts. The superficial mesenchyme develops as the perichondrium.

Once formed cartilage tissue enlarges both by **interstitial growth**, involving mitotic division of preexisting chondroblasts, and by **appositional growth**, which involves chondroblast differentiation from progenitor cells in the

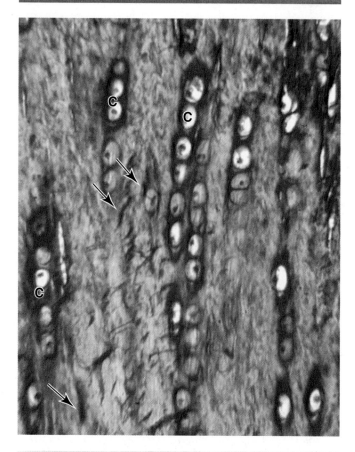

FIGURE **7–5** Fibrocartilage.

Fibrocartilage varies histologically in different structures but is always essentially a mixture of hyaline cartilage and dense connective tissue.

In a small region of intervertebral disc, the axially arranged aggregates of chondrocytes (**C**) are seen to be surrounded by small amounts of matrix and separated by larger regions with dense collagen and scattered fibroblasts with elongated nuclei (arrows). (×250; Picrosirius-hematoxylin)

perichondrium (Figure 7–2b). In both cases matrix synthesis contributes most volumetric growth of the cartilage. Appositional growth of cartilage becomes more important during postnatal development, although as described in Chapter 8 interstitial growth in cartilaginous regions within long bones allows increasing length of these structures. Cartilage at the surfaces of articular joints often becomes eroded, with cell and matrix replacement reliant on the remaining cells since such joints lack perichondrium to add cells by appositional growth.

Except in young children, damaged cartilage undergoes slow and often incomplete **repair**, primarily dependent on cells from the perichondrium, which invade the injured area and produce new cartilage. In damaged areas the perichondrium produces a scar of dense connective tissue instead of forming new cartilage. As mentioned earlier the poor capacity of cartilage for repair or regeneration is due in part to its avascularity and low metabolic rate.

FIGURE **7–6** Chondrogenesis.

Diagrams here depict the major stages of embryonic cartilage formation, or **chondrogenesis**.

(a) Mesenchyme represents the precursor for all types of cartilage.

(b) Mitosis and initial cell differentiation produce a tissue with condensations of rounded cells called **chondroblasts**.

(c) Chondroblasts then separate from one another by their production of the various matrix components, which collectively swell with water and form the very extensive ECM.

(d) Multiplication of chondroblasts within the matrix gives rise to isogenous cell aggregates surrounded by a condensation of territorial matrix. In mature cartilage, this interstitial mitotic activity ceases and all chondrocytes typically become more widely separated by their production of matrix.

FIGURE **7–7** Chondrocytes in growing cartilage.

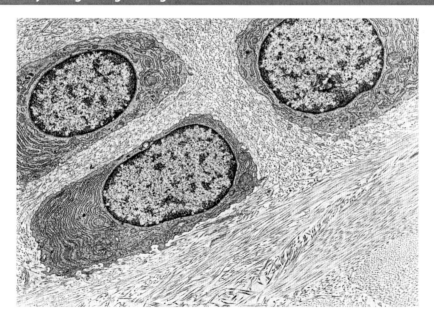

This TEM of **fibrocartilage** shows **chondrocytes** with abundant RER actively secreting the collagen-rich matrix. Bundles of **collagen fibrils**, sectioned in various orientations, predominate around the chondrocytes of this fibrocartilage, with collagen types I and II both present. Chondrocytes in growing hyaline and elastic cartilage have more prominent Golgi complexes and synthesize abundant proteoglycans in addition to collagen. (×3750)

Cartilage SUMMARY OF KEY POINTS

- Cartilage is a **tough**, **resilient** type of connective tissue that structurally supports certain soft tissues, notably in the respiratory tract, and provides cushioned, low-friction surfaces in joints.
- Cells of cartilage, **chondrocytes**, make up a small percentage of the tissue's mass, which is mainly a flexible mass of **extracellular matrix (ECM)**.
- Chondrocytes lie embedded within **lacunae** surrounded by the ECM.
- Cartilage ECM typically includes **collagen** as well as abundant **proteoglycans**, notably **aggrecan**, which bind a large amount of **water**.
- Cartilage always **lacks blood vessels**, lymphatics and nerves, but usually has a surrounding dense connective tissue **perichondrium** that is vascularized.
- There are three major forms of cartilage: (1) **hyaline cartilage**, (2) **elastic cartilage**, and (3) **fibrocartilage**.

Hyaline Cartilage

- The ECM of hyaline cartilage appears **homogenous and glassy**, rich in fibrils of type II collagen and aggrecan complexes with bound water.
- The ECM has less collagen and more proteoglycan immediately around the lacunae, producing slight staining differences in this **territorial matrix**.
- Chondrocytes occur **singly** or in small, mitotically derived **isogenous groups**.
- **Perichondrium** is usually present, but not with hyaline cartilage of articular surfaces or the epiphyses of growing long bones.

Elastic Cartilage

- Elastic cartilage resembles hyaline cartilage in its chondrocytes and major ECM components, but its matrix includes **abundant elastic fibers**, visible with special stains, which increase the tissue's **flexibility**.
- Elastic cartilage provides flexible support for the external ear as well as certain structures of the middle ear and larynx; it always includes surrounding **perichondrium**.

Fibrocartilage

- Fibrocartilage contains varying **combinations of hyaline cartilage** in variable amounts of **dense connective tissue**.
- Histologically it consists of small **chondrocytes** in a hyaline matrix, usually layered with larger areas of bundled **type I collagen** with scattered **fibroblasts**.
- Fibrocartilage provides very **tough**, **strong support** at tendon insertions and in **intervertebral discs** and certain other joints.

Cartilage Formation, Growth, & Repair

- All forms of cartilage develop from embryonic **mesenchyme**.
- Cartilaginous structures grow by mitosis of existing **chondroblasts** in lacunae (**interstitial growth**) or formation of new chondroblasts peripherally from progenitor cells in the perichondrium (**appositional growth**).
- Repair or replacement of injured cartilage occurs very slowly and ineffectively, due in part to the tissue's **avascularity** and **low metabolic rate**.

Cartilage ASSESS YOUR KNOWLEDGE

1. The molecular basis for the shock absorbing properties of cartilage involves which of the following?
   a. Electrostatic interaction of proteoglycans with type IV collagen
   b. Ability of glycosaminoglycans to bind anions
   c. Noncovalent binding of glycosaminoglycans to protein cores
   d. Sialic acid residues in the glycoproteins
   e. Hydration of glycosaminoglycans

2. What distinguishes cartilage from most other connective tissues?
   a. Its extracellular matrix is rich in collagen.
   b. Its predominant cell type is a mesenchymal derivative.
   c. Its predominant cell type secretes both fibers and proteoglycans.
   d. It lacks blood vessels.
   e. It functions in mechanical support.

3. Which feature is typical of elastic cartilage?
   a. Primary skeletal tissue in the fetus
   b. No identifiable perichondrium
   c. Found in intervertebral discs
   d. Most widely distributed cartilage type in the body
   e. Collagen is mainly type II

4. Which area in cartilage is relatively collagen-poor and proteoglycan-rich?
   a. Fibrocartilage
   b. Territorial matrix
   c. Epiphyseal plate
   d. Interterritorial matrix
   e. Perichondrium

5. What is the source of the mesenchymal progenitor cells activated for the repair of hyaline cartilage of accident-damaged costal cartilages?
   a. Perichondrium
   b. Adjacent loose connective tissue
   c. Bone of the adjacent rib(s) and sternum
   d. Chondrocytes of the injured cartilage
   e. Stem cells circulating with blood

6. How does articular cartilage differ from most other hyaline cartilage?
   a. It undergoes mainly appositional growth.
   b. It contains isogenous groups of chondrocytes.
   c. It lacks a perichondrium.
   d. Its matrix contains aggrecan.
   e. It is derived from embryonic mesenchyme.

7. Which step occurs first in chondrogenesis?

    a. Appositional growth
    b. Conversion of chondroblasts to chondrocytes
    c. Formation of mesenchymal condensations
    d. Interstitial growth
    e. Secretion of collagen-rich and proteoglycan-rich matrix

8. Osteoarthritis is characterized by the progressive erosion of articular cartilage. The matrix metalloproteinases involved in this erosion primarily act on which matrix component?

    a. Aggrecan
    b. Link proteins
    c. Network-forming collagen
    d. Fibril-forming collagen
    e. Chondronectin

9. A 28-year-old woman visits the family medicine clinic complaining of loss of the sense of smell, nosebleeds, problems with swallowing, and hoarseness. She admits to "casual, social use" of cocaine on a regular basis since her sophomore year of college. A complete examination of her nose with a speculum and otoscope shows severe rhinitis (inflammation). There is also perforation and collapse of the nasal cartilage resulting in a "saddle nose" deformity. Erosions in the enamel of her front teeth are noted. The breakdown of the nasal cartilage releases collagen fibers primarily of which type?

    a. Type I
    b. Type II
    c. Type III
    d. Type IV
    e. Type VII

10. A 66-year-old man who suffered from severe osteoarthritis is referred to an orthopedic surgeon for replacement of his right knee. He had been actively involved in both high school and intercollegiate football and had continued running until about the age of 45 as a form of relaxation and exercise. With the patient's permission, the removed joint is used by investigators performing a proteomic analysis of different joint tissues. The meniscus was found to contain almost exclusively type I collagen and aggrecan was undetectable. What is the most likely explanation for this result?

    a. The meniscus normally consists of dense regular connective tissue, which contains primarily type I collagen.
    b. The meniscus normally consists of fibrocartilage, which contains only type I collagen.
    c. The meniscus had undergone repeated rounds of repair due to wear-and-tear during which its hyaline cartilage component was replaced by dense connective tissue.
    d. Osteoarthritic injury in the knee resulted in the chondrocytes of the meniscus switching from expression of genes for type II collagen to type I collagen.
    e. Elastic cartilage is normally replaced by fibrocartilage during aging and this process can be accelerated by exercise.

Answers: 1e, 2d, 3e, 4b, 5a, 6c, 7c, 8d, 9b, 10c

8 Bone

A s the main constituent of the adult skeleton, bone tissue (Figure 8–1) provides solid support for the body, protects vital organs such as those in the cranial and thoracic cavities, and encloses internal (medullary) cavities containing bone marrow where blood cells form. Bone (or osseous) tissue also serves as a reservoir of calcium, phosphate and other minerals, storing or releasing these ions in a controlled fashion to maintain constant concentrations in body fluids.

In addition, bones form a system of levers that multiply the forces generated during skeletal muscle contraction and transform them into bodily movements. This mineralized tissue therefore confers mechanical and metabolic functions to the skeleton.

Bone is a specialized connective tissue composed of calcified extracellular material, the **bone matrix**, and following three major cell types (Figure 8–2):

- **Osteocytes** (Gr. *osteon*, bone + *kytos*, cell), which become localized in cavities (**lacunae**) between bone matrix layers (**lamellae**), with cytoplasmic processes in small **canaliculi** (L. *canalis*, canal) extending into the matrix (Figure 8–1b)
- **Osteoblasts** (*osteon* + Gr. *blastos*, germ), growing cells which synthesize and secrete the organic components of the matrix
- **Osteoclasts** (*osteon* + Gr. *klastos*, broken), giant, multinucleated cells involved in removing calcified bone matrix and remodeling bone tissue.

Because metabolites cannot diffuse through the calcified matrix of bone, the exchanges between osteocytes and blood capillaries depend on communication through the very thin, cylindrical spaces of the canaliculi.

Both the internal and external surfaces of all bones have coverings of connective tissue containing osteogenic cells—**endosteum** on the internal surface surrounding the marrow cavity and **periosteum** on the outer surface.

Because of its hardness bone cannot be sectioned routinely. Immersion in a decalcifying solution softens bone matrix, allowing sectioning after paraffin embedding. Alternatively, embedding bone in plastic polymers after fixation can permit sectioning with a specialized microtome.

› BONE CELLS

Osteoblasts

Originating from mesenchymal stem cells, **osteoblasts** produce the organic components of bone matrix, including type I collagen fibers, proteoglycans, and matricellular glycoproteins, such as osteonectin. Deposition of the inorganic components of bone also depends on osteoblast activity. Active osteoblasts occur exclusively at bone matrix surfaces, bound there by integrins and typically forming a single layer of cuboidal cells joined by adherent and gap junctions (Figure 8–3). After completing their synthetic activity, some osteoblasts differentiate as osteocytes entrapped in matrix-bound lacunae, others flatten and cover the matrix surface as **bone lining cells**, and the majority undergo apoptosis.

During the processes of matrix synthesis and calcification, osteoblasts occur as polarized cells with ultrastructural features denoting active protein synthesis and secretion. Secreting matrix components at the cell surface in contact with existing bone matrix, osteoblasts produce a layer of unique collagen-rich material called **osteoid** between the cuboidal cell layer

FIGURE **8–1** Components of bone.

- Diaphysis of humerus
- Central canal
- Osteon
- External circumferential lamellae
- Perforating fibers
- Periosteum
  - Fibrous layer
  - Cellular layer
- Perforating canals
- Central canal

(a) Section of humerus

- Collagen fiber orientation
- Concentric lamellae
- Nerve
- Vein
- Artery
- Canaliculi
- Central canal

Osteon

- Internal circumferential lamellae
- Interstitial lamellae
- Inner circumferential lamellae
- Trabeculae of cancellous bone

- Lacuna
- Osteocyte
- Canaliculi

(b) Compact bone

- Space for bone marrow
- Trabeculae
- Canaliculi opening at surface
- Endosteum
- Osteoclast
- Lamellae
- Osteocyte in lacuna
- Osteoblasts aligned along trabecula of new bone
- Canaliculi opening at surface

(c) Cancellous bone

A schematic overview of the basic features of bone, including the three key cell types: **osteocytes**, **osteoblasts**, and **osteoclasts**; their usual locations; and the typical **lamellar organization** of bone. Osteoblasts secrete the matrix that then hardens by calcification, trapping the differentiating cells now called **osteocytes** in individual **lacunae**. Osteocytes maintain the calcified matrix and receive nutrients from microvasculature in the central canals of the osteons via very small channels called **canaliculi** that interconnect the lacunae. Osteoclasts are monocyte-derived cells in bone required for bone remodeling.

The **periosteum** consists of dense connective tissue, with a primarily fibrous layer covering a more cellular layer. Bone is vascularized by small vessels that penetrate the matrix from the periosteum. **Endosteum** covers all **trabeculae** around the marrow cavities.

FIGURE **8–2** Bone tissue.

Newly formed bone tissue decalcified for sectioning and stained with trichrome in which the collagen-rich ECM appears blue. The tissue is a combination of pale-staining mesenchymal regions (**M**) containing capillaries, fibroblasts, and osteoprogenitor stem cells and variably darker blue regions of normally calcified matrix with varying amounts of collagen and the three major cell types found in all bone tissue.

Bone-forming osteoblasts (**Ob**) differentiate from osteoprogenitor cells in the periosteum and endosteum, and cover the surfaces of existing bone matrix. The osteoblasts secrete **osteoid** rich in collagen type I, but also containing proteoglycans and other molecules. As osteoid undergoes calcification and hardens, it entraps some osteoblasts which then differentiate further as osteocytes (**Oc**) occupying lacunae surrounded by bony matrix. The much less numerous large, multinuclear osteoclasts (**Ocl**), produced by the fusion of blood monocytes, reside on bony surfaces and erode the matrix during bone remodeling. (400×; Mallory trichrome)

FIGURE **8–3** Osteoblasts, osteocytes, and osteoclasts.

(a) Diagram showing the relationship of osteoblasts to the newly formed matrix called "osteoid," bone matrix, and osteocytes. Osteoblasts and most of the larger osteoclasts are part of the endosteum covering the bony trabeculae.

(b) The photomicrograph of developing bone shows the location and morphologic differences between active osteoblasts (**Ob**) and osteocytes (**Oc**). Rounded osteoblasts, derived from progenitor cells in the adjacent mesenchyme (**M**), cover a thin layer of lightly stained osteoid (**Os**) on the surface of the more heavily stained bony matrix (**B**). Most osteoblasts that are no longer actively secreting osteoid will undergo apoptosis; others differentiate either as flattened bone lining cells on the trabeculae of bony matrix or as osteocytes located within lacunae surrounded by bony matrix. (×300; H&E)

and the preexisting bone surface (Figure 8–3). Deposition of calcium salts into this newly formed matrix completes this process of bone appositional growth.

Figure 8–4 diagrams basic aspects of the bone matrix mineralization process. Prominent among the noncollagen proteins secreted by osteoblasts is the vitamin K-dependent polypeptide **osteocalcin**, which together with various glycoproteins binds Ca^{2+} ions and concentrates this mineral locally. Osteoblasts also release membrane-enclosed **matrix vesicles** rich in alkaline phosphatase and other enzymes whose activity raises the local concentration of PO_4^{3-} ions. In the resulting microenvironment with high concentrations of both these ions, matrix vesicles serve as foci for the formation of hydroxyapatite $[Ca_{10}(PO_4)_6(OH)_2]$ crystals, the first visible step in calcification. These crystals grow rapidly by accretion

of more mineral and eventually produce a confluent mass of calcified material embedding the collagen fibers and proteoglycans (Figure 8–4).

FIGURE **8–4** **Mineralization in bone matrix.**

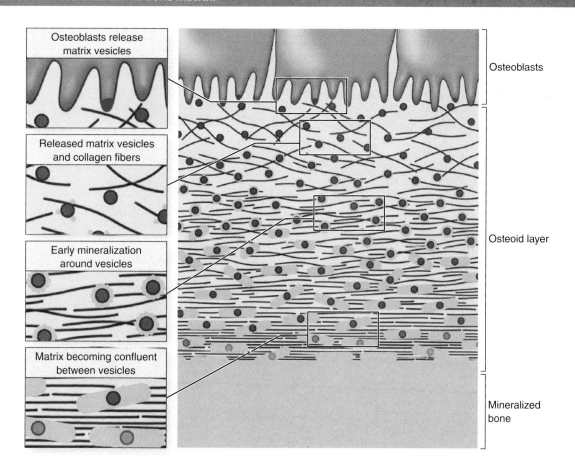

From their surfaces adjacent to the bone matrix, osteoblasts secrete type I collagen, several glycoproteins, and proteoglycans. Some of these factors, notably **osteocalcin** and certain glycoproteins, bind Ca^{2+} with high affinity, raising the local concentration of these ions. Osteoblasts also release very small membrane-enclosed **matrix vesicles** containing alkaline phosphatase and other enzymes. These enzymes remove PO_4^- ions from various matrix macromolecules, creating a high concentration of these ions locally. The high Ca^{2+} and PO_4^- ion concentrations cause calcified nanocrystals to form in and around the matrix vesicles. The crystals grow and mineralize further with formation of small growing masses of calcium hydroxyapatite $[Ca_{10}(PO_4)_6(OH)_2]$, which surround the collagen fibers and all other macromolecules. Eventually, the masses of hydroxyapatite merge as a confluent solid bony matrix as calcification of the matrix is completed.

Osteocytes

As mentioned, some osteoblasts become surrounded by the material they secrete and then differentiate as **osteocytes** enclosed singly within the **lacunae** spaced throughout the mineralized matrix. During the maturation from osteoblasts to osteocytes, the cells extend many long dendritic processes, which also become surrounded by calcifying matrix. These processes thus come to occupy the many canaliculi, 250–300 nm in diameter, radiating from each lacuna (Figures 8–5 and 8–1b).

Exchange of metabolites between osteocytes and blood vessels occurs through the small amount of interstitial fluid in the lacunae and canaliculi between the bone matrix and the osteocytes and their processes. Osteocytes also communicate with one another and ultimately with nearby osteoblasts and bone lining cells via gap junctions at the ends of their processes. These connections between osteocyte processes and nearly all other bone cells form an extensive lacunar-canalicular network that allows osteocytes to serve as mechanosensors detecting the mechanical load on the bone as well as stress- or fatigue-induced microdamage and to trigger remedial activity in osteoblasts and osteoclasts.

Normally the most abundant cells in bone, osteocytes exhibit significantly less RER, smaller Golgi complexes, and more condensed nuclear chromatin than osteoblasts (Figure 8–5a). Osteocytes maintain the calcified matrix and their death causes progressive resorption of adjacent matrix. While sharing most matrix-related activities with osteoblasts, osteocytes also express many different proteins, including factors with paracrine and endocrine effects that help regulate bone remodeling.

❯❯ MEDICAL APPLICATION

The extensive network of osteocyte dendritic processes and other bone cells has been called a "mechanostat," monitoring mechanical loads within bones and signaling cells to adjust ion levels and maintain the adjacent bone matrix accordingly. Resistance **exercise** can produce **increased bone density** and thickness in affected regions, while lack of exercise (or the weightlessness experienced by astronauts) leads to **decreased bone density**, due in part to the lack of mechanical stimulation of the bone cells.

FIGURE **8–5** Osteocytes in lacunae.

(a) TEM showing an osteocyte in a lacuna and two dendritic processes in canaliculi (**C**) surrounded by bony matrix. Many such processes are extended from each cell as osteoid is being secreted; this material then undergoes calcification around the processes, giving rise to canaliculi. (×30,000)

(b) Photomicrograph of bone, not decalcified or sectioned, but ground very thin to demonstrate lacunae and canaliculi. The lacunae and canaliculi (**C**) appear dark and show the communication between these structures through which nutrients derived from blood vessels diffuse and are passed from cell to cell in living bone. (×400; Ground bone)

(c) SEM of nondecalcified, sectioned, and acid-etched bone showing lacunae and canaliculi (**C**). (×400)

(Reproduced with permission from Dr Matt Allen, Indiana University School of Medicine, Indianapolis.)

Osteoclasts

Osteoclasts develop as very large, multinucleated, motile cells (Figure 8–6), essential for matrix resorption during bone growth and remodeling. The large size and multiple nuclei of osteoclasts originate as the cells form by fusion of bone marrow-derived monocytes. Osteoclast development requires two polypeptide factors produced by osteoblasts: macrophage-colony-stimulating factor (M-CSF; discussed with hemopoiesis, see Chapter 13) and the receptor activator of nuclear factor-κB ligand (RANKL). In areas of bone undergoing resorption, osteoclasts on the bone surface lie within enzymatically etched depressions or cavities in the matrix known as **resorption lacunae** (or **Howship lacunae**).

In an active osteoclast, the membrane domain that contacts the bone forms a circular **sealing zone** that binds the cell tightly to the bone matrix and surrounds an area of membrane with many surface projections, called the **ruffled border**. This circumferential sealing zone allows a specialized microenvironment to form between the osteoclast and the matrix in which bone resorption occurs (Figure 8–6b).

Into this subcellular pocket the osteoclast's ruffled border pumps protons to acidify and promote local dissolution of hydroxyapatite and secretes matrix metalloproteinases and other hydrolytic enzymes for the localized digestion of collagen and other matrix proteins. These activities occur with regulation by signaling factors from other nearby bone cells. Osteoblasts activated by parathyroid hormone produce M-CSF, RANKL, and other factors that play important roles controlling formation and activity of osteoclasts.

> **>> MEDICAL APPLICATION**
>
> In the genetic disease **osteopetrosis**, characterized by dense, heavy bones ("marble bones"), the osteoclasts lack ruffled borders and bone resorption is defective. This disorder results in overgrowth and thickening of bones, often with obliteration of the marrow cavities, depressing blood cell formation and causing anemia and the loss of white blood cells. The defective osteoclasts in most patients with osteopetrosis have mutations in genes for the cells' proton-ATPase pumps or chloride channels.

❯ BONE MATRIX

Inorganic materials make up about 50% of the dry weight of bone matrix, with calcium hydroxyapatite most abundant, but bicarbonate, citrate, magnesium, potassium, and sodium ions also found. Significant quantities of noncrystalline calcium phosphate also occur in bone. Water binding the surface of hydroxyapatite crystals facilitates exchange of ions between the mineral and body fluids.

Type I collagen comprises 90% of the organic matter embedded in the calcified matrix,, which also includes small proteoglycans and multiadhesive glycoproteins such as

osteonectin. Calcium-binding proteins, notably osteocalcin, and the phosphatases released from cells in matrix vesicles promote calcification of the matrix. Other tissues rich in type I collagen lack osteocalcin and matrix vesicles and therefore do not normally become calcified.

The association of minerals with collagen fibers during calcification provides the hardness and resistance required for bone function. Following a bone's decalcification by a histologist, its shape is preserved but it becomes soft and pliable like other connective tissues. Because of its high-collagen content, decalcified bone matrix usually appears acidophilic.

❯ PERIOSTEUM & ENDOSTEUM

External and internal surfaces of all bones display connective tissue layers of the periosteum and endosteum, respectively (Figures 8–1a and 8–1c). The **periosteum** resembles the perichondrium of cartilage, with an outer fibrous layer of dense connective tissue containing mostly bundled type I collagen, along with fibroblasts and blood vessels. Bundles of periosteal collagen, called **perforating** (or **Sharpey) fibers**, become embedded in bone matrix and bind the periosteum to the bone. Branches of periosteal blood vessels occupy perforating canals also surrounded by matrix and carry metabolites to and from deeper regions of the bone (Figures 8–1a).

The periosteum's more highly cellular inner layer includes osteoblasts, bone lining cells, and mesenchymal stem cells referred to as **osteoprogenitor cells**. With the potential to proliferate extensively and produce many new osteoblasts, osteoprogenitor cells play a prominent role in bone growth and repair.

Internally, the very thin **endosteum** covers small spicules or **trabeculae** of bony matrix that project into the marrow cavities (Figure 8–1). The endosteum also contains osteoprogenitor cells, osteoblasts, and bone lining cells, but within a sparse, delicate matrix of collagen fibers.

> **>> MEDICAL APPLICATION**
>
> **Osteoporosis**, frequently found in immobilized patients and in postmenopausal women, results from an imbalance in skeletal turnover so that bone resorption exceeds bone formation. This leads to calcium loss from bones and reduced **bone mineral density** (BMD). Individuals at risk for osteoporosis are routinely tested for BMD by **dual-energy x-ray absorptiometry** (DEXA scans).

❯ TYPES OF BONE

Gross observation of a bone in cross section (Figure 8–7) shows a dense area near the surface corresponding to **compact (cortical) bone**, which represents 80% of the total bone mass, and deeper areas with numerous interconnecting cavities, called **cancellous** (aka trabecular or spongy) **bone**,

FIGURE **8–6**   Osteoclasts and their activity.

Osteoclasts represent large multinucleated cells derived by the fusion in bone of several blood-derived monocytes.

(a) Photo of bone showing two osteoclasts (**Ocl**) digesting and resorbing bone matrix (**B**) in relatively large resorption cavities (or Howship lacunae) on the matrix surface. An osteocyte (**Oc**) in its smaller lacuna is also shown. (×400; H&E)

(b) Diagram of an osteoclast, including its circumferential **sealing zone** where integrins tightly bind the cell to the bone matrix. The sealing zone surrounds a **ruffled border** of microvilli and other cytoplasmic projections close to this matrix. The sealed space between the cell and the matrix is acidified to ~pH 4.5 by proton pumps in the ruffled part of the cell membrane and receives secreted matrix metalloproteases and other hydrolytic enzymes. Acidification of the sealed space promotes dissolution of hydroxyapatite from bone and stimulates activity of the protein hydrolases, producing localized matrix resorption. The breakdown products of collagen fibers and other polypeptides undergo endocytosis by osteoclasts and degradation in lysosomes, while Ca^{2+} and other ions are released directly and taken up by the blood.

(c) SEM of a single osteoclast after a few hours culture on a flat substrate of bone. A trench forms on the bone surface by the slowly migrating osteoclast. (×5000)

(Figure 8–6c, reproduced with permission from Alan Boyde, Institute of Dentistry, Queen Mary, University of London.)

FIGURE **8–7** Compact and cancellous bone.

Compact bone

Cancellous bone

Macroscopic photo of a thick section of bone showing the cortical **compact bone** and the lattice of trabeculae in **cancellous bone** at the bone's interior. The small trabeculae that make up highly porous cancellous bone serve as supportive struts, collectively providing considerable strength, without greatly increasing the bone's weight. The compact bone is normally covered externally with periosteum and all trabecular surfaces of the cancellous bone are covered with endosteum. (×10)

At the microscopic level, both compact and cancellous bones typically show two types of organization: mature **lamellar bone**, with matrix existing as discrete sheets, and **woven bone**, newly formed with randomly arranged components.

Lamellar Bone

Most bone in adults, compact or cancellous, is organized as **lamellar bone**, characterized by multiple layers or **lamellae** of calcified matrix 3–7 μm thick, separating lacunae with osteocytes. In cancellous bone, lamellae give rise to projecting spicules or trabeculae. Compact bone has the lamellae organized as parallel sheets or concentrically around a central canal. In each lamella, type I collagen fibers lie in parallel, with the pitch of the fibers' orientation shifted orthogonally (by about 90 degrees) in successive lamellae (Figure 8–1a). This highly ordered organization of collagen within lamellar bone causes birefringence with polarizing light microscopy, the alternating bright and dark layers caused by the changing orientation of collagen fibers in the lamellae (Figure 8–8). Like the orientation of wood fibers in plywood, the highly ordered, alternating organization of collagen fibers in lamellae adds greatly to the strength of lamellar bone.

An **osteon** (or **Haversian system**) refers to the complex of concentric lamellae, typically 100–250 μm in diameter, surrounding a **central canal** that contains small blood vessels, nerves and endosteum (Figures 8–1 and 8–9). Between successive lamellae are lacunae, each containing one osteocyte but all interconnected by the canaliculi with the cells' dendritic processes (Figure 8–9). Processes of adjacent cells contact one another via gap junctions, and all cells of an osteon receive nutrients and oxygen from the vessels in the central canal (Figure 8–1). The outer boundary of each osteon is a layer called the cement line that includes many more noncollagen proteins in addition to mineralized collagen.

Osteons represent long, sometimes bifurcated, cylinders generally parallel to the long axis of the diaphysis, each having 5–20 concentric lamellae around a **central canal** containing small blood vessels. These vessels have continuity with those in adjacent osteons, in the marrow cavity and in the periosteum via transverse **perforating canals** (or **Volkmann canals**), which lack concentric lamellae (Figures 8–1 and 8–10).

constituting about 20% of total bone mass. Table 8–1 summarizes the histological features and important locations of the major types of bone.

In long bones, the bulbous ends or **epiphyses** (Gr. *epiphysis*, an excrescence) develop as cancellous bone with a sponge-like appearance covered by a thin layer of compact cortical bone. Dense compact bone makes up almost all of the long bone's cylindrical part, the **diaphysis** (Gr. *diaphysis*, a growing between), with a thin region of **trabecular** cancellous bone on the inner surface around the central **marrow cavity** (Figure 8–1). Short bones such as those of the wrist and ankle usually have cores of cancellous bone surrounded completely by compact bone. The flat bones that form the calvaria (skullcap) have two layers of compact bone called **plates**, separated by a thicker layer of cancellous bone called the **diploë**.

TABLE **8–1** Summary of bone types and their organization.

Type of Bone	Histological Features	Major Locations	Synonyms
Woven bone, newly calcified	Irregular and random arrangement of cells and collagen; lightly calcified	Developing and growing bones; hard callus of bone fractures	Immature bone; primary bone; bundle bone
Lamellar bone, remodeled from woven bone	Parallel bundles of collagen in thin layers (lamellae), with regularly spaced cells between; heavily calcified	All normal regions of adult bone	Mature bone; secondary bone
Compact bone, ~80% of all lamellar bone	Parallel lamellae or densely packed osteons, with interstitial lamellae	Thick, outer region (beneath periosteum) of bones	Cortical bone
Cancellous bone, ~20% of all lamellar bone	Interconnected thin spicules or trabeculae covered by endosteum	Inner region of bones, adjacent to marrow cavities	Spongy bone; trabecular bone; medullary bone

FIGURE **8–8** Lamellar bone.

Two photographs of the same area of an unstained section of compact bone, showing osteons with concentric lamellae around central canals. Lamellae separated by numerous small, dark lacunae are seen only faintly by bright-field microscopy **(a)**, but they appear as alternating bright and dark bands under the polarizing light microscope **(b)**.

Bright bands are due to birefringence from the highly ordered collagen fibers in a lamella. Alternating bright and dark bands indicate that fibers in successive lamellae have different orientations, an organization that makes lamellar bone very strong. (Both ×100)

(Reproduced with permission from Dr Matt Allen, Indiana University School of Medicine, Indianapolis.)

FIGURE **8–9** An osteon.

Osteons (Haversian systems) constitute most of the compact bone. Shown here is an osteon with four to five concentric lamellae (**L**) surrounding the central canal (**CC**). Osteocytes (**O**) in lacunae communicate with each other and with the central canal and periphery of the osteon through hundreds of dendritic processes located within fine canaliculi (**C**). Compare this with the diagrams in Figure 8–1a, b.

Also shown are the partial, interstitial lamellae (**I**) of an osteon that was eroded when the intact osteon was formed. (Ground bone; ×500)

Central osteon canals and perforating canals arise during remodeling of older compact bone or woven bone.

Scattered among the intact osteons are numerous irregularly shaped groups of parallel lamellae called **interstitial lamellae**, which represent the remains of osteons partially destroyed by osteoclasts during growth and remodeling of bone (Figure 8–10).

Compact bone (eg, in the diaphysis of long bones) also includes parallel lamellae organized as multiple **external circumferential lamellae** immediately beneath the periosteum and fewer **inner circumferential lamellae** around the marrow cavity (Figure 8–1a). The lamellae of these outer and innermost areas of compact bone enclose and strengthen the region between them which contains the vascularized osteons.

Bone remodeling occurs continuously throughout life. In compact bone, remodeling resorbs parts of old osteons and produces new ones. As shown in Figure 8–11, osteoclasts remove old bone and form small, tunnel-like cavities. Such tunnels quickly become invaded by osteoprogenitor cells from the endosteum or periosteum and by sprouting loops of capillaries. Osteoblasts

Interstitial lamellae

First-generation osteons

Second-generation osteons

Third-generation osteons

(a) Transverse perforating (Volkmann) canals (**P**) connecting adjacent osteons are shown in this micrograph of compact lamellar bone. Such canals "perforate" lamellae and provide another source of microvasculature for the central canals of osteons. Among the intact osteons are also found remnants of eroded osteons, seen as irregular interstitial lamellae (**I**). (Ground bone; ×100)

(b) Diagram showing the remodeling of compact lamellar bone with three generations of osteons and their successive

contributions to the formation of interstitial lamellae. The shading indicates that successive generations of osteons have different degrees of mineralization, with the most newly formed being the least mineralized.

Remodeling is a continuous process that involves the coordinated activity of osteoblasts and osteoclasts, with responsibility for adaptations of bone to changes in stress, especially during the body's growth.

FIGURE **8–11** Development of an osteon.

Old bone

Osteoclasts tunneling into old bone

Osteoblast

Endothelial cell

Mesenchymal cell

Growing capillary

Newly calcified bone

Osteoid

Lacunae with osteocytes

Quiescent osteoblast

Cutting cone

Reversal zone

Closing cone

Forming resorption cavity

Resorption cavity

Closing osteon

Osteon

During remodeling of compact bone, osteoclasts act as a cutting cone that tunnels into existing bone matrix. Behind the osteoclasts, a population of osteoblast progenitors enters the newly formed tunnel and lines its walls. The osteoblasts secrete osteoid in a cyclic manner, producing layers of new matrix (lamellae), and trapping some cells (future osteocytes) in lacunae. The

tunnel becomes constricted with multiple concentric layers of new matrix, and its lumen finally exists as only a narrow central canal with small blood vessels. The dashed lines in **(a)** indicate the levels of the structures shown in cross section **(b)**. The photo in **(c)** shows an X-ray image revealing the different degrees of mineralization in osteons and in interstitial lamellae (**I**).

develop, line the wall of the tunnels, and begin to secrete osteoid in a cyclic manner, gradually forming a new osteon with concentric lamellae of bone and trapped osteocytes (Figure 8–11). In healthy adults, 5%–10% of the bone turns over annually.

›› MEDICAL APPLICATION

The antibiotic **tetracycline** is a fluorescent molecule that binds newly deposited osteoid matrix during mineralization with high affinity and specifically labels new bone under the UV microscope (Figure 8–12). This discovery led to methods for measuring the rate of bone growth, an important parameter in the diagnosis of certain bone disorders. In one technique, tetracycline is administered twice to patients, with an intervening interval of 11–14 days. A bone biopsy is then performed, sectioned without decalcification, and examined. Bone formed while tetracycline was present appears as fluorescent lamellae and the distance between the labeled layers is proportional to the rate of bone appositional growth. This procedure is of diagnostic importance in such diseases as **osteomalacia**, in which mineralization is impaired, and **osteitis fibrosa cystica**, in which increased osteoclast activity results in removal of bone matrix and fibrous degeneration.

Woven Bone

Woven bone, characterized by randomly disposed (nonlamellar) calcified type I collagen fibers, represents the first bone tissue to appear in fetal development and during bone fracture repair. Usually a temporary structure, woven bone undergoes remodeling into lamellar bone, except in a very few places in the body, for example, near the sutures of the calvaria and in the insertions of some tendons.

In addition to the irregular, interwoven array of collagen fibers, woven bone typically has a lower mineral content (rendering it more easily penetrated by x-rays) and a higher proportion of osteocytes than mature lamellar bone. These features reflect the facts that immature woven bone forms more quickly but has less strength than lamellar bone.

› OSTEOGENESIS

Bone development or **osteogenesis** occurs by one of two processes:

- **Intramembranous ossification**, in which osteoblasts differentiate directly from mesenchyme and begin secreting osteoid, and

---

FIGURE 8–12   Tetracycline localization of new bone matrix.

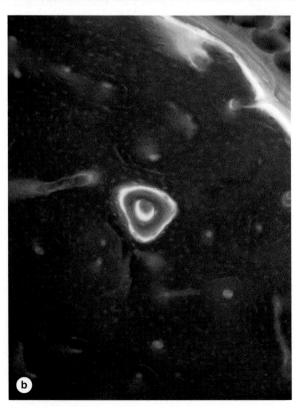

Newly formed bone binds tetracycline, which forms fluorescent complexes with calcium at ossification sites and provides an in vivo tracer by which newly formed bone can be localized. The same group of osteons after tetracycline incorporation in vivo seen first with bright-field microscopy **(a)** and then by fluorescent microscopy **(b)** reveals active ossification in one osteon (center of photo) and in the external circumferential lamellae (upper right).

(Reproduced with permission from Dr Matt Allen, Indiana University School of Medicine, Indianapolis.)

■ **Endochondral ossification**, in which a preexisting matrix of *hyaline cartilage* becomes eroded and invaded by osteoblasts, which then begin osteoid production.

The names refer to the mechanisms by which the bone forms initially; both processes involve initial production of woven bone and its gradual replacement by stronger lamellar bone. During growth of all bones, areas of woven bone, areas of bone resorption, and areas of lamellar bone all exist contiguous to one another.

Intramembranous Ossification

Intramembranous ossification, by which most flat bones begin to form, takes place within condensed sheets ("membranes") of embryonic mesenchymal tissue. Most bones of the skull and jaws, as well as the scapula and clavicle, develop by intramembranous ossification.

Within the condensed mesenchyme, bone formation begins in **ossification centers**, areas in which osteoprogenitor cells arise, proliferate, and form incomplete layers of osteoblasts around a network of developing capillaries. Osteoid secreted by the osteoblasts calcifies as described earlier, forming small irregular areas of woven bone with osteocytes in lacunae and canaliculi (Figure 8–13). Continued matrix secretion and calcification enlarges these areas and leads to the fusion of neighboring ossification centers. The anatomical bone forms gradually during replacement of the woven bone by compact bone enclosing a region of cancellous bone with marrow and larger blood vessels. Regions of the condensed mesenchyme that do not undergo ossification give rise to the endosteum and the periosteum of the new bone.

In cranial flat bones, lamellar bone formation predominates over bone resorption at both the internal and external surfaces. Internal and external plates of compact bone arise, while the central portion (diploë) maintains its cancellous nature. The fontanelles or "soft spots" on the heads of newborn infants represent areas of the skull in which the membranous tissue has not yet ossified.

Endochondral Ossification

Endochondral (Gr. *endon*, within + *chondros*, cartilage) ossification takes place within hyaline cartilage, shaped as a small, initial version, or model, of the developing bone. This type of ossification forms most bones of the body, being especially well studied in long bone formation, where it consists of the sequence of events shown in Figure 8–14.

FIGURE 8–13 Intramembranous ossification.

Two sections of fetal pig mandible developing by intramembranous ossification.

(a) Areas of typical mesenchyme (**M**) and condensed mesenchyme (**CM**) lie adjacent to layers of new osteoblasts (**O**). Some osteoblasts have secreted matrices of bone (**B**), the surfaces of which remain covered by osteoblasts. Between these thin regions of new woven bone are areas with small blood vessels (**V**). (×40; H&E)

(b) At higher magnification, another section shows these same structures, but also includes the developing periosteum (**P**) adjacent to the masses of woven bone that will soon merge to form a continuous plate of bone. The larger mesenchyme-filled region at the top is part of the developing marrow cavity. Osteocytes in lacunae can be seen within the bony matrix. (×100; H&E)

FIGURE **8–14** Osteogenesis of long bones by endochondral ossification.

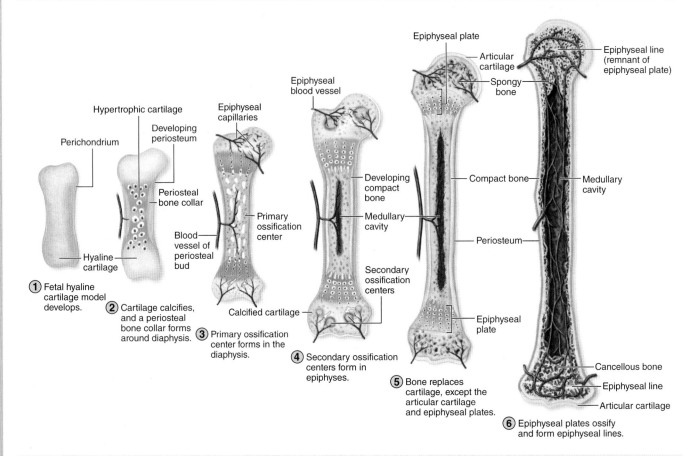

Perichondrium

Hypertrophic cartilage

Developing periosteum

Periosteal bone collar

Hyaline cartilage

Blood vessel of periosteal bud

Epiphyseal capillaries

Primary ossification center

Calcified cartilage

Epiphyseal blood vessel

Developing compact bone

Medullary cavity

Secondary ossification centers

Epiphyseal plate

Articular cartilage

Spongy bone

Compact bone

Periosteum

Epiphyseal plate

Epiphyseal line (remnant of epiphyseal plate)

Medullary cavity

Cancellous bone

Epiphyseal line

Articular cartilage

① Fetal hyaline cartilage model develops.

② Cartilage calcifies, and a periosteal bone collar forms around diaphysis.

③ Primary ossification center forms in the diaphysis.

④ Secondary ossification centers form in epiphyses.

⑤ Bone replaces cartilage, except the articular cartilage and epiphyseal plates.

⑥ Epiphyseal plates ossify and form epiphyseal lines.

This process, by which most bones form initially, begins with embryonic models of the skeletal elements made of hyaline cartilage (**1**).

Late in the first trimester, a bone collar develops beneath the perichondrium around the middle of the cartilage model, causing chondrocyte hypertrophy in the underlying cartilage (**2**).

This is followed by invasion of that cartilage by capillaries and osteoprogenitor cells from what is now the periosteum to produce a **primary ossification center** in the diaphysis (**3**).

Here osteoid deposited by the new osteoblasts, undergoes calcification into woven bone and then remodeling as compact bone. (**4**) Around the time of birth **secondary ossification centers** begin to develop by a similar process in the bone's epiphyses.

During childhood, the primary and secondary ossification centers gradually come to be separated only by the **epiphyseal plate** (**5**) that provides for continued bone elongation.

The two ossification centers do not merge until the epiphyseal plate disappears (**6**) when full stature is achieved.

In this process, ossification first occurs within a **bone collar** produced by osteoblasts that differentiate within the perichondrium (transitioning to periosteum) around the cartilage model diaphysis. The bone collar impedes diffusion of oxygen and nutrients into the underlying cartilage, causing many local chondrocytes to swell up (hypertrophy), compress the surrounding matrix, and initiate its calcification by releasing osteocalcin and alkaline phosphatase. The hypertrophic chondrocytes undergo apoptosis, creating empty spaces within the calcified matrix, while other chondrocytes may transdifferentiate as osteoprogenitor cells. One or more blood vessels from the perichondrium (now the periosteum) penetrate the bone collar, bringing more osteoprogenitor cells to the eroded central region. Along with the vasculature, newly formed osteoblasts move into all available spaces and produce woven bone. The remnants of calcified cartilage at this stage appear basophilic and the new bone appears more acidophilic (Figure 8–15).

This process in the diaphysis forms the **primary ossification center** (Figure 8–14), beginning in many embryonic bones as early as the first trimester. **Secondary ossification centers** appear later at the epiphyses of the cartilage model and develop in a similar manner. During their expansion and remodeling, both the primary and secondary ossification centers produce cavities that are gradually filled with bone marrow and trabeculae of cancellous bone.

FIGURE **8–15** Cells and matrices of a primary ossification center.

A small region of a primary ossification center showing key features of endochondral ossification. Compressed remnants of calcified cartilage matrix (**C**) are basophilic and devoid of chondrocytes. This material becomes enclosed by more lightly stained osteoid and woven bone (**B**) that contains osteocytes in lacunae. The new bone is produced by active osteoblasts (**O**) arranged as a layer on the remnants of old cartilage. (×200; Pararosaniline–toluidine blue)

With the primary and secondary ossification centers, two regions of cartilage remain:

- **Articular cartilage** within the joints between long bones (Figure 8–14), which normally persists through adult life, and
- The specially organized **epiphyseal cartilage** (also called the **epiphyseal plate** or growth plate), which connects each epiphysis to the diaphysis and allows longitudinal bone growth (Figure 8–14).

The epiphyseal cartilage allows growth in bone length and disappears upon completion of bone development at adulthood. Elimination of these epiphyseal plates ("epiphyseal closure") occurs at various times in different bones, being complete by about age 20 in all bones, with further growth in bone length no longer possible. In forensics or through x-ray examination of the growing skeleton, it is possible to determine the "bone age" of a young person by noting which epiphyses have completed closure.

An epiphyseal growth plate shows distinct regions of cellular activity usually described as overlapping but histologically distinct zones (Figures 8–16 and 8–17). Starting with the cartilage farthest from the ossification center in the diaphysis, these include the following:

1. The **zone of reserve** (or **resting**) **cartilage** is typical hyaline cartilage.

2. In the **proliferative zone**, the cartilage cells divide repeatedly, becoming organized into columns parallel to the long axis of the bone, then enlarge and secrete more type II collagen and proteoglycans.

3. The **zone of hypertrophy** contains swollen, terminally differentiated chondrocytes, which compress the matrix into aligned spicules and stiffen it by secretion of type X collagen. Unique to the hypertrophic chondrocytes in developing (or fractured) bone, type X collagen limits diffusion in the matrix and with growth factors promotes vascularization from the adjacent primary ossification center.

4. In the **zone of calcified cartilage**, chondrocytes about to undergo apoptosis release matrix vesicles and osteocalcin to begin matrix calcification by the formation of hydroxyapatite crystals.

5. In the **zone of ossification**, bone tissue first appears. Capillaries and osteoprogenitor cells invade the now vacant chondrocytic lacunae, many of which merge to form the initial marrow cavity. Osteoblasts settle in a layer over the spicules of calcified cartilage matrix and secrete osteoid, which becomes woven bone (Figures 8–16 and 8–17). This woven bone then undergoes remodeling as lamellar bone.

In summary, longitudinal growth of a bone occurs by cell proliferation in the epiphyseal plate cartilage. At the same time, chondrocytes in the diaphysis side of the plate undergo hypertrophy, their matrix becomes calcified, and the cells die. Osteoblasts lay down a layer of new bone on the calcified cartilage matrix. Because these two opposing events (proliferation and destruction) occur at approximately equal rates, the epiphyseal plate does not change thickness but is instead displaced away from the center of the diaphysis as the length of the bone increases.

Growth in the circumference of long bones does not involve endochondral ossification but occurs through the activity of osteoblasts developing from osteoprogenitor cells in the periosteum by a process of **appositional growth**, which begins with formation of the bone collar on the cartilaginous diaphysis. As shown in Figure 8–18, the increasing bone circumference is accompanied by enlargement of the central marrow cavity by the activity of osteoclasts in the endosteum.

FIGURE 8–16   Epiphyseal growth plate: Locations and zones of activity.

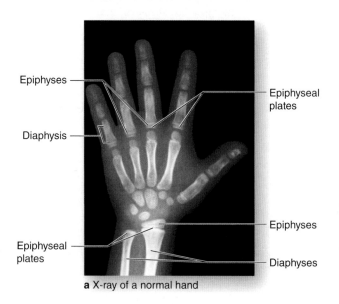

a X-ray of a normal hand

1. Zone of reserve cartilage

2. Zone of proliferation

3. Zone of hypertrophy

4. Zone of calcified cartilage

5. Zone of ossification

b Epiphyseal plate

The large and growing primary ossification center in long bone diaphyses and the secondary ossification centers in epiphyses are separated in each developing bone by a plate of cartilage called the **epiphyseal plate**.

(a) Epiphyseal plates can be identified in an x-ray of a child's hand as marrow regions of lower density between the denser ossification centers. Cells in epiphyseal growth plates are responsible for continued elongation of bones until the body's full size is reached. Developmental activities in the epiphyseal growth plate occur in overlapping zones with distinct histological appearances.

(b) From the epiphysis to the diaphysis, five general zones have cells specialized for the following: (**1**) a reserve of normal hyaline cartilage, (**2**) cartilage with proliferating chondroblasts aligned as axial aggregates in lacunae, (**3**) cartilage in which the aligned cells are hypertrophic and the matrix condensed, (**4**) an area in which the chondrocytes have disappeared and the matrix is undergoing calcification, and (**5**) an ossification zone in which blood vessels and osteoblasts invade the lacunae of the old cartilage, producing marrow cavities and osteoid for new bone. (×100; H&E)

❯❯ MEDICAL APPLICATION

Calcium deficiency in children can lead to **rickets**, a disease in which the bone matrix does not calcify normally and the epiphyseal plate can become distorted by the normal strains of body weight and muscular activity. Ossification processes are consequently impeded, which causes bones to grow more slowly and often become deformed. The deficiency can be due either to insufficient calcium in the diet or a failure to produce the steroid prohormone vitamin D, which is important for the absorption of Ca^{2+} by cells of the small intestine.

In adults, calcium deficiency can give rise to **osteomalacia** (osteon + Gr. *malakia*, softness), characterized by deficient calcification of recently formed bone and partial decalcification of already calcified matrix.

❯ BONE REMODELING & REPAIR

Bone growth involves both the continuous resorption of bone tissue formed earlier and the simultaneous laying down of new bone at a rate exceeding that of bone removal. The sum of osteoblast and osteoclast activities in a growing bone constitutes osteogenesis or the process of bone modeling, which maintains each bone's general shape while increasing its mass. The rate of **bone turnover** is very active in young children, where it can be 200 times faster than that of adults. The adult skeleton is also renewed continuously in a process of **bone remodeling** that involves the coordinated, localized cellular activities for bone resorption and bone formation shown in the diagram of Figure 8–11.

The constant remodeling of bone ensures that, despite its hardness, this tissue remains plastic and capable of adapting its internal structure in the face of changing stresses. A well-known example of bone plasticity is the ability of the positions of teeth in the jawbone to be modified by the lateral pressures produced by orthodontic appliances. Bone forms on the side of the tooth where traction is applied and is resorbed on the opposite side where pressure is exerted. In this way, teeth move within the jaw while the bone undergoes remodeling.

Because it contains osteoprogenitor stem cells in the periosteum, endosteum, and marrow and is well vascularized, bone normally has an excellent capacity for repair. **Bone repair** after a fracture or other damage uses cells, signaling molecules, and processes already active in bone remodeling. Surgically created gaps in bone become filled with new bone, especially when periosteum remains in place. The major

FIGURE **8–17** Details of the epiphyseal growth plate.

(a) At the top of the micrograph, the growth plate (**GP**) shows its zones of hyaline cartilage with chondrocytes at re©(**R**), proliferating (**P**), and hypertrophying (**H**). As the chondrocytes swell, they release alkaline phosphatase and type X collagen, which initiates hydroxyapatite formation and strengthens the adjacent calcifying spicules (**C**) of old cartilage matrix. The tunnel-like lacunae in which the chondrocytes have undergone apoptosis are invaded from the diaphysis by capillaries that begin to convert these spaces into marrow (**M**) cavities. Endosteum with osteoblasts also moves in from the diaphyseal primary ossification center, covering the spicules of calcified cartilage and laying down layers of osteoid to form a matrix of woven bone (**B**). (×40; H&E)

(b) Higher magnification of the upper left region shows more detail of the cells and matrix spicules in the zones undergoing hypertrophy (**H**) and ossification. Staining properties of the matrix clearly change as it is compressed and begins to calcify (**C**), and when osteoid and bone (**B**) are laid down.

The large spaces between the ossifying matrix spicules become the marrow cavity (**M**), in which pooled masses of eosinophilic red blood cells and aggregates of basophilic white blood cell precursors can be distinguished. Still difficult to see at this magnification is the thin endosteum between the calcifying matrices and the marrow. (×100; H&E)

phases that occur typically during bone fracture repair include initial formation of fibrocartilage and its replacement with a temporary **callus** of woven bone, as shown in Figure 8–19.

❯❯ MEDICAL APPLICATION

Bone fractures are repaired by a developmental process involving fibrocartilage formation and osteogenic activity of the major bone cells (Figure 8–19). Bone fractures disrupt blood vessels, causing bone cells near the break to die. The damaged blood vessels produce a localized hemorrhage or hematoma. Clotted blood is removed along with tissue debris by macrophages and the matrix of damaged, cell-free bone is resorbed by osteoclasts.

The periosteum and the endosteum at the fracture site respond with intense proliferation and produce a soft callus of fibrocartilage-like tissue that surrounds the fracture and covers the extremities of the fractured bone.

The fibrocartilaginous callus is gradually replaced in a process that resembles a combination of endochondral and intramembranous ossification. This produces a hard callus of woven bone around the fractured ends of bone.

Stresses imposed on the bone during repair and during the patient's gradual return to activity serve to remodel the bone callus. The immature, woven bone of the callus is gradually resorbed and replaced by lamellar bone, remodeling and restoring the original bone structure.

FIGURE **8–18** Appositional bone growth.

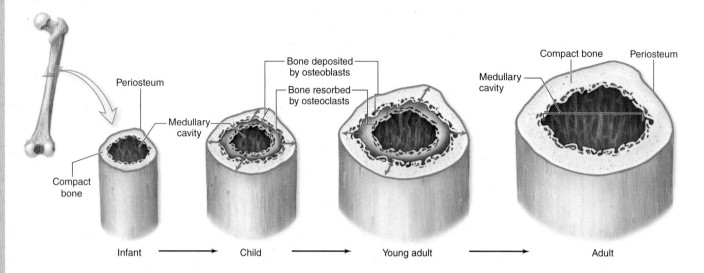

Infant → Child → Young adult → Adult

Bones increase in diameter as new bone tissue is added beneath the periosteum in a process of appositional growth. Also called radial bone growth, such growth in long bones begins with formation of the bone collar early in endochondral ossification. During radial bone growth, formation of new bone at the periosteal surface occurs concurrently with bone removal at the endosteal surface around the large medullary, enlarging this marrow-filled region and not greatly increasing the bone's weight.

❯ METABOLIC ROLE OF BONE

Calcium ions are required for the activity of many enzymes and many proteins mediating cell adhesion, cytoskeletal movements, exocytosis, membrane permeability, and other cellular functions. The skeleton serves as the calcium reservoir, containing 99% of the body's total calcium in hydroxyapatite crystals. The concentration of calcium in the blood (9–10 mg/dL) and tissues remains quite stable generally because of continuous interchange between blood calcium and bone calcium.

The principal mechanism for raising blood calcium levels involves mobilization of ions from hydroxyapatite to

FIGURE **8–19** Main features of bone fracture repair.

(1) A fracture hematoma forms.   **(2)** A fibrocartilaginous (soft) callus forms.   **(3)** A hard (bony) callus forms.   **(4)** The bone is remodeled.

Repair of a fractured bone occurs through several stages but utilizes the cells and mechanisms already in place for bone growth and remodeling. **(1)** Blood vessels torn within the fracture release blood that clots to produce a large fracture hematoma. **(2)** This is gradually removed by macrophages and replaced by a soft fibrocartilage-like mass called procallus tissue. If torn by the break, the periosteum reestablishes its continuity over this tissue. **(3)** The procallus is invaded by regenerating blood vessels and proliferating osteoblasts. In the next few weeks, the fibrocartilage undergoes gradual replacement by woven bone, forming a hard callus throughout the original area of fracture. **(4)** The woven bone is then remodeled as compact and cancellous bone in continuity with the adjacent uninjured areas and fully functional vasculature is reestablished.

interstitial fluid, primarily in cancellous bone. Ca^{2+} mobilization is regulated mainly by paracrine interactions among bone cells, many not well understood, but two polypeptide hormones also target bone cells to influence calcium homeostasis:

- **Parathyroid hormone (PTH)** from the parathyroid glands raises low blood calcium levels by stimulating osteoclasts and osteocytes to resorb bone matrix and release Ca^{2+}. The PTH acts indirectly on osteoclasts; PTH receptors occur on *osteoblasts*, which respond by secreting RANKL and other paracrine factors stimulating osteoclast formation and activity.
- **Calcitonin**, produced within the thyroid gland, can reduce elevated blood calcium levels by opposing the effects of PTH in bone. This hormone directly targets osteoclasts to slow matrix resorption and bone turnover.

>> **MEDICAL APPLICATION**

In addition to PTH and calcitonin, several other hormones act on bone. The anterior lobe of the pituitary synthesizes growth hormone (GH or somatotropin), which stimulates the liver to produce insulin-like growth factor-1 (IGF-1 or somatomedin). IGF has an overall growth-promoting effect, especially on the epiphyseal cartilage. Consequently, lack of growth hormone during the growing years causes **pituitary dwarfism**; an excess of growth hormone causes excessive growth of the long bones, resulting in **gigantism**. Adult bones cannot increase in length even with excess IGF because they lack epiphyseal cartilage, but they do increase in width by periosteal growth. In adults, an increase in GH causes **acromegaly**, a disease in which the bones—mainly the long ones—become very thick.

>> **MEDICAL APPLICATION**

In **rheumatoid arthritis**, chronic inflammation of the synovial membrane causes thickening of this connective tissue and stimulates the macrophages to release collagenases and other hydrolytic enzymes. Such enzymes eventually cause destruction of the articular cartilage, allowing direct contact of the bones projecting into the joint.

> ## JOINTS

Joints represent skeletal regions where adjacent bones become capped and firmly held together by other connective tissues. The type of joint determines the degree of movement between the bones. Joints classified as **synarthroses** (Gr. *syn*, together + *arthrosis*, articulation) allow very limited or no movement and occur as either fibrous and cartilaginous joints, depending on the type of tissue joining the bones. Major subtypes of synarthroses include the following:

- **Synostoses** involve bones linked to other bones and allow essentially no movement. In older adults, synostoses unite the skull bones, which in children and young

adults are held together by **sutures**, or thin layers of dense connective tissue with osteogenic cells.

- **Syndesmoses** join bones by dense connective tissue only. Examples include the interosseous ligament of the inferior tibiofibular joint and the posterior region of the sacroiliac joints.
- **Symphyses** have a thick pad of fibrocartilage between the thin articular cartilage covering the ends of the bones. All symphyses, such as the intervertebral discs and pubic symphysis, occur in the midline of the body.

Intervertebral discs (Figure 8–20) develop as large symphyses between the articular surfaces of successive bony

FIGURE **8–20** Intervertebral disc.

Section of a rat tail showing an intervertebral disc and the two adjacent vertebrae with bone marrow (**BM**) cavities. The disc consists of concentric layers of fibrocartilage, comprising the annulus fibrosus (**AF**), which surrounds the nucleus pulposus (**NP**). The nucleus pulposus contains scattered residual cells of the embryonic notochord embedded in abundant gel-like matrix. The intervertebral discs function primarily as shock absorbers within the spinal column and allow greater mobility within the spinal column. (×40; PSH)

vertebral bodies. Held in place by ligaments these discoid components of the intervertebral joints cushion the bones and facilitate limited movements of the vertebral column. Each disc has an outer portion, the **annulus fibrosus**, consisting of concentric fibrocartilage laminae in which fibroblasts produce orthogonally arranged collagen bundles in adjacent layers. The multiple lamellae of fibrocartilage make up a disc with unusual toughness able to withstand pressures and torsion generated within the vertebral column.

Situated in the center of the annulus fibrosus, a gel-like body called the **nucleus pulposus** allows each disc to function also as a shock absorber (Figure 8–20). The nucleus pulposus consists of a viscous fluid matrix rich in hyaluronan and type II collagen fibers, but also contains scattered, vacuolated cells derived from the embryonic notochord, the only cells of that structure to persist postnatally. Relatively large in children, each nucleus pulposus gradually becomes smaller with age, undergoing partial replacement by fibrocartilage.

Joints classified as **diarthroses** permit free bone movement. Diarthroses (Figure 8–21), such as the elbow and the knee, generally unite long bones and allow great mobility. In a

---

FIGURE 8–21   **Diarthroses or synovial joints.**

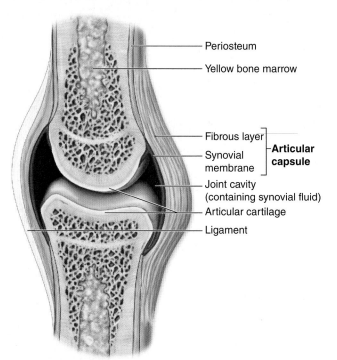

Periosteum
Yellow bone marrow

Fibrous layer ⎤
Synovial membrane ⎦ **Articular capsule**
Joint cavity (containing synovial fluid)
Articular cartilage
Ligament

a Typical synovial joint

b

Diarthroses are joints that allow free movement of the attached bones, such as knuckles, knees, and elbows.

(a) Diagram showing major components of a diarthrosis, including the **articular capsule** continuous with a ligament inserting into the periosteum of both bones; the **joint cavity** containing synovial fluid lubricant; and the ends of epiphyses covered by **articular cartilage**. The **synovial membrane** lines the capsule and produces the synovial fluid.

(b) Longitudinal section through a diarthrosis with the growing bones of a mouse knee, showing the position near the boundaries of the capsule (**C**) of the epiphyseal growth plate (**E**) where endochondral ossification occurs. Also shown are the articular cartilage (**A**) and the folds of synovial membrane (**SM**), which extend prominently into the joint cavity from connective tissue of the capsule for production of synovial fluid. (×10; PSH stain)

FIGURE **8–22** **Synovial membrane.**

The synovial membrane represents a specialized connective tissue lining capsules of synovial joints and contacting the synovial fluid lubricant, which it produces and maintains primarily.

(a) The synovial membrane projects folds into the joint cavity (**JC**) and these contain many small blood vessels (**V**). The joint cavity surrounds the articular cartilage (**AC**). (×100; Mallory trichrome)

(b) Higher magnification of the fold showing a high density of capillaries and two specialized types of cells called **synoviocytes**. Contacting the synovial fluid at the tissue surface are many rounded **macrophage-like synovial cells (type A)** derived from blood monocytes. These cells bind, engulf, and remove tissue debris from synovial fluid. These cells often form a layer at the

tissue surface (**A**) and can superficially resemble an epithelium, but there is no basal lamina and the cells are not joined together by cell junctions. **Fibroblast-like (type B) synovial cells** (**B**) represent mesenchymally derived cells specialized for synthesis of hyaluronan entering the synovial fluid, replenishing it. (×400)

(c) Schematic representation of synovial membrane histology. Among the macrophage-like and fibroblast-like synovial cells are collagen fibers and other typical components of connective tissue. Surface cells have no basement membrane or junctional complexes denoting an epithelium, despite the superficial resemblance. Blood capillaries are fenestrated, which facilitates exchange of substances between blood and synovial fluid.

---

diarthrosis, ligaments and a capsule of dense connective tissue maintain proper alignment of the bones. The capsule encloses a sealed **joint cavity** containing a clear, viscous liquid called **synovial fluid**. The joint cavity is lined, not by epithelium, but by a specialized connective tissue called the **synovial membrane** that extends folds and villi into the joint cavity and produces the lubricant synovial fluid.

In different diarthrotic joints, the synovial membrane may have prominent regions with dense connective tissue or fat. The superficial regions of this tissue however are usually well vascularized, with many porous (fenestrated) capillaries. Besides having cells typical of connective tissue proper and a changing population of leukocytes, this area of a synovial membrane also maintains two specialized cells with distinctly different functions and origins (Figure 8–22):

▪ **Macrophage-like synovial cells**, also called **type A cells**, develop from blood monocytes and remove wear-and-tear debris from the synovial fluid. These modified

macrophages, representing approximately 25% of the cells lining the synovial membrane, have great importance in regulating inflammatory events within diarthrotic joints.

▪ **Fibroblastic synovial cells**, or **type B cells**, produce abundant hyaluronan and smaller amounts of proteoglycans. This material enters the joint cavity with water from the membrane's capillaries to form the synovial fluid, which lubricates the joint, reducing friction on all internal surfaces, and supplies nutrients and oxygen to the articular cartilage.

The collagen fibers of the hyaline articular cartilage have an arched disposition with their tops near the exposed surface which, unlike most hyaline cartilage, also lacks a covering perichondrium (Figure 8–23). This arrangement of collagen helps distribute more evenly the forces generated by pressure on joints. The resilient articular cartilage efficiently absorbs the intermittent mechanical pressures occurring in many joints.

FIGURE 8–23   Articular cartilage.

(a) Articular surfaces of a diarthrosis consists of hyaline cartilage that lacks the usual perichondrium covering (×40; H&E).

(b) The top diagram here shows a small region of articular cartilage in which type II collagen fibers run perpendicular to the tissue surface and then bend gradually in a broad arch. The lower left diagram shows a 3D view of arched collagen fibers in articular cartilage.

Proteoglycan aggregates bound to hyaluronan fill the space among the collagen fibers and form a hydrated megacomplex that acts as a biomechanical spring. When pressure is applied, a small amount of water is forced out of the cartilage matrix into the synovial fluid. When pressure is released, water is attracted back into the interstices of the matrix. Such movements of water occur constantly with normal use of the joint and are essential for nutrition of the articular cartilage and for facilitating the interchange of O_2, CO_2, and metabolites between synovial fluid and chondrocytes.

Bone   SUMMARY OF KEY POINTS

- Bone represents a type of connective tissue with a **calcified** extracellular matrix (ECM), specialized to **support** the body, **protect** many internal organs, and act as the body's **Ca^{2+} reservoir**.

Major Cells & Matrix Components of Bone

- **Osteoblasts** differentiate from (stem) osteoprogenitor cells and secrete components of the initial matrix, called **osteoid**, that allow matrix mineralization to occur.
- Important components of osteoid include type I collagen, the protein **osteocalcin**, which binds Ca^{2+} and **matrix vesicles** with enzymes generating PO_4^-.
- High concentrations of Ca^{2+} and PO_4^- ions cause formation of **hydroxyapatite** crystals, whose growth gradually calcifies the entire matrix.
- **Osteocytes** differentiate further from osteoblasts when they become enclosed within matrix **lacunae** and act to maintain the matrix and detect mechanical stresses on bone.

- Osteocytes maintain communication with adjacent cells via a network of long **dendritic processes** that extend through the matrix via narrow **canaliculi** radiating from each lacuna.
- **Osteoclasts** are very large cells, formed by fusion of several blood monocytes, which locally erode bone matrix during osteogenesis and bone remodeling.

Periosteum & Endosteum

- **Periosteum** is a layer of dense connective tissue on the outer surface of bone, bound to bone matrix by bundles of type I collagen called **perforating** (or **Sharpey**) **fibers**.
- Regions of periosteum adjacent to bone are rich in **osteoprogenitor cells** and **osteoblasts** that mediate much bone growth and remodeling.
- The **endosteum** is a thin layer of active and inactive osteoblasts, which lines all the internal surfaces within bone; osteoblasts here are also required for bone growth.

Types & Organization of Bone (Table 8–1)

- Dense bone immediately beneath the periosteum represents **compact bone**; deep to the compact bone lies **cancellous** (or spongy) **bone** consisting of bony trabeculae or spicules.
- In long bones of the limbs these two types of mature bone tissue occur in both the knobby, bulbous ends, called **epiphyses**, and in the intervening shaft or **diaphysis**.
- Immature bone, called **woven bone**, forms during osteogenesis or repair and has a calcified matrix with randomly arranged collagen fibers.
- By the action of osteoclasts and osteoblasts, woven bone undergoes rapid turnover and is remodeled into **lamellar bone** with new matrix deposited in distinct layers with parallel collagen bundles; both compact and cancellous bone is lamellar bone.
- Most lamellar bone consists of lamellae organized concentrically around small **central canals** containing blood vessels and nerves; this organization is called an **osteon or Haversian system**.
- Within each osteon, osteocytic lacunae occur between the lamellae, with **canaliculi** radiating through the lamellae, which allow all cells to communicate with the central canal.

Osteogenesis

- Bones of the skull and jaws form initially by **intramembranous ossification**, with osteoblasts differentiating directly from progenitor cells in condensed **"membranes" of mesenchyme**.
- All other bones form by **endochondral ossification**, in which osteoprogenitor cells surround and then invade hyaline **cartilage models** of the skeletal elements in the embryo.
- **Primary ossification centers** in diaphyses of fetal long bones form when chondrocytes die after enclosure of the cartilage within a collar of woven bone, creating an initial cavity that is entered by periosteal osteoblasts and vasculature.
- Later, **secondary ossification centers** develop similarly within the epiphyses, with cartilage of the **epiphyseal growth plate** between the primary and secondary ossification sites.
- The growth plates are the key to **bone elongation** during childhood and involve an interrelated series of developing zones.
- A **"resting"** or **reserve zone** of typical hyaline cartilage occurs most distally.
- In an adjacent **zone of proliferation**, chondrocytes undergo mitosis and appear stacked within elongated lacunae.
- The most mature chondrocytes in these lacunae swell up, compress the matrix, and undergo apoptosis in a **zone of hypertrophy** closer to the large primary ossification center.
- Spaces created in the matrix by these events characterize the **zone of cartilage calcification** when they are invaded by osteoblasts, osteoclasts, and vasculature from the primary center.
- In the **zone of ossification**, woven bone is laid down initially by osteoblasts and remodeled into lamellae bone.

- **Appositional bone growth** increases the circumference of a bone by osteoblast activity at the periosteum and is accompanied by enlargement of the medullary marrow cavity.

Bone Growth, Remodeling, & Repair

- **Growth** of bones occurs throughout life, with cells and matrix turning over continuously through activities of osteoblasts and osteoclasts.
- Lamellae and osteons are temporary structures, replaced and rebuilt continuously in a process of **bone remodeling** by which bones change size and shape according to changes in mechanical stress.
- **Bone repair** after fracture or other injury involves the activation of periosteal fibroblasts to produce an initial **soft callus of fibrocartilage-like tissue**.
- The soft callus is gradually replaced by a **hard callus of woven bone** that is soon remodeled to produce stronger lamellar bone.

Metabolic Role of Bone

- Ca^{2+}, a key ion for all cells, is **stored** in bone when dietary calcium is adequate and **mobilized** from bone when dietary calcium is deficient.
- Maintenance of proper **blood calcium levels** involves activity of all three major bone cells and is largely regulated by subtle paracrine interaction among these and other cells.
- Hormones affecting calcium deposition and removal from bone include **PTH**, which indirectly stimulates osteoclasts to elevate levels of calcium in blood, and **calcitonin**, which can inhibit osteoclast activity, lowering blood calcium levels.

Joints

- **Joints** are places where bones meet, or articulate, allowing at least the potential for bending or movement in that portion of the skeleton.
- Joints with very limited or no movement are classified collectively as **synarthroses** and freely mobile joints are called **diarthroses**.
- **Intervertebral discs** represent synarthroses in the vertebral column that cushion adjacent vertebrae.
- Each intervertebral disc consists of a thick outer layer of fibrocartilage forming a tough **annulus fibrosus** and a shock-absorbing inner, gel-like core, the **nucleus pulposus**.
- Diarthroses have a **joint cavity** filled with lubricant **synovial fluid**, enclosed within a tough, fibrous **articular capsule**; ends of the bones involved are covered with hyaline **articular cartilage**.
- Specialized connective tissue of the **synovial membrane** lines the capsule, with folds extended into some areas of the joint cavity.
- **Macrophage-like synovial cells** of the synovial membrane remove wear-and-tear debris from synovial fluid.
- **Fibroblast-like synovial cells** of the synovial membrane synthesize hyaluronan that moves into the synovial fluid with water from local capillaries to lubricate and nourish the articular cartilage.

Bone ASSESS YOUR KNOWLEDGE

1. Which component of bone impedes the distribution of nutrients and oxygen to osteocytes?
   a. ECM
   b. Canaliculi
   c. Periosteum
   d. Cell processes
   e. Haversian canals

2. Which if the following most accurately describes compact bone?
   a. Predominant bone type in the epiphyses of adult long bones
   b. Also known as cancellous bone
   c. Characterized by the presence of osteons
   d. Lines the medullary (marrow) cavity
   e. Forms the diploë in cranial bones

3. In healthy bone, canaliculi are likely to contain which one of the following?
   a. Capillaries
   b. Nerve axons
   c. Osteocytic processes
   d. Osteoid
   e. Osteoclasts in resorption lacunae

4. Which of the following most accurately describes the endosteum?
   a. Composed of two layers: osteogenic and fibrous
   b. Continuous with the joint capsule
   c. Attached to the bone surface by collagen bundles called Sharpey fibers
   d. Lines the medullary cavity
   e. Contains mature osteocytes

5. In the diaphysis of a typical long bone, which of the following structures is in closest proximity to the trabeculae of cancellous bone?
   a. Interstitial lamellae
   b. Osteons
   c. Sharpey fibers
   d. Outer circumferential lamellae
   e. Inner circumferential lamellae

6. Which "zone" of endochondral ossification in the growing femur of an adolescent is the farthest from that bone's secondary ossification center?
   a. Zone of hypertrophy
   b. Zone of reserve cartilage
   c. Zone of calcified cartilage
   d. Zone of ossification
   e. Zone of proliferation

7. The major lubricant for diarthrotic joints is synthesized by cells located in which joint structure?
   a. Nucleus pulposus
   b. Synovial membrane
   c. Articular cartilage
   d. Annulus fibrosus
   e. Fibrous capsule

8. A 25-year-old man presents with persistent joint pain and a history of recurrent fractures of each humerus. His hematocrit and complete blood count (CBC) are normal, but blood calcium levels are high. Hormone levels are all within normal ranges except PTH that exceeds normal by threefold. Which of the following could be prescribed to offset the effects of the elevated PTH?
   a. Vitamin D
   b. Vitamin C
   c. Recombinant RANK ligand
   d. Somatotrophin (growth hormone)
   e. Calcitonin

9. A 42-year-old woman, who has been a type 1 diabetic for 30 years, falls when she trips over the vacuum cleaner hose. She tried to break her fall by placing her hand out to save herself and in the process her wrist was forced backward, breaking her radius near the wrist. Which of the following is produced in the first step in healing this bone injury?
   a. Osteoid
   b. Hematoma
   c. Bony callus
   d. Fibrocartilage
   e. Compact bone

10. A 46-year-old woman presents with pain in the left leg that worsens on weight bearing. An x-ray shows demineralization, and a bone biopsy decalcified with EDTA shows reduction in bone quantity. The patient had undergone menopause at age 45 without estrogen replacement. She reports long-standing diarrhea. In addition, laboratory tests show low levels of vitamin D, calcium, and phosphorus, and elevated alkaline phosphatase. A second bone biopsy was taken but not decalcified, which showed extensive deposition of uncalcified osteoid on all the bone surfaces. On the basis of these data, the best diagnosis would be which of the following?
    a. Osteoporosis
    b. Scurvy
    c. Osteomalacia
    d. Rickets
    e. Hypoparathyroidism

CHAPTER 9

Nerve Tissue & the Nervous System

The human nervous system, by far the body's most complex system, comprises a network of many billion nerve cells (**neurons**), all supported by many more cells called **glial cells**. Each neuron has hundreds of interconnections with other neurons, forming an extremely intricate system for processing information and generating responses.

Neurons and their processes become localized throughout the body as an integrated communications network. Anatomically, the general organization of the nervous system (Figure 9–1) has two major divisions:

- **Central nervous system (CNS)**, consisting of the brain and the spinal cord
- **Peripheral nervous system (PNS)**, composed of the cranial, spinal and peripheral nerves conducting impulses to and from the CNS (sensory and motor nerves, respectively) and **ganglia** consisting of small aggregates of nerve cells outside the CNS

In both central and peripheral nerve tissue, **neurons** typically have numerous long processes for intercellular communication and the various **glial cells** (Gr. *glia*, glue) have shorter, more variable processes involved in many neural activities, neural maintenance, and defense.

Neurons respond to environmental changes (**stimuli**) by altering the ionic gradient that exists across their plasma membranes. All cells maintain such a gradient, also called an electrical potential, but cells that can rapidly change this potential in response to stimuli (eg, neurons, muscle cells, and some gland cells) are said to be **excitable** or irritable. Neurons react promptly to stimuli with a reversal of the ionic gradient (**membrane depolarization**) that generally spreads from the place that received the stimulus and propagates across the neuron's entire plasma membrane. This propagation, called the **action potential**, the **depolarization wave**, or the **nerve impulse**, can travel long distances along the neuronal processes, transmitting such signals to other neurons, muscles, and glands.

By collecting, analyzing, and integrating information in such signals, the nervous system continuously stabilizes the intrinsic conditions of the body (eg, blood pressure, O_2 and CO_2 content, pH, blood glucose levels, and hormone levels) within normal ranges and maintains behavioral patterns (eg, feeding, reproduction, defense, and interaction with other living creatures).

› DEVELOPMENT OF NERVE TISSUE

The nervous system develops from the outermost of the three early embryonic layers, the ectoderm, beginning in the third week of development (Figure 9–2). With signals from the underlying axial structure, the notochord, ectoderm on the mid-dorsal side of the embryo thickens to form the epithelial **neural plate**. The sides of this plate fold upward and grow toward each other medially, and within a few days fuse to form the **neural tube**. Cells of this tube give rise to the entire CNS, including neurons and most glial cells.

FIGURE **9–1**   **The general organization of the nervous system.**

Cerebrum
Cerebellum
Spinal cord
}   **Central nervous system (CNS)**

Cranial nerves
Spinal nerves
Ganglia
}   **Peripheral nervous system (PNS)**

Anatomically the nervous system is divided into the **CNS** and **PNS**, which have the major components shown in the diagram. Functionally the nervous system consists of the following:

1. **Sensory division (afferent)**
   A. **Somatic**—sensory input perceived consciously (eg, from eyes ears, skin, and musculoskeletal structures)
   B. **Visceral**—sensory input *not* perceived consciously (eg, from internal organs and cardiovascular structures)
2. **Motor division (efferent)**
   A. **Somatic**—motor output controlled consciously or voluntarily (eg, by skeletal muscle effectors)
   B. **Autonomic**—motor output *not* controlled consciously (eg, by heart or gland effectors)

The autonomic motor nerves, comprising what is often called the **autonomic nervous system (ANS)**, all have pathways involving two neurons: a **preganglionic neuron** with the cell body in the CNS and a **postganglionic neuron** with the cell body in a ganglion. The ANS has two divisions: (1) The **parasympathetic division**, with its ganglia within or near the effector organs, maintains normal body homeostasis. (2) The **sympathetic division** has its ganglia close to the CNS and controls the body's responses during emergencies and excitement. ANS components located in the wall of the digestive tract are sometimes referred to as the enteric nervous system.

FIGURE **9–2**   **Neurulation in the early embryo.**

Neural groove

Neural folds
Notochord

Neural crest

① Neural folds and neural groove form from the neural plate.

Neural groove

② Neural folds elevate and approach one another.

Neural groove

Ectoderm

Neural crest cells

③ As neural folds prepare to fuse and form the neural tube and dorsal epidermis, neural crest cells loosen, and become mesenchymal.

Neural tube

Neural crest cells

Developing epidermis

④ The mass of neural crest cells initially lies atop the newly formed neural tube.

Stages in the process of **neurulation**, which produces cells of the CNS and PNS, are shown in diagrammatic cross sections of a 3- and 4-week human embryo with the extraembryonic membranes removed. Under an inductive influence from the medial notochord, the overlying layer of ectodermal cells thickens as a bending **neural plate,** with a medial neural groove and lateral neural folds **(1).** All other ectoderm will become epidermis. The plate bends further, making the **neural folds** and **groove** more prominent **(2).** The neural folds rise and fuse at the midline **(3),** converting the groove into the **neural tube (4),** which is large at the cranial end of the embryo and much narrower caudally. The neural tube will give rise to the entire CNS.

As the neural tube detaches from the now overlying ectoderm, many cells separate from it and produce a mass of mesenchymal cells called the **neural crest.** Located initially above the neural tube, neural crest cells immediately begin migrating laterally. Cell derived from the neural crest will form all components of the PNS and contribute to certain non-neural tissues.

As the folds fuse and the neural tube separates from the now overlying surface ectoderm that will form epidermis, a large population of developmentally important cells, the **neural crest**, separates from the neuroepithelium and becomes mesenchymal. Neural crest cells migrate extensively and differentiate as all the cells of the PNS, as well as several other non-neuronal cell types.

❯ NEURONS

Neurons make up the functional units in both the CNS and PNS. Some neuronal components have special names, such as "neurolemma" for the cell membrane. Most neurons have three main parts (Figure 9–3):

- The **cell body** (also called the **perikaryon** or **soma**), which contains the nucleus and most of the cell's organelles and serves as the synthetic or trophic center for the entire neuron.
- The **dendrites**, numerous elongated processes extending from the perikaryon, become specialized to receive stimuli from other neurons at unique sites called **synapses**.
- The **axon** (Gr. *axon*, axis), usually a single long process ending at synapses, develops to generate and conduct nerve impulses to other cells (eg, nerve, muscle, and gland cells).

Axons may also receive information from other neurons, information that mainly modifies the transmission of action potentials to those neurons.

Neurons and their processes or "nerve fibers" show variability in both size and shape, with certain very large cell bodies measuring up to 150 μm in diameter. Other neurons, such as those in the cerebellar granular layer, are among the body's smallest cells.

Figure 9–4 depicts a structural classification of neurons utilizing the number of processes extending from the cell body:

- **Multipolar neurons**, each with one axon and two or more dendrites, occur most commonly.
- **Bipolar neurons**, with one dendrite and one axon, comprise the sensory neurons of the retina, the olfactory epithelium, and the inner ear.
- **Unipolar** or **pseudounipolar neurons**, which include all other sensory neurons, each have a single process that bifurcates close to the perikaryon, with the longer branch extending to a peripheral ending and the other toward the CNS.
- **Anaxonic neurons**, have many dendrites but no true axon and do not produce action potentials, but regulate electrical changes of adjacent CNS neurons.

Histological sections of nervous tissue seldom include all the fine processes associated with cell bodies, making it difficult to classify neurons structurally by microscopic inspection.

Figure 9–1 includes the major functional classifications of nervous components. **Sensory neurons** are **afferent**, receiving stimuli from receptors throughout the body. **Motor neurons** are **efferent**, sending impulses to effector organs such as muscle fibers and glands. **Somatic** motor nerves function under voluntary control and typically innervate skeletal muscle; **autonomic** motor nerves control the involuntary or unconscious activities of glands, cardiac muscle and most smooth muscle.

Interneurons establish relationships among other neurons, forming complex functional networks or **circuits** in the CNS. Interneurons are either multipolar or anaxonic and comprise 99% of all neurons in adults.

In the CNS most neuronal perikarya occur in the **gray matter**, with their axons concentrated in the **white matter**. These terms refer to the general appearance of unstained CNS tissue caused in part by the different densities of nerve cell bodies. In the PNS cell bodies become localized in groups called ganglia and in specific sensory regions, such as the olfactory mucosa, with their axons bundled in **nerves**.

❯❯ MEDICAL APPLICATION

Parkinson disease, a slowly progressing disorder affecting muscular activity, includes characteristic tremors, reduced activity of the facial muscles, loss of balance, and postural stiffness. It is caused by gradual loss by apoptosis of dopamine-producing neurons whose cell bodies lie within the nuclei of the CNS substantia nigra. Parkinson disease is treated with L-**dopa** (L-3,4-dihydroxyphenylalanine), a precursor of dopamine that augments the declining production of this neurotransmitter.

Cell Body (Perikaryon or Soma)

The neuronal **cell body** contains the nucleus and surrounding cytoplasm, exclusive of the cell processes (Figure 9–3). It acts as a trophic center, producing most of the cytoplasm for the processes. Most cell bodies are in contact with a great number of nerve endings conveying excitatory or inhibitory stimuli generated in other neurons. A typical neuron has an unusually large, euchromatic nucleus with a prominent nucleolus, indicating intense synthetic activity.

Cytoplasm of perikarya often includes areas with numerous free polyribosomes and highly developed RER, indicating active production of both cytoskeletal proteins and proteins for transport and secretion. Histologically, such basophilic regions comprise the neurons' **chromatophilic substance** (or **Nissl substance**, **Nissl bodies**) (Figure 9–3). The amount of this material varies with the type and functional state of the neuron, being particularly rich in large nerve cells such as motor neurons (Figure 9–3b). Golgi complexes develop only in the cell body but mitochondria occur throughout the cell, usually appearing abundantly in the axon terminals.

Both perikarya and processes have numerous microtubules, actin filaments and intermediate filaments, with the latter formed by unique protein subunits and called **neurofilaments** in this cell type. Light microscopists also often refer

FIGURE **9–3** Structures of a typical neuron.

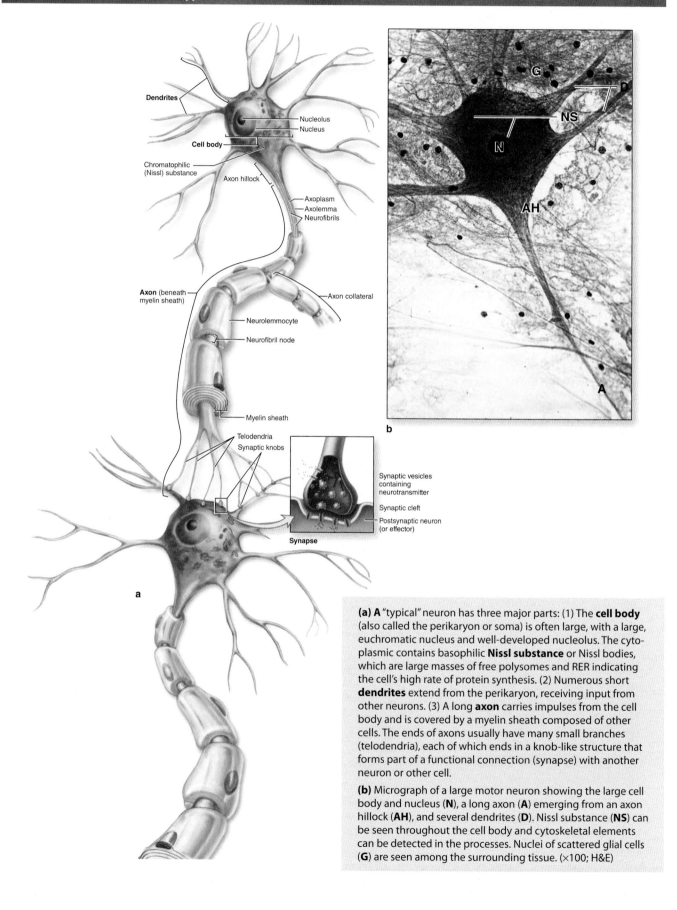

Dendrites

Nucleolus
Nucleus

Cell body

Chromatophilic
(Nissl) substance

Axon hillock

Axoplasm
Axolemma
Neurofibrils

Axon (beneath
myelin sheath)

Axon collateral

Neurolemmocyte

Neurofibril node

Myelin sheath

Telodendria
Synaptic knobs

Synaptic vesicles
containing
neurotransmitter

Synaptic cleft

Postsynaptic neuron
(or effector)

Synapse

a

b

(a) A "typical" neuron has three major parts: (1) The **cell body** (also called the perikaryon or soma) is often large, with a large, euchromatic nucleus and well-developed nucleolus. The cytoplasmic contains basophilic **Nissl substance** or Nissl bodies, which are large masses of free polysomes and RER indicating the cell's high rate of protein synthesis. (2) Numerous short **dendrites** extend from the perikaryon, receiving input from other neurons. (3) A long **axon** carries impulses from the cell body and is covered by a myelin sheath composed of other cells. The ends of axons usually have many small branches (telodendria), each of which ends in a knob-like structure that forms part of a functional connection (synapse) with another neuron or other cell.

(b) Micrograph of a large motor neuron showing the large cell body and nucleus (**N**), a long axon (**A**) emerging from an axon hillock (**AH**), and several dendrites (**D**). Nissl substance (**NS**) can be seen throughout the cell body and cytoskeletal elements can be detected in the processes. Nuclei of scattered glial cells (**G**) are seen among the surrounding tissue. (×100; H&E)

FIGURE **9–4** Structural classes of neurons.

(a) Multipolar neuron

(b) Bipolar neuron

(c) Unipolar neuron

(d) Anaxonic neuron

Neurons can be classified structurally into four main types.

(a) Most neurons, including all motor neurons and most CNS interneurons, are **multipolar**.

(b) Bipolar neurons include sensory neurons of the retina, olfactory mucosa, and inner ear.

(c) All other sensory neurons are **unipolar** or **pseudounipolar**.

(d) The **anaxonic** configuration, found only in certain CNS interneurons, lack true axons and do not produce action potentials, but regulate local electrical changes of adjacent neurons.

to the neurofilaments, cross-linked with certain fixatives and impregnated with silver stains, as neurofibrils. Some nerve cell bodies also contain inclusions of pigmented material, such as lipofuscin, consisting of residual bodies left from lysosomal digestion.

Dendrites

Dendrites (Gr. *dendron*, tree) typically comprise short, small processes emerging and branching off the soma (Figure 9–3). Usually covered with many synapses, dendrites represent the principal neuronal sites for signal reception and processing. The large number and extensive arborization of dendrites allow a single neuron to receive and integrate signals from many other nerve cells. For example, up to 200,000 axonal endings can make functional contact with the dendrites of a single large Purkinje neuron of the cerebellum.

Unlike axons, which maintain a nearly constant diameter, dendrites become much thinner as they branch, with cytoskeletal elements predominating in their distal regions. In the CNS, most synapses on dendrites occur on **dendritic spines**, dynamic membrane protrusions along the small dendritic branches, visualized with silver staining (Figure 9–5) and studied by confocal or electron microscopy. Dendritic spines serve as the initial processing sites for synaptic signals and occur in vast numbers, estimated to be on the order of 10^{11} for cells of the human cerebral cortex. Dendritic spine morphology depends on actin filaments and changes continuously as synaptic connections on neurons undergo modification. Such changes in dendritic spines are fundamentally important for the **neural plasticity** which occurs during embryonic brain development and underlies adaptation, learning, and memory postnatally.

Axons

Most neurons have only one **axon**, typically longer than its dendrites. Axonal processes vary in length and diameter according to the type of neuron. Axons of the motor neurons innervating foot muscles have lengths of nearly a meter, requiring large cell bodies to maintain these axons which contain most of such neurons' cytoplasm. The plasma membrane of the axon is often termed the **axolemma** and its cytoplasmic contents, the **axoplasm**.

Axons originate from a pyramid-shaped region of the perikaryon called the **axon hillock** (Figure 9–3), just beyond which the axolemma has concentrated ion channels that generate the action potential. At this initial segment of the axon,

FIGURE 9–5 Dendrites and dendritic spines.

The large Purkinje neuron in this silver-impregnated section of cerebellum has many dendrites (**D**) emerging from its cell body (**CB**) and forming branches. The small dendritic branches each have many tiny projecting dendritic spines (**DS**) spaced closely along their length, each of which is a site of a synapse with another neuron. Dendritic spines are highly dynamic, the number of synapses changing constantly. (×650; Silver stain)

the various excitatory and inhibitory stimuli impinging on the neuron undergo algebraic summation, resulting in the decision to propagate or not to propagate a nerve impulse.

Axons generally branch less profusely than dendrites but do undergo **terminal arborization** (Figure 9–3). Axons of interneurons and some motor neurons also have a few large branches called **collaterals** that branch further and end with synapses influencing the activity of other neurons. The tip of each small axonal branch shows a dilation called a **terminal bouton** (Fr. *bouton*, button) that contacts another neuron or non-nerve cell at the synapse to initiate an impulse in that cell.

Axoplasm contains mitochondria, microtubules, neurofilaments, and transport vesicles, but very few polyribosomes or cisternae of RER, features that emphasize the dependence of axoplasm on the perikaryon. If an axon is severed from its cell body, its distal part quickly degenerates and undergoes phagocytosis.

Lively bidirectional transport of molecules large and small occurs within axons. Organelles and macromolecules synthesized in the cell body move by **anterograde transport** along axonal microtubules via **kinesin** from the perikaryon to the synaptic terminals. **Retrograde transport** in the opposite direction along the microtubules via **dynein** carries certain other macromolecules, such as material taken up by endocytosis (including viruses and toxins), from the periphery to the cell body. Retrograde transport also permits the study of many neuronal pathways: if peroxidase or another marker is injected into regions with axon terminals, its later distribution throughout the neurons serving such regions can be determined histochemically.

Anterograde and retrograde transports both occur at rates of 50–400 mm/day. A much slower anterograde stream, advancing only a few millimeters per day, involves movement of the axonal cytoskeleton itself. This slow axonal transport corresponds roughly to the rate of axon growth.

Nerve Impulses

A **nerve impulse**, or **action potential**, travels along an axon like a spark moves along an explosive's fuse, consisting of an electrochemical process initiated at the axon hillock when other impulses received at the cell body or dendrites meet a certain threshold. The action potential propagates along the axon as a wave of membrane depolarization produced by **voltage-gated Na⁺ and K⁺ channels** in the axolemma that allow diffusion of these ions into and out of the axoplasm. Around all regions of the neuron the extracellular compartment occurs as a very thin zone formed by enclosing glial cells that also regulate its ionic contents.

In unstimulated neurons ATP-dependent Na-K pumps and other membrane proteins maintain an axoplasmic Na⁺ concentration only one-tenth of that outside the cell and a K⁺ level many times greater than the extracellular concentration. This produces a potential electrical difference across the axolemma of about –65 mV, with the inside negative to the outside. This difference represents the axon's **resting potential**.

❯❯ MEDICAL APPLICATION

Most **local anesthetics** consist of low-molecular-weight molecules that bind to the voltage-gated sodium channels of the axolemma, interfering with sodium ion influx and, consequently, inhibiting the action potential responsible for the nerve impulse.

When the threshold for triggering an impulse is met, channels at the axon's initial segment open and allow a very rapid influx of extracellular Na⁺ that makes the axoplasm positive in relation to the extracellular environment and shifts (depolarizes) the resting potential from negative to positive, to +30 mV. Immediately after the membrane depolarization, the voltage-gated Na⁺ channels close and those for K⁺ open, which rapidly returns the membrane to its resting potential. This cycle of events occurs in less than 1 millisecond.

Depolarization stimulates adjacent portions of the axolemma to depolarize and return immediately to the resting potential, causing a nerve impulse, or wave of depolarization, to move rapidly along the axon. After a refractory period, also measured in milliseconds, the neuron can repeat this process and generate another action potential. Impulses arriving at the synaptic nerve endings promote the discharge of stored neurotransmitter that stimulates or inhibits action potentials in another neuron or non-neural cell.

Synaptic Communication

Synapses (Gr. *synapsis*, union) represent sites where nerve impulses are transmitted from one neuron to another, or from neurons to other effector cells. The structure of a synapse (Figure 9–6) ensures that transmission is unidirectional. Synapses convert an electrical signal (nerve impulse) from the **presynaptic cell** into a chemical signal that affects the **postsynaptic cell**. Most synapses act by releasing **neurotransmitters**, usually small molecules that bind specific receptor proteins to either open or close ion channels or initiate second-messenger cascades. A synapse (Figure 9–6a) has the following components:

- The **presynaptic axon terminal** (or **terminal bouton**) contains mitochondria and numerous **synaptic vesicles**, which release neurotransmitters by exocytosis.

- The **postsynaptic cell membrane** contains receptors for the neurotransmitter, along with ion channels or other mechanisms to initiate a new impulse.
- A 20- to 30-nm-wide intercellular space called the **synaptic cleft** separates these presynaptic and postsynaptic membranes.

At the presynaptic region the nerve impulse briefly opens calcium channels, promoting a Ca^{2+} influx that triggers neurotransmitter release by exocytosis or similar mechanisms. Immediately, the released neurotransmitter molecules diffuse across the synaptic cleft and bind receptors at the postsynaptic region. This produces either an excitatory or an inhibitory effect at the postsynaptic membrane, as follows:

- Neurotransmitters from **excitatory synapses** cause postsynaptic Na^+ channels to open, and the resulting Na^+ influx

FIGURE 9–6 **Major components of a synapse.**

(a) Diagram showing a synapse releasing neurotransmitters by exocytosis from the terminal bouton. Presynaptic terminals always contain many **synaptic vesicles** containing neurotransmitters, numerous **mitochondria**, and smooth ER as a source of new membrane. Some neurotransmitters are synthesized in the cell body and then transported in vesicles to the presynaptic terminal. Upon arrival of a nerve impulse, voltage-regulated Ca^{2+} channels permit Ca^{2+} entry, which triggers neurotransmitter release into the synaptic cleft. Excess membrane accumulating at the presynaptic region as a result of exocytosis is recycled by clathrin-mediated endocytosis, which is not depicted here.

(b) The TEM shows a large presynaptic terminal (T_1) filled with synaptic vesicles and asymmetric electron-dense regions around 20- to 30-nm-wide synaptic clefts (**arrows**). The postsynaptic membrane contains the neurotransmitter receptors and mechanisms to initiate an impulse at the postsynaptic neuron. The postsynaptic membrane on the right is part of a dendrite (**D**), associated with fewer vesicles of any kind, showing this to be an axodendritic synapse. On the lower left is another presynaptic terminal (T_2), suggesting an axoaxonic synapse with a role in modulating activity of the other terminal. (×35,000) triggers depolarization in the postsynaptic neuron or effector cell resembling that initiated at the axon hillock.

- At **inhibitory synapses** neurotransmitters open Cl⁻ or other anion channels, causing influx of anions and **hyperpolarization** of the postsynaptic cell, making its membrane potential more negative and more resistant to depolarization.

Interplay between excitatory and inhibitory effects on postsynaptic cells allows synapses to process neuronal input and fine-tune the reaction of the effector cell. Impulses passing from presynaptic neurons to postsynaptic cells usually undergo modification at the synapse by similar connections there with other neurons (Figure 9–6b). The response in postsynaptic neurons results from the summation of activity at hundreds of synapses on that cell. Figure 9–7 depicts three common morphological types of synapses occurring between CNS neurons.

The chemical transmitter used at neuromuscular junctions and some synapses in the CNS is **acetylcholine**. Within the CNS other major categories of neurotransmitters include the following:

- Certain **amino acids** (often modified), such as glutamate and γ-aminobutyrate (GABA),
- **Monoamines**, such as serotonin (5-hydroxytryptamine or 5-HT) and **catecholamines**, such as dopamine, all of which are synthesized from amino acids, and
- Small **polypeptides**, such as endorphins and substance P.

Table 9–1 summarizes important actions of these and other common neurotransmitters. Different receptors and second messenger systems often occur for the same transmitter, greatly multiplying the possible effects of these molecules. After their release transmitters undergo quick removal by enzymatic breakdown, by glial activity, or by endocytotic recycling involving presynaptic membrane receptors.

❯❯ MEDICAL APPLICATION

Levels of neurotransmitters in the synaptic cleft and available for binding postsynaptic receptors are normally regulated by several local mechanisms. **Selective serotonin reuptake inhibitors (SSRIs)**, a widely used class of drugs for treatment of depression and anxiety disorders, were designed to augment levels of this neurotransmitter at the postsynaptic membrane of serotonergic CNS synapses by specifically inhibiting its reuptake at the presynaptic membrane.

❯ GLIAL CELLS & NEURONAL ACTIVITY

Glial cells, about 10 times more abundant than neurons in the mammalian brain, support neuronal survival and activities in many ways. Like neurons, most glial cells develop from progenitor cells of the embryonic neural plate. In the CNS glial cells surround both the neuronal cell bodies, which are often larger than the glial cells, and the processes of axons and dendrites between neurons. Except around the larger blood vessels, the CNS has only a very small amount of connective tissue and collagen. Glial cells substitute for cells of connective tissue in some respects, supporting neurons and creating immediately around those cells microenvironments optimized for neuronal activity. The fibrous intercellular network of CNS tissue may superficially resemble collagen by light microscopy, but represents the web of fine cellular processes emerging from neurons and glial cells. Collectively such intercellular processes comprise the CNS **neuropil** (Figure 9–8).

As shown schematically in Figure 9–9, six major categories of glial cells occur, four in the CNS and two in the PNS. Table 9–2 summarizes their main functions, locations, and origins.

Oligodendrocytes

Oligodendrocytes (Gr. *oligos*, small, few + *dendron*, tree + *kytos*, cell) extend many processes, each of which becomes sheetlike and wraps repeatedly around a portion of a nearby CNS axon (Figure 9–9a). During this wrapping most cytoplasm gradually moves out of the growing extension, leaving multiple compacted layers of cell membrane collectively termed as **myelin**. An axon's full length becomes covered by the action of many oligodendrocytes. The resulting **myelin sheath** electrically insulates the axon and creates the microenvironment that facilitates rapid transmission of nerve impulses. Found only in the CNS, oligodendrocytes represent the predominant glial cells in white matter, which appears white because of the lipid concentrated in the wrapped membrane sheaths. The processes and sheaths remain largely undetectable by routine light microscope staining in which oligodendrocytes usually appear as small cells with rounded, condensed nuclei and unstained cytoplasm (Figure 9–8a).

Astrocytes

Also unique to the CNS **astrocytes** (Gr. *astro-*, star + *kytos*) have numerous long radiating, branching processes (Figures 9–9a and 9–10). Proximal regions of the astrocytic processes bear reinforcing bundles of intermediate filaments made of **glial fibrillary acid protein (GFAP)**, which serves as a unique marker for this glial cell. Distally the processes lack GFAP and form a vast network of delicate terminals, not readily seen by light microscopy, contacting synapses and other structures. Terminal processes of a single astrocyte typically occupy a volume much larger than its perikaryon and associate with up to two million synaptic sites.

Astrocytes originate from progenitor cells in the embryonic neural tube and represent by far the most numerous glial cells of the brain, as well as the most diverse, structurally and functionally. **Fibrous astrocytes**, with long delicate processes, are abundant in white matter; those with many shorter processes, so-called **protoplasmic astrocytes**, predominate in the gray matter. Astrocytes communicate directly with one another via gap junctions, forming a very large cellular network for the coordinated regulation of their various activities

FIGURE **9–7** Types of synapses.

Axosomatic synapse

Axon

Cell body

Axodendritic synapse

Dendrite

Axon

Dendritic spine

Axoaxonic synapse

Axons

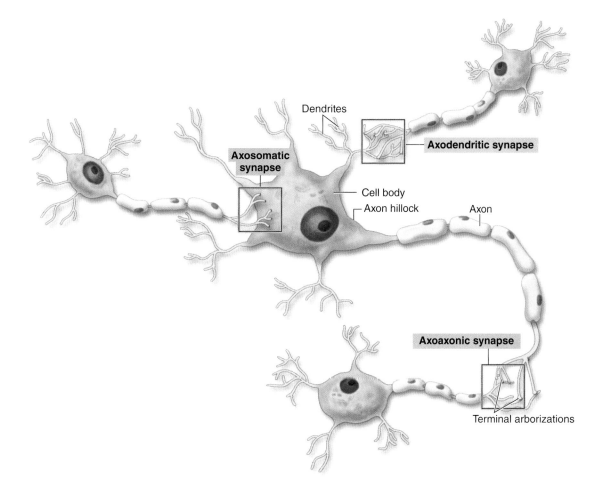

Dendrites

Axodendritic synapse

Axosomatic synapse

Cell body

Axon hillock

Axon

Axoaxonic synapse

Terminal arborizations

The diagrams show three common morphologic types of synapses. Branched axon terminals usually associate with and transmit a nerve impulse to another neuron's cell body (or soma) or a dendritic spine. These types of connections are termed an **axosomatic synapse** and an **axodendritic synapse**, respectively. Less frequently, an axon terminal forms a synapse with an axon terminal of another neuron; such an **axoaxonic synapse** functions to modulate synaptic activity in the other two types.

All three morphologic types of synapses have the features of all true synapses: a presynaptic axon terminal that releases a transmitter; a postsynaptic cell membrane with receptors for the transmitter; and an intervening synaptic cleft.

Synaptic structure usually cannot be resolved by light microscopy, although components such as dendritic spines may be shown with special techniques (Figure 9–5).

TABLE 9–1	Common neurotransmitters and their actions.
Neurotransmitter	**Description/Action**
ACETYLCHOLINE (ACh)	
$H_3C—N^+—CH_2—CH_2—O—C—CH_3$ with three CH_3 groups	Chemical structure significantly different from that of other neurotransmitters; active in CNS and in both somatic and autonomic parts of PNS; binds to ACh receptors (cholinergic receptors) in PNS to open ion channels in postsynaptic membrane and stimulate muscle contraction
AMINO ACIDS	
$NH_2—CH_2—C$ with O, OH, and R groups	Molecules with both carboxyl (—COOH) and amine (—NH$_2$) groups and various R groups; act as important transmitters in the CNS
Glutamate	Excites activity in neurons to promote cognitive function in the brain (learning and memory); most common neurotransmitter in the brain; opens Na$^+$ channels
Gamma-aminobutyric acid (GABA)	Synthesized from glutamate; primary inhibitory neurotransmitter in the brain; also influences muscle tone; opens or closes various ion channels
Glycine	Inhibits activity between neurons in the CNS, including retina; opens Cl$^-$ channels
MONOAMINES	
$NH_2—CH_2—CH$ with OH, Aromatic ring, OH, OH	Molecules synthesized from an amino acid by removing the carboxyl group and retaining the single amine group; also called biogenic amines
Serotonin or 5-hydroxytryptamine (5-HT)	Has various functions in the brain related to sleep, appetite, cognition (learning, memory), and mood; modulates actions of other neurotransmitters
Catecholamines	A distinct group of monoamines
Dopamine	Produces inhibitory activity in the brain; important roles in cognition (learning, memory), motivation, behavior, and mood; opens K$^+$ channels, closes Ca^{2+} channels
Norepinephrine (noradrenaline)	Neurotransmitter of PNS (sympathetic division of autonomic nervous system) and specific CNS regions
Epinephrine (adrenaline)	Has various effects in the CNS, especially the spinal cord, thalamus, and hypothalamus
NEUROPEPTIDES	
Tyr—Gly—Gly—Phe—Met	Small polypeptides act as signals to assist in and modulate communication among neurons in the CNS
Enkephalin	Helps regulate response to noxious and potentially harmful stimuli
Neuropeptide Y	Involved in memory regulation and energy balance (increased food intake and decreased physical activity)
Somatostatin	Inhibits activities of neurons in specific brain areas
Substance P	Assists with pain information transmission into the brain
Cholecystokinin (CCK)	Stimulates neurons in the brain to help mediate satiation (fullness) and repress hunger
Beta-endorphin	Prevents release of pain signals from neurons and fosters a feeling of well-being
Neurotensin	Helps control and moderate the effects of dopamine
OTHERS	
Adenosine	Also part of a nucleotide, inhibits activities in certain CNS neurons
Nitric oxide	Involved in learning and memory; relaxes muscle in the digestive tract; important for relaxation of smooth muscle in blood vessels (vasodilation)

FIGURE 9–8 Neurons, neuropil, and the common glial cells of the CNS.

(a) Most neuronal cell bodies (**N**) in the CNS are larger than the much more numerous glial cells (**G**) that surround them. The various types of glial cells and their relationships with neurons are difficult to distinguish by most routine light microscopic methods. However, oligodendrocytes have condensed, rounded nuclei and unstained cytoplasm due to very abundant Golgi complexes, which stain poorly and are very likely represented by the cells with

those properties seen here. The other glial cells seen here similar in overall size, but with very little cytoplasm and more elongated or oval nuclei, are mostly astrocytes. Routine H&E staining does not allow neuropil to stand out well. (×200; H&E)

(b) With the use of gold staining for neurofibrils, neuropil (**Np**) is more apparent. (×200; Gold chloride and hematoxylin)

in different brain regions. The highly variable and dynamic processes mediate most of these glial cells' many functions.

Functions attributed to astrocytes of various CNS regions include the following:

- Extending processes that associate with or cover synapses, affecting the formation, function, and plasticity of these structures,
- Regulating the extracellular ionic concentrations around neurons, with particular importance in buffering extracellular K⁺ levels,
- Guiding and physically supporting movements and locations of differentiating neurons during CNS development,
- Extending fibrous processes with expanded **perivascular feet** that cover capillary endothelial cells and modulate blood flow and help move nutrients, wastes, and other metabolites between neurons and capillaries (Figure 9–9a),
- Forming a barrier layer of expanded protoplasmic processes, called the **glial limiting membrane**, which lines the meninges at the external CNS surface, and
- Filling tissue defects after CNS injury by proliferation to form an **astrocytic scar**.

Ependymal Cells

Ependymal cells develop as columnar or cuboidal cells of the ependyma, which lines the fluid-filled ventricles of the brain and the central canal of the spinal cord (Figures 9–9a and 9–11). In some CNS locations, the apical ends of ependymal cells have cilia, which facilitate the movement of cerebrospinal fluid (CSF), and long microvilli likely involved in absorption.

Ependymal cells adhere to one another by apical junctional complexes like those of epithelial cells. However, unlike a true epithelium, the ependyma lacks a basal lamina. Instead, the basal ends of ependymal cells become elongated and extend branching processes into the adjacent neuropil.

Microglia

Microglia, consisting of small cell bodies from which radiate many long, branched processes (Figures 9–9a and 9–12), are less numerous than oligodendrocytes or astrocytes but nearly as common as neurons in some CNS regions. Evenly

FIGURE **9–9** Glial cells of the CNS and PNS.

Neuron

Myelinated axon

Myelin sheath (cut)

Oligodendrocyte

Astrocyte

Perivascular feet

Capillary

Ependymal cell

Ventricle of brain

Microglial cell

Functions of Astrocyte

1. Forms part of the blood-brain barrier
2. Regulates interstitial fluid composition
3. Provides structural support and organization to the central nervous system (CNS)
4. Assists with neuronal development
5. Replicates to occupy space of dying neurons

Functions of Ependymal Cell

1. Lines ventricles of brain and central canal of spinal cord
2. Assists in production and circulation of cerebrospinal fluid (CSF)

Functions of Microglial Cell

1. Phagocytic cells that move through the CNS
2. Protects the CNS by engulfing infectious agents and other potential harmful substances

Functions of Oligodendrocyte

1. Myelinates and insulates CNS axons
2. Allows faster action potential propagation along axons in the CNS

(a)

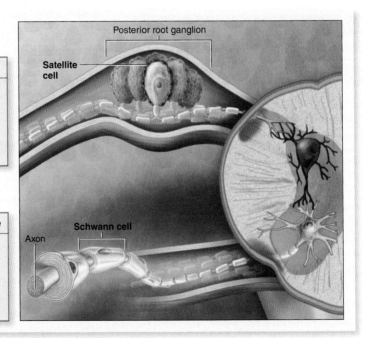

Functions of Satellite Cell

1. Electrically insulates PNS cell bodies.
2. Regulates nutrient and waste exchange for cell bodies in ganglia

Functions of Neurolemmocyte

1. Surround and insulate PNS axons and myelinate those having large diameters
2. Allows for faster action potential propagation along an axon in the PNS

Posterior root ganglion

Satellite cell

Schwann cell

Axon

(b)

(a) There are four major kinds of glial cells in the CNS: **oligoden-drocytes, astrocytes, ependymal cells,** and **microglial cells.** The interrelationships of these cells are shown diagrammatically here and their most important functions are summarized in the boxes.

(b) Two glial cells occur in the PNS: **Schwann cells** (sometimes called neurolemmocytes), which surround peripheral nerve fibers, and **satellite cells,** which surround the nerve cell bodies and are thus found only in ganglia. Major functions of these cells are indicated.

TABLE **9–2**	Origin, location, and principal functions of neuroglial cells.		
Glial Cell Type	**Origin**	**Location**	**Main Functions**
Oligodendrocyte	Neural tube	CNS	Myelin production, electrical insulation
Astrocyte	Neural tube	CNS	Structural and metabolic support of neurons, especially at synapses; repair processes
Ependymal cell	Neural tube	Line ventricles and central canal of CNS	Aid production and movement of CSF
Microglia	Bone marrow (monocytes)	CNS	Defense and immune-related activities
Schwann cell	Neural crest	Peripheral nerves	Myelin production, electrical insulation
Satellite cells (of ganglia)	Neural crest	Peripheral ganglia	Structural and metabolic support for neuronal cell bodies

distributed throughout specific regions of gray and white matter, the microglial cell bodies remain relatively static while their processes continuously probe and interact with neuropil, synapses, and other cells in an area up to 10-fold that of the cell body. Phagocytosing debris from damaged synapses, myelin, or apoptosis, microglial cells also constitute the major mechanism of immune defense in the CNS, removing any microbial invaders and secreting several immunoregulatory factors. Unlike other glial cells, microglia originate not from neural progenitor cells, but mostly from embryonic yolk sac monocytes with minimal input from circulating marrow-derived monocytes. Microglia belong to the family of tissue-resident macrophages and other antigen-presenting cells (Table 5–2) and are especially long-lived thanks in part to support from astrocytes.

Nuclei of microglial cells can often be recognized in routine hematoxylin and eosin (H&E) preparations by their small, dense, slightly elongated structure, which contrasts with the

FIGURE **9–10** Astrocytes.

(a) Astrocytes are the most abundant glial cells of the CNS and are characterized by numerous cytoplasmic processes (**P**) radiating from the glial cell body or soma (**S**). Astrocytic processes are not seen with routine light microscope staining but are easily seen after gold staining. Morphology of the processes allows astrocytes to be classified as fibrous (relatively few and straight processes) or protoplasmic (numerous branching processes), but functional differences between these types are not clear. (×500; Gold chloride)

(b) All astrocytic processes contain intermediate filaments of GFAP, and antibodies against this protein provide a simple method to stain these cells, as seen here in a fibrous astrocyte (**A**) and its processes. The small pieces of other GFAP-positive

processes in the neuropil around this cell give an idea of the density of this glial cell and its processes in the CNS. Astrocytes form part of the blood-brain barrier (BBB) and help regulate entry of molecules and ions from blood into CNS tissue. Capillaries at the extreme upper right and lower left corners are enclosed by GFAP-positive perivascular feet (**PF**) at the ends of numerous astrocytic processes. (×500; Anti-GFAP immunoperoxidase and hematoxylin counterstain)

(c) A length of capillary (**C**) is shown here completely covered by silver-stained terminal processes extending from astrocytes (**A**). (×400; Rio Hortega silver)

FIGURE **9–11** Ependymal cells.

Ependymal cells are epithelial-like cells that form a single layer lining the fluid-filled ventricles and central canal of the CNS.

(a) Lining the ventricles of the cerebrum, columnar ependymal cells (**E**) extend cilia and microvilli from the apical surfaces into the ventricle (**V**). These modifications help circulate the CSF and monitor its contents. Ependymal cells have junctional complexes at their apical ends like those of epithelial cells but lack a basal lamina. The cells' basal ends are tapered, extending processes that branch and penetrate some distance into the adjacent neuropil (**N**). Other areas of ependyma are responsible for production of CSF. (×100; H&E)

(b) Ependymal cells (**E**) lining the central canal (**C**) of the spinal cord help move CSF in that CNS region. (×200; H&E)

larger, spherical, more lightly stained nuclei of other glial cells. Immunohistochemistry using antibodies against cell surface antigens of immune cells clearly demonstrates microglial processes. When activated by CNS damage or infection, microglia retract their processes, proliferate, and assume the morphologic characteristics and functions of antigen-presenting cells (see Chapter 14).

FIGURE **9–12** Microglial cells.

Microglia are monocyte-derived, antigen-presenting cells of the CNS, less numerous than astrocytes but nearly as common as neurons and evenly distributed in both gray and white matter. By immunohistochemistry, here using a monoclonal antibody against human leukocyte antigens (HLA) of immune-related cells, the short branching processes of microglia can be seen. Routine staining demonstrates only the small dark nuclei of the cells.

Unlike other glia of the CNS, microglia are not interconnected; they are motile cells, constantly used in immune surveillance of CNS tissues. When activated by products of cell damage or by invading microorganisms, the cells retract their processes, begin phagocytosing the damage- or danger-related material, and behave as antigen-presenting cells. (×500; Antibody against HLA-DR and peroxidase)

(Reproduced with permission from Wolfgang Streit, Department of Neuroscience, University of Florida College of Medicine, Gainesville.)

›› MEDICAL APPLICATION

In **multiple sclerosis** (MS) an autoimmune mechanism damages the myelin sheaths surrounding axons, which interferes with the activity of the affected neurons and produces various neurologic problems. T lymphocytes and microglia, which phagocytose and degrade myelin debris, play major roles in progression of this disease. In MS, destructive actions of these cells exceed the capacity of oligodendrocytes to produce myelin and repair the myelin sheaths.

Schwann Cells

Schwann cells (named for 19th-century German histologist Theodor Schwann), sometimes called neurolemmocytes, occur only in the PNS and differentiate from precursors in the neural crest. Schwann cells represent the counterparts to oligodendrocytes of the CNS, having trophic interactions with axons and most importantly forming their **myelin sheaths**. However, unlike an oligodendrocyte, a Schwann cell extends only a single process forming myelin around a portion of one axon. Figure 9–9b shows a series of Schwann cells sheathing the full length of an axon, in a process described more fully below with peripheral nerves.

FIGURE 9–13 Satellite cells around neurons of ganglia in the PNS.

Satellite cells become very closely associated with neuronal cell bodies in sensory and autonomic ganglia of the PNS and support these cells in various ways.

(a) Nuclei of the many satellite cells (**S**) surrounding the perikarya of neurons (**N**) in an autonomic ganglion can be seen by light microscopy, but their cytoplasmic extensions are too thin to see with H&E staining. These long-lived neurons commonly accumulate brown lipofuscin (**L**). (×560; H&E)

(b) Immunofluorescent staining of satellite cells (**S**) reveals the cytoplasmic sheets extending from these cells and surrounding the neuronal cell bodies (**N**). The layer of satellite cells around each soma is continuous with the myelin sheath around the axon. Like the effect of Schwann cells on axons, satellite glial cells insulate, nourish, and regulate the microenvironment of the neuronal cell bodies. (×600; Rhodamine red-labeled antibody against glutamine synthetase)

(Reporoduced with permission from Menachem Hanani, Laboratory of Experimental Surgery, Hadassah Medical Center, Hebrew University of Jerusalem, Israel.)

Satellite Cells of Ganglia

Also derived from the embryonic neural crest, small **satellite cells** form a thin, intimate glial layer around each large neuronal cell body in the ganglia of the PNS (Figures 9–9b and 9–13). Satellite cells exert a trophic or supportive effect on these neurons, insulating, nourishing, and regulating their microenvironments.

› CENTRAL NERVOUS SYSTEM

The major structures comprising the CNS are the cerebrum, cerebellum, and **spinal cord** (Figure 9–1). The CNS is completely covered by connective tissue layers, the meninges, but CNS tissue contains very little collagen or similar material, making it relatively soft and easily damaged by injuries affecting the protective skull or vertebral bones. Most CNS neurons and their functional organization are more appropriately covered in neuroscience rather than histology courses, but certain important cells and basic topics will be introduced here.

Many structural features of CNS tissues can be seen in unstained, freshly dissected specimens. Many regions show organized areas of **white matter** and **gray matter**, differences caused by the differential distribution of lipid-rich myelin. The main components of white matter are myelinated axons (Figure 9–14), often grouped together as **tracts**, and the myelin-producing oligodendrocytes. Astrocytes and microglia are also present, but very few neuronal cell bodies. Gray matter contains abundant neuronal cell bodies, dendrites, astrocytes, and microglial cells, and is where most synapses occur. Gray matter makes up the thick cortex or surface layer of both the cerebrum and the cerebellum; most white matter is found in deeper regions. Deep within the brain are localized, variously shaped darker areas called the **cerebral nuclei**, each containing large numbers of aggregated neuronal cell bodies.

In the folded **cerebral cortex**, neuroscientists recognize six layers of neurons with different sizes and shapes. The most conspicuous of these cells are the efferent **pyramidal neurons** (Figure 9–15). Neurons of the cerebral cortex function in the integration of sensory information and the initiation of voluntary motor responses.

The sharply folded **cerebellar cortex** coordinates muscular activity throughout the body and is organized with three layers (Figure 9–16):

- A thick outer **molecular layer** has much neuropil and scattered neuronal cell bodies.
- A thin middle layer consists only of very large neurons called **Purkinje cells** (named for the 19th-century Czech histologist Jan Purkinje). These are conspicuous even in H&E-stained sections, and their dendrites extend throughout the molecular layer as a branching basket of nerve fibers (Figures 9–16c and d).
- A thick inner **granular layer** contains various very small, densely packed neurons (including granule cells, with diameters of only 4-5 μm) and little neuropil.

In cross sections of the **spinal cord**, the white matter is peripheral and the gray matter forms a deeper, H-shaped mass (Figure 9–17). The two anterior projections of this gray

FIGURE **9–14** White versus gray matter.

A cross section of H&E-stained spinal cord shows the transition between white matter (left region) and gray matter (right). The gray matter has many glial cells (**G**), neuronal cell bodies (**N**), and neuropil; white matter also contains glia (**G**) but consists mainly of axons (**A**) whose myelin sheaths were lost during preparation, leaving the round empty spaces shown. Each such space surrounds a dark-stained spot that is a small section of the axon. (×400)

FIGURE **9–15** Cerebral cortex.

(a) Important neurons of the cerebrum are the pyramidal neurons (**P**), which are arranged vertically and interspersed with numerous smaller glial cells, mostly astrocytes, in the eosinophilic neuropil. (×200; H&E)

(b) From the apical ends of pyramidal neurons (**P**), long dendrites extend in the direction of the cortical surface, which can be best seen in thick silver-stained sections in which only a few other protoplasmic astrocytes (**A**) cells are seen. (×200; Silver)

FIGURE **9–16** Cerebellum.

(a) The cerebellar cortex is convoluted with many distinctive small folds, each supported at its center by tracts of white matter in the cerebellar medulla (**M**). Each fold has distinct molecular layers (**ML**) and granular layers (**GL**). (×6; Cresyl violet)

(b) Higher magnification shows that the granular layer (**GL**) immediately surrounding the medulla (**M**) is densely packed with several different types of very small rounded neuronal cell bodies. The outer molecular layer (**ML**) consists of neuropil with fewer, much more scattered small neurons. At the interface of these two regions, a layer of large Purkinje neuron (**P**) perikarya can be seen. (×20; H&E)

(c) A single intervening layer contains the very large cell bodies of unique Purkinje neurons (**P**), whose axons pass through the granular layer (**GL**) to join tracts in the medulla and whose multiple branching dendrites ramify throughout the molecular layer (**ML**). Dendrites are not seen well with H&E staining. (×40; H&E)

(d) With appropriate silver staining dendrites from each large Purkinje cell (**P**) are shown to have hundreds of small branches, each covered with hundreds of dendritic spines. Axons from the small neurons of the granular layer are unmyelinated and run together into the molecular layer where they form synapses with the dendritic spines of Purkinje cells. (×40; Silver)

FIGURE **9–17** Spinal cord.

Lumbar

The spinal cord varies slightly in diameter along its length but in cross section always shows bilateral symmetry around the small, CSF-filled central canal (**C**). Unlike the cerebrum and cerebellum, gray matter makes up the center of the spinal cord, forming a roughly H-shaped structure that consists of two posterior (**P**) horns (sensory) and two anterior (**A**) (motor) horns, all joined by the gray commissure around the central canal.

(a) The gray matter contains abundant astrocytes and large neuronal cell bodies, especially those of motor neurons in the ventral horns.

(b) The white matter surrounds the gray matter and contains primarily oligodendrocytes and tracts of myelinated axons

running along the length of the cord. (Center ×5, a, b ×100; All silver-stained)

(c) With H&E staining, the large motor neurons (**N**) of the ventral horns show large nuclei, prominent nucleoli, and cytoplasm rich in Nissl substance, all of which indicate extensive protein synthesis to maintain the axons of these cells that extend great distances.

(d) In the white commissure ventral to the central canal, tracts (**T**) run lengthwise along the cord, seen here in cross section with empty myelin sheaths surrounding axons, as well as small tracts running from one side of the cord to the other. (Both ×200; H&E)

matter, the **anterior horns**, contain cell bodies of very large motor neurons whose axons make up the ventral roots of spinal nerves. The two **posterior horns** contain interneurons, which receive sensory fibers from neurons in the spinal (dorsal root) ganglia. Near the middle of the cord, the gray matter surrounds a small **central canal**, which develops from the lumen of the neural tube, is continuous with the ventricles of the brain, is lined by ependymal cells, and contains CSF.

Meninges

The skull and the vertebral column protect the CNS, but between the bone and nervous tissue are membranes of connective tissue called the **meninges**. Three meningeal layers are distinguished: the dura, arachnoid, and pia maters (Figures 9–18 and 9–19).

Dura Mater

The thick external **dura mater** (L. *dura mater*, tough mother) consists of dense irregular connective tissue organized as an outer periosteal layer continuous with the periosteum of the skull and an inner meningeal layer. These two layers are usually fused, but along the superior sagittal surface and other specific

areas around the brain, they separate to form the blood-filled **dural venous sinuses** (Figure 9–19). Around the spinal cord, the dura mater is separated from the periosteum of the vertebrae by the **epidural space**, which contains a plexus of thin-walled veins and loose connective tissue (Figure 9–18). The dura mater may be separated from the arachnoid by formation of a thin subdural space.

Arachnoid

The **arachnoid** (Gr. *arachnoeides*, spider web-like) has two components: (1) a sheet of connective tissue in contact with the dura mater and (2) a system of loosely arranged trabeculae composed of collagen and fibroblasts, continuous with the underlying pia mater layer. Surrounding these trabeculae is a large, sponge-like cavity, the **subarachnoid space**, filled with CSF. This fluid-filled space helps cushion and protect the CNS from minor trauma. The subarachnoid space communicates with the ventricles of the brain where the CSF is produced.

The connective tissue of the arachnoid is said to be avascular because it lacks nutritive capillaries, but larger blood vessels run through it (Figures 9–18 and 9–19). Because the

---

FIGURE 9–18 Spinal cord and meninges.

a   Anterior view

(a) A diagram of the spinal cord indicates the relationship of the three meningeal layers of connective tissue: the innermost **pia mater**, the **arachnoid**, and the **dura mater**. Also depicted are the blood vessels coursing through the subarachnoid space and the nerve rootlets that fuse to form the posterior and anterior roots of the spinal nerves. The posterior root ganglia contain the cell bodies of sensory nerve fibers and occupy intervertebral foramina (not shown).

(b) Section of an area near the anterior median fissure showing the tough dura mater (**D**). Surrounding the dura, the epidural space (not shown) contains cushioning adipose tissue and vascular plexuses. The subdural space (**SD**) is an artifact created by

separation of the dura from underlying tissue. The middle meningeal layer is the thicker weblike arachnoid mater (**A**) containing the large subarachnoid space (**SA**) and connective tissue trabeculae (**T**). The subarachnoid space is filled with CSF and the arachnoid acts as a shock-absorbing pad between the CNS and bone. Fairly large blood vessels (**BV**) course through the arachnoid. The innermost pia mater (**P**) is thin and is not clearly separate from the arachnoid; together, they are sometimes referred to as the pia-arachnoid or the leptomeninges. The space between the pia and the white matter (**WM**) of the spinal cord here is an artifact created during dissection; normally the pia is very closely applied to a layer of astrocytic processes at the surface of the CNS tissue. (×100; H&E)

FIGURE **9–19** Meninges around the brain.

The **dura, arachnoid, and pia maters** also surround the brain and as shown here the relationships among the cranial meninges are similar to those of the spinal cord. The diagram includes **arachnoid villi**, which are outpocketings of arachnoid away from the brain, which penetrate the dura mater and enter blood-filled **venous sinuses** located within that layer. The arachnoid villi function in releasing excess CSF into the blood. Blood vessels from the arachnoid branch into smaller arteries and veins that enter brain tissue carrying oxygen and nutrients. These small vessels are initially covered with pia mater, but as capillaries, they are covered only by the perivascular feet of astrocytes.

arachnoid has fewer trabeculae in the spinal cord, it can be more clearly distinguished from the pia mater in that area. The arachnoid and the pia mater are intimately associated and are often considered a single membrane called the pia-arachnoid.

In some areas, the arachnoid penetrates the dura mater and protrudes into blood-filled dural venous sinuses located there (Figure 9–19). These CSF-filled protrusions, which are covered by the vascular endothelial cells lining the sinuses, are called **arachnoid villi** and function as sites for absorption of CSF into the blood of the venous sinuses.

Pia Mater

The innermost **pia mater** (L. *pia mater*, tender mother) consists of flattened, mesenchymally derived cells closely applied to the entire surface of the CNS tissue. The pia does not directly contact nerve cells or fibers, being separated from the neural elements by the very thin superficial layer of astrocytic processes (the glial limiting membrane, or glia limitans), which adheres firmly to the pia mater. Together, the pia mater and the layer of astrocytic end feet form a physical barrier separating CNS tissue from CSF in the subarachnoid space (Figure 9–19).

Blood vessels penetrate CNS tissue through long **perivascular spaces** covered by pia mater, although the pia disappears when the blood vessels branch to form the small capillaries. However, these capillaries remain completely covered by the perivascular layer of astrocytic processes (Figures 9–9a and 9–10c).

Blood-Brain Barrier

The **blood-brain barrier** (BBB) is a functional barrier that allows much tighter control than that in most tissues over the passage of substances moving from blood into the CNS tissue. The main structural component of the BBB is the **capillary endothelium**, in which the cells are tightly sealed together with well-developed occluding junctions, with little or no transcytosis activity, and surrounded by the basement membrane. The **limiting layer of perivascular astrocytic feet**, which closely envelops the basement membrane of the continuous capillaries in most CNS regions (Figures 9–9 and 9–10c), also contributes to the BBB and further regulates passage of molecules and ions from blood to brain.

The BBB protects neurons and glia from bacterial toxins, infectious agents, and other exogenous substances, and helps maintain the stable composition and constant balance of ions in the interstitial fluid required for normal neuronal function. The BBB is not present in regions of the hypothalamus where plasma components are monitored, in the posterior pituitary that releases hormones, or in the choroid plexus where CSF is produced.

Choroid Plexus

The **choroid plexus** consists of highly vascular tissue, elaborately folded and projecting into the large ventricles of the brain (Figure 9–20a). It is found in the roofs of the third and fourth ventricles and in parts of the two lateral ventricular walls, all regions in which the ependymal lining directly contacts the pia mater.

Each villus of the choroid plexus contains a thin layer of well-vascularized pia mater covered by cuboidal ependymal cells (Figure 9–20b). The function of the choroid plexus is to remove water from blood and release it as the **CSF**. CSF is clear, contains Na⁺, K⁺, and Cl⁻ ions but very little protein, and its only cells are normally very sparse lymphocytes. It is produced continuously and it completely fills the ventricles, the central canal of the spinal cord, the subarachnoid and perivascular spaces. It provides the ions required for CNS neuronal activity and in the arachnoid serves to help absorb mechanical shocks. Arachnoid villi (Figure 9–19) provide the main pathway for absorption of CSF back into the venous circulation. There are very few lymphatic vessels in CNS tissue.

FIGURE **9–20** Choroid plexus.

The choroid plexus consists of ependyma and vascularized pia mater and projects many thin folds from certain walls of the ventricles.

(a) Section of the bilateral choroid plexus (**CP**) projecting into the fourth ventricle (**V**) near the cerebellum. (×12; Kluver-Barrera stain)

(b) At higher magnification each fold of choroid plexus is seen to be well-vascularized with large capillaries (**C**) and covered by a continuous layer of cuboidal ependymal cells (**E**). (×150)

(c) The choroid plexus is specialized for transport of water and ions from the blood plasma across the capillary endothelium and ependymal layer and into the brain ventricles as cerebrospinal fluid (CSF).

A decrease in the absorption of CSF or a blockage of out-flow from the ventricles during fetal or postnatal develop-ment results in the condition known as **hydrocephalus** (Gr. *hydro*, water + *kephale*, head), which promotes a progressive enlargement of the head followed by mental impairment.

› PERIPHERAL NERVOUS SYSTEM

The main components of the peripheral nervous system (PNS) are the **nerves, ganglia**, and **nerve endings**. Periph-eral nerves are bundles of nerve fibers (axons) individually surrounded by Schwann cells and connective tissue.

Nerve Fibers

Nerves are analogous to tracts in the CNS, containing axons enclosed within sheaths of glial cells specialized to facilitate axonal function. In peripheral nerves, axons are sheathed by **Schwann cells** or neurolemmocytes (Figure 9–9b). The sheath may or may not form myelin around the axons, depending on their diameter.

Myelinated Fibers

As axons of large diameter grow in the PNS, they are engulfed along their length by a series of differentiating neurolemmo-cytes and become **myelinated nerve fibers**. The plasma membrane of each covering Schwann cell fuses with itself at an area termed the mesaxon and a wide, flattened process of the cell continues to extend itself, moving circumferentially around the axon many times (Figure 9–21). The multiple lay-ers of Schwann cell membrane unite as a thick **myelin sheath**. Composed mainly of lipid bilayers and membrane proteins, myelin is a large lipoprotein complex that, like cell membranes, is partly removed by standard histologic procedures (Figures 9–14 and 9–17d). Unlike oligodendrocytes of the CNS, a Schwann cell forms myelin around only a portion of one axon.

FIGURE **9–21** **Myelination of large-diameter PNS axons.**

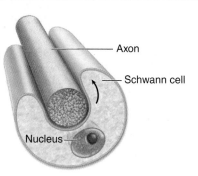

① A Schwann cell becomes aligned along a portion of the axon and extends a wide cytoplasmic process to encircle it.

Axon

Schwann cell

Nucleus

② The growing process completely encloses the axonal portion and continues to extend spirally around it, always in immediate contact with the axon.

Mesaxon

③ Multiple such spiral wrappings become compacted layers of cell membrane (myelin) as cytoplasm leaves the growing process.

Cytoplasm of the Schwann cell

Compacting myelin layers

④ The mature Schwann cell myelin sheath has up to 100 lamellae, with most cytoplasm in the outermost layer with the cell body.

Myelin sheath

Schwann cell nucleus

A Schwann cell (neurolemmocyte) engulfs one portion along the length of a large-diameter axon. The processes of the Schwann cell encircling the axon fuse their cell membranes, forming a paired, parallel structure called the mesaxon. The process in direct contact with the axonal surface elongates greatly, moves most of its cytoplasm toward the Schwann cell nucleus, and wraps itself repeatedly around the axon to form multiple, com-pacted layers. The Schwann cell membrane wrappings constitute the myelin sheath, with the Schwann cell body always on its outer surface. The myelin layers are very rich in lipid and provide insulation and facilitate formation of action potentials along the axolemma.

With high-magnification TEM, the myelin sheath appears as a thick electron-dense axonal covering in which the concentric membrane layers may be visible (Figure 9–22). The prominent electron-dense layers visible ultrastructurally in the sheath, the **major dense lines**, represent the fused, protein-rich cytoplasmic surfaces of the Schwann cell membrane. Along the myelin sheath, these surfaces periodically separate slightly to allow transient movement of cytoplasm for

FIGURE **9–22** Ultrastructure of myelinated and unmyelinated fibers.

Cross section of PNS fibers in the TEM reveals differences between myelinated and unmyelinated axons. Large axons (**A**) are wrapped in a thick myelin sheath (**M**) of multiple layers of Schwann cell membrane.

The inset shows a portion of myelin at higher magnification in which the major dense lines of individual membrane layers can be distinguished, as well as the neurofilaments (**NF**) and microtubules (**MT**) in the axoplasm (**A**). At the center of the photo is a Schwann cell showing its active nucleus (**SN**) and Golgi-rich cytoplasm (**SC**). At the right is an axon around which myelin is still forming (**FM**).

Unmyelinated axons (**UM**) are much smaller in diameter, and many such fibers may be engulfed by a single Schwann cell (**SC**). The glial cell does not form myelin wrappings around such small axons but simply encloses them. Whether it forms myelin or not, each Schwann cell is surrounded, as shown, by an external lamina containing type IV collagen and laminin like the basal laminae which underlie epithelia. (×28,000, inset ×70,000)

(Reproduced with permission from Dr Mary Bartlett Bunge, The Miami Project to Cure Paralysis, University of Miami Miller School of Medicine, Miami, FL.)

membrane maintenance; at these **myelin clefts** (or Schmidt-Lanterman clefts), the major dense lines temporarily disappear (Figure 9–23). Faintly seen ultrastructurally in the light staining layers are the intraperiod lines that represent the apposed outer bilayers of the Schwann cell membrane.

Membranes of Schwann cells have a higher proportion of lipids than do other cell membranes, and the myelin sheath serves to insulate axons and maintain a constant ionic microenvironment most suitable for action potentials. Between adjacent Schwann cells on an axon, the myelin sheath shows small **nodes of Ranvier** (or **nodal gaps**, Figures 9–9b, 9–23, and 9–24), where the axon is only partially covered by interdigitating Schwann cell processes. At these nodes, the axolemma is exposed to ions in the interstitial fluid and has a much higher concentration of voltage-gated Na^+ channels, which renew the action potential and produce **saltatory conduction** (L. *saltare*, to jump) of nerve impulses, their rapid movement from node to node. The length of axon ensheathed by one Schwann cell, the **internodal segment**, varies directly with axonal diameter and ranges from 300 to 1500 μm.

Unmyelinated Fibers

Unlike the CNS where many short axons are not myelinated at all but course among other neuronal and astrocytic processes, the smallest diameter axons of peripheral nerves are still enveloped within simple folds of Schwann cells (Figure 9–25). These very small **unmyelinated fibers** do not however undergo multiple wrapping to form a myelin sheath (Figure 9–21). In unmyelinated nerves, each Schwann cell can enclose portions of many axons with small diameters. Without the thick myelin sheath, nodes of Ranvier are not seen along unmyelinated nerve fibers. Moreover, these small-diameter axons have evenly distributed voltage-gated ion channels; their impulse conduction is not saltatory and is much slower than that of myelinated axons.

Nerve Organization

In the PNS, nerve fibers are grouped into bundles to form **nerves**. Except for very thin nerves containing only unmyelinated fibers, nerves have a whitish, glistening appearance because of their myelin and collagen content.

Axons and Schwann cells are enclosed within layers of connective tissue (Figures 9–24, 9–26, and 9–27). Immediately around the external lamina of the Schwann cells is a thin layer called the **endoneurium**, consisting of reticular fibers, scattered fibroblasts, and capillaries. Groups of axons with Schwann cells and endoneurium are bundled together as **fascicles** by a sleeve of **perineurium**, containing flat fibrocytes with their edges sealed together by tight junctions. From two to six layers of these unique connective tissue cells regulate diffusion into the fascicle and make up the **blood-nerve barrier** that helps maintain the fibers' microenvironment. Externally, peripheral nerves have a dense, irregular fibrous coat called the **epineurium**, which extends deeply to fill the space between fascicles.

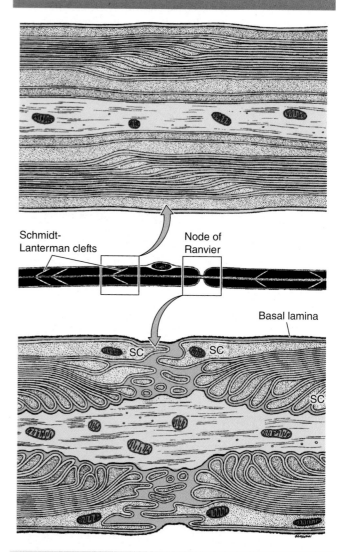

FIGURE 9–23 Myelin maintenance and nodes of Ranvier.

Schmidt-Lanterman clefts

Node of Ranvier

Basal lamina

SC

SC

SC

The *middle* diagram shows schematically a myelinated peripheral nerve fiber as seen under the light microscope. The axon is enveloped by the myelin sheath, which, in addition to membrane, contains some Schwann cell cytoplasm in spaces called **Schmidt-Lanterman or myelin clefts** between the major dense lines of membranes.

The *upper* diagram shows one set of such clefts ultrastructurally. The clefts contain Schwann cell cytoplasm that was not displaced to the cell body during myelin formation. This cytoplasm moves slowly along the myelin sheath, opening temporary spaces (the clefts) that allow renewal of some membrane components as needed for maintenance of the sheath.

The *lower* diagram depicts the ultrastructure of a single node of Ranvier or nodal gap. Interdigitating processes extending from the outer layers of the **Schwann cells (SC)** partly cover and contact the axolemma at the nodal gap. This contact acts as a partial barrier to the movement of materials in and out of the periaxonal space between the axolemma and the Schwann sheath. The basal or external lamina around Schwann cells is continuous over the nodal gap. The axolemma at nodal gaps has abundant voltage-gated Na^+ channels important for impulse conductance in these axons.

FIGURE 9–24 Node of Ranvier and endoneurium.

A longitudinally oriented nerve shows one node of Ranvier (**N**) with the axon visible. Collagen of the sparse endoneurium (**En**), blue in this trichrome stain, surrounds the Schwann cells and a capillary (**C**). At least one Schwann cell nucleus (**S**) is also clearly seen. (×400; Mallory trichome)

Very small nerves consist of one fascicle (Figure 9–28). Small nerves can be found in sections of many organs and often show a winding disposition in connective tissue.

Peripheral nerves establish communication between centers in the CNS and the sense organs and effectors (muscles,

FIGURE 9–25 Unmyelinated nerves.

Unmyelinated axons

① Schwann cell starts to envelop multiple axons.

Schwann cell

Axons

② The unmyelinated axons are enveloped by the Schwann cell, but there are *no* myelin sheath wraps around each axon.

Schwann cell nucleus

Unmyelinated axon

Schwann cell

During development of small-diameter unmyelinated nerves, portions of several axons are engulfed by one Schwann cell. Subsequently, the axons are separated and each typically becomes enclosed within its own fold of Schwann cell surface. No myelin is formed by wrapping. Small-diameter axons utilize action potentials whose formation and maintenance do not depend on the insulation provided by the myelin sheath required by large-diameter axons.

glands, etc). They generally contain both afferent and efferent fibers. **Afferent** fibers carry information from internal body regions and the environment to the CNS. **Efferent** fibers carry impulses from the CNS to effector organs commanded by these centers. Nerves possessing only sensory fibers are called **sensory nerves**; those composed only of fibers carrying impulses to the effectors are called **motor nerves**. Most nerves have both sensory and motor fibers and are called **mixed nerves**, usually also with both myelinated and unmyelinated axons.

Ganglia

Ganglia are typically ovoid structures containing neuronal cell bodies and their surrounding glial satellite cells supported by delicate connective tissue and surrounded by a denser capsule. Because they serve as relay stations to transmit nerve impulses, at least one nerve enters and another exits from each ganglion. The direction of the nerve impulse determines whether the ganglion will be a **sensory** or an **autonomic** ganglion.

Sensory Ganglia

Sensory ganglia receive afferent impulses that go to the CNS. Sensory ganglia are associated with both cranial nerves (cranial ganglia) and the dorsal roots of the spinal nerves (spinal ganglia). The large neuronal cell bodies of ganglia (Figure 9–29) are associated with thin, sheetlike extensions of small glial **satellite cells** (Figures 9–9b and 9–13). Sensory ganglia are supported by a distinct connective tissue capsule and an internal framework continuous with the connective tissue layers of the nerves. The neurons of these ganglia are pseudounipolar and relay information from the ganglion's nerve endings to the gray matter of the spinal cord via synapses with local neurons.

FIGURE 9–26 Peripheral nerve connective tissue: Epi-, peri-, and endoneurium.

(a) The diagram shows the relationship among these three connective tissue layers in large peripheral nerves. The epineurium (**E**) consists of a dense superficial region and a looser deep region that contains the larger blood vessels.

(b) The micrograph shows a small vein (**V**) and artery (**A**) in the deep epineurium (**E**). Nerve fibers (**N**) are bundled in fascicles. Each fascicle is surrounded by the perineurium (**P**), consisting of a few layers of unusual squamous fibroblastic cells that are all joined at the peripheries by tight junctions. The resulting blood-nerve barrier helps regulate the microenvironment inside the fascicle. Axons and Schwann cells are in turn surrounded by a thin layer of endoneurium. (×140; H&E)

(c) As shown here and in the diagram, septa (**S**) of connective tissue often extend from the perineurium into larger fascicles. The

endoneurium (**En**) and lamellar nature of the perineurium (**P**) are also shown at this magnification, along with some adjacent epineurium (**E**). (×200; PT)

(d) SEM of small, transversely cut nerve showing a single fascicle surrounded by distinct **perineurium** and packed with delicate **endoneurium** in which are located a few axons with myelin sheaths and many unmyelinated axons, all shown at higher magnification in the next figure. Endoneurium also contains sparse capillaries with tightly joined cells, another part of the blood-nerve barrier controlling release of substances from plasma into the axonal microenvironment. Dense, irregular connective tissue of the **epineurium** surrounds the perineurium and larger blood vessels (on far right of photo). A fragment of epineurium lies across the cut fascicle here. (×400)

Autonomic Ganglia

Autonomic (Gr. *autos,* self + *nomos,* law) nerves affect the activity of smooth muscle, the secretion of some glands, heart rate, and many other involuntary activities by which the body maintains a constant internal environment (**homeostasis**).

Autonomic ganglia are small bulbous dilations in autonomic nerves, usually with multipolar neurons. Some are located within certain organs, especially in the walls of the digestive tract, where they constitute the **intramural ganglia**. The capsules of these ganglia may be poorly defined among

FIGURE **9–27** Peripheral nerve ultrastructure.

This low-magnification TEM shows a fibroblast (**F**) surrounded by collagen (**C**) in the epineurium and three layers of flattened cells in the perineurium (**P**) that form another part of the blood-nerve barrier. Inside the perineurium, the endoneurium (**En**) is rich in reticulin fibers (**RF**) that surround all Schwann cells. Nuclei of two Schwann cells (**SC**) of myelinated axons (**A**) are visible as well as many unmyelinated axons (**UM**) within Schwann cells. (×1200)

the local connective tissue. A layer of satellite cells also envelops the neurons of autonomic ganglia (Figure 9–29), although these may also be inconspicuous in intramural ganglia.

Autonomic nerves use two neuron circuits. The first neuron of the chain, with the **preganglionic fiber**, occurs in the CNS. Its axon forms a synapse with **postganglionic fibers** of the second multipolar neuron in the chain located in a peripheral ganglion system. The chemical mediator present in the synaptic vesicles of all preganglionic axons is acetylcholine.

As indicated earlier, autonomic nerves make up the **autonomic nervous system**. This has two parts: the **sympathetic** and the **parasympathetic divisions**. Neuronal cell bodies of preganglionic sympathetic nerves develop in the thoracic and lumbar segments of the spinal cord and those of the parasympathetic division are in the medulla and midbrain and in the sacral portion of the spinal cord. Sympathetic second neurons

occur in small ganglia along the vertebral column, while second neurons of the parasympathetic series are found in very small ganglia always located near or within the effector organs, for example in the walls of the stomach and intestines. Parasympathetic ganglia may lack distinct capsules altogether, perikarya and associated satellite cells simply forming a loosely organized plexus within the surrounding connective tissue.

› NEURAL PLASTICITY & REGENERATION

Despite its general stability, the nervous system exhibits neuronal differentiation and formation of new synapses even in adults. Embryonic development of the nervous system produces an excess of differentiating neurons, and the cells which do not establish correct synapses with other neurons are eliminated by apoptosis. In adult mammals after an injury, the neuronal circuits may be reorganized by the growth of neuronal processes, forming new synapses to replace ones lost by injury. Thus, new communications are established with some degree of functional recovery. This **neural plasticity** and reformation of processes are controlled by several growth factors produced by both neurons and glial cells in a family of proteins called **neurotrophins**.

Neuronal stem cells are present in the adult CNS, located in part among the cells of the ependyma, which can supply new neurons, astrocytes, and oligodendrocytes. Fully differentiated, interconnected CNS neurons cannot temporarily disengage these connections and divide to replace cells lost by injury or disease; the potential of neural stem cells to allow tissue regeneration and functional recovery within the CNS components is a subject of intense investigation. Astrocytes do proliferate at injured sites and these growing cells can interfere with successful axonal regeneration in structures such as spinal cord tracts.

In the histologically much simpler peripheral nerves, injured axons have a much greater potential for regeneration and return of function. If the cell bodies are intact, damaged or severed PNS axons can regenerate as shown in the sequence of diagrams in Figure 9–30. Distal portions of axons, isolated from their source of new proteins and organelles, degenerate; the surrounding Schwann cells dedifferentiate, shed the myelin sheaths, and proliferate within the surrounding layers of connective tissue. Cellular debris including shed myelin is removed by blood-derived macrophages, which also secrete neurotrophins to promote anabolic events of axon regeneration.

The onset of regeneration is signaled by changes in the perikaryon that characterize the process of **chromatolysis**: the cell body swells slightly, Nissl substance is initially diminished, and the nucleus migrates to a peripheral position within the perikaryon. The proximal segment of the axon close to the wound degenerates for a short distance, but begins to grow again distally as new Nissl substance appears and debris is removed. The new Schwann cells align to serve as guides for

FIGURE **9–28** Small nerves.

Small nerves can be seen in sections from most organs.

(a) In cross section, an isolated, resin-embedded nerve is seen to have a thin perineurium (**P**), one capillary (**C**), and many large axons (**A**) associated with Schwann cells (**S**). A few nuclei of fibroblasts can be seen in the endoneurium between the myelinated fibers. (×400; PT)

(b) In longitudinal sections, the flattened nuclei of endoneurial fibroblasts (**F**) and more oval nuclei of Schwann cells (**S**) can be distinguished. Nerve fibers are held rather loosely in the endoneurium and in low-magnification longitudinal section are seen to be wavy rather than straight. This indicates a slackness of fibers within the nerve, which allows nerves to stretch slightly during body movements with no potentially damaging tension on the fibers. (×200; H&E)

(c) In sections of mesentery and other tissues, a highly wavy or tortuous disposition of a single small nerve (**N**) will be seen as multiple oblique or transverse pieces as the nerve enters and leaves the area in the section. (×200; H&E)

(d) Often, a section of small nerve will have some fibers cut transversely and others cut obliquely within the same fascicle, again suggesting the relatively unrestrained nature of the fibers within the endoneurium (**E**) and perineurium (**P**). (×300; H&E)

the regrowing axons and produce polypeptide factors that promote axonal outgrowth. Motor axons reestablish synaptic connections with muscles and function is restored.

›› MEDICAL APPLICATION

Regeneration of peripheral nerves is functionally efficient only when the fibers and the columns of Schwann cells are directed properly. In a mixed nerve, if regenerating sensory fibers grow into columns formerly occupied by motor fibers connected to motor end plates, the function of the muscle will not be reestablished. When there is an extensive gap between the distal and proximal segments of cut or injured peripheral nerves or when the distal segment disappears altogether (as in the case of amputation of a limb), the newly growing axons may form a swelling, or **neuroma**, that can be the source of spontaneous pain.

FIGURE **9–29** Ganglia.

(a) A sensory ganglion (**G**) has a distinct connective tissue capsule (**C**) and internal framework continuous with the epineurium and other components of peripheral nerves, except that no perineurium is present and that there is no blood-nerve barrier function. Fascicles of nerve fibers (**F**) enter and leave these ganglia. (×56; Kluver-Barrera stain)

(b) Higher magnification shows the small, rounded nuclei of glia cells called satellite cells (**S**) which produce thin, sheetlike

cytoplasmic extensions that completely envelop each large neuronal perikaryon. (×400; H&E)

(c) Sympathetic ganglia are smaller than most sensory ganglia but similar in having large neuronal cell bodies (**N**), some containing lipofuscin (**L**). Sheets from satellite cells (**S**) enclose each neuronal cell body with morphology slightly different from that of sensory ganglia. Autonomic ganglia generally have less well-developed connective tissue capsules (**C**) than sensory ganglia. (×400; H&E)

FIGURE 9–30 Regeneration in peripheral nerves.

a 　**b** 2 weeks 　**c** 3 weeks 　**d** 3 months

In an injured or cut peripheral nerve, proximal axon segments can regenerate from their cut ends after a delay. The main changes that take place in an injured nerve fiber are shown here.

(a) Normal nerve fiber, with its perikaryon, extensive RER (Nissl substance), and effector cell (muscle).

(b) When the axon is injured, the RER is greatly reduced initially and the nerve fiber distal to the injury degenerates along with its myelin sheath. Debris is phagocytosed by macrophages (shown in purple).

(c) In the following weeks after injury, muscle fiber shows denervation atrophy, but Schwann cells proliferate to form a compact cord penetrated by the regrowing axon. The axon grows at the rate of 0.5–3 mm/d.

(d) After some months, the nerve fiber regeneration is successful and functional connections with the muscle fiber are restored.

Nervous System　SUMMARY OF KEY POINTS

Development of Nerve Tissue

- Nervous tissue develops in the early embryo when the dorsal ectoderm **neural plate** folds lengthwise to form the **neural tube**, the precursor of the CNS, and releases **neural crest cells**, precursors for much of the PNS.

Neurons

- There are many kinds of **neurons**, but all consist of a **cell body (perikaryon)** containing the nucleus, a long cytoplasmic extension called the **axon**, and one or more shorter processes called **dendrites**.
- Neurons use the common cell property of **excitability** to produce and move an **action potential (nerve impulse)** along the axon to excite another neuron or other effector cell.

- Such nerve communication is transmitted to another neuron or effector cell via a **synapse**, where **neurotransmitter** is released at the **presynaptic membrane** and binds receptors on the **postsynaptic cell**, initiating a new action potential there.

Glial Cells

- **Glial cells (glia)**, required to support neurons in many ways, consist of six major types:
  - **Oligodendrocytes** wrap flattened processes around portions of axons in the CNS, forming **myelin sheaths** that insulate the axons and facilitate nerve impulses.
  - **Astrocytes**, the most numerous cell of the CNS, all produce hundreds of processes to enclose and provide regulated microenvironments for neuronal perikarya, synapses, and capillaries.

- **Ependymal cells** are epithelial-like cells, lacking basement membranes, which line the fluid-filled cerebral ventricles and central canal of the spinal cord.
- **Microglia** differs from all other glial cells in originating from blood monocytes, not from neural tissue precursors; they mediate immune defense activity within the CNS.
- **Schwann cells (neurolemmocytes)** enclose all axons in nerves of the PNS, producing **myelin sheaths** around large-diameter axons, whose impulse conductivity is augmented at the **nodes of Ranvier** between successive Schwann cells.
- **Satellite cells** are located within PNS **ganglia**, aggregated sensory or autonomic neuronal cell bodies, where they enclose each perikaryon and regulate its microenvironment.

Central Nervous System

- Within the brain and spinal cord, regions rich in neuronal perikarya and astrocytes comprise the **gray matter** and regions containing tracts of myelinated axons comprise **white matter**.
- Hundreds of different neurons make up the CNS; large, unique **Purkinje neurons** characterize the cortex of the cerebellum, and layers of small **pyramidal neurons** form the cerebral cortex.
- The CNS is completely enclosed by three connective tissue layers called **meninges**: (1) the tough external **dura mater**; (2) the middle **arachnoid layer**; and (3) the delicate **pia mater** that directly contacts neural tissue.
- The **arachnoid layer** contains much **CSF**, which helps **cushion** the CNS within its bony enclosure.
- The **choroid plexus** consists of elaborate folds of vascularized **pia mater** covered by **ependyma** that project from walls of the cerebral ventricles; the water is removed from capillaries and transferred into the ventricles as **CSF**.
- In most CNS regions, neurons are also protected by the blood-brain barrier, consisting of the **perivascular feet of astrocytic processes** and the nonfenestrated capillary endothelial cells' **tight junctions**.

Peripheral Nervous System

- **Peripheral nerves** consist of axons from motor neurons (in the spinal cord), sensory neurons, and autonomic neurons (in ganglia); all the axons are enclosed within a series of **Schwann cells**, but only large (myelinated) axons have myelin sheaths and nodes of Ranvier.
- **Endoneurium** is a thin connective tissue layer immediately surrounding Schwann cells in peripheral nerves, containing a few nonfenestrated capillaries and much reticulin.
- Groups of axons (with Schwann cells and endoneurium) are surrounded by **perineurium**, consisting of layered, squamous fibroblastic cells joined by **tight junctions** to make a **blood-nerve barrier**.
- In large peripheral nerves, groups of axons are subdivided as **fascicles**, each of which is surrounded by perineurium.
- Surrounding the perineurium is a thick, outermost layer of dense irregular connective tissue, the **epineurium**.
- **Ganglia**, which can be either sensory or autonomic, contain neuronal cell bodies and their **satellite cells** and are surrounded by connective tissue continuous with that of nerves.

Neural Plasticity & Regeneration

- Certain regions of the CNS, such as near the ependyma, retain rare **neural stem and progenitor cells** that allow some replacement of neurons throughout life; **neural plasticity** involving formation and remodeling of synaptic connections is also prevalent throughout life.
- The complexity and distances of the neuronal and glial interconnections with the CNS make regeneration and restoration of function within this tissue after major injury very difficult.
- The more simply organized peripheral nerves have better capacity for **axonal regeneration**, a process involving reactivation of the perikaryon, Schwann cells, and macrophages.

Nervous System ASSESS YOUR KNOWLEDGE

1. Which of the following is characteristic of the chromatophilic material called Nissl substance in neural tissue?

   a. Found throughout neurons
   b. Site of mRNA translation for proteins of the axolemma
   c. Most abundant in unipolar neurons
   d. Becomes more abundant as an individual gets older
   e. An example of intermediate filament proteins

2. Which of the following events occurs immediately after an action potential reaches a synapse at an axon terminal?

   a. Vesicle fusion with the presynaptic terminal membrane
   b. Calcium ion influx at the presynaptic terminal
   c. Neurotransmitter binding to receptors on the postsynaptic membrane
   d. Neurotransmitter release into the synaptic cleft
   e. Binding of the neurotransmitter at the presynaptic terminal

3. A report from a hospital pathology laboratory indicates that a microscope slide with a small specimen of neural tissue contains "numerous GFAP-positive" cells. What is the most likely source of this specimen?

   a. A region of white matter
   b. A sensory ganglion
   c. An autonomic ganglion
   d. A region of gray matter
   e. Pia mater

4. In the choroid plexus, water from capillaries is transported directly into the cerebrospinal fluid by what structure(s)?

   a. Ependyma
   b. Astrocytes
   c. Cells of the arachnoid mater
   d. Lining of the central canal
   e. Microglial cells

5. What term applies to collections of neuronal cell bodies (somata) in the central nervous system?

   a. Ganglia
   b. Neuroglia
   c. Nodes
   d. White matter
   e. Nuclei

6. Which structure contains trabeculae around which cerebrospinal fluid (CSF) flows?

   a. Arachnoid mater
   b. Ependyma
   c. Dura mater
   d. Pia mater
   e. Gray matter

7. Which of the following is a characteristic of the connective tissue layer that surrounds individual fascicles in large peripheral nerves?

   a. A delicate region of connective tissue in contact with Schwann cells
   b. Called the dura mater
   c. Important as part of the blood-nerve barrier in the nerve
   d. Rich in myelin
   e. The thickest sheath of connective tissue in the nerve

8. A 35-year-old woman presents with weakness and spasticity in the lower left extremity, visual impairment and throbbing in the left eye, and difficulties with balance, fatigue, and malaise. There is an increase in CSF protein, elevated gamma globulin, and moderate pleocytosis. MRI confirms areas of demyelination in the anterior corpus callosum. Imaging identifies plaques that are hyperintense on T2-weighted and fluid-attenuated inversion recovery (FLAIR) images, and hypointense on T1-weighted scans. Which of the following cells are specifically targeted in her condition?

   a. Microglia
   b. Oligodendrocytes
   c. Astrocytes
   d. Schwann cells
   e. Multipolar neurons

9. A 22-year-old man receives a severe, traumatic compression injury to his radial nerve during a motorcycle crash. He shows an advancing Tinel sign. Which one of the following characterizes regeneration of axons after this nerve injury?

   a. It occurs in the absence of motor nerve action potentials.
   b. It occurs at a rate of about 100 mm/d.
   c. It occurs in the segment distal to the site of axon damage.
   d. It occurs by a process that involves Schwann cell proliferation.
   e. It occurs in conjunction with degeneration and phagocytosis of the endoneurium.

10. A 2-year-old boy presents with hearing impairment, poliosis (a white shock of hair), complete heterochromia and sectoral heterochromia, hypertelorism, a low hairline with eyebrows that touch in the middle, white pigmentation of the skin, and suspected neurologic deficits. He is diagnosed with Waardenburg syndrome with a mutation in the *PAX-3* gene that affects neural crest differentiation. Which of the following structures would most likely also be affected in this patient?

   a. Purkinje cells
   b. Pyramidal neurons
   c. Ventral horns of the spinal cord
   d. Astrocytes
   e. Neurons and satellite cells of the spinal ganglion

10 Muscle Tissue

Muscle tissue, the fourth basic tissue type with epithelia, connective tissues, and nervous tissue, consists of cells that optimize the universal cell property of **contractility**. As in all cells, actin microfilaments and associated proteins generate the forces necessary for muscle contraction, which drives movement within organ systems, of blood, and of the body as a whole. Essentially all muscle cells originate from embryonic mesoderm and differentiate by elongation and abundant synthesis of the myofibrillar proteins actin and myosin.

Three generally different types of muscle tissue develop based on their morphologic and functional characteristics (Figure 10–1), with the structure of each well adapted to its physiologic role.

- **Skeletal muscle** contains bundles of very long, multinucleated cells with cross-striations and produces quick, forceful contractions, usually under voluntary control.
- **Cardiac muscle** also has cross-striations but consists of less elongated, often branched cells bound to one another at structures called **intercalated discs**, unique to cardiac muscle. Contraction is involuntary, vigorous, and rhythmic.
- **Smooth muscle** comprises collections of fusiform cells, which lack striations and generate slow, involuntary contractions.

In all types of muscle contraction involves the sliding interaction of thick myosin filaments along thin actin filaments. The forces necessary for this sliding are generated by other proteins affecting the weak interactions in the bridges between actin and myosin.

As with neurons, muscle specialists refer to certain muscle cell components with special names. The cytoplasm of muscle cells often becomes **sarcoplasm** (Gr. *sarkos*, flesh + *plasma*, thing formed), smooth ER is the **sarcoplasmic reticulum**, and the muscle cell membrane is called the **sarcolemma** (*sarkos* + Gr. *lemma*, husk).

> **>> MEDICAL APPLICATION**
>
> The variation in diameter of muscle fibers depends on factors such as the specific muscle, age, gender, nutritional status, and physical training of the individual. Exercise enlarges the skeletal musculature by stimulating formation of new myofibrils and growth in the diameter of individual muscle fibers. This process, characterized by increased cell volume, is called **hypertrophy** (Gr. *hyper*, above + *trophe*, nourishment).
>
> Tissue growth by an increase in the number of cells is termed **hyperplasia** (hyper + Gr. *plasis*, molding), which takes place very readily in smooth muscle, where cells have not lost the capacity to divide by mitosis.

❯ SKELETAL MUSCLE

Skeletal (or **striated**) **muscle** consists of **muscle fibers**, which are long, cylindrical multinucleated cells with diameters of 10–100 μm and lengths up to several centimeters. During embryonic skeletal muscle development, mesenchymal myoblasts (L. *myo*, muscle) fuse to form multinucleated myotubes, each surrounded and bound by an external (or basal) lamina. Myotubes then mature further as striated muscle fibers (Figure 10–2). The highly organized contractile apparatus begins to fill the sarcoplasm, while nuclei elongate and localize peripherally just under the sarcolemma, a characteristic nuclear site unique to skeletal muscle fibers. A small population of reserve progenitor cells called muscle **satellite cells** remains adjacent to most fibers of mature skeletal muscle, between the sarcolemma and the external lamina.

FIGURE **10–1** Three types of muscle.

(a) Skeletal muscle   **(b)** Cardiac muscle   **(c)** Smooth muscle

Key features shown in light micrographs and diagrams.

(a) Skeletal muscle contains large, elongated, multinucleated fibers with strong, quick, voluntary contractions.

(b) Cardiac muscle consists of irregular branched cells bound together longitudinally by intercalated discs and shows strong, involuntary contractions.

(c) Smooth muscle comprises groups of smaller, fusiform cells with weak, involuntary contractions. (a, b: ×200; c: ×300; All H&E)

Organization of a Skeletal Muscle

Thin layers of connective tissue surround and organize the contractile fibers in all three types of muscle, becoming particularly well-developed in skeletal muscle (Figures 10–3 and 10–4). The concentric organization given by these supportive layers resembles that in large peripheral nerves.

■ The **epimysium**, an external sheath of dense irregular connective tissue, surrounds the entire muscle. Septa of this tissue extend inward, carrying the larger nerves, blood vessels, and lymphatics of the muscle.

■ The **perimysium** occurs as a thin connective tissue layer immediately surrounding each bundle of muscle fibers termed a **fascicle** (Figure 10–3). A fascicle of muscle fibers makes up a functional unit in which the fibers work together most efficiently. Nerves, blood vessels, and lymphatics penetrate the perimysium to supply each fascicle.

■ Within each fascicle a very thin, delicate layer of reticular fibers and scattered fibroblasts, the **endomysium**, envelops the external lamina of individual muscle fibers. In addition to nerve fibers, capillaries form a rich network in the endomysium bringing O$_2$ to the muscle fibers (Figure 10–5).

Collagen in the external lamina and these connective tissue layers serves to transmit the mechanical forces generated by the contracting muscle fibers, and individual muscle fibers seldom extend from one end of a muscle to the other.

All three layers plus the dense irregular connective tissue of the deep fascia, which overlies the epimysium, have continuity with the dense regular connective tissue of a tendon at **myotendinous junctions**, which join a muscle to bone, skin, or another muscle (Figures 10–3 and 10–4c). Ultrastructural studies show that in these transitional regions, bundles of collagen fibers from the tendon become inserted among muscle fibers and associate directly with complex infoldings of sarcolemma.

Organization Within Muscle Fibers

Longitudinally sectioned skeletal muscle fibers display striations of alternating light and dark bands (Figure 10–6a). The highly organized sarcoplasm consists largely of long cylindrical filament bundles called **myofibrils** running parallel to the fiber's long axis (Figure 10–6b). The dark stripes on the myofibrils comprise the **A bands** (*an*isotropic or birefringent in polarized light microscopy); the light ones are the **I bands** (*iso*tropic, do not alter polarized light). In the TEM (Figure 10–6c)

FIGURE **10–2** Development of skeletal muscle.

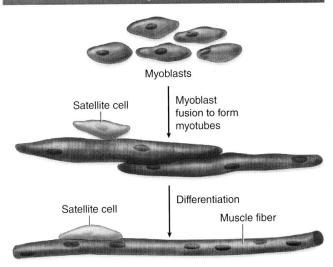

Myoblasts

Satellite cell

Myoblast fusion to form myotubes

Satellite cell

Differentiation

Muscle fiber

Skeletal muscle begins to differentiate when a subset of mesenchymal cells, called **myoblasts**, align and fuse together to make longer, multinucleated tubes called **myotubes**. Myotubes synthesize the proteins that assemble as myofilaments and gradually begin to show cross-striations by light microscopy. Differentiation continues, producing functional muscle fibers, with the nuclei displaced against the sarcolemma.

Part of the myoblast population does not fuse and differentiate, but remains as a group of mesenchymal cells called muscle **satellite cells** located on the external surface of muscle fibers. Satellite cells proliferate and produce new muscle fibers following muscle injury.

FIGURE **10–3** Organization of skeletal muscle.

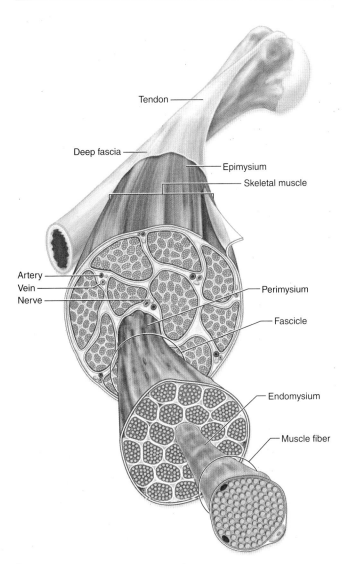

Tendon

Deep fascia

Epimysium

Skeletal muscle

Artery
Vein
Nerve

Perimysium

Fascicle

Endomysium

Muscle fiber

A thick layer of dense connective tissue called the **epimysium**, continuous with fascia and the tendon binding muscle to bone, encloses each skeletal muscle entirely. Large muscles contain several **fascicles** of muscle tissue, each wrapped in a thin layer of connective tissue, the **perimysium**. Within fascicles, individual muscle fibers (elongated multinuclear cells) exist surrounded by a delicate connective tissue layer, the **endomysium**.

each I band appears bisected by a darker transverse line, the **Z disc** (Ger. *zwischen*, between).

The functional subunit of the myofibril is the **sarcomere**, the force-generating and load-bearing apparatus of muscle fibers. Sarcomeres extend from Z disc to Z disc (Figure 10–6c) and average about 3 μm in length in resting muscle. Myofibrils, typically with diameters of only 1–2 μm, consist of an end-to-end repetitive arrangement of sarcomeres, with sarcoplasmic reticulum and most other organelles located between the myofibrils (Figure 10–7). The lateral registration of sarcomeres in adjacent myofibrils causes the entire muscle fiber to exhibit the characteristic pattern of transverse striations.

The A and I banding pattern of sarcomeres is due mainly to the regular arrangement of thick and thin **myofilaments**, composed of **myosin** and **F-actin**, respectively. Each myofibril comprises thousands of symmetrically arranged thick and thin myofilaments (Figure 10–7).

The thick myosin filaments are 1.5-μm long and 15-nm wide; they occupy the A band at the middle region of the sarcomere. **Myosin**, a large protein complex (~500 kDa), has two identical heavy chains and two pairs of light chains. Myosin heavy chains are thin, rodlike motor proteins (150 nm long and 2–3 nm thick) twisted together as the myosin tails (Figure 10–7).

Globular projections containing the four myosin light chains form a head at one end of each heavy chain. The myosin heads contain binding sites for actin, to form transient crossbridges between the thick and thin filaments, and for ATP, catalyzing energy release (**actomyosin ATPase activity**). Several hundred myosin complexes make up each thick filament, arranged with their rodlike portions aligned and their globular heads directed toward either end (Figure 10–7a).

FIGURE **10–4** Skeletal muscle.

(a) A cross section of striated muscle demonstrating all three layers of connective tissue and cell nuclei. The endomysium (**En**) surrounds individual muscle, and perimysium (**P**) encloses a group of muscle fibers comprising a fascicle. A thick epimysium (**E**) surrounds the entire muscle. All three of these tissues contain collagen types I and III (reticulin). (×200; H&E)

(b) An adjacent section immunohistochemically stained for laminin, which specifically stains the external laminae of the muscle fibers, surrounded by endomysium. (×400; Immunoperoxidase)

(c) Longitudinal section of a **myotendinous junction**. Tendons develop together with skeletal muscles and join muscles to the periosteum of bones. The dense collagen fibers of a tendon (**T**) are continuous with those in the connective tissue around muscle fibers (**M**), forming a strong unit that allows muscle contraction to move other structures. (×400; H&E)

FIGURE **10–5** Capillaries of skeletal muscle.

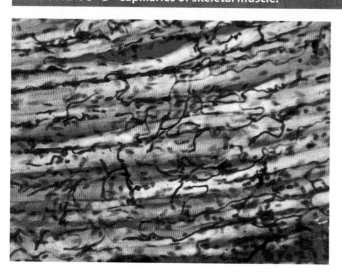

The blood vessels of this muscle were injected with a dark plastic polymer before tissue processing and longitudinal sectioning to reveal a rich network of capillaries in the endomysium surrounding muscle fibers. (×200; Giemsa with polarized light)

FIGURE **10–6** Striated skeletal muscle in longitudinal section.

Longitudinal sections reveal the striations characteristic of skeletal muscle.

(a) Parts of three muscle fibers are separated by very thin endomysium that includes one fibroblast nucleus (**F**). Muscle nuclei (**N**) are found against the sarcolemma. Along each fiber thousands of dark-staining **A** bands alternate with lighter **I** bands. (×200; H&E)

(b) At higher magnification, each fiber is seen to have three or four myofibrils, with their striations slightly out of alignment with one another. Myofibrils consist of cylindrical bundles of thick and thin myofilaments filling most of each muscle fiber. (×500; Giemsa)

(c) TEM showing one contractile unit (**sarcomere**) in the long series that comprises a myofibril. Its middle consists of an electron-dense **A** band bisected by a narrow, less dense region called the **H** zone. On each side of the A band the two lighter-stained **I** bands occur, each bisected by a dense **Z disc** marking one end of the sarcomere. Mitochondria (**M**), glycogen granules and small cisternae of SER occur around the Z discs. (×24,000)

(Figure 10-6c, reproduced with permission from Dr. Mikel H. Snow.)

The thin, double helical F-actin filaments, each 1.0 μm long and only 8 nm wide, run between the thick filaments. The G-actin monomers comprising these filaments each contain a binding site for myosin (Figure 10–7b). The thin filaments also have two tightly associated regulatory proteins (Figure 10–7b):

- **Tropomyosin**, a 40-nm-long coil of two polypeptide chains located in the groove between the two twisted actin strands, and
- **Troponin**, a complex of three subunits: TnT, which attaches to tropomyosin; TnC, which binds Ca^{2+}; and TnI, which regulates the actin-myosin interaction.

Troponin complexes attach at specific sites regularly spaced along each tropomyosin molecule.

Figure 10–8 shows the overall organization of important myofibril components. I bands consist only of the portions of the thin filaments that do not overlap the thick filaments in the A bands, explaining why I bands show lighter staining and electron density than A bands. Actin filaments are anchored on the Z disc by the actin-binding protein **α-actinin** and exhibit opposite polarity on each side of this disc (Figure 10–8c). An important accessory protein in I bands is **titin** (3700 kDa), the largest protein in the body. With both scaffolding and elastic properties, titin supports the ends of thick myofilaments and connects them to the Z disc (Figure 10–8c). Another large accessory protein, nebulin, binds each thin myofilament laterally, helps anchor them to α-actinin, and specifies the length of the actin polymers during myogenesis.

The A bands contain both the thick filaments and the overlapping portions of thin filaments. Close observation of the A band shows at its middle the presence of a lighter zone, called the H zone, which corresponds to a region with only the rodlike portions of the myosin molecules and no thin filaments (Figure 10–8c). Bisecting the H zone is the M line (Ger. *mitte*, middle; Figure 10–8d), containing a myosin-binding protein **myomesin** that holds the thick filaments in place, and **creatine kinase**. This enzyme catalyzes transfer of phosphate groups from phosphocreatine, a storage form of high-energy phosphate groups, to ADP, helping to supply ATP for muscle contraction.

Despite the many proteins present in sarcomeres, myosin and actin together represent over half of the total protein in striated muscle. The overlapping arrangement of thin and thick filaments within sarcomeres produces in TEM cross sections hexagonal patterns of structures, which were important in determining the functional organization of the filaments and other proteins in the myofibril (Figures 10–8b and 10–8e).

Sarcoplasmic Reticulum & Transverse Tubule System

In skeletal muscle fibers, the membranous smooth ER, called **sarcoplasmic reticulum**, contains pumps and other proteins for Ca^{2+} sequestration and surrounds the myofibrils (Figure 10–9). Calcium release from cisternae of the sarcoplasmic reticulum through voltage-gated Ca^{2+} channels is triggered by membrane depolarization produced by a motor nerve.

FIGURE **10–7** Molecules composing thin and thick filaments.

a Thick filament

b Thin filament

Myofilaments, which include both thick and thin filaments, consist of contractile protein arrays bundled within myofibrils.

(a) A thick myofilament, overall diameter 15 nm, contains 200–500 molecules of **myosin**.

(b) A thin filament, diameter 8 nm, contains **F-actin**, **tropomyosin**, and **troponin**. Figure 10-8 depicts the positional relationships between thick and thin myofilaments as well as their relative sizes.

Triggering simultaneous Ca²⁺ release from sarcoplasmic reticulum throughout the muscle fiber to produce uniform contraction of all myofibrils depends on long tubular infoldings of the sarcolemma called **transverse** or **T-tubules** (Figures 10–9 and 10–10). These fingerlike invaginations of cell membrane penetrate deeply into the sarcoplasm and encircle each myofibril near the aligned A- and I-band boundaries of sarcomeres.

Adjacent to each T-tubule are expanded **terminal cisternae** of sarcoplasmic reticulum. In longitudinal TEM sections this complex of a T-tubule with two terminal cisternae constitutes a **triad** (Figures 10–9 and 10–10). The triad complex allows depolarization of the sarcolemma in a T-tubule to affect the sarcoplasmic reticulum and trigger its release of Ca²⁺ ions around the thick and thin filaments, which initiates contraction of sarcomeres.

Mechanism of Contraction

Figure 10–11 summarizes the key molecular events of muscle contraction. During this process, neither the thick nor the thin

filaments change their length. Contraction occurs as the overlapping thin and thick filaments of each sarcomere slide past one another.

Contraction is induced when an action potential arrives at a synapse, the **neuromuscular junction (NMJ)**, and is transmitted along the T-tubules to terminal cisternae of the sarcoplasmic reticulum to trigger Ca²⁺ release. In a resting muscle the myosin heads cannot bind actin because the binding sites are blocked by the troponin-tropomyosin complex on the F-actin filaments. Calcium ions released upon neural stimulation bind troponin, changing its shape and moving tropomyosin on the F-actin to expose the myosin-binding active sites and allow crossbridges to form. Binding actin produces a conformational change or pivot in the myosins, which pulls the thin filaments farther into the A band, toward the Z disc (Figure 10–11).

Energy for the myosin head pivot that pulls actin comes from hydrolysis of ATP bound to the myosin heads, after which myosin binds another ATP and detaches from actin. In the continued presence of Ca²⁺ and ATP, these attach-pivot-detach events occur in repeating cycles, each about

FIGURE **10–8** Structure of a myofibril: A series of sarcomeres.

(a) The diagram shows that each muscle fiber contains several parallel bundles called **myofibrils**.

(b) Each myofibril consists of a long series of sarcomeres, separated by Z discs and containing thick and thin filaments which overlap in certain regions.

(c) Thin filaments are actin filaments with one end bound to the protein α-**actinin** in the Z disc. Thick filaments consist of bundled myosins, which span the entire A band and bind at the bundle's middle to proteins of the M line. Each end of the thick filament associates with a very large protein called **titin**, which has spring-like domains and crosses the I bands to attach at the Z disc.

(d) The molecular organization and different protein densities within the sarcomeres leads to staining differences causing the dark- and light-staining bands visible by light microscopy and TEM. (×28,000)

(e) With the TEM an oblique section of myofibrils includes both **A** and **I** bands and shows hexagonal patterns that indicate the relationships between thin and thick myofilaments and other proteins, as shown in part **b** of this figure. Thin and thick filaments assemble with each myosin bundle in contact with six actin filaments. Mitochondria in cross section and SER cisternae occur between the myofibrils. (×45,000)

FIGURE 10–9 Organization of a skeletal muscle fiber.

Skeletal muscle fibers consist mainly of myofibrils. Each myofibril extends the length of the fiber, surrounded by parts of the sarcoplasmic reticulum. The sarcolemma has deep invaginations called T-tubules, each of which becomes associated with two terminal cisternae of the sarcoplasmic reticulum. A T-tubule and its two associated terminal cisternae comprise a "triad" of small spaces along the surface of the myofibrils.

50 milliseconds, which rapidly shorten the sarcomere and contract the muscle (Figures 10–11 and 10–12). A single muscle contraction results from hundreds of these cycles.

When the neural impulse stops and levels of free Ca²⁺ ions diminish, tropomyosin again covers the myosin-binding sites on actin and the filaments passively slide back and sarcomeres return to their relaxed length (Figure 10–11). In the complete absence of ATP, the actin-myosin crossbridges become stable, which accounts for the rigidity of skeletal muscles (**rigor mortis**) that occurs as mitochondrial activity stops after death.

Innervation

Myelinated motor nerves branch out within the perimysium, where each nerve gives rise to several unmyelinated terminal twigs that penetrate the endomysium and form synapses with individual muscle fibers. Schwann cells enclose the small axon branches and cover their points of contact with the muscle cells (Figure 10–13); the external lamina of the Schwann cell fuses with that on the sarcolemma. Each axonal branch forms a dilated termination situated within a trough on the muscle cell surface, forming part of the synapses termed neuromuscular junctions or **motor end plates (MEPs)** (Figure 10–13). As in all synapses, the axon terminal contains mitochondria and numerous synaptic vesicles; here the vesicles contain the neurotransmitter **acetylcholine**. A **synaptic cleft** lies between axon and muscle in these junctions. Adjacent to the synaptic cleft, the sarcolemma is thrown into numerous deep **junctional folds**, which provide for greater postsynaptic surface area and more transmembrane acetylcholine receptors.

When a **nerve action potential** reaches the MEP, acetylcholine is liberated from the axon terminal, diffuses across the cleft, and binds to its receptors in the folded sarcolemma. The **acetylcholine receptor** contains a nonselective cation channel that opens upon neurotransmitter binding, allowing influx of cations, depolarizing the sarcolemma, and producing the **muscle action potential**. Acetylcholine quickly dissociates from its receptors, and free neurotransmitter is removed from the synaptic cleft by the extracellular enzyme **acetylcholinesterase**, preventing prolonged contact of the transmitter with its receptors.

FIGURE **10–10** Transverse or T-tubule system and triads.

Transverse tubules represent invaginations of the sarcolemma that penetrate deeply into the muscle fiber around all myofibrils.

(a) TEM cross section of fish muscle shows portions of two fibers and the endomysium (**E**) between them. Several transverse or T-tubules (**T**) occur here, perpendicular to the fiber surface, penetrating between myofibrils (**M**). (×50,000)

(b) Higher-magnification TEM of skeletal muscle in longitudinal section shows four membranous triads (**Tr**) cut transversely near the **A**-band-**I**-band junctions. Each triad consists of a central

transverse tubule (**T**) and two adjacent terminal cisterns (**TC**) extending from the sarcoplasmic reticulum. The **Z** disc appears centrally located here. Besides the triad elements, sarcoplasm surrounding the myofibril also contains dense glycogen granules (**G**).

Components of the triad allow cyclic release of Ca^{2+} from SR cisternae and its sequestration again which occurs during muscle contraction and relaxation.

Figure 10–11 begins with a diagram showing the functional association between SR cisternae and T-tubules. (×90,000)

As discussed with Figure 10–11, the muscle action potential moves along the sarcolemma and along T-tubules, which penetrate deeply into sarcoplasm. At triads the depolarization signal triggers the release of Ca^{2+} from terminal cisterns of the sarcoplasmic reticulum, initiating the contraction cycle.

An axon from a single motor neuron can form MEPs with one or many muscle fibers. Innervation of single muscle fibers by single motor neurons provides precise control of muscle activity and occurs, for example, in the extraocular muscles for eye movements. Larger muscles with coarser movements have motor axons that typically branch profusely and innervate 100 or more muscle fibers. In this case, the single axon and all the muscle fibers in contact with its branches make up a **motor unit**. Individual striated muscle fibers do not show graded contraction—they contract either all the way or not at all. To vary the force of contraction, the fibers within a muscle fascicle do not all contract at the same time. With large muscles composed of many motor units, the firing of a single motor axon will generate tension proportional to the number of muscle fibers it innervates. Thus, the number of motor units and their variable size control the intensity and precision of a muscle contraction.

Table 10–1 summarizes key features of skeletal muscle cells, connective tissue, contraction, and innervation.

⟩⟩ MEDICAL APPLICATION

Myasthenia gravis is an autoimmune disorder that involves circulating antibodies against proteins of acetylcholine receptors. Antibody binding to the antigenic sites interferes with acetylcholine activation of their receptors, leading to intermittent periods of skeletal muscle weakness. As the body attempts to correct the condition, junctional folds of sarcolemma with affected receptors are internalized, digested by lysosomes, and replaced by newly formed receptors. These receptors, however, are again made unresponsive to acetylcholine by similar antibodies, and the disease follows a progressive course. The extraocular muscles of the eyes are commonly the first affected.

Muscle Spindles & Tendon Organs

Striated muscles and myotendinous junctions contain sensory receptors that act as proprioceptors (L. *proprius*, one's own + *capio*, to take), providing the central nervous system (CNS) with data from the musculoskeletal system. Among the muscle fascicles are stretch detectors known as **muscle spindles**, approximately 2 mm long and 0.1 mm wide (Figure 10–14a). A muscle spindle is encapsulated by modified perimysium,

FIGURE **10–11** Events of muscle contraction.

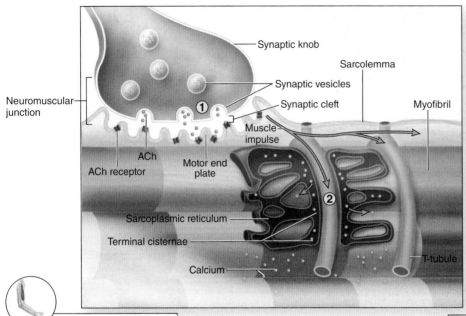

Synaptic knob

Sarcolemma

Synaptic vesicles

Myofibril

Neuromuscular junction

Synaptic cleft

①

Muscle impulse

②

ACh

Motor end plate

ACh receptor

Sarcoplasmic reticulum

Terminal cisternae

T-tubule

Calcium

① A nerve impulse triggers release of ACh from the synaptic knob into the synaptic cleft. ACh binds to ACh receptors in the motor end plate of the neuromuscular junction, initiating a muscle impulse in the sarcolemma of the muscle fiber.

② As the muscle impulse spreads quickly from the sarcolemma along T tubules, calcium ions are released from terminal cisternae into the sarcoplasm.

Active sites blocked

⑤ When the impulse stops, calcium ions are actively transported into the sarcoplasmic reticulum, tropomyosin re-covers active sites, and filaments passively slide back to their relaxed state.

Actin

Troponin

Active site

Tropomyosin

Calcium

Crossbridge

③ Calcium ions bind to troponin. Troponin changes shape, moving tropomyosin on the actin to expose active sites on actin molecules of thin filaments. Myosin heads of thick filaments attach to exposed active sites to form crossbridges.

Active site

Calcium

Thin filament

Thick filament

ATP → ADP + P

④ Myosin heads pivot, moving thin filaments toward the sarcomere center. ATP binds myosin heads and is broken down into ADP and P. Myosin heads detach from thin filaments and return to their prepivot position. The repeating cycle of *attach-pivot-detach-return* slides thick and thin filaments past one another. The sarcomere shortens and the muscle contracts. The cycle continues as long as calcium ions remain bound to troponin to keep active sites exposed.

FIGURE **10–12** Sliding filaments and sarcomere shortening in contraction.

a Relaxed skeletal muscle

b Contracted skeletal muscle

Diagrams and TEM micrographs show sarcomere shortening during skeletal muscle contraction. **(a)** In the relaxed state the sarcomere, I band, and H zone exist at their expanded length. The springlike action of titin molecules, which span the I band, helps pull thin and thick filaments past one another in relaxed muscle.

(b) During muscle contraction, the Z discs at the sarcomere boundaries are drawn closer together moved toward the ends of thick filaments in the A band. **(c)** During contraction the I bands become increasingly narrow and the titin molecules increasingly compressed.

with concentric layers of flattened cells, containing interstitial fluid and a few thin muscle fibers filled with nuclei and called **intrafusal fibers** (Figure 10–14). Several sensory nerve axons penetrate each muscle spindle and wrap around individual intrafusal fibers. Muscle spindles detect changes in length (distension) of the surrounding (extrafusal) muscle fibers caused by body movements and the sensory nerves relay this information to the spinal cord. Different types of sensory and intrafusal fibers mediate reflexes of varying complexity to help maintain posture and to regulate the activity of opposing muscle groups involved in motor activities such as walking.

A similar role is played in myotendenous junctions by **Golgi tendon organs**, much smaller encapsulated structures that enclose sensory axons penetrating among the collagen bundles (Figure 10–14a). Tendon organs detect changes in tension within tendons produced by muscle contraction and

act to inhibit motor nerve activity if tension becomes excessive. Because both of these proprioceptors detect increases in tension, they help regulate the amount of effort required to perform movements that call for variable amounts of muscular force.

›› MEDICAL APPLICATION

Dystrophin is a large actin-binding protein located just inside the sarcolemma of skeletal muscle fibers, which is involved in the functional organization of myofibrils. Research on **Duchenne muscular dystrophy** revealed that mutations of the dystrophin gene can lead to defective linkages between the cytoskeleton and the extracellular matrix (ECM). Muscle contractions can disrupt these weak linkages, causing the atrophy of muscle fibers typical of this disease.

FIGURE **10–13** The neuromuscular junction (NMJ).

Before terminating in a skeletal muscle, each motor axon bundled in the nerve subdivides into many branches, each of which forms a synapse with a different muscle fiber.

(a) Silver staining can reveal the nerve bundle (**NB**), the terminal axonal twigs, and the motor end plates (**MEPs**, also called neuromuscular junctions or NMJ) on striated muscle fibers (**S**). (×1200)

(b) An SEM shows the branching ends of a motor axon, each covered by an extension of the last Schwann cell and expanded terminally as an MEP embedded in a groove in the external lamina of the muscle fiber.

(c) Diagram of the enclosed portion of the SEM indicating key features of a typical MEP: synaptic vesicles of acetylcholine (**ACh**), a synaptic cleft, and a postsynaptic membrane. This membrane, the sarcolemma, has many folds increasing the number of ACh receptors at the MEP. Receptor binding initiates muscle fiber depolarization, which propagates to the deeper myofibrils via the T-tubules.

TABLE **10–1**	Important comparisons of the three types of muscle.		
	Skeletal Muscle	**Cardiac Muscle**	**Smooth Muscle**
Fibers	Single multinucleated cells	Aligned cells in branching arrangement	Single small, closely packed fusiform cells
Cell/fiber shape and size	Cylindrical, 10–100 μm diameter, many cm long	Cylindrical, 10–20 μm diameter, 50–100 μm long	Fusiform, diameter 0.2–10 μm, length 50–200 μm
Striations	Present	Present	Absent
Location of nuclei	Peripheral, adjacent to sarcolemma	Central	Central, at widest part of cell
T tubules	Center of triads at A-I junctions	In dyads at Z discs	Absent; caveolae may be functionally similar
Sarcoplasmic reticulum (SR)	Well-developed, with two terminal cisterns per sarcomere in triads with T tubule	Less well-developed, one small terminal cistern per sarcomere in dyad with T tubule	Irregular smooth ER without distinctive organization
Special structural features	Very well-organized sarcomeres, SR, and transverse tubule system	Intercalated discs joining cell, with many adherent and gap junctions	Gap junctions, caveolae, dense bodies
Control of contraction	Troponin C binds Ca^{2+}, moving tropomyosin and exposing actin for myosin binding	Similar to that of skeletal muscle	Actin-myosin binding occurs with myosin phosphorylation by MLCK triggered when calmodulin binds Ca^{2+}
Connective tissue organization	Endomysium, perimysium, and epimysium	Endomysium; subendocardial and subpericardial CT layers	Endomysium and less-organized CT sheaths
Major locations	Skeletal muscles, tongue, diaphragm, eyes, and upper esophagus	Heart	Blood vessels, digestive and respiratory tracts, uterus, bladder, and other organs
Key function	Voluntary movements	Automatic (involuntary) pumping of blood	Involuntary movements
Efferent innervation	Motor	Autonomic	Autonomic
Contractions	All-or-none, triggered at motor end plates	All-or-none, intrinsic (beginning at nodes of conducting fibers)	Partial, slow, often spontaneous, wavelike and rhythmic
Cell response to increased load	Hypertrophy (increase in fiber size)	Hypertrophy	Hypertrophy and hyperplasia (increase in cell/fiber number)
Capacity for regeneration	Limited, involving satellite cells mainly	Very poor	Good, involving mitotic activity of muscle cells

Skeletal Muscle Fiber Types

Skeletal muscles such as those that move the eyes and eyelids need to contract rapidly, while others such as those for bodily posture must maintain tension for longer periods while resisting fatigue. These metabolic differences are possible because of varied expression in muscle fibers of contractile or regulatory protein isoforms and other factors affecting oxygen delivery and use. Classification of different skeletal muscle fiber types utilizes (1) their maximal rate of contraction (fast or slow) and (2) their major pathway for ATP synthesis (oxidative phosphorylation or glycolysis). Fast versus slow rates of fiber contraction are due largely to myosin isoforms with different maximal rates of ATP hydrolysis.

Histochemical staining can identify fibers with differing amounts of "fast" and "slow" ATPases (Figure 10–15). Other histological features reflecting metabolic differences among muscle fibers include the density of surrounding capillaries, the number of mitochondria, and levels of glycogen and

FIGURE **10–14** Sensory receptors associated with skeletal muscle.

Capsule

Intrafusal muscle fibers — Muscle spindle

Stretch receptor

Afferent nerve fibers

Extrafusal muscle fiber

Golgi tendon organ

Tendon

a

b

(a) The diagram shows both a **muscle spindle** and a **tendon organ**. Muscle spindles have **afferent sensory** and **efferent motor** nerve fibers associated with modified muscle fibers called **intrafusal fibers**. The size of the spindle is here exaggerated relative to the extrafusal fibers to show better the nuclei packed in the intrafusal fibers. Both types of sensory receptors provide the CNS with information concerning degrees of stretch and tension within the musculoskeletal system.

(b) A TEM cross section near the end of a muscle spindle shows the capsule (**C**), lightly myelinated axons (**MA**) of a sensory nerve, and the intrafusal muscle fibers (**MF**). These thin fibers differ from the ordinary skeletal muscle fibers in having very few myofibrils. Their many nuclei can either be closely aligned (nuclear chain fibers) or piled in a central dilation (nuclear bag fibers) as shown in (a). Muscle satellite cells (**SC**) also occur within the external lamina of the intrafusal fibers. (×3600)

(Figure 10-14b, reproduced with permission from Dr. Mikel H. Snow.)

myoglobin, a globular sarcoplasmic protein similar to hemoglobin that contains iron atoms and allows for O_2 storage.

Each of these features exists as a continuum in skeletal muscle fibers, but fiber diversity is divided into three major types:

- **Slow oxidative** muscle fibers, adapted for slow contractions over long periods without fatigue, have many mitochondria, many surrounding capillaries, and much myoglobin, all features that make fresh tissue rich in these fibers dark or red in color.
- **Fast glycolytic** fibers are specialized for rapid, short-term contraction, having few mitochondria or capillaries and depending largely on anaerobic metabolism of glucose derived from stored glycogen, features which make such fibers appear white. Rapid contractions lead to rapid fatigue as lactic acid produced by glycolysis accumulates.
- **Fast oxidative-glycolytic** fibers have physiological and histological features intermediate between those of the other two types.

Table 10–2 summarizes these and other characteristics of the three skeletal muscle fiber types. The metabolic type of each fiber is influenced by the rate of impulse conduction along its motor nerve supply, making all fibers of a motor unit similar. Most skeletal muscles receive motor input from multiple nerves and contain a mixture of fiber types (Figure 10–15). Determining the fiber types in needle biopsies of skeletal muscle helps in the diagnosis of specific myopathies (*myo* + Gr. *pathos*, suffering), motor neuron diseases, and other causes of muscle atrophy. Different fiber types also exist in cardiac muscle at various locations within the heart and in smooth muscle of many organs.

› **CARDIAC MUSCLE**

During embryonic development, mesenchymal cells around the primitive heart tube line up into chainlike arrays. Rather than fusing into multinucleated cells/fibers as in developing skeletal muscle, the aligned **cardiac muscle** cells form fibers

FIGURE **10–15** Skeletal muscle fiber types.

Transverse section of a skeletal muscle stained histochemically for myosin ATPase at acidic pH, which reveals activity of
the "slow" ATPase and shows the distribution of the three main
fiber types. Slow oxidative (**SO**) or type I fibers have high levels
of acidic ATPase activity and stain the darkest. Fast glycolytic
(**FG**) or type IIb fibers stain the lightest. Fast oxidative-glycolytic
(**FOG**) or type IIa fibers show intermediate staining between the
other two types (×40). ATPase histochemistry of unfixed, cryostat
section, pH 4.2.

TABLE **10–2** | Major characteristics of skeletal muscle fiber types.

	Slow, Oxidative Fibers (Type I)	Fast, Oxidative-Glycolytic Fibers (Type IIa)	Fast, Glycolytic Fibers (Type IIb)
Mitochondria	Numerous	Numerous	Sparse
Capillaries	Numerous	Numerous	Sparse
Fiber diameter	Small	Intermediate	Large
Size of motor unit	Small	Intermediate	Large
Myoglobin content	High (red fibers)	High (red fibers)	Low (white fibers)
Glycogen content	Low	Intermediate	High
Major source of ATP	Oxidative phosphorylation	Oxidative phosphorylation	Anaerobic glycolysis
Glycolytic enzyme activity	Low	Intermediate	High
Rate of fatigue	Slow	Intermediate	Fast
Myosin-ATPase activity	Low	High	High
Speed of contraction	Slow	Fast	Fast
Typical major locations	Postural muscles of back	Major muscles of legs	Extraocular muscles

having complex cell-cell junctions with abundant interdigitating processes (Figure 10–16). Myocardial cells within one such fiber often branch and join with cells in adjacent fibers. Consequently, the heart consists of tightly knit bundles of cells, interwoven in spiraling layers that provide for a characteristic wave of contraction that resembles wringing out of the heart ventricles.

Mature cardiac muscle cells are 15–30 μm in diameter and 85–120 μm long, with a striated banding pattern comparable to that of skeletal muscle. Unlike skeletal muscle, however, each cell of the cardiac muscle fiber usually has only one centrally located nucleus. A delicate sheath of endomysium with a rich capillary network surrounds each fiber. A thicker perimysium separates bundles and layers of cardiac muscle fibers and in specific areas (described in Chapter 11) forms larger masses of fibrous connective tissue comprising the "cardiac skeleton."

Their mode of development produces a unique structural characteristic of cardiac muscle: **intercalated discs** seen as transverse lines crossing the fibers at irregular intervals where the myocardial cells join. These represent the interdigitated faces between adjacent cells and include many junctional complexes (Figure 10–16). The transverse regions of these irregular, step-like discs are highly interdigitated and contain many **desmosomes** and adhesive strips called **fascia adherens** junctions, which together provide strong intercellular adhesion during the cells' constant contractile activity. The laterally oriented regions of each step-like intercalated disc run parallel to the myofibrils and include numerous **gap junctions**, which provide ionic continuity between the cells. These regions serve as "electrical synapses," promoting rapid impulse conduction through many cardiac muscle cells simultaneously and contraction of many adjacent cells as a unit.

The structure and function of the contractile apparatus in cardiac muscle cells are essentially the same as in skeletal muscle (Figure 10–17). Mitochondria occupy up to 40% of the cell volume, higher than in slow oxidative skeletal muscle fibers. Fatty acids, the major fuel of the heart, are stored as triglycerides in small lipid droplets. Glycogen granules as well as perinuclear lipofuscin pigment granules may also occur.

Muscle of the heart ventricles is much thicker than that of the atria, reflecting its role in pumping blood through the cardiovascular system. Well-developed T-tubules in ventricular muscle fibers have large lumens and penetrate the sarcoplasm in the vicinity of the myofibrils' Z discs. In atrial muscle, T-tubules are much smaller or entirely absent. Sarcoplasmic reticulum is less well-organized in cardiac compared to skeletal muscle fibers. The junctions between its terminal cisterns and T-tubules typically involve only one structure of each type, forming profiles called **dyads** rather than triads in TEM sections. Components of this cardiac muscle transverse tubule system have the same basic functions as their counterparts in skeletal muscle.

Cardiac muscle fiber contraction occurs intrinsically and spontaneously, as evidenced by the continued contraction of myocardial cells in tissue culture. As with skeletal muscle fibers, contraction of individual myocardial fibers is all-or-none. Impulses for rhythmic contraction (or heartbeat) are regulated and coordinated locally by nodes of unique myocardial fibers specialized for this activity, as discussed in Chapter 11. Autonomic innervation at the nodes of conducting cells modify the contraction rate, with the sympathetic nerve supply accelerating and the parasympathetic supply decreasing the frequency of impulses.

Secretory granules about 0.2–0.3 μm in diameter occur near atrial muscle nuclei, associated with small Golgi complexes (Figure 10–17b). These granules release the peptide hormone atrial natriuretic factor (ANF), which acts on target cells in the kidney to affect Na^+ excretion and water balance. Thus, contractile cells of the heart's atria also serve an endocrine function.

Table 10–1 summarizes key features of cardiac muscle cells, with comparisons to those of skeletal muscle.

> ## ❯❯ MEDICAL APPLICATION
>
> The most common injury sustained by cardiac muscle occurs due to **ischemia**, lack of oxygen when coronary arteries undergo gradual occlusion during cardiovascular disease. Lacking muscle satellite cells, adult mammalian cardiac muscle has little potential to regenerate after injury. However, certain fish and amphibians, as well as newborn mice, do form new muscle when the heart is partially removed, despite the lack of satellite cells. Research on the possibility of mammalian **heart muscle regeneration** builds on work with the animal models, focusing primarily on the potential of mesenchymal stem cells to form new, site-specific muscle.

❯ SMOOTH MUSCLE

Smooth muscle becomes specialized for slow, steady contraction under the influence of autonomic nerves and various hormones. This type of muscle represents a major component of blood vessels and of the digestive, respiratory, urinary, and reproductive systems. Fibers of smooth muscle (also called **visceral muscle**) develop as elongated, tapering, and nonstriated cells, each enclosed by an external lamina and a network of type I and type III collagen fibers comprising the endomysium (Figure 10–18).

Smooth muscle cells/fibers range in length from 20 μm in small blood vessels to 500 μm in the pregnant uterus. At each cell's central, broadest part, where its diameter is 5–10 μm, lies a single elongated nucleus. The cells stain uniformly along their lengths and close packing is achieved with the narrow ends of each cell adjacent to the broad parts of neighboring cells. With this arrangement, cross sections of smooth muscle show a range of cell diameters, with only the largest cell profiles containing nuclei (Figures 10–18 and 10–19a). All adjacent cells/fibers possess abundant gap junctions. The borders of the cell become scalloped when smooth muscle contracts and the nucleus becomes distorted (Figure 10–20). Mitochondria,

FIGURE **10–16** Cardiac muscle: Intercalated discs.

(a)

Desmosome

Intercalated disc

Openings of transverse tubules

Intercalated disc

Gap junction

Cardiac muscle cell

Sarcolemma

Nucleus

Mitochondrion

Myofibril

(a) The diagram of cardiac muscle cells indicates their characteristic features. The fibers consist of separate cells joined in a series at the **intercalated discs**, which TEM reveals to have step-like structures. The transverse regions of the discs are highly interdigitated and have abundant **desmosomes** and other adherent junctions for firm adhesion (upper box in diagram), while longitudinal regions of the discs have numerous **gap junctions** (lower box).

Cardiac muscle cells show central nuclei and myofibrils which are usually sparser and less well-organized than those of skeletal muscle. The cells are often branched, allowing the fibers to interweave in a complicated, more helical arrangement within fascicles, which helps produce an efficient, wringing contraction mechanism for emptying the heart.

(b) Light microscopy of cardiac muscle in longitudinal section show euchromatic nuclei (**N**) in the center of the muscle fibers

and widely spaced intercalated discs (**I**) that cross the fibers. These irregular intercalated discs should not be confused with the repetitive, much more closely spaced striations (**S**), which are like those of skeletal muscle but less well-defined. A few elongated nuclei of fibroblasts in endomysium are also present. (×200; H&E)

(c) TEM showing an intercalated disc with a step-like structure between adjacent cardiac muscle cells. As shown here transverse disc regions have many short, interdigitating processes with numerous electron-dense desmosomes (**D**) and adherent junctions called **fascia adherens (F)** which provide firm adhesion between the cells. Abundant in the latera regions of the disc, gap junctions (**G**) join the cells physiologically. The sarcoplasm has numerous mitochondria (**M**) and myofibrillar structures like those of skeletal muscle but slightly less organized. (×65,000)

FIGURE **10–17** Cardiac muscle ultrastructure.

(a) TEM of cardiac muscle shows abundant mitochondria (**M**) and rather sparse sarcoplasmic reticulum (**SR**) in the areas between myofibrils. Compared to those of skeletal muscle, T-tubules here become less well organized and usually associate with one expanded terminal cistern of SR, forming dyads (**D**) rather than the triads. Functionally, these structures are similar in these two muscle types. (×30,000)

(b) Muscle cells from the heart atrium show the presence of membrane-bound granules (**G**), mainly aggregated at the nuclear poles. These granules occur most abundantly in muscle cells of

the right atrium (~600 per cell), but smaller quantities also appear in the left atrium and the ventricles. The atrial granules contain the precursor of a polypeptide hormone, **atrial natriuretic factor (ANF)**. ANF targets cells of the kidneys to bring about sodium and water loss (natriuresis and diuresis). This hormone thus opposes the actions of aldosterone and antidiuretic hormone, whose effects on kidneys result in sodium and water conservation. (×10,000)

(Figure 10-17b, reproduced with permission from Dr J.C. Nogueira, Department of Morphology, Federal University of Minas Gerais, Belo Horizonte, Brazil.)

polyribosomes, RER, and Golgi apparatus vesicles occur concentrated near the cell nucleus. Smooth muscle cell surfaces often display numerous small plasmalemma invaginations resembling caveolae.

The fibers have rudimentary sarcoplasmic reticulum but lack T-tubules, the latter unnecessary in these smaller, tapering cells bearing many gap junctions. The **caveolae** of smooth muscle cells contain the major ion channels controlling Ca^{2+} release from sarcoplasmic cisternae that initiates contraction of myofibrils. The characteristic contractile activity of smooth muscle involves myofibrillar arrays of actin and myosin organized differently from those of striated muscle. In smooth muscle cells, bundles of thin and thick myofilaments crisscross the sarcoplasm obliquely. The myosin filaments have a less regular arrangement among the thin filaments and fewer cross bridges than in striated muscle. Moreover, thin filaments of smooth muscle lack troponin and have tropomyosin of uncertain function. Here these proteins are replaced in the contractile apparatus with two others, **calmodulin** and Ca^{2+}-sensitive **myosin light-chain kinase (MLCK)**, respectively.

The contraction mechanism itself, however, basically resembles that in striated muscle.

As shown in Figure 10–20, the actin myofilaments insert into anchoring cytoplasmic and plasmalemma-associated **dense bodies**, which contain α-actinin and serve functionally like the Z discs of striated and cardiac muscle. An elaborate array of 10 nm intermediate filaments composed of desmin and attached to the dense bodies also occur in smooth muscle cells. The dense bodies include cadherins of desmosomes linking adjacent smooth muscle cells. Dense bodies in smooth muscle cells thus serve as points for transmitting the contractile force not only within the cells, but also between adjacent cells (Figure 10–20). The endomysium and other connective tissue layers help combine the force generated by the smooth muscle fibers into a concerted action, for example, peristalsis in the intestine.

Smooth muscle contraction occurs without voluntary motor control and its fibers typically lack well-defined neuromuscular junctions. Contraction is usually stimulated by autonomic nerves, but in the gastrointestinal tract control of

FIGURE **10–18** Smooth muscle.

Cells or fibers of smooth muscle consist of long, tapering structures with elongated nuclei centrally located at the cell's widest part.

(a) In most of the digestive tract and other similar structures smooth muscle becomes organized into two layers which contract in a coordinated manner to produce a wave that moves the tract's contents in a process termed **peristalsis**. In smooth muscle of the small intestine wall cut in cross section, cells of the inner circular (**IC**) layer are cut lengthwise, and cells of the outer longitudinal layer (**OL**) are cut transversely. Only some nuclei (arrows) of the latter cells occur in the plane of section, causing many cells to appear devoid of nuclei. (×140; H&E)

(b) Section of smooth muscle in bladder shows interwoven bundles of muscle fibers in cross section (**XS**) and longitudinal section (**LS**) with the same fascicle. Abundant collagen occurs in the branching perimysium (**P**), but the endomysium can barely be seen by routine staining. (×140; Mallory trichrome)

(c) Section stained only for reticulin reveals the thin endomysium around each fiber, with more reticulin in the connective tissue of small arteries (**A**). Reticulin fibers associated with the basal laminae of smooth muscle cells help hold the cells together as a functional unit during the slow, rhythmic contractions of this tissue. (×200; Silver)

smooth muscle activity also involves various paracrine secretions and in the uterus oxytocin from the pituitary gland.

Axons of autonomic nerves passing through smooth muscle have periodic swellings or varicosities that lie in close contact with muscle fibers. Synaptic vesicles in the varicosities release a neurotransmitter, usually acetylcholine or norepinephrine, which diffuses and binds receptors in the sarcolemmae of muscle cells. Little or no specialized structure defines such synaptic junctions. As in cardiac muscle, stimulation is propagated to more distant fibers via gap junctions that allow all the smooth muscle cells to contract synchronously or in a coordinated manner.

In addition to contractile activity, smooth muscle cells also supplement fibroblast activity, synthesizing collagen, elastin, and proteoglycans, with a major influence on the ECM in tissues with many such cells. Active synthesis of ECM by the small cells/fibers of smooth muscle may reflect less specialization for strong contractions than in skeletal and cardiac muscle and resembles this synthetic function in other contractile cells, such as myofibroblasts and pericytes.

Table 10–1 summarizes key histologic and functional features of smooth muscle, with comparisons to those of skeletal and cardiac muscle.

FIGURE 10–19 Smooth muscle ultrastructure.

(a) TEM of a transverse section of smooth muscle showing several cells sectioned at various points along their lengths, yielding profiles of various diameters with only the largest here containing a nucleus. Thick and thin filaments do not get organized into myofibril bundles and there are few mitochondria **(M)**. A sparse external lamina surrounds each cell and dark reticular fibers appear abundantly in the ECM. A small unmyelinated nerve **(N)** is also seen between the cells. (×6650)

(b) Longitudinal section showing several dense bodies **(DB)** in the cytoplasm and at the cell membrane. Both thin filaments and intermediate filaments attach to the dense bodies. Near the nucleus **(N)** are mitochondria, glycogen granules, and Golgi complexes. In both photos the cell membranes show invaginations called caveolae **(C)** with various membrane proteins for cell signaling and for regulating uptake and release of Ca²⁺ from sarcoplasmic reticulum. (×9000)

FIGURE 10–20 Smooth muscle contraction.

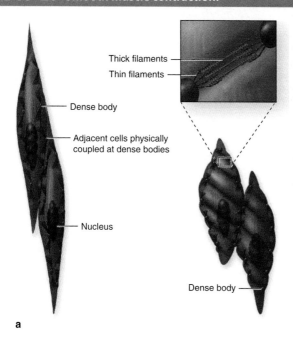

Thick filaments
Thin filaments
Dense body
Adjacent cells physically coupled at dense bodies
Nucleus
Dense body

a

b

Most molecules that allow contraction are similar in the three types of muscle, but the contractile filaments of smooth muscle are oriented at oblique angles to the long axis of the cell, resulting in a twisting of the smooth muscle cells during contraction.

(a) The diagram shows that thin filaments attach to **dense bodies** located at the cell membrane and deep in the cytoplasm, with the connection mediated by α-actinin in the dense bodies. Dense bodies also serve as attachment sites for intermediate filaments and for intercellular adhesive junctions. This arrangement of both

the cytoskeleton and contractile apparatus allows the multicellular tissue to contract as a unit, providing better efficiency and force.

(b) Micrograph showing a contracted **(C)** region of smooth muscle, with contraction decreasing the cell length and deforming the nuclei. The long nuclei of individual muscle fibers assume a corkscrew shape when the fibers contract, reflecting the cell twisting with contraction. Connective tissue **(CT)** of the perimysium outside the muscle fascicle is stained blue here. (×240; Mallory trichrome)

>> **MEDICAL APPLICATION**

Benign tumors called **leiomyomas** commonly develop from smooth muscle fibers but are seldom problematic. They most frequently occur in the wall of the uterus, where they are more commonly called **fibroids** and where they can become sufficiently large to produce painful pressure and unexpected bleeding.

REGENERATION OF MUSCLE TISSUE

The three types of adult muscle have different potentials for regeneration after injury, also summarized in Table 10–1.

In skeletal muscle, although the multinucleated cells cannot undergo mitosis, the tissue can still display limited regeneration. The sparse population of mesenchymal **satellite cells** lying inside the external lamina of each muscle fiber serve as the source of regenerating cells. Satellite cells occur as inactive, reserve myoblasts that persist after muscle differentiation.

After injury, the normally quiescent satellite cells become activated, proliferating, and fusing to form new skeletal muscle fibers. A similar activity of satellite cells has been implicated in muscle growth after extensive exercise, a process in which they fuse with existing fibers to increase muscle mass beyond that which occurs by cell/fiber hypertrophy. Following major traumatic injuries, scarring and excessive connective tissue growth interferes with skeletal muscle regeneration.

Cardiac muscle lacks satellite cells and shows very little regenerative capacity beyond early childhood. Defects or damage (eg, infarcts) to heart muscle are generally replaced by proliferating fibroblasts and growth of connective tissue, forming only myocardial scars.

Smooth muscle, composed of simpler and smaller mononucleated cells, can undertake a more active regenerative response. After injury, viable smooth muscle cells undergo mitosis and replace the damaged tissue. As discussed in Chapter 11, contractile pericytes from the walls of small blood vessels participate in the repair of vascular smooth muscle.

Muscle Tissue SUMMARY OF KEY POINTS

- Three major types of muscle occur: (1) **skeletal** or striated muscle, (2) **cardiac** muscle, and (3) **smooth** or visceral muscle.
- **Skeletal muscle cells** are very **long, multinucleated fibers**, cylindrically shaped and with **diameters up to 100 μm**.
- The **sarcolemma** of each fiber is surrounded by an external lamina and thin connective tissue, **endomysium**, containing capillaries.

Organization of Skeletal Muscle Fibers

- Groups of fibers called **fascicles** are surrounded by **perimysium**; all fascicles are enclosed within a dense connective tissue **epimysium**.
- Internally, each muscle fiber is filled with myofibrils, composed of thousands of **thick myosin filaments** and **thin actin filaments**, highly organized into contractile units called **sarcomeres**.
- Within sarcomeres, thick and thin filaments **interdigitate**; globular myosin heads project from the thick filaments toward the F-actin filaments, which are associated with **tropomyosin** and **troponin**.
- Sarcomeres are separated by **Z discs** that bisect the **light-staining I bands** that contain mainly the thin filaments attached to **α-actinin** in the Z disc.
- Between the two I bands of a sarcomere is the **dark-staining A band** with the thick myosin filaments; alternating light and dark bands appear as microscopic **striations** along the fibers.

Sarcoplasmic Reticulum & Transverse Tubule System

- In the sarcoplasm between parallel myofibrils are **mitochondria** and cisternae of smooth ER, called the **sarcoplasmic reticulum (SR)** specialized for **Ca²⁺ sequestration and release**.
- At each sarcomere, two **terminal cisterns of SR** contact a deep invagination of the sarcolemma called a **transverse** or **T-tubule**, forming a **triad** that triggers Ca²⁺ release when the sarcolemma is depolarized.

Mechanism of Contraction

- **Ca²⁺ binding to troponin** causes **tropomyosin to change shape** and allow the **myosin heads to bind the actin** subunits, forming **crossbridges** between thick and thin filaments.
- The myosin heads then pivot with **ATP hydrolysis**, which pulls the thin filaments along the thick filaments.

- With Ca²⁺ and ATP present, a **contraction cycle** ensues in which **myosin heads repeatedly attach, pivot, detach, and return**, causing the **filaments to slide past one another**, shortening the sarcomere.
- When the membrane **depolarization ends**, Ca²⁺ **is again sequestered**, ending contraction and allowing the sarcomeres to lengthen again as the **muscle relaxes**.
- Synapses of motor axons with skeletal muscle are called **MEPs, NMJs**, or **myoneural junctions**; the neurotransmitter is **acetylcholine**.
- A motor axon may form many terminal branches, each ending on an MEP of a muscle fiber; all fibers innervated by branches of that axon comprise a **motor unit**.

Muscle Spindles & Tendon Organs

- These are both **sensory proprioceptors** in which sensory **axons wrap around intrafusal fibers** in small, specialized fascicles or around **myotendinous collagen bundles**, respectively.

Muscle Fiber Types

- Skeletal muscles contain fibers classified into three main physiological types: (1) **slow, oxidative** (type I); (2) **fast, intermediate oxidative-glycolytic** (type IIa); and (3) **fast, glycolytic** (type IIb).

Cardiac Muscle

- **Cardiac muscle fibers** are **striated**, but they consist of **individual cylindrical cells**, often branched, each containing one (or two) **central nuclei** and linked by adherent and gap junctions at prominent **intercalated discs**.
- **Sarcomeres** of cardiac muscle resemble those of skeletal muscle structurally and functionally.
- Contraction of cardiac muscle is **intrinsic** at nodes of **impulse-generating pacemaker muscle fibers**; autonomic nerves regulate the rate of contraction.

Smooth Muscle

- **Smooth muscle fibers** are individual **small, fusiform (tapering) cells**, linked by numerous gap junctions.
- **Thin and thick filaments** in smooth muscle fibers do not form sarcomeres, and **no striations** are present.

- Thin actin filaments attach to α-actinin located in **dense bodies** that are located throughout the sarcoplasm and near the sarcolemma; contraction causes cells to shorten individually.
- Sarcoplasmic reticulum is less well-organized in smooth muscle fibers, and there is **no transverse tubule system**.
- Troponin is lacking in smooth muscle; proteins controlling the sliding filaments here include **myosin light-chain kinase (MLCK)** and the Ca²⁺-binding protein **calmodulin**.

Regeneration of Muscle Tissue

- Repair and regeneration can occur in **skeletal muscle** because of a population of **reserve muscle satellite cells** that can proliferate, fuse, and form new muscle fibers.
- Cardiac muscle **lacks satellite cells** and has little capacity for regeneration.
- Regeneration is rapid in smooth muscle because the cells/fibers are small and relatively less differentiated, which allow **renewed mitotic activity** after injury.

Muscle Tissue ASSESS YOUR KNOWLEDGE

1. The basal lamina of a muscle fiber is part of which structure?
   a. Perimysium
   b. Epimysium
   c. Fascia
   d. Endomysium
   e. Sarcoplasmic reticulum

2. With the transmission electron microscope skeletal muscle fibers can be seen to contain structures called triads. What do the two lateral components of a triad represent?
   a. Attachment sites for thick myofilaments
   b. Sites for calcium sequestration and release
   c. Sites for impulse conduction into the fiber
   d. Sites for ATP production
   e. Sites for synthesis of proteins to be secreted outside the cell

3. Which characteristic is unique to cardiac muscle?
   a. Contain centrally located nuclei
   b. Striated
   c. Often branched
   d. Multinucleated
   e. Lack T-tubules

4. In smooth muscle, calcium released by the smooth ER initiates contraction by binding to what protein?
   a. Actin
   b. Calmodulin
   c. Desmin
   d. Myosin light chain kinase
   e. Tropomyosin

5. Which feature typifies T-tubules?
   a. Evaginations of the sarcoplasmic reticulum
   b. Sequester calcium during muscle relaxation, releasing it during contraction
   c. Carry depolarization to the muscle fiber interior
   d. Overlie the A-I junction in cardiac muscle cells
   e. Rich supply of acetylcholine receptors

6. Which characteristic is unique to smooth muscle?
   a. T-tubules lie across Z lines.
   b. Each thick filament is surrounded by six thin filaments.
   c. Thin filaments attach to dense bodies.
   d. Cells are multinucleated.
   e. Cells have centrally located nuclei.

7. In one type of muscle, numerous gap junctions, desmosomes, and adherens junctions are specifically localized in which structures?
   a. Myofilaments
   b. Dense bodies
   c. Sarcomeres
   d. Neuromuscular spindles
   e. Intercalated discs

8. A 66-year-old man who lives alone has a severe myocardial infarction and dies during the night. The medical examiner's office is called the following morning and describes the man's body as being in *rigor mortis*. This state of *rigor mortis* is due to which one of the following?
   a. Inhibition of Ca²⁺ leakage from the extracellular fluid and sarcoplasmic reticulum
   b. Enhanced retrieval of Ca²⁺ by the sarcoplasmic reticulum
   c. Failure to disengage tropomyosin and troponin from the myosin active sites
   d. Absence of ATP preventing detachment of the myosin heads from actin
   e. Increased lactic acid production

9. A 5-year-old boy sustains a small tear in his gastrocnemius muscle when he is involved in a bicycle accident. Regeneration of the muscle will occur through which of the following mechanisms?
   a. Dedifferentiation of muscle cells into myoblasts
   b. Differentiation of muscle satellite cells
   c. Fusion of damaged myofibers to form new myotubes
   d. Hyperplasia of existing muscle fibers
   e. Differentiation of fibroblasts to form myoblasts

10. A healthy 32-year-old man lifts weights regularly as part of his workout. In one of his biceps muscle fibers at rest, the length of the I band is 1.0 μm and the A band is 1.5 μm. Contraction of that muscle fiber results in a 10% shortening of the length of the sarcomere. What is the length of the A band after the shortening produced by muscle contraction?
    a. 1.50 μm
    b. 1.35 μm
    c. 1.00 μm
    d. 1.90 μm
    e. 0.45 μm

11 The Circulatory System

The circulatory system pumps and directs blood cells and substances carried in blood to all tissues of the body. It includes both the blood and lymphatic vascular systems, and in an adult the total length of its vessels reaches an estimate between 100,000 and 150,000 kilometers. The **blood vascular system**, or **cardiovascular system** (Figure 11–1), consists of the following structures:

- The **heart** propels blood through the system and is surrounded by the **pericardium**, a fibrous sac lined by serous mesothelium.
- **Arteries**, a series of vessels efferent from the heart that become smaller as they branch into the various organs, carry blood to the tissues.
- **Capillaries**, the smallest vessels, correspond to the sites of O_2, CO_2, nutrient, and waste product exchange between blood and tissues. Together with the smallest arterial and venous branches carrying blood to and from them, capillaries in almost every organ form a complex network of thin, anastomosing tubules called the **microvasculature** or microvascular bed.
- **Veins** result from the convergence of venules into a system of larger channels which continue enlarging as they approach the heart, toward which they carry the blood to be pumped again.

As shown in Figure 11–1, two major divisions of arteries, microvasculature, and veins make up the **pulmonary circulation**, where blood receives oxygen in the lungs, and the **systemic circulation**, where blood delivers nutrients and removes wastes in tissues throughout the body.

The **lymphatic vascular system**, introduced with the discussion of interstitial fluid in Chapter 5, begins with the **lymphatic capillaries**, which consist of thin-walled, closed-ended tubules carrying lymph and merging to create vessels of steadily increasing size. The largest lymph vessels connect with the blood vascular system, emptying into the large veins near the heart. This returns fluid from tissue spaces all over the body to the blood.

The internal surface of all components of the blood and lymphatic systems has a lining of simple squamous epithelium called **endothelium**. As the interface between blood and the organs, vascular endothelial cells have crucial physiologic and medical importance. Not only must endothelial cells maintain a selectively permeable, antithrombogenic (inhibitory to clot formation) barrier, they also determine when and where white blood cells leave the circulation for the interstitial space of tissues and secrete a variety of paracrine factors for vessel dilation, constriction, and growth of adjacent cells.

❯ HEART

Cardiac muscle in the four chambers of the heart wall contracts rhythmically, pumping the blood through the circulatory system (Figure 11–2). The right and left **ventricles** propel blood to the pulmonary and systemic circulations, respectively; right and left **atria** receive blood from the body and the pulmonary veins, respectively. The walls of all four heart chambers consist of three major layers: the internal endocardium, the middle myocardium, and the external epicardium.

- The **endocardium** comprises the lining **endothelium**, its supporting layer of fibroelastic connective tissue with scattered smooth muscle fibers, and a deeper layer of connective tissue (continuous with that of the myocardium and often called the **subendocardial layer**) surrounding variable numbers of modified cardiac muscle fibers that make up the heart's impulse conducting system (Figure 11–3).

FIGURE **11–1** The cardiovascular system.

Systemic circulation (black arrows)

① Oxygenated blood flows from the left atrium to the left ventricle and then is pumped into the aorta.

② Blood passes from the aorta into elastic arteries and then into muscular arteries before entering arterioles.

③ Blood in arterioles enters systemic capillaries for exchange of gases and nutrients.

④ Deoxygenated blood exits capillary beds into venules and then into veins.

⑤ Deoxygenated blood is conducted to either the superior or inferior vena cava and then enters the right atrium of the heart.

Pulmonary circulation (yellow arrows)

⑥ Blood flows from the right atrium to the right ventricle and is then pumped into the pulmonary trunk.

⑦ The pulmonary trunk conducts deoxygenated blood into pulmonary arteries to the lungs.

⑧ The blood passes through smaller and smaller arteries before entering pulmonary capillaries for gas exchange.

⑨ Oxygenated blood exits the lung via a series of progressively larger veins that merge to form the pulmonary veins.

⑩ Pulmonary veins drain into the left atrium.

⑪ The cycle repeats.

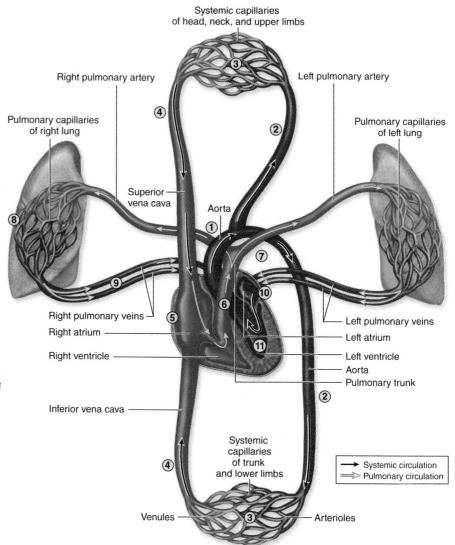

The cardiovascular system consists of the **heart, arteries, veins,** and **microvascular beds** and moves blood throughout the body along two routes: the **systemic circulation** and the **pulmonary circulation**. In the larger systemic circulation (black arrows), blood is pumped from the left side of the heart into the aorta and then through other arteries supplying the multiple microvascular beds with systemic capillaries in most organs and regions of both the upper and lower body, and finally back to the right side of the heart in veins.

In the pulmonary circulation (yellow arrows), the right side of the heart pumps blood through pulmonary arteries into the lungs for oxygenation in the local microvasculature of pulmonary capillaries, and then back to the left side of the heart via pulmonary veins.

In the resting human body approximately 70% of the blood is moving through the systemic circulation, about 18% through the pulmonary circulation, and 12% through the heart.

■ The **myocardium** consists mainly of typically contractile cardiac muscle fibers arranged spirally around each heart chamber. Because pumping blood through the systemic and pulmonary circulations requires strong force, the myocardium becomes much thicker in the walls of the ventricles than the atria (Figure 11–2). Moreover, the wall of the left ventricle develops about three times thicker than that of the right ventricle because the left side must produce sufficient force to propel blood through the much larger systemic circulation with its multiple capillary beds (Figures 11–1 and 11–2).

■ The **epicardium** consists of a simple squamous **mesothelium** supported by a layer of loose connective tissue containing blood vessels and nerves (Figure 11–4). The epicardium corresponds to the **visceral layer of the pericardium**, the membrane surrounding the heart.

FIGURE **11–2** Overview of the heart.

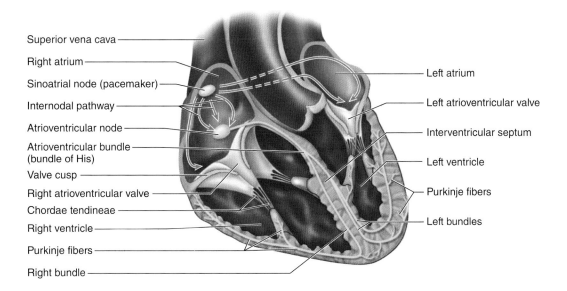

Superior vena cava

Right atrium

Sinoatrial node (pacemaker)

Internodal pathway

Atrioventricular node

Atrioventricular bundle (bundle of His)

Valve cusp

Right atrioventricular valve

Chordae tendineae

Right ventricle

Purkinje fibers

Right bundle

Left atrium

Left atrioventricular valve

Interventricular septum

Left ventricle

Purkinje fibers

Left bundles

As seen in the diagram the human heart has two **atria** and two **ventricles**, with the myocardium of the ventricular walls thicker than that of the atria. The **valves** basically consist of connective tissue flaps anchored in the heart's dense connective tissue, or **cardiac skeleton**, concentrated at the regions shown in white. This fibrous tissue includes the chordae tendineae, cords which extend from the cusps of both atrioventricular valves and attach to papillary muscles, preventing the valves from turning inside-out during ventricular contraction. Valves and cords are covered by the nonthrombogenic endothelium.

Yellow depicts parts of the cardiac **conducting system**, which initiates the electrical impulse for contraction (heartbeat) and spreads it through the ventricular myocardium. Both the **sino-atrial (SA) node (pacemaker)** in the right atrial wall, and the **atrioventricular (AV) node** in the floor of the right atrium, consist of myocardial tissue difficult to distinguish histologically from surrounding cardiac muscle. The AV node is continuous with a specialized bundle of cardiac muscle fibers, the **AV bundle** (of His), which gives rise to right and left bundle branches that run along the interventricular septum to the apex of the heart. At the apex the bundle branches subdivide further as **conducting (Purkinje) fibers**, which extend into myocardium of the ventricles.

Where the large vessels enter and leave the heart, the epicardium continues and reflects back as the **parietal layer** lining the pericardium. During heart movements, its underlying structures are cushioned by deposits of adipose tissue in the epicardium, and friction within the pericardium is prevented by lubricant fluid secreted by serous cells in both mesothelial layers.

Within these major layers, the heart contains other structures important for its overall function in moving blood. Prominent dense irregular connective tissue making up the fibrous **cardiac skeleton** separates the musculature of the atria from that of the ventricles, forms part of the interventricular and interatrial septa, and extends into the valve cusps and their chordae tendineae attachments (Figures 11–2 and 11–5). Various regions of the cardiac skeleton have the following functions:

- Surrounding, anchoring, and supporting all heart valves,
- Providing firm points of insertion for cardiac muscle in the atria and ventricles, and
- Helping coordinate the heartbeat by acting as electrical insulation between atria and ventricles.

In both the subendocardial layer and the adjacent myocardium, modified cardiac muscle cells make up the impulse **conducting system of the heart**, specialized to generate and conduct waves of depolarization stimulating rhythmic contractions in adjacent myocardial fibers. This system (Figure 11–2) consists of two nodes of specialized myocardial tissue in the right atrial wall: the **sinoatrial (SA) node** (or **pacemaker**) and the **atrioventricular (AV) node**, from which the **AV bundle** (bundle of His) emerges.

Located in the right atrial wall near the superior vena cava, the SA node is a 6- to 7-mm³ region of less contractile cardiac muscle cells with smaller size, fewer myofibrils, and fewer typical intercalated disks than the neighboring contractile fibers. Impulses initiated by these cells move along myocardial fibers of both atria, stimulating their contraction. When the impulses reach the slightly smaller AV node, located in the floor of the right atrium near the AV valve and composed of cells resembling those of the SA node, they stimulate depolarization in myocytes there. From the AV node, conducting myocytes are grouped into the AV bundle, which passes through an opening in the cardiac skeleton into the interventricular septum where

FIGURE 11–3 Endocardium, myocardium, and fibers of the subendocardial conducting network.

The lining layer of the heart, the **endocardium**, includes the surface endothelium (**En**), a supporting layer of fibroelastic connective tissue, and a deeper layer of connective tissue surrounding variable amounts of cardiac muscle specialized for impulse conduction. The deep layer is also called the **subendocardial layer** and is continuous with connective tissue of the myocardium.

(a) The subendocardial layer of connective tissue (**SEn**) in the ventricles surrounds Purkinje fibers (**P**) of the heart's impulse conducting network. This develop as modified cardiac muscle fibers

joined by intercalated disks, becoming specialized for impulse conduction rather than contraction. Containing glycogen but relatively few organelles and peripheral myofibrils, Purkinje fibers typically stain slightly paler than contractile muscle fibers (**M**).

(b) In the atrial walls conducting Purkinje-like fibers (**P**) often occupy most of the subendocardial layer, lying close to the endothelium (**En**), and merging with the contractile fibers of the myocardium (**M**), with the latter organized into many partially separated bundles and muscles. (Both ×200; H&E)

it splits into left and right bundles of myocytes located within the myocardium and subendocardial layer.

At the apex of the heart, these bundles subdivide further into a subendocardial conducting network of cardiac muscle fibers, usually called **Purkinje fibers**. These appear as pale-staining fibers, larger than the adjacent contractile fibers, with sparse, peripheral myofibrils, and much glycogen (Figure 11–3). Purkinje fibers mingle distally with contractile muscle fibers of each ventricle and trigger waves of contraction through both ventricles simultaneously.

Both parasympathetic and sympathetic neural components innervate the heart. Ganglionic nerve cells and nerve fibers develop in regions close to the SA and AV nodes, where they affect heart rate and rhythm, such as during physical exercise and emotional stress. Stimulation of the parasympathetic division (vagus nerve) slows the heartbeat, whereas stimulation of the sympathetic nerve accelerates activity of the pacemaker. Between fibers of the myocardium afferent free nerve endings occur that register pain, such as the discomfort called

angina pectoris that occurs when partially occluded coronary arteries cause local oxygen deprivation.

❯❯ MEDICAL APPLICATION

Abnormalities in the structure of heart valves can be produced by developmental defects, scarring after certain infections, or cardiovascular problems such as hypertension. Such abnormal valves may not close tightly, allowing slight regurgitation and backflow of blood. This produces an abnormal heart sound referred to as a **heart murmur**. If the valve defect is severe, the heart will have to work harder to circulate the normal amount of blood, eventually enlarging to accommodate the increased workload. Defective heart valves often may be repaired surgically or replaced by an artificial valve or one from a large animal donor. Because such valve replacements lack a complete endothelial covering, the patients require exogenous anticoagulant agents to prevent thrombus formation at these sites.

FIGURE 11–4 Epicardium or visceral pericardium.

The external tunic of the heart, the epicardium, contains the coronary vessels nourishing the heart, along with considerable adipose tissue. This section of atrium shows part of the myocardium (**M**) and epicardium (**Ep**). The epicardium consists of loose connective tissue (**CT**) containing autonomic nerves (**N**) and variable amounts of fat (**F**). The epicardium represents the visceral layer of the pericardium and has a simple mesothelium covering (**Mes**) which also lines the pericardial space. The mesothelial cells secrete a lubricant fluid that prevents friction as the beating heart contacts the parietal pericardium on the other side of the pericardial cavity. (×100; H&E)

FIGURE 11–5 Valve leaflet and cardiac skeleton.

The fibrous **cardiac skeleton** consists of dense irregular connective tissue, primarily in the endocardium (**En**), which anchors the valves and surrounds the two atrioventricular canals, maintaining their proper shape. The micrograph shows a section through a cusp of an **atrioventricular valve** (arrow) and attached chordae tendineae (**CT**). These structures are largely dense connective tissue (**C**) covered with a thin layer of endothelium. The collagen-rich connective tissue of the valves stains pale blue here and is continuous with the fibrous ring of connective tissue at the base of the valves which fills the endocardium between the atrium (**A**) and ventricle (**V**). Part of the thick ventricular myocardium (**M**) also appears here. (×20; Masson trichrome

›› TISSUES OF THE VASCULAR WALL

In addition to their endothelial lining, walls of all blood vessels except capillaries contain smooth muscle and connective tissue. The amount and arrangement of all these tissues in vessels depend on **mechanical factors**, primarily blood pressure, and **metabolic factors** reflecting the local needs of tissues.

The specialized epithelium, termed **endothelium**, acts as a semipermeable barrier between two major internal body compartments: the blood and the interstitial tissue fluid. Vascular endothelial cells develop as squamous, polygonal, and elongated cells with their long axes in the direction of blood flow. Endothelium with its basal lamina become highly differentiated to mediate and actively monitor the bidirectional exchange of molecules by simple and active diffusion, receptor-mediated endocytosis, transcytosis, and other mechanisms discussed in Chapter 4.

Besides their key role in metabolite exchanges between blood and tissues, endothelial cells exert several other functions:

- The endothelium presents a **nonthrombogenic surface** on which blood will not clot and actively secretes agents that control local clot formation (such as heparin, tissue plasminogen activator, and von Willebrand factor).
- The cells regulate local **vascular tone and blood flow** by secreting various factors stimulating smooth muscle contraction (such as endothelin-1 and angiotensin-converting enzyme [ACE]) or relaxation (including nitric oxide [NO] and prostacyclin).
- Endothelium has several roles in **inflammation and local immune responses**. In venules, endothelial cells induce specific white blood cells to adhere and migrate across the endothelium at sites of injury or infection. Under those conditions **P-selectin** appears very rapidly on the luminal surface when unique elongated granules, called **Weibel–Palade bodies**, fuse with the cell membrane for selectin exocytosis. As described further in Chapter 12, adhesion to selectins represents the first step in the activation of white blood cells specifically where they are needed. Endothelial cells also secrete various factors called **interleukins** that affect the activity of local white blood cells during inflammation.
- Under various conditions, endothelial cells also secrete a variety of **growth factors**, including proteins promoting proliferation of specific white blood cell lineages and cells that make up the vascular wall.

Growth factors such as vascular endothelial growth factor (VEGF) stimulate formation of the vascular system from embryonic mesenchyme (**vasculogenesis**), help maintain the vasculature in adults, and promote capillary sprouting and outgrowth from small existing vessels (**angiogenesis**) during normal growth, during tissue repair and regeneration, and in tumors and other pathological conditions. In both processes other growth factors, called **angiopoietins**, stimulate endothelial cells to recruit smooth muscle cells and fibroblasts to form the other tissues of the vascular wall.

The normal vascular endothelium is antithrombogenic, allowing adhesion of no blood cells or platelets and preventing blood clot formation. When endothelial cells of the microvasculature are damaged by tissue injury, collagen is exposed in the subendothelial tissues and induces the aggregation of blood platelets. These platelets release factors, which initiate a cascade of events that produce fibrin from circulating plasma fibrinogen. An intravascular clot, or **thrombus** (plural, thrombi), with a fibrin framework quickly forms to stop blood loss from the damaged vessels.

From large thrombi, solid masses called **emboli** (singular, embolus) may detach and be carried by the blood to obstruct distant vessels. In both cases, vascular flow may be blocked, producing a potentially life-threatening condition. Thus, the integrity of the endothelial layer preventing contact between platelets and the subendothelial connective tissue is an important antithrombogenic mechanism.

Individuals in the initial stages of medical conditions involving thrombus formation, such as myocardial infarct, stroke, or pulmonary embolism, are treated intravenously with tissue plasminogen activator, commonly abbreviated as tPA. This is a serine protease that breaks down fibrin and quickly dissolves the clot.

Smooth muscle fibers arranged helically in layers occur in the walls of all vessels larger than capillaries. In arterioles and small arteries, the smooth muscle cells have connections through many more gap junctions, permitting vasoconstriction and vasodilation of key importance in regulating the overall blood pressure.

Connective tissue components appear within vascular walls in variable amounts and proportions based on local functional requirements. Collagen fibers occur in the subendothelial layer, between the smooth muscle layers, and in the outer covering. Elastic fibers provide the resiliency required for the vascular wall to expand under pressure. Elastin becomes a major component in large arteries where it forms parallel lamellae, regularly distributed between the muscle layers. Variations in the amount and composition of ground substance components such as proteoglycans and hyaluronate also contribute to the physical and metabolic properties of the wall in different vessels, especially affecting their permeability.

The walls of all blood vessels larger than the microvasculature have many components in common and similar organization. Branching of such vessels produces reductions in their size and gradual changes in the composition of the vascular wall. Transitions such as those from "small arteries" to "arterioles" most often occur gradually, making classification of some vessels problematic. However, all these larger vessels have walls with three concentric layers, or tunics (L. *tunica*, coat), as shown with the diagrams in Figure 11–6 and in the micrographs of Figures 11–7 through 11–9.

- The innermost tunica **intima** consists of the endothelium and a thin subendothelial layer of loose connective tissue

sometimes containing smooth muscle fibers (Figure 11–7). In arteries, the intima includes a thin layer of elastin, the **internal elastic lamina**, with holes allowing better diffusion of substances from blood deeper into the wall.
- The tunica **media**, the middle layer, consists chiefly of concentric layers of helically arranged smooth muscle cells (Figures 11–6 and 11–7). Interposed among the muscle fibers are variable amounts of elastic fibers and elastic lamellae, reticular fibers, and proteoglycans, all produced by the smooth muscle cells. In arteries, the media may also have an external elastic lamina separating it from the outermost tunic.
- The outer **adventitia**, or tunica externa, contains connective tissue consisting principally of type I collagen and elastic fibers (Figures 11–7 and 11–8). The adventitia is continuous with and bound to the stroma of the organ through which the blood vessel runs.

Just as the heart wall has its own coronary vasculature to supply nutrients and O_2 locally, large vessels usually have **vasa vasorum** ("vessels of the vessel"): arterioles, capillaries, and venules in the adventitia and outer part of the media (Figure 11–8). Vasa vasorum provide metabolites to cells in those tunics in larger vessels with walls too thick to be nourished solely by diffusion from the blood in their lumens. Luminal blood alone does provide the needs of cells in the intima. Because they carry deoxygenated blood, large veins commonly have more vasa vasorum than arteries.

The adventitia of larger vessels also contains a network of unmyelinated autonomic nerve fibers, the vasomotor nerves (Figure 11–8), which release the vasoconstrictor norepinephrine. Reflecting its function, this innervation is more abundant in arteries than in veins.

› VASCULATURE

Large blood vessels and those of the microvasculature branch frequently and undergo gradual transitions into structures with different histologic features and functions. For didactic purposes vessels are classified arbitrarily as the types discussed here and listed in Table 11–1.

Elastic Arteries

Elastic arteries include the aorta, the pulmonary artery, and their largest branches; all these large vessels also make up the so-called **conducting arteries** because their major role is simply to move blood to smaller arteries. As shown in Figure 11–7a the most prominent feature of elastic arteries is the very thick tunica media in which elastic lamellae alternate with layers of smooth muscle fibers. The adult aorta has about 50 elastic lamellae (more in hypertensive individuals).

The tunica intima is well developed, with many smooth muscle cells in the subendothelial connective tissue, and often shows folds in cross section because of the vessel's contraction with loss of blood pressure at death (Figure 11–8). Between the intima and the media lies the internal elastic lamina,

FIGURE **11–6** Walls of arteries and veins.

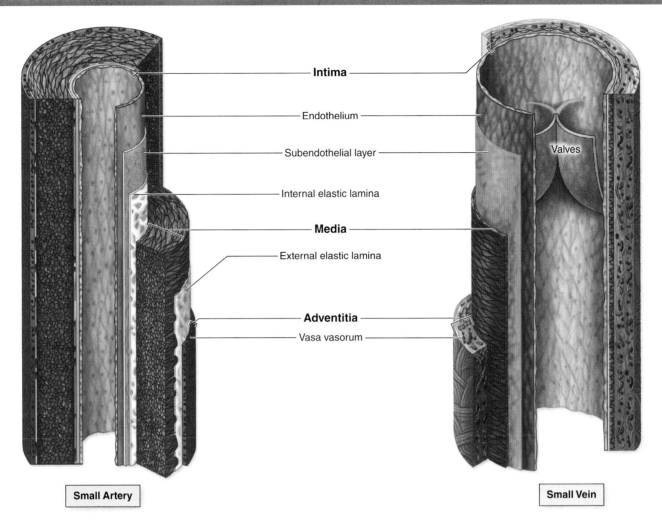

Intima

Endothelium

Subendothelial layer

Internal elastic lamina

Media

External elastic lamina

Adventitia

Vasa vasorum

Valves

Small Artery

Small Vein

Walls of both arteries and veins have three tunics called the **intima, media,** and **adventitia** (or externa), which correspond roughly to the heart's endocardium, myocardium, and epicardium. An artery has a thicker media and relatively narrow lumen.

A vein has a larger lumen, with its adventitia as the thickest layer. At regular intervals the intima of veins develops folds that act as valves that prevent back-flow of blood. Capillaries have only an endothelium, with no subendothelial layer or other tunics.

usually better defined than the elastic laminae of the media (Figures 11–7a and 11–9). The relatively thin adventitia contains vasa vasorum.

The numerous elastic laminae of these arteries contribute to their important function of making blood flow more uniform. During ventricular contraction (systole), blood moves through the arteries forcefully, stretching the elastin and distending the wall within limits set by its content of collagen. When the ventricles relax (diastole), ventricular pressure drops to a low level, and the elastin layers rebound passively, helping to maintain arterial pressure. The aortic and pulmonary valves prevent backflow of blood into the heart, so blood continues the flow away from the heart during this rebound. Arterial blood pressure and blood velocity decrease and become less variable as the distance from the heart increases.

❯❯ MEDICAL APPLICATION

Atherosclerosis (Gr. *athero*, gruel or porridge, and *scleros*, hardening) represents a disease of elastic arteries and large muscular arteries that may play a role in nearly half of all deaths in developed parts of the world. It is initiated by damaged or dysfunctional endothelial cells oxidizing low-density lipoproteins (LDLs) in the tunica intima, which induces adhesion, penetration, and activation of monocytes to remove the modified LDL. Lipid-filled macrophages (called **foam cells**) accumulate and, along with the free LDL, produce a pathologic sign of early atherosclerosis called **fatty streaks**. During disease progression, these develop into **fibro-fatty plaques**, or **atheromas**, consisting of a gruel-like mix of smooth muscle cells, lymphocytes, collagen fibers, and necrotic regions

FIGURE **11–7** Tunics of the vascular wall.

Comparison of the three major layers or tunics in the largest artery and vein. **(a)** Aorta, **(b)** vena cava. Simple squamous endothelial cells (arrows) line the intima (**I**) which also has subendothelial connective tissue and in arteries is separated from the media by an internal elastic lamina (**IEL**), a structure absent in all but the largest veins. The media (**M**) contains many elastic lamellae and elastic fibers (**EF**) alternating with layers of smooth muscle. The media becomes much thicker in large arteries than veins, with relatively more elastin. Elastic fibers also occur in the outer tunica adventitia (**A**), which is relatively thicker in large veins. Vasa vasorum (**V**) are seen in the adventitia of the aorta. The connective tissue of the adventitia always merges with the irregular connective tissue around it. (Both ×122; Elastic stain)

of lipid, debris, and foam cells. Predisposing factors include dyslipidemia (>3:1 ratios of LDL to HDL [high-density lipoprotein]), hyperglycemia of diabetes, hypertension, and the presence of toxins introduced by smoking.

In elastic arteries, atheromas produce localized destruction within the wall, weakening it and causing arterial bulges or **aneurysms**, which can rupture. In smaller muscular arteries such as the coronary arteries, atheromas can occlude blood flow to downstream vessels, leading to ischemic heart disease.

Arterial Sensory Structures

Carotid sinuses consist of slight dilations of the bilateral internal carotid arteries where they branch from the (elastic) common carotid arteries; they act as important **baroreceptors** monitoring arterial blood pressure. At these sinuses, the tunica media thins, allowing greater distension when blood pressure rises, and the adventitia contains many sensory nerve endings from cranial nerve IX, the glossopharyngeal nerve. The brain's vasomotor centers process these afferent impulses and adjust vasoconstriction, maintaining normal blood pressure. Functionally similar baroreceptors present in the aortic

FIGURE **11–8** Vasa vasorum.

The adventitia of the larger arteries contains a supply of micro-vasculature to bring O_2 and nutrients to local cells located too far from the lumen to be nourished by blood there. These arterioles (**A**), capillaries, and venules (**V**) constitute the vasa vasorum (vessels of vessels). The adventitia of large arteries is also supplied more sparsely with small sympathetic nerves (**N**) for control of vasoconstriction. Above the adventitia in this section can be seen muscle fibers (**SM**) and elastic lamellae (**E**) in the media. (×100; H&E)

FIGURE **11–9** Elastic artery.

The largest arteries contain considerable elastic material and expand with blood when the heart contracts. A transverse section through part of a large elastic artery shows a thick media (**M**) consisting largely of many well-developed elastic lamellae. Strong pressure of blood pulsating into such arteries during systole expands the arterial wall, reducing the pressure, and allowing strong blood flow to continue during diastole. The intima (**I**) of the empty aorta typically displays small folds, and the adventitia (**A**) consists of dense irregular connective tissue. (×200; PT)

arch transmit signals pertaining to blood pressure via cranial nerve X, the vagus nerve.

Histologically more complex **chemoreceptors** that monitor blood CO_2 and O_2 levels, as well as its pH, occur in the **carotid bodies** and in the **aortic bodies**, located in the walls of the carotid sinuses and aortic arch, respectively. These structures are parts of the autonomic nervous system called **paraganglia** with rich capillary networks. The capillaries are closely surrounded by large, neural crest-derived **glomus cells**, filled with dense-core vesicles containing dopamine, acetylcholine, and other neurotransmitters and supported by smaller satellite cells (Figure 11–10). Ion channels in the glomus cell membranes respond to stimuli in the arterial blood, primarily hypoxia (low O_2), hypercapnia (excess CO_2), or acidosis, by activating release of neurotransmitters. Sensory fibers branching from the glossopharyngeal nerve form

synapses with the glomus cells and signal appropriate brain centers to initiate cardiovascular and respiratory adjustments to correct the condition.

Muscular Arteries

The muscular arteries, also called distributing arteries, distribute blood to the organs and help regulate blood pressure by contracting or relaxing the smooth muscle in the media. The intima has a thin subendothelial layer and a prominent internal elastic lamina (Figure 11–11). The media may contain up to 40 layers of large smooth muscle cells interspersed with a variable number of elastic lamellae (depending on the size of the vessel). An external elastic lamina is present only in the larger muscular arteries. The adventitial connective tissue

TABLE 11–1	Size ranges, major features, and important roles of major blood vessel types.				
Type of Vessel	**Outer Diameter (Approx. Range)**	**Intima**	**Media**	**Adventitia**	**Roles in Circulatory System**
Elastic arteries	>10 mm	Endothelium; connective tissue with smooth muscle	Many elastic lamellae alternating with smooth muscle	Connective tissue, thinner than media, with vasa vasorum	Conduct blood from heart and with elastic recoil help move blood forward under steady pressure
Muscular arteries	10-1 mm	Endothelium; connective tissue with smooth muscle, internal elastic lamina prominent	Many smooth muscle layers, with much less elastic material	Connective tissue, thinner than media; vasa vasorum may be present	Distribute blood to all organs and maintain steady blood pressure and flow with vasodilation and constriction
Small arteries	1-0.1 mm	Endothelium; connective tissue less smooth muscle	3–10 layers of smooth muscle	Connective tissue, thinner than media; no vasa vasorum	Distribute blood to arterioles, adjusting flow with vasodilation and constriction
Arterioles	100-10 μm	Endothelium; no connective tissue or smooth muscle	1–2 layers of smooth muscle	Very thin connective tissue layer	Resist and control blood flow to capillaries; major determinant of systemic blood pressure
Capillaries	10-4 μm	Endothelium only	A few pericytes only	None	Exchange metabolites by diffusion to and from cells
Venules (postcapillary, collecting, and muscular)	10-100 μm	Endothelium; no valves	Pericytes and scattered smooth muscle cells	None	Drain capillary beds; site of leukocyte exit from vasculature
Small veins	0.1-1 mm	Endothelium; connective tissue with scattered smooth muscle fibers	Thin, 2–3 loose layers of smooth muscle cells	Connective tissue, thicker than media	Collect blood from venules
Medium veins	1-10 mm	Endothelium; connective tissue, with valves	3–5 more distinct layers of smooth muscle	Thicker than media; longitudinal smooth muscle may be present	Carry blood to larger veins, with no backflow
Large veins	>10 mm	Endothelium; connective tissue, smooth muscle cells; prominent valves	>5 layers of smooth muscle, with much collagen	Thickest layer, with bundled longitudinal smooth muscle	Return blood to heart

contains lymphatic capillaries, vasa vasorum, and nerves, all of which may penetrate to the outer parts of the media.

Arterioles

Muscular arteries branch repeatedly into smaller and smaller arteries, until reaching a size with only three or four layers of medial smooth muscle. The smallest arteries branch further as **arterioles**, which have only one or two smooth muscle layers; these indicate the beginning of an organ's **microvasculature** (Figures 11–12 and 11–13) where exchanges between blood and tissue fluid occur. Arterioles are generally less than 0.1 mm in diameter, with lumens approximately as wide as the wall is thick (Figure 11–14). The subendothelial layer is very thin, elastic laminae are absent, and the media consists of the circularly arranged smooth muscle cells. In both small arteries and arterioles, the thin adventitia is inconspicuous.

Arterioles almost always branch to form anastomosing networks of capillaries that surround the parenchymal cells of the organ. At the ends of arterioles, the smooth muscle fibers act as sphincters and produce periodic blood flow into capillaries (Figure 11–13). Muscle tone normally keeps arterioles partially closed, resisting blood flow, which makes these vessels the major determinants of systemic blood pressure.

FIGURE **11–10** Cells and capillaries in a glomus body.

Specialized regions in the walls of certain elastic arteries contain tissues acting as chemoreceptors that provide information to the brain regarding blood chemistry. The glomus bodies comprise two small (0.5-5 mm diameter) ganglion-like structures found near the common carotid arteries. They contain many large capillaries (**C**) intermingled with clusters of large glomus cells (**G**) filled with vesicles of various neurotransmitters. Supportive satellite cells (**S**) with elongated nuclei sheath each glomus cell, which form synaptic connections with sensory fibers. The chemoreceptive glomus cells detect significant changes in the blood CO_2, O_2, or H^+ concentrations and release neurotransmitters that activate the sensory nerve to relay this information to the brain. (×400; PT)

❯❯ MEDICAL APPLICATION

Blood pressure depends on cardiac output and the total peripheral resistance to blood flow, which is mostly due to the resistance of arterioles. **Hypertension** or elevated blood pressure may occur secondarily to renal or endocrine problems, but is more commonly essential hypertension, due to a wide variety of mechanisms that increase arteriolar constriction.

As depicted in Figure 11–15 arterioles in certain tissues and organs can deviate from this simple path to accommodate various specialized functions. For example, thermoregulation by the skin involves arterioles that can bypass capillary

FIGURE **11–11** Muscular artery.

With distance from the heart, arteries gradually have relatively less elastin and more smooth muscle in their walls. Most arteries large enough to have names are of the muscular type. A transverse section through a muscular (medium caliber) artery shows a slightly folded intima with only sparse connective tissue between the endothelial cells (**E**) and internal elastic lamina (**IEL**). Multiple layers of smooth muscle (**SM**) in the media are thicker than the elastic lamellae and fibers with which they intersperse. The adventitia contains vasa vasorum (**V**). (×100; H&E)

networks and connect directly to venules. In these **arteriovenous shunts** (or arteriovenous anastomoses) the media and adventitia become thicker and richly innervated by sympathetic and parasympathetic nerve fibers. The autonomic fibers control the degree of vasoconstriction at the shunts, regulating blood flow through the capillary beds. Increased capillary blood flow in the skin allows more heat dissipation from the body while reduced capillary blood flow conserves heat, both important functions when the environmental temperature is hot or cold, respectively.

Venous **portal systems** represent another important alternative microvascular pathway (Figure 11–15) in which

FIGURE **11–12** Microvasculature.

Arterioles (**A**), capillaries (**C**), and venules (**V**) comprise the microvasculature where, in almost every organ, molecular exchange takes place between blood and the interstitial fluid of the surrounding tissues. Lacking media and adventitia tunics and with diameters of only 4–10 μm, capillaries (**C**) in paraffin sections can be recognized by nuclei adjacent to small lumens or by highly eosinophilic red blood cells in the lumen. As described in Figure 5–20, not all interstitial fluid formed at capillary beds is reabsorbed and drained via venules; the excess becomes **lymph** and collects in thin-walled, irregularly shaped lymphatic vessels (**L**), such as those seen in connective tissue and smooth muscle here. (×200; H&E)

FIGURE **11–13** Microvascular bed structure and perfusion.

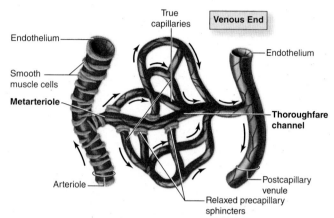

(a) **Sphincters relaxed; capillary bed well perfused**

(b) **Sphincters contracted; blood bypasses capillary bed**

Arterioles supplying a capillary bed typically form smaller branches called **metarterioles** in which the **smooth muscle cells** localize in bands that act as **precapillary sphincters**. The distal portion of the metarteriole, sometimes called a **thoroughfare channel**, lacks smooth muscle cells and merges with the **postcapillary venule**. Branching from the metarteriole and thoroughfare channel are the smallest vessels, **true capillaries**, which lack smooth muscle cells (although pericytes may be present). The precapillary sphincters regulate blood flow into the network of true capillaries.

Part (**a**) depicts a well-perfused capillary bed with all the sphincters relaxed and open; (**b**) shows a capillary bed with the blood shunted away by contracted sphincters. At any given moment, most sphincters are at least partially closed, and blood enters the capillary bed in a pulsatile manner for maximally efficient exchange of nutrients, wastes, O_2, and CO_2 across the endothelium. Except in the pulmonary circulation (Figure 11–1), blood enters the microvasculature well oxygenated and leaves poorly oxygenated.

blood flows through two successive capillary beds separated by a **portal vein**. This arrangement allows for hormones or nutrients picked up by the blood in the first capillary network to be delivered most efficiently to cells around the second capillary bed before the blood returns to the heart for general distribution. The best examples are the hepatic portal system of the liver and the hypothalamic-hypophyseal portal system in the anterior pituitary gland, both of which have major physiologic importance.

Capillary Beds

Capillaries permit and regulate metabolic exchanges between blood and surrounding tissues. These smallest blood vessels

always function in networks called **capillary beds**, whose size and overall shape conforms to that of the structure supplied. The density of the capillary bed relates directly to the metabolic activity of the tissues. Tissues with high metabolic rates, such as the kidney, liver, and striated muscle, have abundant

FIGURE **11–14** Arterioles.

(a) Arterioles are microvessels with an intima (**I**) consisting only of endothelium (**E**), in which the cells may have rounded nuclei. They have media (**M**) tunics with only one or two layers of smooth muscle, and usually thin, inconspicuous adventitia (**A**). (×350; Masson trichrome

(b) Three arterioles (**A**) of various sizes and a capillary (**C**) are shown here. (×400; H&E)

(c) A large mesenteric arteriole cut obliquely and longitudinally clearly shows the endothelial cells (arrow heads) and one or two layers of smooth muscle cells (**M**) cut transversely. Adventitia merges imperceptibly with neighboring connective tissue. (×300; PT)

FIGURE **11–15** Comparison of the simple microvascular pathway with arteriovenous shunts and portal systems.

Most capillary beds simply receive blood from arterioles and drain into venules, but alternative pathways occur in certain organs. In skin, blood flow can be varied according to the external temperature by **arteriovenous (AV) shunts**, or anastomoses, commonly coiled, which directly connect the arterial and venous systems and temporarily bypass the capillary beds.

In **venous portal systems**, one capillary bed drains into a vein which then directly branches again into another capillary bed. This arrangement allows molecules entering the blood in the first set of capillaries to be delivered quickly and at high concentrations to surrounding tissues at the second capillary bed, with particular importance in the anterior pituitary gland and liver.

Not shown are **arterial portal systems** (afferent arteriole → capillaries → efferent arteriole), which occur in the kidney (Chapter 19).

capillaries; the opposite is true of tissues with low metabolic rates, such as smooth muscle and dense connective tissue.

Capillary beds receive blood preferentially from one or more terminal arteriole branches called **metarterioles**, which are continuous with **thoroughfare channels** connected to the **postcapillary venules** (Figure 11–13). Capillaries branch from the metarterioles, which are encircled by scattered smooth muscle cells, and converge into the thoroughfare channels, which lack muscle. As described with Figure 11–13 the metarteriole muscle cells act as **precapillary sphincters** that contract and relax cyclically, with 5–10 cycles per minute, causing blood to pass through capillary beds in a pulsatile manner. When the sphincters are closed, blood flows directly from the metarterioles and thoroughfare channels into postcapillary venules.

FIGURE **11–16** Capillary with pericytes.

Capillaries consist only of an endothelium rolled as a tube, across which molecular exchange occurs between blood and tissue fluid. **(a)** Capillaries normally become associated with perivascular contractile cells called **pericytes (P)** which have a variety of functions. The more flattened nuclei belong to endothelial cells. (×400; H&E of a spread mesentery preparation)

(b) TEM of a capillary cut transversely, showing the nucleus of one thin capillary endothelial cell (**E**). Endothelial cells form the capillary lumen (**L**), become covered by a basal lamina (**BL**), and bind one another tightly with junctional complexes (**J**). One pericyte (**P**) is shown, surrounded by its own basal lamina (**BL**) and extending processes around the endothelial cells. (×13,000)

Capillaries consist of a simple layer of **endothelial cells** rolled up as a tube surrounded by basement membrane (Figure 11–16). The average diameter of capillaries varies from 4 to 10 μm, which allows transit of blood cells only one at a time, and their individual length seldom exceeds 50 μm. These minute vessels make up over 90% of the body's vasculature, with a total length of more than 100,000 km and a total surface area of approximately 5000 m². Because of the cyclical opening and closing of the sphincters, most capillaries are essentially empty at any given time, with only about 5% (~300 mL in an adult) of the total blood volume moving through these structures. Their thin walls, extensive surface area, and slow, pulsatile blood flow optimize capillaries for the exchange of water and solutes between blood and tissues.

In addition to the endothelial cell properties mentioned earlier in this chapter, capillary cells have many features specialized for molecular transfer by mechanisms ranging from simple diffusion to transcytosis. The average thickness of the cells is only 0.25 μm and their nuclei are often distinctively curved to accommodate the very small tubular structure (Figure 11–10). The cytoplasm contains mitochondria and most other organelles, as well as a typically large population of membranous vesicles. Along with the basal lamina, junctional complexes between the cells maintain the tubular structure, with variable numbers of tight junctions having an important role in capillary permeability.

Major structural differences occur in capillaries of organs with various functions, permitting very different levels of metabolic exchange. Capillaries generally fall into one of three histological types, depending on the continuity of the endothelial cells and the basement membrane (Figures 11–17 through 11–20).

- **Continuous capillaries** (Figure 11–17a) have many tight, well-developed occluding junctions between slightly overlapping endothelial cells, which provide for continuity along the endothelium and well-regulated metabolic exchange across the cells. This represents the most common type of capillary and is found in muscle, connective tissue, lungs, exocrine glands, and nervous tissue. Ultrastructural studies show numerous vesicles indicating transcytosis of macromolecules in both directions across the endothelial cell cytoplasm.

- **Fenestrated capillaries** (Figure 11–17b) have a sieve-like structure that allows more extensive molecular exchange across the endothelium. Here numerous small circular openings or fenestrations (L. *fenestra*, window), approximately 80 nm in diameter, completely penetrate the endothelial cells. Some such fenestrations have very thin diaphragms of proteoglycans (Figure 11–19); others may represent membrane invaginations during transcytosis that temporarily involve both sides of the very thin cells. The basement membrane of these cells, however, covers the fenestrations and lacks perforations. Fenestrated capillaries occur in organs with rapid interchange of substances between tissues and the blood, such as the kidneys, intestine, choroid plexus, and endocrine glands.

- **Discontinuous capillaries**, commonly called **sinusoids** (Figure 11–17c), permit maximal exchange of macromolecules as well as allow easier movement of cells

FIGURE **11–17** Types of capillaries.

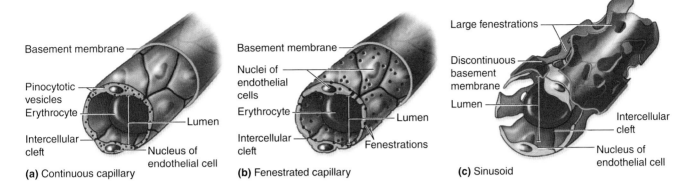

(a) Continuous capillary

(b) Fenestrated capillary

(c) Sinusoid

The vessels between arterioles and venules occur as one of three types. **(a) Continuous capillaries**, the most common type, have tight, occluding junctions sealing the intercellular clefts between all the endothelial cells to produce minimal fluid leakage. All molecules exchanged across the endothelium must cross the cells by diffusion or transcytosis.

(b) Fenestrated capillaries also have tight junctions, but perforations (fenestrations) through the endothelial cells themselves allow greater exchange across the endothelium. The basement membrane

is continuous in both these capillary types. Fenestrated capillaries abound in organs where molecular exchange with the blood is important, such as endocrine organs, intestinal walls, and choroid plexus.

(c) Sinusoids, or discontinuous capillaries, usually have a wider diameter than the other types and have discontinuities between the endothelial cells, large fenestrations through the cells, and a partial discontinuous basement membrane. Sinusoids develop in organs where exchange of macromolecules and cells occurs readily between tissue and blood, such as in bone marrow, liver, and spleen.

between tissues and blood. The endothelium here shows large perforations and irregular intercellular clefts, forming a discontinuous layer with spaces both between and through the cells. Unlike other capillaries, basement membranes of sinusoids also have many discontinuities.

Moreover, sinusoids have much larger diameters, often 30–40 μm, than other capillaries, which slow blood flow. Sinusoidal capillaries of this type develop in the liver, spleen, some endocrine organs, and bone marrow (Figure 11–20).

FIGURE **11–18** Continuous capillary.

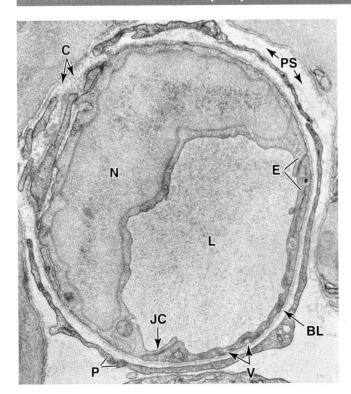

Continuous capillaries exert the tightest control over what molecules leave and enter the capillary lumen (**L**). This TFM shows a continuous capillary in transverse section with a prominent endothelial cell nucleus (**N**). Tight or occluding junctions occur abundantly in the junctional complexes (**JC**) at overlapping folds between the endothelial cells (**E**). Numerous transcytotic vesicles (**V**) are also evident. All material that crosses continuous capillary endothelium must pass *through* the cells, usually by diffusion or transcytosis.

Around the capillary are a basal lamina (**BL**) and thin cytoplasmic extensions from pericytes (**P**). Collagen fibers (**C**) and other extracellular material characterize the narrow perivascular space (**PS**). (×10,000)

FIGURE **11–19** Fenestrated capillary.

Fenestrated capillaries become specialized for uptake of molecules such as hormones in endocrine glands or for outflow of molecules such as in the kidney's filtration system. TEM of a transversely sectioned fenestrated capillary in the peritubular region of the kidney shows many typical fenestrae closed by diaphragms (arrows), with a continuous basal lamina surrounding the endothelial cell (**BL**). In this cell, the Golgi apparatus (**G**), nucleus (**N**), and centrioles (**C**) can also be seen. Fenestrated capillaries allow a freer exchange of molecules than continuous capillaries and occur in the intestinal wall, kidneys, and endocrine glands. (×10,000) (*Reproduced with permission from Dr Johannes Rhodin, Department of Cell Biology, New York University School of Medicine.*)

At various locations along continuous capillaries and postcapillary venules are mesenchymal cells called **pericytes** (Gr. *peri*, around + *kytos*, cell), with long cytoplasmic processes that partly surround the endothelial layer. Pericytes secrete many ECM components and form their own basal lamina, which fuses with the basement membrane of the endothelial cells (Figure 11–16). Well-developed cytoskeletal networks of myosin, actin and tropomyosin indicate that pericytes also dilate or constrict capillaries, helping to regulate blood flow in some organs. Within the CNS pericytes help maintain the endothelial blood-brain barrier. After injuries, pericytes proliferate and differentiate to form smooth muscle and other cells in new vessels reestablishing the microvasculature. In many organs the pericyte population also includes mesenchymal stem cells important for regeneration of other tissues.

❯❯ MEDICAL APPLICATION

The **hyperglycemia** or excessive blood sugar that occurs with diabetes commonly leads to **diabetic microangiopathy**, a diffuse thickening of capillary basal laminae and concomitant decrease in metabolic exchange at these vessels, particularly in the kidneys, retina, skeletal muscle, and skin.

FIGURE **11–20** Sinusoidal capillary.

Sinusoidal capillaries or sinusoids generally have much greater diameters than most capillaries and are specialized not only for maximal molecular exchange between blood and surrounding tissue, but also for easy movement of blood cells across the endothelium. The bone marrow sinusoid (**S**) shown here occurs in tissue containing adipocytes (**A**) and masses of hematopoietic cells (**H**). The endothelial cells become very thin, with cell nuclei more difficult to find than in smaller capillaries. Ultrastructurally, sinusoidal capillaries display large fenestrations through the cells and large discontinuities between the cells and through the basal lamina. (×200; H&E)

Venules

The transition from capillaries to venules occurs gradually. Postcapillary venules (Figure 11–21a) resemble capillaries with pericytes but larger, ranging in diameter from 15 to 20 μm. As described with blood in Chapter 12, postcapillary venules represent the microvascular component in which white blood cells adhere to endothelium and leave the circulation at sites of infection or tissue damage.

Postcapillary venules converge into larger **collecting venules** that have more distinct contractile cells. With increasing size venules develop medial tunics with two or three smooth muscle layers and become **muscular venules**. A characteristic feature of all venules is the large lumen diameter compared to the overall thinness of the wall (Figure 11–21).

Veins

Veins carry blood back to the heart from microvasculature all over the body. Blood entering veins is under very low pressure and moves toward the heart by contraction of the smooth muscle fibers in the media and by external compressions from surrounding skeletal muscles and other organs. Most veins are classified as **small** or **medium veins** (Figure 11–22), with diameters of 10 mm or less (Table 11–1). These veins are usually located close and parallel to corresponding muscular arteries. The tunica intima is usually thin, the media has small bundles of smooth muscle cells mixed with a network of

FIGURE **11–21** Venules.

A series of increasingly larger and more organized venules lie between capillaries and veins.

(a) Compared to arterioles (**A**), postcapillary venules (**V**) have large lumens surrounded only by an intima of simple endothelial cells, with occasional pericytes (**P**). (×400; Toluidine blue [TB]

(b) Larger collecting venules (**V**) have much greater diameters than arterioles (**A**), but the wall remains very thin, consisting of an endothelium with more numerous pericytes or smooth muscle cells. (×200; H&E)

(c) The muscular venule cut lengthwise here has a better-defined tunica media, with smooth muscle (**M**) in some areas, a thin intima

(**I**) of endothelial cells (**E**), and a more distinct adventitia (**Ad**). Part of an arteriole (**A**) shows a thicker wall than the venule. (×200; Masson trichrome)

As discussed with white blood cells in Chapter 12, postcapillary venules represent important sites in the vasculature where these cells leave the circulation to become functional in the interstitial space of surrounding tissues when such tissues are inflamed or infected.

(d) A postcapillary venule (**V**) from an infected organ shows several round, white blood cells adhering to and migrating across the intima. (×200; H&E)

reticular fibers and delicate elastic fibers, and the collagenous adventitial layer is thick and well developed.

The big venous trunks, paired with elastic arteries close to the heart, make up the **large veins** (Figure 11–7b). These have distinct intimal layers, but relatively thin media with alternating smooth muscle and connective tissue. In large veins the tunica adventitia is thicker than the media and frequently contains longitudinal bundles of smooth muscle. Both

the media and adventitia contain elastic fibers, and an internal elastic lamina like those of arteries may be present.

Valves represent an important feature of large and medium veins. These consist of thin, paired folds of tunica intima projecting across the lumen, rich in elastic fibers and covered on both sides by endothelium (Figures 11–22 and 11–23). Such valves, especially numerous in veins of the legs, help keep the flow of venous blood directed toward the heart.

FIGURE **11–22** Veins.

Veins usually travel as companions to arteries and are classified as small, medium, or large based on size and development of the tunics.

(a) The small vein (**V**) shows a relatively large lumen compared to the small muscular artery (**A**) with its thick media (**M**) and adventitia (**Ad**). The wall of a small vein is very thin, containing only two or three layers of smooth muscle. (×200; H&E)

(b) This oblique section of a small vein includes a valve (arrow). Valves occur as thin folds of intima projecting well into the lumen, which act to prevent backflow of blood. (×200; Aldehyde fuchsin & van Gieson)

(c) A medium vein (**MV**) shows a thicker wall but still less prominent than that of the accompanying muscular artery (**MA**). Both the media and adventitia are better developed, but the vein wall often displays floppy folds around the relatively large lumen (×100; Aldehyde fuchsin & van Gieson).

(d) Micrograph of a medium vein contains blood and shows valve folds (arrows). (×200; Masson trichrome)

›› MEDICAL APPLICATION

Junctions between endothelial cells of postcapillary venules are the loosest of the microvasculature. This facilitates trans-endothelial migration of leukocytes at these locations during **inflammation**, as well as a characteristic loss of fluid here during the inflammatory response, leading to tissue **edema**.

› LYMPHATIC VASCULAR SYSTEM

In addition to the blood vasculature, the body has a system of very thin-walled channels, the **lymphatic capillaries**, which collect excess interstitial fluid from the tissue spaces as **lymph** and return it to the blood. Like interstitial fluid, lymph is usually rich in lightly staining proteins but does not normally contain red blood cells, although lymphocytes and other

FIGURE **11–23** **Wall of large vein with valve.**

Large veins have a muscular media layer (**M**), usually very thin compared to the surrounding adventitia (**A**) of dense irregular connective tissue. The wall is often folded as shown here, with the intima (**I**) projecting into the lumen as a valve (**V**) composed of the subendothelial connective tissue with endothelium on both sides. (×100; PT)

white blood cells normally appear there (Figure 11–24a). With exceptions such as the bone marrow and most of the CNS, most tissues with blood microvasculature also contain lymphatic capillaries (or lymphatics).

Lymphatic capillaries originate locally as tubes of very thin endothelial cells, which lack tight junctions and rest on a discontinuous basal lamina. Fine anchoring filaments of collagen extend from the basal lamina to the surrounding

FIGURE **11–24** **Lymphatic capillary.**

Lymphatic capillaries drain interstitial fluid produced when the plasma forced from the microvasculature by hydrostatic pressure does not all return to blood by the action of osmotic pressure.

(a) Micrograph shows a lymphatic capillary filled with this fluid called lymph (**L**). Lymphatics are blind-ended vessels with a wall of very thin endothelial cells (**E**) and are quite variable in diameter (10-50 μm). Lymph is rich in proteins and other material and often stains somewhat better than the surrounding ground substance, as seen here. (×200; Mallory trichrome)

(b) Diagram indicating more details about lymphatics, including the **openings between the endothelial cells**. The openings are held in place by **anchoring filaments** containing elastin, and are covered by extensions of the endothelial cells. **Interstitial fluid** enters primarily via these openings, and the endothelial folds prevent backflow of lymph into tissue spaces. Lymphatic endothelial cells are typically larger than those of blood capillaries.

FIGURE 11–25 Lymphatic vessels and valve.

Lymphatic vessels form by the merger of lymphatic capillaries, but their walls remain extremely thin. **(a)** Cross section shows a lymphatic vessel (**LV**) near a venule (**V**), whose wall is thick by comparison. Lymphatic vessels normally do not contain red blood cells, which provides another characteristic distinguishing them from venules. (×200; Mallory trichrome)

(b) Lymphatic vessel (**LV**) in muscle cut longitudinally shows a valve, the structure responsible for the unidirectional flow of lymph. The solid arrow indicates the direction of the lymph flow, and the dashed arrows show how the valves prevent lymph back-flow. The lower small lymphatic vessel represents a lymphatic capillary with a wall consisting only of endothelium. (×200; PT)

connective tissue, preventing collapse of the vessels. Interstitial fluid enters lymphatic capillaries by flowing between endothelial cells and by transcytosis. Specific domains of adjacent endothelial cells also lack hemidesmosome connections to the basal lamina and extend into the lumen to form leaflets of valves facilitating fluid entry and preventing most backflow of lymph (Figure 11–24b).

Lymphatic capillaries converge into larger **lymphatic vessels** with thin walls and increasing amounts of connective tissue and smooth muscle that never form clearly distinct outer tunics (Figure 11–25). Like veins, lymphatic vessels have valves comprised of complete intimal folds. Interposed in the path of these larger lymphatic vessels are **lymph nodes**, where lymph is processed by cells of the immune system (discussed in Chapter 14). In histological sections, lymphatic vessels often appear dilated with lymph. As in veins, lymphatic circulation depends on external forces (eg, contraction of surrounding skeletal muscle), with the valves keeping lymph flow unidirectional.

Lymphatic vessels ultimately converge as two large trunks, the **thoracic duct** and the **right lymphatic duct**, which empty lymph back into the blood. The thoracic duct connects with the blood circulatory system near the junction of the left internal jugular vein with the left subclavian vein, whereas the right lymphatic duct enters near the confluence of the right subclavian vein and the right internal jugular vein. The structure of these largest lymphatic vessels somewhat resembles that of small veins. The relatively underdeveloped adventitia contains vasa vasorum and a neural network.

Besides gathering interstitial fluid as lymph and returning it to the blood, the lymphatic vascular system represents a major distributor of lymphocytes, antibodies, and other immune components that are carried through many organs to and from lymph nodes and other lymphoid tissues.

❯❯ MEDICAL APPLICATION

Lymphatics and larger lymphatic vessels are clinically important because (among other reasons) they facilitate the spread of pathogens, parasites, and malignant cells in the body. Surgical removal of lymph nodes, standard procedure to determine the occurrence of cancer metastasis, can disrupt the lymphatic drainage and produce swelling or **lymphedema**, in tissues of the affected region.

The Circulatory System SUMMARY OF KEY POINTS

Heart

- The heart has three major layers: (1) the inner **endocardium** of endothelium and subendothelial connective tissue; (2) the **myocardium** of cardiac muscle; and (3) the **epicardium**, connective tissue with many adipocytes and covered by mesothelium.
- The **cardiac conducting system** stimulates rhythmic contractions and consists of modified cardiac muscle fibers forming the **sinoatrial (SA) and atrioventricular (AV) nodes**, the **atrioventricular bundle (of His)**, left and right bundle branches, and **Purkinje fibers**.
- **Purkinje fibers**, located in the subendocardial layer of both ventricles, are distinguished from contractile fibers by their greater diameter, abundant glycogen, and more sparse bundles of myofibrils.
- Masses of dense irregular connective tissue make up the **cardiac skeleton**, which surrounds the bases of all heart valves, separates the atria from the ventricles, and provides insertions for cardiac muscle.

Vasculature

- Macroscopically visible blood vessels have three major layers or **tunics**: (1) The **intima** includes the endothelium, connective tissue, and an internal elastic lamina in larger vessels; (2) the **media** contains alternating layers of smooth muscle and collagen or elastic lamellae; and (3) the **adventitia** (or externa) contains connective tissue, small vessels (**vasa vasorum**), and nerves.
- Throughout the vasculature, **endothelial cells** do not simply line the heart and vessels; they actively produce factors that prevent blood clotting, factors that cause adjacent smooth muscle cells to contract or relax, and factors that initiate inflammation at sites of damage or infection.
- Artery classification relies on their size and wall composition: (1) **large elastic arteries**, with fenestrated elastic laminae in the thick tunica media; (2) **muscular, medium-sized arteries**; and (3) **small arteries**, with fewer than 10 layers of smooth muscle in the media.
- A **microvasculature** too small for surgical manipulation permeates most organs and consists of (1) **arterioles**, with one to three smooth muscle layers; (2) **capillaries**, consisting only of an intima endothelial layer; and (3) **venules**, with large lumens and thin walls, which drain capillaries.
- Terminal arterioles branch into **metarterioles**, in which smooth muscle **sphincters** contract to resist blood flow and relax cyclically

to allow pulsatile flow of blood into an anastomosing **capillary bed**, where **metabolic exchange** with surrounding cells occurs.

- Capillaries are classified as three structural and functional types, with features that allow different degrees of molecular or even cellular exchange: (1) **continuous capillaries** with many tight junctions so that all exchange must occur through the cells; (2) **fenestrated capillaries** with small pores or fenestrations through the cells; and (3) **discontinuous capillaries**, or **sinusoids**, with larger lumens, large spaces between the endothelial cells, and a discontinuous basal lamina.
- Capillary beds generally drain into **venules**, the last segment of the microvasculature; **postcapillary venules** are the sites at which white blood cells enter damaged or infected tissues.
- The endothelium of continuous capillaries and postcapillary venules is frequently surrounded by thin cells called **pericytes**, which contract to facilitate blood flow, and which can give rise to smooth muscle and connective tissue during microvascular remodeling or repair.
- Two alternative microvascular pathways include **arteriovenous anastomoses**, or **AV shunts**, in which arterioles can bypass a capillary bed, and **venous portal systems**, in which venules draining a capillary bed quickly branch again to form another capillary bed.
- **Small, medium, and large veins**, all with lumen diameters exceeding the thickness of the wall, carry blood back to the heart, with intimal **valves** preventing backflow, and have increasingly well-developed tunics.

Lymphatic Vessels

- Interstitial fluid not pulled into venules by colloidal osmotic pressure drains as **lymph** into blind vessels called **lymphatics**, or **lymphatic capillaries**, which have very thin endothelial cell walls with spaces between the cells.
- Lymphatics converge into larger, thin-walled **lymphatic vessels** in which lymph is propelled by movements of surrounding muscles and organs, with intimal **valves** keeping the flow unidirectional.
- The largest lymphatic vessels, the **thoracic duct** and **right lymphatic duct**, both with walls having tunics like those of veins, return lymph to the circulatory system by joining veins near the heart.

The Circulatory System ASSESS YOUR KNOWLEDGE

1. Vasa vasorum serve a function analogous to that of which of the following?
   a. Valves
   b. Basal lamina
   c. Coronary arteries
   d. Endothelial diaphragms
   e. Arterioles

2. What tissue is directly associated with and extends into the heart valves?
   a. Myocardium
   b. Epicardium
   c. Atrioventricular bundle of His
   d. Cardiac skeleton
   e. Pericardium

3. Which of the following is true for ventricles?
   a. Located at the base of the heart
   b. Myocardial cells contain abundant granules
   c. Receive blood directly from the venae cavae and pulmonary veins
   d. Walls contain Purkinje fibers of the right and left branches from the atrioventricular bundle
   e. Contain more elastic fibers than the atria

4. Individuals with Marfan syndrome have mutations in the fibrillin gene and commonly experience aortic aneurisms. What portion of the arterial wall is most likely to be affected by the malformed fibrillin?
   a. Endothelium
   b. Tunica intima
   c. Tunica media
   d. Tunica adventitia
   e. Vasa vasorum

5. Which description is true of continuous capillaries?
   a. Unusually wide lumens
   b. Most common in both brain and muscle
   c. Abundant fenestrations
   d. Lack a complete basement membrane
   e. Phagocytic cells often seen inserted in the intercellular clefts

6. Which of the following is true of pericytes?
   a. Are associated with the basal lamina of capillary endothelial cells
   b. Have similar histological features as contractile cells of the myocardium
   c. Form a layer of cells joined by gap junctions
   d. Are terminally differentiated
   e. Capable of forming multinucleated muscle fibers

7. During light microscopic examination of a tissue, you note a vessel that has no smooth muscle but a large amount of connective tissue at its periphery. Which of the following vessels are you examining?
   a. Arteriole
   b. Venule
   c. Elastic artery
   d. Capillary
   e. Large vein

8. A 43-year-old woman notices a lump in her left breast which upon pathological examination of a needle biopsy is diagnosed as stage 3 adenocarcinoma of the mammary gland. She elects to have a single mastectomy and the surgeon also removes several axillary lymph nodes to be examined to determine the tumor's state of metastasis. The patient recovers well from the surgery, but at a 6-month follow-up visit at the clinic her upper left arm is seen to be swollen and the surgeon prescribes a bandage wrap for "lymph edema." This condition likely resulted from which of the following?
   a. Angiogenesis from arterial branches that brought blood to the left breast
   b. Growth of cancer cells and blockage of lymphatic drainage from the left arm
   c. Surgical disruption of the left arm's lymphatic drainage by removal of lymph nodes
   d. Surgical damage to the thoracic duct during lymph node removal
   e. Hypertrophy of the vessels in the upper arm to accommodate blood otherwise flowing to the left breast

9. A 66-year-old man diagnosed with type II diabetes 10 years earlier presents with an aching pain in the muscles of his lower extremities. He says the pain is relieved by rest and worsened by physical activity. His lower limbs appear cold, pale, discolored, and he has a sore on the skin of his left heel. He has a weak tibial pulse on both sides and poor skin filling from dermal capillaries. The problems with blood distribution in this patient's leg are most likely associated with what vascular structures?
   a. Veins and venules
   b. Arterioles
   c. Branches of the aorta
   d. Lymphatic vessels
   e. Ventricles

10. A 62-year-old man of African descent presents with exercise-induced angina. His serum cholesterol is 277 mg/dL (normal <200), LDL is 157 (normal <100), HDL is 43 (normal >35), and triglycerides 170 (normal <150). His body mass index (BMI) is 34 and his coronary risk ratio is 6.84 (normal <5). Cardiac catheterization reveals an occlusion of the left anterior descending and the origin of the right coronary artery. This disease process initially involved which one of the following?
    a. Smooth muscle cell proliferation
    b. Formation of an intimal plaque
    c. Intimal thickening through addition of collagen and elastin
    d. Adventitial proliferation of fibroblasts
    e. Injury to endothelial cells

12 Blood

Blood represents a fluid connective tissue consisting of cells and liquid extracellular material called **plasma**. Propelled mainly by rhythmic contractions of the heart, 5 or 6 L of blood in an average adult move unidirectionally within the closed circulatory system. The so-called **formed elements** circulating in the plasma are **erythrocytes** (red blood cells), **leukocytes** (white blood cells [WBCs]) and **platelets**.

When blood leaves the circulatory system, either in a test tube or into the extracellular matrix (ECM) surrounding blood vessels, plasma proteins react with one another to yield a localized clot, which includes formed elements and releases a viscous, yellowish liquid called **serum**. Serum contains cellular growth factors and other proteins secreted by platelets during clot formation, which give serum biological properties very different from those of plasma.

Figure 12–1 shows that when a tube of collected blood, blocked from clotting by the addition of anticoagulants (eg, heparin or citrate), undergoes centrifugation it produces layers reflecting its composition. Erythrocytes comprise the sedimented material, called **hematocrit**, about 44% of the total blood volume in healthy adults.

The straw-colored supernatant comprising 55% at the top half of the centrifugation tube represents **plasma**, three or four times more viscous than water. A thin gray-white layer called the **buffy coat** between the plasma and hematocrit, only 1% of the volume, consists of leukocytes and platelets, both less dense than erythrocytes.

Blood is a distributing vehicle, transporting O_2, CO_2, metabolites, hormones, and other substances to cells throughout the body. Blood O_2 binds the erythrocyte protein hemoglobin and as shown in Figure 12–2 is much more abundant in arterial than in venous blood. Blood CO_2, in addition to being hemoglobin-bound, moves dissolved in plasma, some as HCO_3^-. Blood distributes nutrients from their sites of synthesis or absorption in the gut and collects metabolic residues in tissues throughout the body for removal from the blood by the excretory organs. Hormone distribution in blood permits the exchange of chemical messages between distant organs regulating normal organ function. Blood also participates in heat distribution, the regulation of body temperature, and the maintenance of acid-base and osmotic balance.

Leukocytes have diverse functions and collectively make up the body's chief defense against infection. Generally spherical and inactive while suspended in circulating blood, leukocytes cross the wall of venules, become motile, migrate into the tissues, and display their defensive capabilities when they arrive at sites of infection or inflammation.

❯ COMPOSITION OF PLASMA

Normal plasma, at pH 7.4, contains high and low molecular weight substances which make up about 7% of its volume. As summarized in Table 12–1 the dissolved components comprise mostly a specific set of plasma proteins, but also include nutrients, respiratory gases, nitrogenous wastes, hormones, and inorganic ions or **electrolytes**. Through the capillary walls, the low-molecular-weight components are in equilibrium with the interstitial fluid of tissues. The plasma composition usually serves to indicate well the mean composition of bodily extracellular fluids.

The major plasma proteins include the following:

- **Albumin**, the most abundant plasma protein, is synthesized in the liver and serves primarily to maintain the osmotic pressure of the blood.
- **Globulins (α- and β-globulins)**, a diverse group produced by the liver and other cells, includes transferrin and other transport factors; fibronectin; prothrombin and other coagulation factors; lipoproteins and other proteins entering blood from tissues.

FIGURE **12–1** Composition of whole blood.

A tube of blood after centrifugation (center) has nearly half of its volume represented by erythrocytes in the bottom half of the tube, a percentage called the **hematocrit**. Between the sedimented erythrocytes and the supernatant light-colored plasma is a thin layer of leukocytes and platelets called the **buffy coat**. The concentration ranges of erythrocytes, platelets, and leukocytes in normal blood are included here, along with the **differential count** or percent range for each type of leukocyte represented in the buffy coat. A cubic millimeter of blood is equivalent to a microliter (μL). (Complete blood count [CBC] values in this chapter are those used by the US National Board of Medical Examiners.)

- **Immunoglobulins** (**antibodies** or **γ-globulins**) secreted by plasma cells in many locations.
- **Fibrinogen**, the largest plasma protein (340 kD), also made in the liver, polymerizes during clotting as insoluble, cross-linked fibers of fibrin that block blood loss from small vessels.
- **Complement proteins** constitute a defensive system important in inflammation and destruction of microorganisms.

FIGURE **12–2** Blood O$_2$ content in each type of blood vessel.

The amount of O$_2$ in blood (the O$_2$ pressure) is highest in arteries and lung capillaries and decreases in tissue capillaries, where exchange of O$_2$ and CO$_2$ occurs between blood and tissues.

TABLE **12–1**	The composition of blood plasma.
Plasma Component (Percentage of Plasma)	**Functions**
Water (~92% of plasma)	Is the solvent in which formed elements are suspended and proteins and solutes are dissolved
Plasma proteins (~7% of plasma)	All proteins serve to buffer against pH changes
Albumin (~58% of plasma proteins)	Exerts osmotic force to retain fluid within the microvasculature
	Contributes to blood's viscosity
	Binds and transports some fatty acids, electrolytes, hormones, and drugs
Globulins (~37% of plasma proteins)	α-Globulins transport lipids and some metal ions
	β-Globulins transport iron ions and lipids in bloodstream
	γ-Globulins are antibodies with various immune functions
Fibrinogen (~4% of plasma proteins)	Participates in blood coagulation (clotting); precursor of fibrin
Regulatory proteins (>1% of plasma proteins)	Consists of enzymes, proenzymes, hormones, and the complement system
Other Solutes (~1% of Blood Plasma)	
Electrolytes (eg, sodium, potassium, calcium, chloride, iron, bicarbonate, and hydrogen)	Help establish and maintain membrane potentials, maintain pH balance, and regulate osmosis (control of the percentages of water and salt in the blood)
Nutrients (eg, amino acids, glucose, cholesterol, vitamins, fatty acids)	Energy source; precursor for synthesizing other molecules
Respiratory gases (eg, oxygen: >2% dissolved in plasma, 98% bound to hemoglobin within erythrocytes; and carbon dioxide: ~7% dissolved in plasma, ~27% bound to hemoglobin within erythrocytes, ~66% converted to HCO_3^-)	Oxygen is needed for aerobic cellular respiration; carbon dioxide is a waste product produced by cells during this process
Wastes (breakdown products of metabolism) (eg, lactic acid, creatinine, urea, bilirubin, ammonia)	Waste products serve no function in the blood plasma; they are merely being transported to the liver and kidneys where they can be removed from the blood

❯ BLOOD CELLS

Blood cells are best studied histologically in a thin smear of blood on a slide, prepared as shown in Figure 12–3. In such films the cells become clearly visible and distinct from one another, facilitating observation of cell nuclei and general cytoplasmic features. Blood smears are routinely stained with mixtures of acidic (eosin) and basic (methylene blue) dyes, but may also contain dyes called azures with better ability to stain cytoplasmic granules containing charged proteins and proteoglycans. Azurophilic granules produce metachromasia in stained leukocytes like that of mast cells in connective tissue. Some of these special stains, such as Giemsa and Wright stain, are named after hematologists who introduced their own modifications into the original mixtures.

Erythrocytes

Erythrocytes (red blood cells or RBCs) are terminally differentiated cells, lacking nuclei and filled completely with the O_2-carrying protein hemoglobin. RBCs are the only blood cells whose function does not require them to leave the vasculature.

Normal human erythrocytes suspended in an isotonic medium invariably form flexible biconcave discs (Figure 12–4), about 7.5 μm in diameter, 2.6-μm thick at the rim, but only 0.75-μm thick in the center. Because of their uniform dimensions and presence in most tissue sections, RBCs can often serve as an internal standard allowing histologists to estimate the size of other nearby cells or structures.

> **❯❯ MEDICAL APPLICATION**
>
> **Anemia** is the condition of having a concentration of erythrocytes below the normal range. With fewer RBCs per milliliter of blood, tissues may be unable to receive adequate O_2. Symptoms of anemia include lethargy, shortness of breath, fatigue, skin pallor, and heart palpitations. **Sickle cell anemia** results from a homozygous mutation causing an amino acid substitution in hemoglobin, which renders the mature RBCs deformed and slightly rigid (Figure 12–5) and can lead to capillary blockage.
>
> An increased concentration of erythrocytes in blood (**erythrocytosis** or **polycythemia**) may be a physiologic adaptation found, for example, in individuals who live at high altitudes, where O_2 tension is low. Elevated hematocrit increases blood viscosity, putting strain on the heart, and, if severe, can impair circulation through the capillaries.

The biconcave shape provides a large surface-to-volume ratio, facilitating gas exchange. The normal concentration of erythrocytes in blood is approximately 3.9–5.5 million per microliter (μL, or mm³) in women and 4.1–6.0 million/μL in men.

Erythrocytes are normally quite flexible, permitting them to bend and adapt to the small diameters and irregular turns of capillaries. Observations in vivo show that at acute angles of

FIGURE **12–3** Preparing a blood smear.

Withdraw blood

Stain

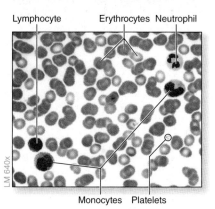

Lymphocyte   Erythrocytes   Neutrophil

LM 640x

Monocytes   Platelets

① Prick finger and collect a small amount of blood using a micropipette.

② Place a drop of blood on a slide.

③a Using a second slide, pull the drop of blood across the first slide's surface, leaving a thin layer of blood on the slide.

③b After the blood dries, apply a stain briefly and rinse. Place a coverslip on top.

④ When viewed under the microscope, blood smear reveals the components of the formed elements.

branching capillaries erythrocytes with normal adult hemoglobin frequently assume a cuplike shape. In larger vessels within the microvasculature, RBCs may adhere to one another loosely in stacks called rouleau (Figure 12–4c), particularly in conditions of low flow velocity or increased plasma viscosity.

The erythrocyte plasmalemma, because of its ready availability, is the best-known cell membrane. It consists of about 40% lipid, 10% carbohydrate, and 50% protein. Most of the latter represent integral membrane proteins (see Chapter 2), including ion channels, the anion transporter called **band 3 protein**, and

FIGURE **12–4** Normal human erythrocytes.

Sectional view

~.75 μm   ~2.6 μm

b   ~7.5 μm

Rouleaux   Erythrocytes

(a) Pseudocolored SEM micrograph of normal **erythrocytes** with each side concave. (×1800)

(b) Diagram of an **erythrocyte** giving the cell's dimensions. The biconcave shape provides the cell a very high surface-to-volume ratio and places most hemoglobin close to the cell surface, both qualities that provide maximally efficient O$_2$ transport. This shape

also contributes to erythrocyte flexibility, allowing them to bend easily to pass through small capillaries.

(c) In small blood vessels erythrocytes may also stack up in loose aggregates called rouleau. The standard 7.5 μm diameter of RBCs allows one to estimate that the venule shown here is approximately 15 μm in diameter. (×250; H&E)

FIGURE **12–5** Sickle cell erythrocyte.

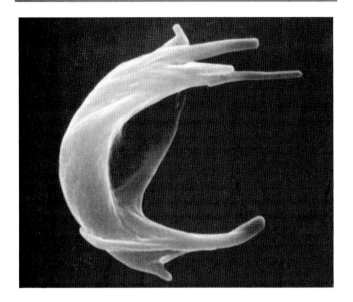

A single nucleotide substitute in the hemoglobin gene produces a version of the protein that polymerizes to form rigid aggregates, leading to greatly misshapen cells with reduced flexibility. In individuals homozygous for the mutated *HbS* gene this can lead to greater blood viscosity and poor microvascular circulation, both features of sickle cell disease. (×6500)

glycophorin A. The glycosylated extracellular domains of the two latter proteins include antigenic sites which form the basis for the ABO blood typing system. Several peripheral proteins are associated with the inner surface of the membrane, including both **spectrin**, dimers of which make a lattice bound to underlying actin filaments, and **ankyrin**, which anchors the spectrin lattice to the glycophorins and band 3 proteins. This submembranous meshwork helps to stabilize the cell membrane, maintain cell shape, and provide the cell elasticity required for passage through capillaries.

Mature erythrocyte cytoplasm lacks all organelles, being completely filled with **hemoglobin**, the tetrameric O_2-carrying protein that accounts for the cells' uniform acidophilia. When bound with O_2 or CO_2, hemoglobin forms oxyhemoglobin or carbaminohemoglobin, respectively. The reversibility of these combinations is the basis for the protein's gas-transporting capacity.

Erythrocytes undergo terminal differentiation (discussed in Chapter 13), which includes loss of the nucleus and organelles shortly before the cells move from bone marrow into the circulation. Lacking mitochondria, erythrocytes rely on anaerobic glycolysis for their minimal energy needs. Lacking nuclei, they cannot replace defective proteins.

Human erythrocytes normally survive in the circulation for about 120 days. By this time, defects in the membrane's cytoskeletal lattice or ion transport systems begin to produce swelling or other shape abnormalities, as well as changes in the cells' surface oligosaccharide complexes. Senescent or worn-out RBCs displaying such changes are recognized and removed from circulation, mainly by macrophages in the spleen, liver, and bone marrow.

Leukocytes

Leukocytes (white blood cells or WBCs) leave the blood and migrate to the tissues where they become functional and perform various activities related to immunity. Hematologists divide leukocytes into two major groups, **granulocytes** and **agranulocytes**, based on the number and density of their cytoplasmic granules (Table 12–2). All appear rather spherical while suspended in blood plasma, but become amoeboid and motile after leaving the blood vessels, attaching to a substrate, and entering the ECM of the tissue. The estimated sizes mentioned here refer to WBCs in blood smears, where the cells may spread and appear slightly larger than their size in circulating blood.

Granulocytes possess two major types of abundant cytoplasmic granules: lysosomes (often called **azurophilic granules** in WBCs) and **specific granules** that have specialized functions and bind neutral, acidic, or basic stains, which allows their classification as **neutrophils, eosinophils**, and **basophils**. As indicated in Figure 12–1 and Table 12–2, the granulocytes all also have **polymorphic nuclei** with two or more distinct (almost separated) lobes.

All granulocytes represent terminally differentiated cells with a life span of only a few days after they leave the bloodstream. Their rough ER and Golgi complexes are now poorly developed, and with few mitochondria they depend largely on glycolysis for energy. Most granulocytes die by apoptosis in the connective tissue and billions of neutrophils alone do so each day in healthy adults. The resulting cellular debris undergoes removal by other cells, notably macrophages, and like all apoptotic cell death does not itself elicit an inflammatory response.

Agranulocytes contain essentially no specific granules and only scattered azurophilic granules (lysosomes). This group includes all **lymphocytes** and **monocytes**. Their nuclei are spherical or indented, but not lobulated. Figure 12–1 and Table 12–2 summarize the sizes, structural features, major functions, and differential count (or percentage of all leukocytes) for each leukocyte type.

All leukocytes play key roles in the constant defense against invading microorganisms and in repair of injured tissues, and many can specifically leave the microvasculature locally where infection and injury occur. At such sites various sources release factors called **cytokines** that loosen intercellular junctions in the endothelium of local postcapillary venules (Figure 12–6). Simultaneously, the cell adhesion protein **P-selectin** appears on the endothelial cells' luminal surfaces after exocytosis from Weibel-Palade bodies in these cells. The surfaces of neutrophils and other leukocytes

TABLE 12–2	Leukocytes: Numbers, structural features, and major functions.

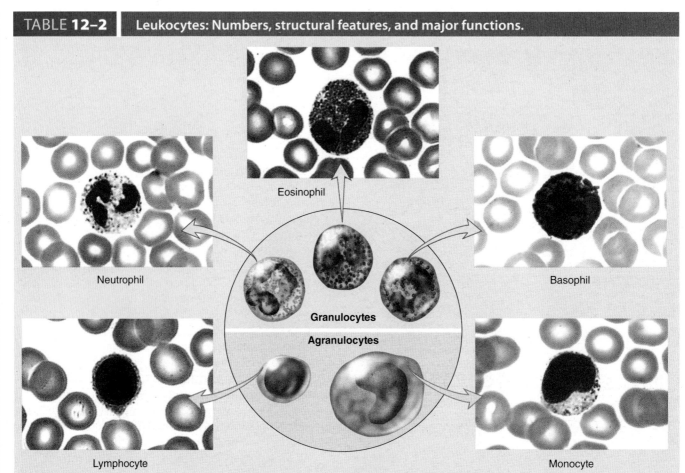

Type	Nucleus	Specific Granules[a]	Differential Count[b] (%)	Life Span Outside the Blood	Major Functions
Granulocytes					
Neutrophils	3–5 lobes	Faint/light pink	50–70	1–4 d	Kill and phagocytose bacteria
Eosinophils	Bilobed	Red/dark pink	1–4	1–2 wk	Kill helminthic and other parasites; modulate local inflammation
Basophils	Bilobed or S-shaped	Dark blue/purple	0.5–1	1–3 d	Modulate inflammation, release histamine during allergy
Agranulocytes					
Lymphocytes	Rather spherical	(none)	20–40	Hours to many years	Effector and regulatory cells for adaptive immunity
Monocytes	Indented or C-shaped	(none)	2–8	Hours to years	Precursors of macrophages and other mononuclear phagocytic cells

[a]Color with routine blood smear stains. There are typically 4500–11,000 total leukocytes/μL of blood in adults, higher in infants and young children.

[b]The percentage ranges given for each type of leukocyte are those used by the US National Board of Medical Examiners. The value for neutrophils includes 3%–5% circulating, immature band forms.

All micrographs ×1600.

FIGURE **12–6** Diagram of events involving leukocytes in a postcapillary venule at sites of inflammation.

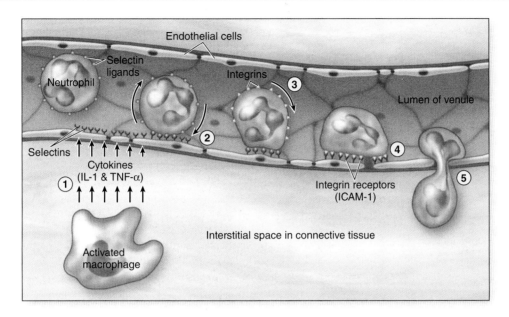

Locations in connective tissue with infection or injuries require the rapid immigration of various leukocytes to initiate cellular events to remove invading microorganisms and for tissue repair. The cytokines and cell binding proteins target various leukocytes and are best known for neutrophils, in which the major initial events of migration during inflammation occur as follows:

1. Local macrophages activated by bacteria or tissue damage release **proinflammatory cytokines** such as interleukin-1 (IL-1) or tumor necrosis factor-α (TNF-α) that signal endothelial cells of nearby postcapillary venules to rapidly insert glycoprotein **selectins** on the luminal cell surfaces.
2. Passing neutrophils with appropriate cell surface glycoproteins bind the selectins, which causes such cells to adhere loosely to the endothelium and "roll" slowly along its surface.
3. Exposure to these and other cytokines causes expression of new **integrins** on the rolling leukocytes and expression

of the integrin ligand **ICAM-1** (intercellular adhesion molecule-1) on the endothelial cells, as well as selectively downregulating junctional complexes in the endothelium, loosening these cells.
4. Integrins and their ligands provide firm endothelial adhesion of neutrophils to the endothelium, allowing the leukocytes to receive further stimulation from the local cytokines.
5. Neutrophils become motile, probe the endothelium with pseudopodia, and, being attracted by other local injury-related factors called chemokines, finally migrate by **diapedesis** between the loosened cells of the venule. Rapid transendothelial migration of neutrophils is facilitated by the cells' elongated and segmented nuclei. All leukocytes first become functional in the ECM after extravasation from the circulation by this process.

display glycosylated ligands for P-selectin, and their interactions cause cells flowing through the affected venules to slow down, like rolling tennis balls arriving at a surface with Velcro. Other cytokines stimulate these now slowly rolling leukocytes to express integrins and other adhesion factors that produce firm attachment to the endothelium (see Figure 11–21d). In a process called **diapedesis** (Gr. *dia*, through + *pedesis*, to leap), these leukocytes squeeze through the openings between the endothelial cells, migrate out of the venules into the surrounding tissue, and crawl directly to the site of injury or microbial invasion. The attraction of neutrophils to bacteria involves chemical mediators in a type of **chemotaxis**, which causes leukocytes to accumulate rapidly where their defensive actions are specifically needed.

The number of leukocytes in the blood varies according to age, sex, and physiologic conditions, with healthy adults having 4500–11,000 leukocytes per microliter of blood.

Neutrophils (Polymorphonuclear Leukocytes)

Neutrophils constitute 50%–70% of circulating leukocytes, a figure that includes slightly immature forms released to the circulation. Typically, 12–15 μm in diameter in blood smears, mature neutrophils have nuclei with two to five distinct lobes linked by thin nuclear extensions (Table 12–2; Figure 12–7). In females, the inactive X chromosome in neutrophils may appear as a drumstick-like appendage on one of the nuclear lobes (Figure 12–7c). Neutrophils remain inactive and spherical while circulating but become amoeboid and very dynamic

FIGURE 12–7 Neutrophils.

(a) In blood smears, **neutrophils** can be identified by their multilobulated nuclei, with lobules held together by very thin strands. Given this feature, the cells are often called **polymorphonuclear leukocytes**, PMNs, or just **polymorphs**. The cells are dynamic and the nuclear shape appears to change frequently. (×1500; Giemsa)

(b) **Neutrophils** typically have diameters ranging from 12 to 15 μm, approximately twice that of the surrounding erythrocytes. The cytoplasmic granules are relatively sparse and have heterogeneous, generally pale staining properties and do not obscure the nucleus. (×1500; Giemsa)

(c) **Neutrophils** from females often have the condensed X chromosome appearing as a drumstick appendage from a nuclear lobe (arrow). (×1500; Wright)

during diapedesis and upon adhering to ECM substrates such as collagen fibers.

Neutrophils usually represent the first leukocytes to arrive at sites of infection, where they actively pursue bacterial cells using chemotaxis and remove the invaders or their debris by phagocytosis during the early phase of inflammation.

The cytoplasmic granules of neutrophils provide the cells' functional activities and as mentioned, exist as two main types (Figure 12–8). **Azurophilic primary granules** or lysosomes are large, dense vesicles with a major role in both killing and degrading microorganisms after phagocytosis. They contain proteases and antibacterial proteins, including the following:

- **Myeloperoxidase** (MPO), which generates hypochlorite and other agents toxic to bacteria,
- **Lysozyme**, which degrades components of bacterial cell walls, and
- **Defensins**, small cysteine-rich proteins that bind and disrupt the cell membranes of many types of bacteria and other microorganisms.

Several kinds of **neutrophil defects**, often genetic in origin, can affect function of these cells, for example, by decreasing adhesion to the wall of venules, by causing the absence of specific granules, or with deficits in certain factors of the azurophilic granules. Individuals with such disorders typically experience more frequent and more persistent bacterial infections, although macrophages and other leukocytes may substitute for certain neutrophil functions.

Specific secondary granules appear as smaller and less dense vesicles, staining faintly pink, and have diverse functions, including secretion of various ECM-degrading enzymes such as collagenases, delivery of additional bactericidal proteins to phagolysosomes, and insertion of new cell membrane components.

After clearing microorganisms early in inflammation, more neutrophils arrive locally and undertake supportive roles in the events initiating restoration of the tissue's normal microenvironment. These neutrophils release **proresolving mediators**, various proteins and specialized lipids that promote resolution of inflammation, as well as polypeptide **chemokines** and **cytokines**, which attract and regulate the activities of other leukocytes and local cells.

Neutrophils contain glycogen which the glycolytic pathway breaks down into glucose to yield energy. The citric acid cycle is less important, consistent with the paucity of mitochondria in these cells. Neutrophils' capacity for dynamic activities in an anaerobic environment allows them to operate killing bacteria and helping to clean up debris in poorly oxygenated environments, most importantly in damaged tissue lacking normal microvasculature.

Neutrophils are short-lived cells with a half-life of 6–8 hours in the circulation and a life span of 1–4 active days in connective tissues before undergoing apoptosis.

Neutrophils look for bacteria to engulf by pseudopodia and internalize them in vacuoles called **phagosomes**. Immediately thereafter, specific granules fuse with and discharge their contents into the phagosomes that are then acidified by proton pumps. Azurophilic granules then discharge their enzymes into this acidified vesicle, killing and digesting the engulfed microorganisms.

During phagocytosis, a burst of O_2 consumption leads to the formation of superoxide anions (O_2^-) and hydrogen peroxide (H_2O_2). O_2^- is a short-lived, highly reactive free radical that, together with MPO and halide ions, forms a powerful microbial killing system inside the neutrophils. Besides the activity of lysozyme cleaving cell wall peptidoglycans to kill certain bacteria, the protein lactoferrin avidly binds iron, a crucial element in bacterial nutrition whose lack of availability then causes bacteria to die. A combination of these mechanisms will kill most microorganisms, which are then digested by lysosomal enzymes. Apoptotic neutrophils, bacteria, semidigested material, and tissue fluid form a viscous, usually yellow collection of fluid called **pus**.

FIGURE **12–8** Neutrophil ultrastructure.

A TEM of a sectioned human **neutrophil** reveals the two types of cytoplasmic granules: the small, pale, more variably stained specific granules (**S**) and the larger, electron-dense azurophilic granules (**A**).

Specific granules undergo exocytosis during and after diapedesis, releasing many factors with various activities, including enzymes to digest ECM components and bactericidal factors.

Azurophilic granules represent modified lysosomes with components to kill engulfed bacteria.

Lobes of the nucleus (**N**) associate closely with the small, central Golgi apparatus (**G**). Rough ER and mitochondria are relatively sparse because the cell utilizes anaerobic glycolysis and has little synthetic activity in circulation or after activation. (×25,000)

Several neutrophil hereditary dysfunctions have been described. In one of them, actin does not polymerize normally, reducing neutrophil motility. With an NADPH oxidase deficiency, there is a failure to produce H_2O_2 and hypochlorite, reducing the cells' microbial killing power. Children with such dysfunctions can experience more persistent bacterial infections.

Eosinophils

Eosinophils occur far less commonly than neutrophils, constituting only 1%–4% of leukocytes. In blood smears, this cell is about the same size as a neutrophil or slightly larger, but with a characteristic bilobed nucleus (Table 12–2; Figure 12–9). The abundance of large, acidophilic specific granules typically staining pink or red make up their main identifying characteristic.

Ultrastructurally, the eosinophil's-specific granules are seen to be oval shaped with flattened crystalloid cores (Figure 12–9c) containing **major basic proteins (MBP)**, an arginine-rich factor that accounts for the granule's acidophilia and constitutes up to 50% of the total granule protein. MBPs, along with eosinophilic peroxidase, other enzymes and toxins, act to kill parasitic worms or helminths. Eosinophils also modulate inflammatory responses by releasing chemokines, cytokines, and proresolving lipid mediators, all important in inflammatory responses triggered by allergies. The number of circulating eosinophils increases during both helminthic infections and allergic reactions. These leukocytes also specifically phagocytose antigen-antibody complexes from interstitial fluid.

Eosinophils occur more abundantly in connective tissue of the intestinal lining and at sites of chronic inflammation, such as lung tissues of asthma patients.

FIGURE **12–9** Eosinophils.

Eosinophils are about the same size as neutrophils but have simpler bilobed nuclei and more abundant coarse cytoplasmic granules. The cytoplasm is usually filled with brightly eosinophilic specific granules, but also includes some azurophilic granules.

(a) Micrograph shows an eosinophil (**E**) next to a neutrophil (**N**) and a small lymphocyte (**L**). (×1500; Wright)

(b) Even with granules filling the cytoplasm, the two nuclear lobes of **eosinophils** often appear clearly. (×1500; Giemsa)

(c) Ultrastructurally, a sectioned **eosinophil** distinctly shows the unique eosinophilic granules (**EG**), as oval structures with disc-shaped electron-dense, crystalline cores. These granules, along with a few lysosomes and mitochondria (**M**), fill the cytoplasm around the bilobed nucleus (**N**). (×20,000)

›› MEDICAL APPLICATION

An increase in the number of eosinophils in blood (**eosinophilia**) is associated with allergic reactions and helminthic infections. In patients with such conditions, eosinophils are found in the connective tissues underlying epithelia of the bronchi, gastrointestinal tract, uterus, and vagina, and surrounding any parasitic worms present. In addition, these cells produce substances that modulate inflammation by inactivating the leukotrienes and histamine produced by other cells. Corticosteroids (hormones from the adrenal cortex) produce a rapid decrease in the number of blood eosinophils, probably by interfering with their release from the bone marrow into the bloodstream.

Basophils

Basophils also have diameters of 12–15 μm, but make up less than 1% of circulating leukocytes and are therefore rare in normal blood smears. The nucleus characteristically displays two irregular lobes, but the large specific granules overlying the nucleus often obscure its shape.

The specific granules (0.5 μm in diameter) typically stain purple with the basic dye of blood smear stains and are fewer, larger, and more irregularly shaped than the granules of other granulocytes (Table 12–2; Figure 12–10). The strong basophilia of the granules is due to the presence of **heparin** and other sulfated GAGs. Basophilic specific granules also contain much **histamine** and various other mediators of inflammation, including platelet activating factor, eosinophil chemotactic factor, and the enzyme phospholipase A that catalyzes an initial step in producing lipid-derived inflammatory factors called **leukotrienes**.

By migrating into connective tissues basophils appear to transiently supplement the functions of mast cells, described in Chapter 5. Like mast cells basophils have surface **receptors for immunoglobulin E (IgE)** and secrete heparin and histamine in response to various antigens and allergens.

FIGURE **12–10** Basophils.

(a–c) Basophils are also approximately the same size as neutrophils and eosinophils, but they have large, strongly basophilic specific granules that most often obstruct the appearance of the nucleus, which usually has two large irregular lobes. Basophils are also the least abundant type of granulocyte in the circulation. (a and b: ×1500, Wright; c: ×1500, Giemsa)

(d) A TEM of a sectioned **basophil** reveals the single bilobed nucleus (**N**) and the large, electron-dense specific basophilic granules (**B**). Basophils exert many activities modulating the immune response and inflammation and have many functional similarities with mast cells, which develop as normal, longer-term residents of connective tissue. (×25,000)

>> MEDICAL APPLICATION

In some individuals a second exposure to a strong allergen, such as that delivered in a bee sting, may produce an intense, adverse systemic response. Basophils and mast cells may rapidly degranulate, producing vasodilation in many organs, a sudden drop in blood pressure, and other effects comprising a potentially lethal condition called **anaphylaxis** or **anaphylactic shock**.

Basophils and mast cells also are central to immediate or **type 1 hypersensitivity**. In some individuals, substances such as certain pollen proteins or specific proteins in food are allergenic, that is, elicit production of specific IgE antibodies, which then bind to receptors on mast cells and immigrating basophils. Upon subsequent exposure, the allergen combines with the receptor-bound IgE molecules, causing them to cross-link and aggregate on the cell surfaces and triggering rapid exocytosis of the cytoplasmic granules. Release of the inflammatory mediators in this manner can result in **bronchial asthma**, cutaneous **hives**, **rhinitis**, **conjunctivitis**, or **allergic gastroenteritis**.

Lymphocytes

By far the most numerous type of agranulocyte in normal blood smears, **lymphocytes** make up a leukocyte family with spherical nuclei (Table 12–2; Figure 12–11). Typically the smallest leukocytes, lymphocytes constitute approximately one-third of all these cells. Although they are morphologically similar, mature lymphocytes can be subdivided into functional groups by distinctive surface molecules (called "cluster of differentiation" or **CD markers**) distinguished using antibodies with immunocytochemistry or flow cytometry. Major classes include **B lymphocytes**, helper and cytotoxic **T lymphocytes** (CD4$^+$ and CD8$^+$, respectively), and **natural killer (NK) cells**. These and other types of lymphocytes have diverse roles in immune defenses against invading microorganisms, certain parasites, and abnormal cells. T lymphocytes, unlike B cells and all other circulating leukocytes, differentiate outside the bone marrow in the thymus. Discussion of the immune system in Chapter 14 includes the formation and major functions of lymphocytes.

FIGURE **12–11** Lymphocytes.

Lymphocytes are agranulocytes and lack all specific granules characteristic of granulocytes. Lymphocytes circulating in blood generally range in size from 6 to 15 μm in diameter and are sometimes classified arbitrarily as small, medium, and large.

(a) The most numerous **small lymphocytes** shown here are slightly larger than the neighboring erythrocytes and have only a thin rim of cytoplasm surrounding the spherical nucleus. (×1500; Giemsa)

(b) Medium lymphocytes are distinctly larger than erythrocytes. (×1500; Wright)

(c) Large lymphocytes, much bigger than erythrocytes, may represent activated cells that have returned to the circulation. (×1500; Giemsa)

(d) Ultrastructurally, a **medium-sized lymphocyte** is seen to be mostly filled with a euchromatic nucleus (**N**) surrounded by cytoplasm containing mitochondria (**M**), free polysomes, and a few dark lysosomes (azurophilic granules). (×22,000)

The size of each lymphocyte reflects the cell's state of maturation and immune activation.

Although generally small, circulating lymphocytes have a wider range of sizes than most leukocytes. The smallest, newly released lymphocytes have diameters similar to those of RBCs; medium and large lymphocytes are 9-18 μm in diameter, with the latter representing activated lymphocytes or NK cells. Immature lymphocytes characteristically have spherical nuclei with highly condensed chromatin and only a thin surrounding rim of scant cytoplasm, making them easily distinguishable from granulocytes. Larger lymphocytes have larger, slightly indented nuclei and more, slightly basophilic, cytoplasm with a few azurophilic granules, mitochondria, free polysomes, and other organelles (Figure 12–11d).

Lymphocytes vary in life span according to their specific functions; some live only a few days and others survive in the circulating blood or other tissues for many years.

❯❯ MEDICAL APPLICATION

Given their central roles in immunity, lymphocytes are obviously important in many diseases. **Lymphomas** are a group of disorders involving neoplastic proliferation of lymphocytes or the failure of these cells to undergo apoptosis. Although often slow-growing, all lymphomas are considered malignant because they can very easily become widely spread throughout the body.

Monocytes

Monocytes are the precursor cells of macrophages, osteoclasts, microglia, and other cells of the **mononuclear phagocyte system** in connective tissue of nearly all organs (see Chapter 5). Circulating monocytes have diameters of 12–15 μm and have characteristic nuclei that are large and usually distinctly indented or C-shaped (Figure 12–12). The chromatin appears less condensed than in lymphocytes and typically stains lighter than that of large lymphocytes. Cells of the mononuclear phagocyte system arise in developing organs from monocytes formed in the embryonic yolk sac and are supplemented throughout life by monocytes from the bone marrow. All monocyte-derived cells serve as key antigen-presenting cells with important roles in immune defense as well as tissue repair.

The cytoplasm of the monocyte is basophilic and contains many small lysosomal azurophilic granules, some of which are at the limit of the light microscope's resolution. These granules become distributed throughout the cytoplasm, giving it a bluish-gray color in stained smears. Mitochondria and small areas of rough ER also occur, along with a Golgi apparatus involved in lysosome formation (Figure 12–12e).

FIGURE 12–12 Monocytes.

Monocytes are large agranulocytes with diameters from 12 to 20 μm circulating as precursors to macrophages and other cells of the mononuclear phagocyte system.

(a–d) Micrographs of **monocytes** showing their distinctive nuclei that are indented, kidney-shaped, or C-shaped. (a: ×1500, Giemsa; b–d: ×1500, Wright)

(e) Ultrastructurally the cytoplasm of a **monocyte** shows a Golgi apparatus (**G**), mitochondria (**M**), and lysosomes or azurophilic granules (**A**). Rough ER remains poorly developed and there are some free polysomes (**R**). (×22,000)

(Figure 12–12e, reproduced with permission from D. F. Bainton and M. G. Farquhar, Department of Pathology, University of California, San Francisco, CA.)

Platelets

Blood **platelets** (or **thrombocytes**) consist of very small non-nucleated, membrane-bound cell fragments, only 2–4 µm in diameter (Figure 12–13a). As described in Chapter 13, platelets originate by separation from the ends of cytoplasmic processes extending from giant polyploid bone marrow cells called **megakaryocytes**. Platelets promote blood clotting and help repair minor tears or leaks in the walls of small

FIGURE **12–13** Platelets.

Platelets are cell fragments 2-4 µm in diameter derived from megakaryocytes in bone marrow. Their primary function involves rapid release of their granules' contents upon contact with collagen (or other ECM material outside of the endothelium) to begin the process of clot formation and reduce blood loss from the vasculature.

(a) In a blood smear **platelets** (arrows) are often found as aggregates. Individually they show a lightly stained **hyalomere** region surrounding a more darkly stained central **granulomere** region containing membrane-enclosed granules. (×1500; Wright)

(b) Ultrastructurally a **platelet** shows a system of microtubules and actin filaments near the periphery, called the **marginal bundle (MB)**, which forms as the platelet pinches off from megakaryocyte (see Chapter 13) and helps maintain its shape. An open canalicular system (**OCS**) of invaginating membrane vesicles continuous with the plasmalemma facilitates rapid degranulation upon activation and Ca^{2+} release. The central granulomere region contains small dense delta granules (**δG**), larger and more numerous alpha granules (**αG**), and glycogen (**G**). (×40,000)

(Figure 12–13b, reproduced with permission from Dr M. J. G. Harrison, Middlesex Hospital and University College London, UK.)

blood vessels, preventing loss of blood from the microvasculature. Normal platelet counts range from 150,000 to 400,000/μL (mm³) of blood. Circulating platelets have a life span of about 10 days.

In stained blood smears, platelets often appear in clumps. Each individual platelet is generally discoid, with a very lightly stained peripheral zone, the **hyalomere**, and a darker-staining central zone rich in granules, called the **granulomere**. A sparse glycocalyx surrounding the platelet plasmalemma is involved in adhesion and activation during blood coagulation.

Ultrastructural analysis (Figure 12–13b) reveals a peripheral **marginal bundle** of microtubules and microfilaments, which helps to maintain the platelet's shape. Also, in the hyalomere are two systems of membrane channels. An **open canalicular system** of vesicles connects with invaginations of the plasma membrane and may facilitate platelets' uptake of factors from plasma. A less prominent set of irregular tubular vesicles, the dense tubular system, derives from the ER and stores Ca^{2+} ions. Together, these two membranous systems facilitate the extremely rapid exocytosis of proteins from platelets (degranulation) upon their adhesion to collagen or other substrates outside the vascular endothelium.

Besides specific granules, the central granulomere has a sparse population of mitochondria and glycogen particles (Figure 12–13b). Electron-dense **delta granules (δG)**, 250–300 nm in diameter, contain ADP, ATP, and serotonin (5-hydroxytryptamine) taken up from plasma. **Alpha granules (αG)** are larger (300–500 nm in diameter) and contain platelet-derived growth factor (PDGF), platelet factor 4, and several other platelet-specific proteins. Most of the stained granules seen in platelets with the light microscope represent alpha granules.

The role of platelets in controlling blood loss (hemorrhage) and in wound healing can be summarized as follows:

- **Primary aggregation:** Disruptions in the microvascular endothelium, which are very common, allow the platelet glycocalyx to adhere to collagen in the vascular basal lamina. Thus, a **platelet plug** forms as a first step to stop bleeding (Figure 12–14).
- **Secondary aggregation:** Platelets in the plug release a specific adhesive glycoprotein and ADP, which induce further platelet aggregation and increase the size of the platelet plug.
- **Blood coagulation:** During platelet aggregation **fibrinogen** from plasma, **von Willebrand factor** and other proteins released from the damaged endothelium, and **platelet factor 4** from platelet granules promote the sequential interaction (cascade) of plasma proteins, giving rise to a **fibrin** polymer that forms a three-dimensional network of fibers trapping RBCs and more platelets to form a **blood clot**, or **thrombus** (Figure 12–14). Platelet factor 4 is a chemokine for monocytes, neutrophils, and fibroblasts, and platelet-derived growth factor (PDGF) stimulates fibroblast proliferation and growth.

FIGURE 12–14 Platelet aggregation, degranulation, and fibrin clot formation.

(a) SFM showing the fibrin clot surrounding local erythrocytes immediately after minor trauma to vessels of the microvasculature, which happens routinely in active individuals thanks to the activity of **platelets**. Upon contact with collagen in the vascular basement membrane, platelets aggregate, swell, and disintegrate to release factors triggering formation of a fibrin meshwork **(F)** that traps erythrocytes and other blood cells. Recruiting more platelets, such a clot is enlarged to block blood loss from the small vessel. (Aggregated platelets in various states of degranulation are shown in the next photo.) After repair of the vessel wall, fibrin clots are gradually removed by proteolysis due primarily to locally generated plasmin, a non-specific protease. (×4000)

(b) Platelets aggregate at the onset of clot formation. This TEM section shows platelets in a platelet plug adhering to collagen **(C)**. Upon adhering to collagen, platelets are activated and their granules undergo exocytosis into the open canalicular system, which facilitates extremely rapid release of factors involved in blood coagulation. With their contents completely released, the degranulated platelets **(arrows)** remain as part of the aggregate until the clot is removed. Several other key proteins for blood coagulation occur in the plasma and are secreted locally from adjacent endothelial cell processes **(EP)**. Part of an erythrocyte **(E)** is seen at the right. (×7500)

- **Clot retraction:** The clot initially bulges into the blood vessel lumen, but soon contracts slightly due to the activity of platelet-derived actin and myosin.
- **Clot removal:** Protected by the clot, the endothelium and surrounding tunic are restored with new tissue, after which the clot is removed, mainly dissolved by the proteolytic enzyme **plasmin**, formed through the local action of **plasminogen activators** from the endothelium on **plasminogen** from plasma.

> **» MEDICAL APPLICATION**
>
> **Aspirin** and other nonsteroidal anti-inflammatory agents have an inhibitory effect on platelet function and blood coagulation because they block the local prostaglandin synthesis, which is needed for platelet aggregation, contraction, and exocytosis at sites of injury. **Bleeding disorders** result from abnormally slow blood clotting. One such disease directly related to a defect in the platelets is a rare autosomal recessive **glycoprotein Ib deficiency**, involving a factor on the platelet surface needed to bind subendothelial collagen and begin the cascade of events leading to clot formation.

Blood SUMMARY OF KEY POINTS

- **Plasma** makes up the liquid portion of circulating blood, while the cells and platelets comprise the **formed elements**; upon clotting, some proteins are removed from plasma and others are released from platelets, forming a new liquid termed **serum**.
- Important protein components of plasma include **albumin**, diverse **α- and β-globulins**, proteins of the **complement** system, and **fibrinogen**, all of which are secreted within the liver, as well as the **immunoglobulins**.
- **RBCs** or **erythrocytes**, which make up the **hematocrit** portion (~45%) of a blood sample, are **enucleated, biconcave discs** 7.5 μm in diameter, filled with **hemoglobin** for the uptake, transport, and release of O_2, and with a normal life span of about **120 days**.
- **WBCs** or **leukocytes** are broadly grouped as **granulocytes** (neutrophils, eosinophils, basophils) or **agranulocytes** (lymphocytes, monocytes).
- All leukocytes become active outside the circulation, specifically leaving the microvasculature in a process involving cytokines, selective adhesion, changes in the endothelium, and **transendothelial migration** or **diapedesis**.
- All granulocytes have specialized lysosomes called **azurophilic granules** and smaller **specific granules** with proteins for various cell-specific functions.
- **Neutrophils**, the most abundant type of leukocyte, have **polymorphic, multilobed nuclei**, and faint pink cytoplasmic granules that contain many factors for highly efficient phagolysosomal killing and removal of bacteria.

- **Eosinophils** have bilobed nuclei and eosinophilic-specific granules containing factors for destruction of helminthic parasites and for modulating inflammation.
- **Basophils**, the rarest type of circulating leukocyte, have irregular bilobed nuclei and resemble mast cells with strongly basophilic-specific granules containing factors important in allergies and chronic inflammatory conditions, including **histamine**, **heparin**, **chemokines**, and various **hydrolases**.
- **Lymphocytes**, agranulocytes with many functions as T and B cell subtypes in the immune system, range widely in size, depending on their activation state, and have roughly spherical nuclei with little cytoplasm and few organelles.
- **Monocytes** are larger agranulocytes with distinctly indented or C-shaped nuclei, circulating as precursors of macrophages and other cells of the **mononuclear phagocyte system**.
- **Platelets** are small (2–4 μm) cell fragments derived from **megakaryocytes** in bone marrow, with a **marginal bundle** of actin filaments, **alpha granules** and **delta granules**, and an **open canalicular system** of membranous vesicles; rapid degranulation on contact with collagen triggers blood clotting.

Blood ASSESS YOUR KNOWLEDGE

1. Which biochemical component of the erythrocyte cell surface is primarily responsible for determining blood type (eg, the A-B-O system).
   a. Fatty acid
   b. Carbohydrate
   c. Nucleic acid
   d. Protein
   e. Cholesterol

2. What cell in circulating blood is the precursor to microglia and most antigen-presenting cells?
   a. Eosinophil
   b. Basophil
   c. Lymphocyte
   d. Monocyte
   e. Mast cell

3. What is the approximate life span of a circulating erythrocyte?
   a. 8 days
   b. 20 days
   c. 5 weeks
   d. 4 months
   e. 1 year

4. Which cell type has cytoplasmic granules that contain heparin and histamine?
   a. Eosinophils
   b. Basophils
   c. Lymphocytes
   d. Monocytes
   e. Neutrophils

5. A differential cell count of a blood smear from a patient with a parasitic infection is likely to reveal an increase in the circulating numbers of which cell type?

    a. Neutrophils
    b. Lymphocytes
    c. Monocytes
    d. Basophils
    e. Eosinophils

6. Which of the following blood cells differentiate outside of the bone marrow?

    a. Neutrophils
    b. Basophils
    c. Eosinophils
    d. T lymphocytes
    e. Megakaryocytes

7. Examination of a normal peripheral blood smear reveals a cell more than twice the diameter of an erythrocyte with a kidney-shaped nucleus. These cells are less than 10% of the total leukocytes. Which of the following cell types is being described?

    a. Monocyte
    b. Basophil
    c. Eosinophil
    d. Neutrophil
    e. Lymphocyte

8. A 43-year-old anatomy professor is working in her garden, pruning rose bushes without gloves, when a thorn deeply penetrates her forefinger. The next day the area has become infected. She removes the tip of the thorn, but there is still pus remaining at the wound site. Which of the following cells function in the formation of pus?

    a. Cells with spherical nuclei and scant cytoplasm
    b. Biconcave cells with no nuclei
    c. Cells with bilobed nuclei and many acidophilic cytoplasmic granules
    d. Very small, cell-like elements with no nuclei but many granules
    e. Cells with polymorphic, multilobed nuclei

9. A 35-year-old woman's physician orders laboratory blood tests. Her fresh blood is drawn and centrifuged in the presence of heparin as an anticoagulant to obtain a hematocrit. From top to bottom, the fractions resulting from centrifugation are which of the following?

    a. Serum, packed erythrocytes, and leukocytes
    b. Leukocytes, erythrocytes, and serum proteins
    c. Plasma, buffy coat, and packed erythrocytes
    d. Fibrinogen, platelets, buffy coat, and erythrocytes
    e. Albumin, plasma lipoproteins, and erythrocytes

10. A hematologist diagnoses a 34-year-old woman with idiopathic thrombocytic purpura (ITP). Which of the following symptoms/characteristics would one expect in this patient?

    a. Normal blood count
    b. Hypercoagulation
    c. Decreased clotting time
    d. Abnormal bruising
    e. Light menstrual periods

CHAPTER 13 Hemopoiesis

Mature blood cells have a relatively short life span and require continuous replacement with new cells from precursors developing during **hemopoiesis** (Gr. *haima*, blood + *poiesis*, a making). In the early embryo these blood cells arise in the **yolk sac** mesoderm. In the second trimester hemopoiesis (also called **hematopoiesis**) occurs primarily in the developing **liver**, with the spleen playing a minor role (Figure 13–1). Skeletal elements begin to ossify and **bone marrow** develops in their medullary cavities, so in the third-trimester marrow of specific bones becomes the major hemopoietic organ.

Throughout childhood and adult life, erythrocytes, granulocytes, monocytes, and platelets continue to form from stem cells located in bone marrow. The origin and maturation of these cells are termed, respectively, **erythropoiesis** (Gr. *erythros*, red + *poiesis*), **granulopoiesis**, **monocytopoiesis**, and **thrombocytopoiesis**. As described in Chapter 14 on the immune system, **lymphopoiesis** or lymphocyte development occurs in the marrow and in the lymphoid organs to which precursor cells migrate from marrow.

This chapter describes the stem and progenitor cells of hemopoiesis, the histology of bone marrow, the major stages of red and white blood cell differentiation, and platelet formation.

› STEM CELLS, GROWTH FACTORS, & DIFFERENTIATION

As discussed in Chapter 3, stem cells represent **pluripotent** cells capable of asymmetric division and self-renewal. Some of their daughter cells develop as specific, irreversibly committed progenitor cells, and other daughter cells remain as a small pool of slowly dividing stem cells.

Hemopoietic stem cells can be isolated by using fluorescence-labeled antibodies to mark specific cell surface antigens and passing the cell population through a fluorescence-activated cell-sorting (FACS) instrument. Research on hemopoietic stem cells utilizes experimental techniques permitting analysis in vivo and in vitro.

In vivo techniques include injecting the bone marrow of normal donor mice with their own hematopoietic cells destroyed by radiation. In these animals only, the transplanted bone marrow cells produce hematopoietic colonies in the bone marrow and spleen, simplifying studies of this process. This work led to the clinical use of bone marrow transplants to treat potentially lethal hemopoietic disorders.

In vitro techniques using semisolid tissue culture media containing substances produced by marrow stromal cells allow identification and study of cytokines promoting hemopoietic cell growth and differentiation.

Hemopoietic Stem Cells

All blood cells arise from a single type of pluripotent **hemopoietic stem cell** in the bone marrow that can give rise to all the blood cell types (Figure 13–2). These pluripotent stem cells remain rare, proliferate slowly, and first give rise in marrow to two major lineages of progenitor cells with restricted potentials (committed to produce specific blood cells): one for **lymphoid cells** (lymphocytes) and another for **myeloid cells** (Gr. *myelos*, marrow). Myeloid cells include granulocytes, monocytes, erythrocytes, and megakaryocytes. As described in Chapter 14 on the immune system, the lymphoid progenitor cells migrate from the bone marrow to the thymus or the lymph nodes, spleen, and other lymphoid structures, where they proliferate and differentiate.

The local cells and extracellular matrix (ECM) of the hemopoietic organs supply these requirements and together create the niches in which stem cells reside and progenitor cells develop.

Hemopoietic growth factors, often called **colony-stimulating factors (CSF)** or cytokines, typically are glycoproteins that stimulate proliferation of progenitor and precursor cells and promote cell differentiation and maturation within specific lineages. Cloning the genes for several important hematopoietic growth factors has significantly advanced study of blood formation and permitted the production of clinically useful factors for patients with hemopoietic disorders. Table 13–1 presents the major activities, target cells, and sources of several well-characterized cytokines supporting hemopoiesis.

FIGURE **13–1** Shifting locations of hemopoiesis during development and aging.

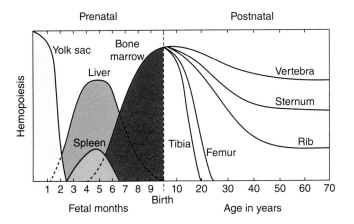

Hemopoiesis, or blood cell formation, first occurs in a mesodermal cell population of the embryonic yolk sac and shifts during the second trimester mainly to the developing liver, before becoming concentrated in newly formed bones during the last 2 months of gestation. Hemopoietic bone marrow occurs in many locations through puberty, but then becomes increasingly restricted to components of the axial skeleton.

Progenitor & Precursor Cells

The progenitor cells for blood cells are often called **colony-forming units (CFUs)** because they give rise to colonies of only one cell type when cultured in vitro or injected into an irradiated spleen. As shown in Figure 13–2, four major types of progenitor cells/CFUs exist:

- Erythroid lineage of erythrocytes,
- Thrombocytic lineage of megakaryocytes for platelet formation,
- Granulocyte-monocyte lineage of all three granulocytes and monocytes, and
- Lymphoid lineage of B lymphocytes, T lymphocytes, and natural killer cells.

Each progenitor cell lineage produces precursor cells (or blasts) that gradually assume the morphologic characteristics of the mature, functional cell types they will become (Figure 13–2). In contrast, stem and progenitor cells cannot be morphologically distinguished and simply resemble large lymphocytes. While stem cells divide at a rate only sufficient to maintain their relatively small population, progenitor and precursor cells divide more rapidly, producing large numbers of differentiated, mature cells (3×10^9 erythrocytes and 0.85×10^9 granulocytes/kg/d in human bone marrow). Figure 13–3 shows graphically the changing potential and activities of cells during hemopoiesis.

Hemopoiesis depends on a microenvironment, or niche, with specific endocrine, paracrine, and juxtacrine factors.

>> MEDICAL APPLICATION

Hemopoietic growth factors are important products of biotechnology companies. They are used clinically to increase marrow cellularity and blood cell counts in patients with conditions such as severe anemia or during chemo- or radiotherapy, which lower white blood cell counts (leukopenia). Such cytokines may also increase the efficiency of marrow transplants by enhancing cell proliferation, enhance host defenses in patients with infectious and immunodeficient diseases, and improve treatment of some parasitic diseases.

> BONE MARROW

Under normal conditions, the production of blood cells in the bone marrow adjusts to the body's needs, increasing its activity several-fold in a very short time. Bone marrow occurs in the medullary canals of long bones and in the small cavities of cancellous bone, with two types based on their appearance at gross examination: blood-forming **red bone marrow**, whose color arises from its abundant blood and hemopoietic cells, and **yellow bone marrow**, filled with adipocytes that exclude most hemopoietic cells. In the newborn all bone marrow is red and active in blood cell production, but as a child grows most marrow changes gradually to the yellow variety. Under certain conditions, such as severe bleeding or hypoxia, yellow marrow can revert to red.

Red bone marrow (Figure 13–4) encompasses a reticular connective tissue **stroma** (Gr. *stroma*, bed) with **hemopoietic cords** or **islands** of differentiating cells interposed with **sinusoidal capillaries**. The stroma develops as a meshwork of specialized fibroblastic cells called **stromal cells** (also called **reticular** or **adventitial cells**) and a delicate web of reticular fibers supporting the hemopoietic cells and macrophages. Its ECM also contains collagen type I, proteoglycans, fibronectin, and laminin, the latter glycoproteins interacting with integrins to hold cells on the matrix. Red marrow also represents a site where older, defective erythrocytes undergo phagocytosis by macrophages, which then reprocess heme-bound iron for delivery to newly differentiating erythrocytes.

FIGURE **13–2** Origin and differentiative stages of blood cells.

The rare pluripotent hemopoietic stem cells divide slowly, maintain their own population, and give rise to two major cell lineages of progenitor cells: the myeloid and lymphoid stem cells. The myeloid lineage includes precursor cells (blasts) for erythropoiesis, thrombopoiesis, granulopoiesis, and monocytopoiesis, all in the bone marrow.

The lymphoid lineage forms B and T lymphocytes and related cells called natural killer cells, with the later differentiative stages occurring in lymphoid organs. Erythropoietin (EPO), colony-stimulating factors (CSF), cytokines, and growth factors promote growth and differentiation throughout these developmental processes.

FIGURE **13–3** Major changes in developing hemopoietic cells.

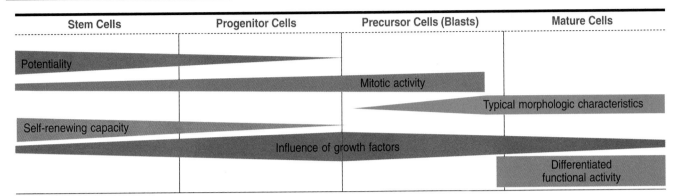

As blood cells in each lineage develop, the stem cells' pluri-potentiality and capacity for self-renewal become restricted. Progenitor and precursor cells undergo more rapid mitotic activity than their stem cells but then terminally differentiate with characteristic morphological features that underlie specific functional properties. Within each lineage, specific protein and glycoprotein growth factors and cytokines promote the growth and development.

TABLE **13–1** Major hemopoietic cytokines (growth factors or colony-stimulating factors).

Cytokine	Major Activities and Target Cells[a]	Important Sources
Stem cell factor (SCF)	Mitogen for all hemopoietic progenitor cells	Stromal cells of bone marrow
Erythropoietin (EPO)	Mitogen for all erythroid progenitor and precursor cells, also promoting their differentiation	Peritubular endothelial cells of the kidney; hepatocytes
Thrombopoietin (TPO)	Mitogen for megakaryoblasts and their progenitor cells	Kidney and liver
Granulocyte-macrophage colony-stimulating factor (GM-CSF)	Mitogen for all myeloid progenitor cells	Endothelial cells of bone marrow and T lymphocytes
Granulocyte colony-stimulating factor (G-CSF or filgrastim)	Mitogen for neutrophil precursor cells	Endothelial cells of bone marrow and macrophages
Monocyte colony-stimulating factor (M-CSF)	Mitogen for monocyte precursor cells	Endothelial cells of marrow and macrophages
Interleukin-1 (IL-1)	Regulates activities and cytokine secretion of many leukocytes and other cells	Macrophages and T helper cells
Interleukin-2 (IL-2)	Mitogen for activated T and B cells; promotes differentiation of NK cells	T helper cells
Interleukin-3 (IL-3)	Mitogen for all granulocyte and megakaryocyte progenitor cells	T helper cells
Interleukin-4 (IL-4)	Promotes development of basophils and mast cells and B-lymphocyte activation	T helper cells
Interleukin-5 (IL-5) or eosinophil differentiation factor (EDF)	Promotes development and activation of eosinophils	T helper cells
Interleukin-6 (IL-6)	Mitogen for many leukocytes; promotes activation of B cells and regulatory T cells	Macrophages, neutrophils, local endothelial cells
Interleukin-7 (IL-7)	Major mitogen for all lymphoid stem cells	Stromal cells of bone marrow

[a]Most of the cytokines listed here target all the cells of specific lineages, including the progenitor cells and the precursor cells that are committed and maturing but still dividing. Many promote both mitosis and differentiation in target cells.

FIGURE 13–4　Red bone marrow (active in hemopoiesis).

Red bone marrow contains adipocytes but is primarily active in hemopoiesis, with several cell lineages usually present. It can be examined histologically in sections of bones or in biopsies, but its cells can also be studied in smears. Marrow consists of capillary sinusoids running through a stroma of specialized, fibroblastic stromal cells, and an ECM meshwork with reticular fibers. Stromal cells produce the ECM; both stromal and bone cells secrete various CSFs, creating the microenvironment for hemopoietic stem cell maintenance, proliferation, and differentiation.

(a) Sections of red bone marrow include trabeculae (**T**) of cancellous bone, adipocytes (**A**), and blood-filled sinusoids (**S**) between hemopoietic cords (**C**) or islands of developing blood cells. (×140; H&E)

(b) At higher magnification the flattened nuclei of sinusoidal endothelial cells (**E**) can be distinguished, as well as the variety of densely packed hemopoietic cells in the cords (**C**) between the sinusoids (**S**) and adipocytes (**A**). Most stromal cells and specific cells of the hemopoietic lineages are difficult to identify with certainty in routinely stained sections of marrow. (×400; H&E)

The hematopoietic niche in marrow includes the stroma, osteoblasts, and megakaryocytes. Between the hematopoietic cords run the sinusoids, with discontinuous endothelium allowing newly differentiated blood cells and platelets ready access to the circulation (Figure 13–5).

❯ MATURATION OF ERYTHROCYTES

A mature cell is one differentiated to the stage at which it can carry out its specific functions. Erythrocyte maturation represents terminal cell differentiation involving hemoglobin synthesis and formation of a small, enucleated, biconcave corpuscle. Several major changes take place during **erythropoiesis** (Figures 13–6 and 13–7). Cell and nuclear volumes decrease, while the nucleoli gradually disappear. Chromatin density increases until the nucleus becomes pyknotic and finally undergoes extrusion from the cell. A gradual decrease in the number of polyribosomes (basophilia) coincides with a simultaneous increase in the amount of hemoglobin, a highly eosinophilic protein. Mitochondria and other organelles steadily disappear.

Erythropoiesis requires approximately a week and involves three to five cell divisions between the progenitor cell stage and the release of functional cells into the circulation. The glycoprotein **erythropoietin**, an essential growth

FIGURE **13–5** Sinusoidal endothelium in active marrow.

Mature, newly formed erythrocytes, leukocytes, and platelets in bone marrow enter the circulation by passing through the discontinuous sinusoidal endothelium. All leukocytes cross the sinusoid's wall by their own activity, but the nonmotile erythrocytes cannot migrate through actively and enter the circulation pushed by a pressure gradient across the wall. Megakaryocytes form thin processes (proplatelets) that also pass through such endothelial apertures and liberate platelets at their tips.

factor produced by cells in the kidneys, stimulates erythrocyte growth and production of mRNA for hemoglobin.

The distinct erythroid progenitor cell, the **proerythroblast**, occurs as a large cell with loose, lacy chromatin, nucleoli, and basophilic cytoplasm (Figure 13–6). The next slightly smaller stage is the early **basophilic erythroblast**, with cytoplasmic basophilia and a more condensed nucleus. The basophilia indicates the large number of free polysomes synthesizing hemoglobin. During the next stage, cell volume shrinks further, density of polysomes decreases, and some cytoplasmic areas become filled with hemoglobin. These changes generate both basophilic and acidophilic cytoplasmic regions, leading to the name **polychromatophilic erythroblast**. Cell and nuclear volumes continue to condense and basophilia gradually disappears, yielding cells with uniformly acidophilic cytoplasm—the **orthochromatophilic erythroblasts** (sometimes called normoblasts). Late in this stage, the pyknotic cell nucleus undergoes ejection and phagocytosis by macrophages. For a few days, the cell retains a few polyribosomes which, when treated with the dye brilliant cresyl blue, appear as a faintly stained network, leading to the name **reticulocytes** for this stage. (Figure 13–7b). These cells enter the circulation (where they may constitute 1% of the red blood cells), where they quickly lose the remaining polyribosomes and mature as erythrocytes.

FIGURE **13–6** Summary of erythrocyte maturation.

The color change in the cytoplasm shows the continuous decrease in basophilia and the increase in hemoglobin concentration from proerythroblast to erythrocyte. A gradual decrease in nuclear volume and an increase in chromatin condensation also occur, followed by extrusion of the pyknotic nucleus. The times indicate the average duration of each cell type. In the graph 100% represents the highest recorded concentrations of hemoglobin and RNA.

FIGURE 13–7   Erythropoiesis: Major erythrocyte precursors.

(a) Micrographs showing a very large and scarce proerythroblast (**P**), a slightly smaller basophilic erythroblast (**B**) with very basophilic cytoplasm, typical and late polychromatophilic erythroblasts (**Pe** and **LPe**) with both basophilic and acidophilic cytoplasmic regions, and a small orthochromatophilic erythroblast (**Oe**) with cytoplasm nearly like that of the mature erythrocytes in the field. (All ×1400; Wright)

(b) Micrograph containing **reticulocytes** (arrows), representing cells that have lost their nuclei but have not yet completely lost the polyribosomes used to synthesize globin, as demonstrated by a stain for RNA. (×1400; Brilliant cresyl blue)

》 MATURATION OF GRANULOCYTES

Granulopoiesis involves cytoplasmic changes dominated by synthesis of proteins for the **azurophilic granules** and **specific granules**. Production of these proteins in the rough ER and the prominent Golgi apparatus occurs in two stages (Figure 13–8). First to form are the azurophilic granules, which contain lysosomal hydrolases, stain with basic dyes, and are generally similar in all three types of granulocytes. Golgi activity then changes to package proteins for the specific granules, whose contents differ in each of the three types of granulocytes and endow each type with different properties (see Chapter 12). In sections of bone marrow, cords of granulopoietic cells can be distinguished from erythropoietic cords by their granule-filled cytoplasm (Figure 13–9).

FIGURE 13–8   Granulopoiesis: Formation of granules.

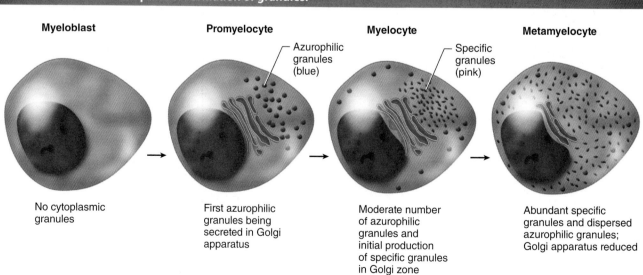

Myeloblast	Promyelocyte	Myelocyte	Metamyelocyte
No cytoplasmic granules	First azurophilic granules being secreted in Golgi apparatus	Moderate number of azurophilic granules and initial production of specific granules in Golgi zone	Abundant specific granules and dispersed azurophilic granules; Golgi apparatus reduced

In the sequence of cytoplasmic events during the maturation of granulocytes from **myeloblasts**, modified lysosomes or azurophilic granules develop first at the **promyelocyte** stage and then the specific granules of particular cell types form at the **myelocyte** stage. All granules are fully dispersed at the **metamyelocyte** stage when indentation of the nucleus begins.

FIGURE **13–9** Developing erythrocytes and granulocytes in marrow.

Precursor cells of different hemopoietic lineages develop side by side with some intermingling as various cell islands or cords in the bone marrow. This plastic section of red bone marrow shows mitotic figures (arrows) and fairly distinct regions of **erythropoiesis** and **granulopoiesis**. Most immature granulocytes are in the myelocyte stage: their cytoplasm contains large, dark-stained azurophilic granules and small, less darkly stained specific granules. The large white areas shown peripherally indicate fat cells. (×400; Giemsa)

FIGURE **13–10** Granulopoiesis: Major granulocyte precursors.

Two micrographs from smears of bone marrow show the major cells of the neutrophilic granulocyte lineage. Typical precursor cells shown are labeled as follows: myeloblast (**MB**); promyelocyte (**1**); myelocytes (**2**); late myelocyte (**3**); metamyelocytes (**4**); band cells (**5**); nearly mature segmented neutrophils (**6**). Some of the early stages show faint nucleoli (**N**). Inset: Eosinophilic myelocytes (**EM**) and metamyelocytes (**EMm**) with their specific granules having distinctly different staining. These and cells of the basophilic lineage resemble the developing neutrophils, except for their specific staining granules and lack of the stab cell stage. Also seen among the erythrocytes of these marrow smears are some orthochromatophilic erythroblasts (**Oe**), a small lymphocyte (**L**), and a cell in mitosis (arrow). (All ×1400; Wright)

The **myeloblast** represents the most immature recognizable cell in the myeloid series (Figures 13–2 and 13–10). Typically, these have finely dispersed chromatin and faint nucleoli. The next stage of **promyelocytes** includes basophilic cytoplasm and developing azurophilic granules with lysosomal enzymes and myeloperoxidase. Different promyelocytes activate different sets of genes, resulting in lineages for the three types of granulocytes (Figure 13–2). The first visible sign of this differentiation appears at the **myelocyte** stage (Figure 13–11), in which specific granules gradually increase in number and eventually occupy most of the cytoplasm at the **metamyelocyte** stage. These neutrophilic, basophilic, and eosinophilic metamyelocytes mature with further condensation of their nuclei. Before its complete maturation, the neutrophilic granulocyte passes through an intermediate stage, the **band cell** (Figure 13–10), in which the nucleus becomes elongated but not yet polymorphic.

⟩⟩ MEDICAL APPLICATION

The appearance of large numbers of immature neutrophils (band cells) in the blood, sometimes called a "shift to the left," is clinically significant, usually indicating a bacterial infection.

Most granulocytes are neutrophils and the total time required for a myeloblast to produce mature, circulating neutrophils ranges from 10 to 14 days. Five mitotic divisions normally occur during the myeloblast, promyelocyte, and neutrophilic myelocyte stages. As diagrammed in Figure 13–12, developing and mature neutrophils exist in four functionally and anatomically defined compartments: (1) the granulopoietic compartment in active marrow, (2) storage as mature cells in marrow until release, (3) the circulating population, and (4) a population undergoing margination, a process in which neutrophils loosely adhere and transiently accumulate along the endothelial surface in venules and small veins. Margination of neutrophils in some organs can persist for several hours and is not always followed by the cells' emigration from the microvasculature.

FIGURE **13–11** Neutrophilic myelocyte.

At the myelocyte stage lysosomes (azurophilic granules) have formed and production of specific secretory granules has begun. This micrograph shows ultrastructurally a peroxidase-stained section of a neutrophilic myelocyte with cytoplasm containing both large, peroxidase-positive azurophilic granules (**AG**) and smaller specific granules (**SG**) not staining for peroxidase. The peroxidase reaction product appears only in mature azurophilic granules and not in the rough ER (**RER**) or Golgi cisternae (**GC**) near the centriole (**C**) and nucleus (**N**). (×15,000)

(*Reproduced with permission from Dr Dorothy F. Bainton, Department of Pathology, University of California at San Francisco.*)

At sites of injury or infection neutrophils and other granulocytes enter the connective tissues by migrating through intercellular junctions between endothelial cells of postcapillary venules in diapedesis (see Figure 12-6). Inflamed connective tissues thus represent a fifth neutrophil compartment, where the cells are activated, live for a few days and then die by apoptosis regardless of whether they have performed their major function of bacterial phagocytosis.

❯❯ MEDICAL APPLICATION

Changes in the number of neutrophils in the blood must be evaluated by taking all their compartments into consideration. Thus, **neutrophilia**, an increase in the number of circulating neutrophils, does not necessarily imply an increase in granulopoiesis. Intense muscular activity or the administration of epinephrine can cause neutrophils in the marginating compartment to move into the circulating compartment, producing neutrophilia even though granulopoiesis has not

FIGURE **13–12** Compartments of neutrophils in the body.

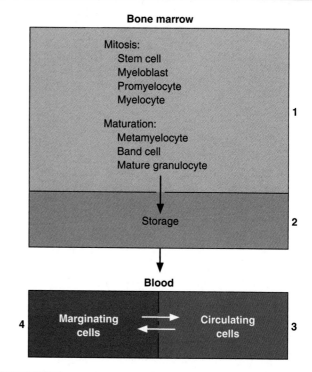

Neutrophils exist in at least four anatomically and temporally distinct compartments, whose sizes reflect the number of cells:

(1) The **granulopoietic region** in bone marrow is where progenitor cell development occurs.

(2) A **storage** (reserve) compartment, also in red marrow, acts as a buffer system capable of releasing large numbers of mature neutrophils as needed. Trillions of neutrophils typically move from marrow to the bloodstream every day.

(3) A **circulating** compartment exists throughout the blood.

(4) A **marginating** compartment consists of sites where neutrophils stop circulating and accumulate at least temporarily at the endothelial surface of venules and small veins.

The marginating and circulating compartments are about equal in size, with a constant interchange of cells between them. The half-life of cells in these two compartments is less than 10 hours. The granulopoietic and storage compartments together include cells in approximately the first 14 days of their existence and are about 10 times larger than the circulating and marginating compartments.

Neutrophils become active and functional only after their migration from venules into the ECM of infected or injured tissues.

increased. However, glucocorticoids (adrenal hormones) such as cortisone increase the mitotic activity of neutrophil precursors, and this also increases the blood count of neutrophils.

Transitory neutrophilia may also result from liberation of greater numbers of neutrophils from the medullary storage compartment and is typically followed by a recovery period during which no neutrophils are released.

The neutrophilia that occurs during bacterial infections is due to an increase in production of neutrophils and a shorter duration of these cells in the medullary storage compartment. In such cases, immature forms such as **band** or **stab cells,** neutrophilic metamyelocytes, and even myelocytes may appear in the bloodstream. The neutrophilia occurring during infection is typically of much longer duration than that resulting from intense muscular activity.

MATURATION OF AGRANULOCYTES

The precursor cells of monocytes and lymphocytes do not show specific cytoplasmic granules or nuclear lobulation, both of which facilitate the distinction of cells in the granulopoietic series. Monocytes and lymphocytes in smear preparations are classified mainly based on size and nuclear shape.

Monocytes

The **monoblast** develops as a committed progenitor cell virtually identical to the myeloblast morphologically. Continued differentiation leads to the **promonocyte**, a large cell (up to 18 μm in diameter) with basophilic cytoplasm and a large, slightly indented nucleus with euchromatin and nucleoli (Figures 13–2 and 12–12). Promonocytes divide twice as they develop into **monocytes**. Differentiating monocytes contain extensive RER and large Golgi complexes forming lysosomes, which appear as fine azurophilic granules at maturity. Monocytes typically circulate in blood for several hours and enter tissues where they mature as **macrophages** (or other phagocytic cells) and function for up to several months.

Lymphocytes

As discussed with the immune system (see Chapter 14), circulating lymphocytes originate mainly in the thymus and in the peripheral lymphoid organs (eg, spleen, lymph nodes, and tonsils). However, lymphocyte progenitor cells originate in bone marrow. Some of the new lymphocytes in marrow migrate to the thymus where they acquire the properties of T lymphocytes. Subsequently, T lymphocytes migrate and populate specific regions of peripheral lymphoid organs. Other lymphocytes arising in bone marrow remain there and differentiate into B lymphocytes, which then move to peripheral lymphoid organs where they inhabit and multiply within their own niches.

The first identifiable progenitor of lymphoid cells, the **lymphoblast**, is a large cell capable of dividing two or three times to form **lymphocytes** (Figures 13–2 and 12–11). As lymphocytes develop, cell size decreases as the amount of cytoplasm is reduced. In the bone marrow and in the thymus, these cells synthesize the specific cell surface proteins characterizing B or T lymphocytes, respectively. Mature and functionally active B and T cells are generally larger than newly formed lymphocytes. During differentiation subsets of lymphocytes acquire additional distinctive cell surface and other proteins, detectable immunocytochemically and used to sort the specific lymphocytic types.

ORIGIN OF PLATELETS

The small, membrane-enclosed formed elements called **platelets** or thrombocytes originate by fragmentation from mature **megakaryocytes** (Gr. *megas*, big + *karyon*, nucleus, + *kytos*), which in turn differentiate from **megakaryoblasts** in a process driven by **thrombopoietin**. The megakaryoblast is 25–50 μm in diameter, with basophilic cytoplasm and a large ovoid or kidney-shaped nucleus (Figure 13–13), often with several nucleoli. Before differentiating these cells undergo endomitosis, with repeated rounds of DNA replication not separated by cell divisions, resulting in highly polyploid nuclei (ranging from 8N to 64N).

The polyploid megakaryocytes exist as giant cells, up to 150 μm in diameter, and the large nuclei display irregular lobes with coarse chromatin. Their cytoplasm contains numerous mitochondria, a well-developed RER, and an extensive Golgi apparatus from which arise the conspicuous specific granules of platelets (see Chapter 12). Best seen in bone marrow, megakaryocytes also occur in the interstitial tissue of the spleen and lungs, most often closely associated with vascular sinusoids or capillaries.

In forming platelets megakaryocytes rapidly extend several long (>100 μm), wide (2-4 μm) branching processes called **proplatelets**, which penetrate adjacent microvascular endothelium and project into the circulating blood (Figure 13–5). Internally, proplatelets have a framework of actin filaments and loosely bundled, mixed polarity microtubules along which membrane vesicles and specific granules are transported. A loop of microtubules at the distal end of the proplatelet forms a teardrop-shaped enlargement, and this cytoplasm is rapidly pinched off to form each platelet, with its characteristic marginal bundle of microtubules and microfilaments surrounding

FIGURE **13–13** Megakaryoblast and megakaryocytes.

(a) Megakaryoblasts (**Mb**) occur as very large, fairly rare cells in bone marrow, with highly basophilic cytoplasm. (×1400; Wright)

(b) Megakaryoblasts undergo endomitosis (DNA replication without intervening cell divisions), becoming polyploid as they differentiate into megakaryocytes (**M**), which are even larger but with less intensely basophilic cytoplasm. (×1400; Wright)

(c) Micrograph of sectioned bone marrow in which a megakaryocyte (**M**) lies next to a sinusoid (**S**). (×400; Giemsa) Megakaryocytes produce all the characteristic components of platelets (membrane vesicles, specific granules, marginal microtubule bundles, etc.) and in a complex process extend many long, branching pseudopodia-like projections called **proplatelets**, from the ends of which platelets pinch off almost fully formed.

cytoplasmic granules and vesicles of the open canalicular system (Figure 12–13b).

During proplatelet growth, microtubules polymerize in both directions. Proplatelet elongation depends on both this polymerization and dynein-based sliding of microtubules past one another. Mature megakaryocytes also display numerous invaginations of plasma membrane called **demarcation membranes** ramifying throughout the cytoplasm (Figure 13–14). These were formerly considered "fracture lines" or "perforations" for the release of platelets but are now thought to represent a membrane reservoir facilitating continuous, rapid proplatelet elongation. From the proplatelets each megakaryocyte's cytoplasm gets apportioned into a few thousand platelets, after which the remainder of the cell undergoes apoptosis and removal by macrophages.

❯❯ MEDICAL APPLICATION

Some bleeding disorders result from **thrombocytopenia**, a reduction in the number of circulating platelets. One cause of thrombocytopenia is **ineffective megakaryopoiesis** resulting from deficiencies of folic acid or vitamin B_{12}. In different types of **thrombocytopenic purpura** (L. purple, the color of small spots or petechiae in the skin from poorly inhibited bleeding), platelet function is compromised, usually by autoimmune reactions.

FIGURE **13–14** Megakaryocyte ultrastructure.

This TEM of a megakaryocyte shows the lobulated nucleus (**N**), numerous cytoplasmic granules (**G**), and an extensive cytoplasmic system of (demarcation membranes) (**D**), which likely represent a membranous reservoir facilitating the very rapid elongation of numerous proplatelets extending from the megakaryocyte surface. (×10,000)

Hemopoiesis SUMMARY OF KEY POINTS

- **Pluripotent stem cells** for blood cell formation, or **hemopoiesis**, occur in the bone marrow of children and adults.
- **Progenitor cells**, committed to forming each type of mature blood cell, proliferate and differentiate within microenvironmental niches of **stromal cells**, other cells, and ECM with specific growth factors.
- These progenitor cells are also known as **CFUs** and the growth factors are also called **CSFs** or cytokines.
- **Red bone marrow** is active in hemopoiesis; **yellow bone marrow** consists mostly of adipose tissue.
- **Erythropoietic islands** or cords within marrow contain the red blood cell lineage: **proerythroblasts**, **erythroblasts** with succeeding developmental stages called **basophilic**, **polychromatophilic**, and **orthochromatophilic** that reflect the cytoplasmic transition from RNA-rich to hemoglobin-filled.
- At the last stage of erythropoiesis cell nuclei are extruded, producing **reticulocytes** that still contain some polyribosomes but are released into the circulation.

- **Granulopoiesis** includes **myeloblasts**, which have large nuclei and relatively little cytoplasm; **promyelocytes**, in which lysosomal **azurophilic granules** develop; **myelocytes**, in which **specific granules** for one of the three types of granulocytes form; and **metamyelocytes**, in which the characteristic changes in nuclear morphology occur.
- Immature neutrophilic metamyelocytes called **band (stab) cells** are released prematurely when the compartment of circulating neutrophils becomes depleted due to bacterial infections.
- **Monoblasts** produce **monocytes** in red marrow, but **lymphoblasts** give rise to **lymphocytes** primarily in the lymphoid tissues in processes involving acquired immunity.
- **Megakaryocytes**, large polyploid cells of red bone marrow, produce **platelets**, or **thrombocytes**, by releasing them from the ends of cytoplasmic processes called **proplatelets**.
- All these **formed elements** of blood enter the circulation by crossing the **discontinuous endothelium** of sinusoids in the red marrow.

Hemopoiesis ASSESS YOUR KNOWLEDGE

1. In which of the following cells involved in erythropoiesis does hemoglobin synthesis begin?
   a. Orthochromatic erythroblast
   b. Polychromatophilic erythroblast
   c. Reticulocyte
   d. Basophilic erythroblast
   e. Proerythroblast

2. Which of the following can be used to describe megakaryocytes?
   a. Multinucleated
   b. Formed by fusion of haploid cells
   c. Precursors to bone marrow macrophages
   d. A minor but normal formed element found in the circulation
   e. Possess dynamic cell projections from which one type of formed element is released

3. Which cytoplasmic components are the main constituents of the dark precipitate that forms in reticulocytes upon staining with the dye cresyl blue?
   a. Golgi complexes
   b. Hemoglobin
   c. Nucleoli
   d. Nuclear fragments
   e. Polyribosomes

4. Which process occurs during granulopoiesis but not during erythropoiesis?
   a. Cells lose their capacity for mitosis.
   b. Euchromatin content increases.
   c. Nucleus becomes increasingly lobulated.
   d. Overall cell diameter decreases.
   e. Overall nuclear diameter decreases.

5. What fate often awaits granulocytes that have entered the marginating compartment?
   a. Undergo mitosis
   b. Crossing the wall of a venule to enter connective tissue
   c. Cannot reenter the circulation
   d. Differentiate into functional macrophages
   e. Begin to release platelets

6. What is the earliest stage at which specific granulocyte types can be distinguished from one another?
   a. Myelocyte
   b. Band form
   c. Reticulocyte
   d. Metamyelocyte
   e. Promyelocyte

7. Which cell type is capable of further mitosis after leaving the hemopoietic organ in which it is formed?
   a. Basophil
   b. Eosinophil
   c. Reticulocyte
   d. Lymphocyte
   e. Neutrophil

8. Shortly after her birth a baby is diagnosed with a mutation in the erythropoietin receptor gene which leads to familial erythrocytosis (familial polycythemia). During the seventh to ninth months of fetal development, the primary effect on her red blood cell production was in which of the following?

   a. Liver
   b. Yolk sac
   c. Spleen
   d. Thymus
   e. Bone marrow

9. A 54-year-old man presents with recurrent breathlessness and chronic fatigue. After routine tests followed by a bone marrow biopsy, he is diagnosed with lymphocytic leukemia. Chemotherapy is administered to remove the cancerous cells, which also destroys the precursor cells of erythrocytes. To reestablish the erythrocytic lineage, which of the following cells should be transplanted?

   a. Reticulocytes
   b. Orthochromatophilic erythroblasts
   c. Megakaryoblasts
   d. Basophilic erythroblasts
   e. Metamyelocytes

10. A smear of blood from a 70-year-old leukemia patient reveals a larger than normal population of cells that have large, round nuclei with one or two nucleoli. The cytoplasm of these cells shows azurophilic granules. Which of the following forms of leukemia would you suspect?

    a. Promyelocytic leukemia
    b. Basophilic leukemia
    c. Lymphoblastic leukemia
    d. Stem cell leukemia
    e. Eosinophilic leukemia

14 The Immune System & Lymphoid Organs

The **immune system** provides various defenses or **immunity** against infectious agents ranging from viruses to multicellular parasites. Histologically, this system consists of a large, diverse population of leukocytes located within every tissue of the body and **lymphoid organs** interconnected only by the blood and lymphatic circulation. Immunity obviously has tremendous medical importance, one part of which focuses on autoimmune diseases in which immune cells function abnormally and attack molecular components of the body's own organs.

Immunologists recognize two partially overlapping lines of defense against invaders and/or other abnormal, potentially harmful cells: **innate immunity** and **adaptive immunity**. Innate immunity encompasses a wide variety of nonspecific effector mechanisms which evolved much earlier than adaptive defenses. Important cells mediating innate immunity include most of the granulocytes and certain other leukocytes described in Chapters 12 and 13. Conversely, adaptive immunity develops to target specific microbial invaders, depends on lymphocytes and **antigen-presenting cells (APCs)** discussed in this chapter, and produces memory cells that permit a very rapid response if that specific microbe appears again.

The lymphocytes and APCs for adaptive immunity become localized throughout the body in the blood, lymph, epithelia and connective tissues. Lymphocytes develop initially in **primary lymphoid organs** (the thymus and bone marrow), but most lymphocyte activation and proliferation occur in **secondary lymphoid organs** (the lymph nodes, the spleen, and diffuse lymphoid tissue found in the mucosa of the digestive system, including the tonsils, Peyer patches, and appendix). The immune cells located diffusely in the digestive, respiratory, or urogenital mucosae collectively comprise the **mucosa-associated lymphoid tissue (MALT)**. Proliferating B lymphocytes in the secondary structures of MALT arrange themselves in small spherical **lymphoid nodules**. The wide distribution of immune system cells and the constant traffic of lymphocytes through the blood, lymph, connective tissues, and secondary lymphoid structures provide the body with an elaborate and efficient system of surveillance and defense (Figure 14–1).

» INNATE & ADAPTIVE IMMUNITY

The system of defenses termed **innate immunity** involves immediate, nonspecific actions, including **physical barriers** such as the skin and mucous membranes of the gastrointestinal, respiratory, and urogenital tracts that prevent easy microbial penetration of the host body. Bacteria, fungi, and parasites that manage to breach these barriers quickly get removed by **neutrophils** and other leukocytes in the epithelia or adjacent connective tissue. **Toll-like receptors (TLRs)** on leukocytes allow the recognition and binding of surface components on such invaders. Other leukocytes orchestrate additional defenses at sites of penetration. **Natural killer (NK) cells** destroy various unhealthy host cells, including those infected with virus or bacteria, as well as certain potentially tumorigenic cells.

Leukocytes and specific cells of the tissue barriers also produce a wide variety of antimicrobial chemicals that contribute importantly to innate immunity, including the following:

- **Hydrochloric acid (HCl)** and **organic acids** in specific regions, which lower the pH locally to either kill entering microorganisms directly or inhibit their growth;

FIGURE 14–1 **The lymphoid organs and main paths of lymphatic vessels.**

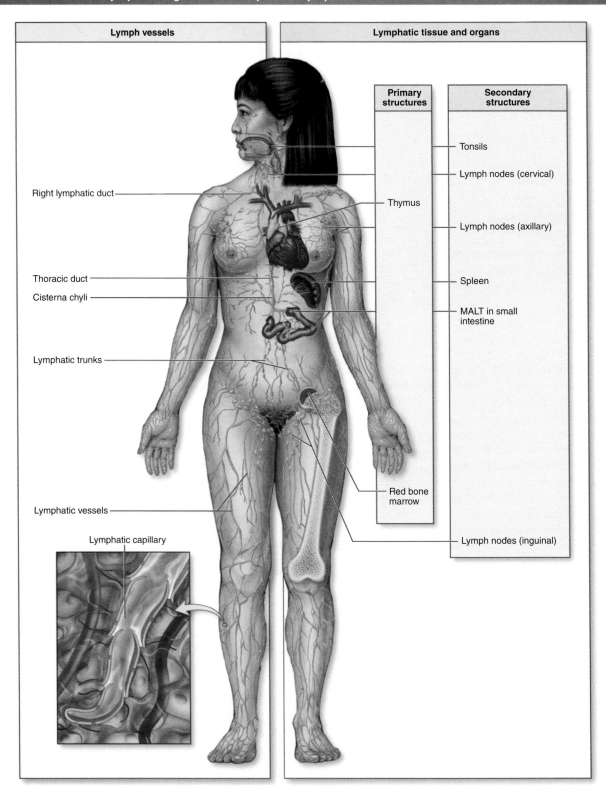

| Lymph vessels | Lymphatic tissue and organs |

Primary structures

Secondary structures

- Right lymphatic duct
- Thoracic duct
- Cisterna chyli
- Lymphatic trunks
- Lymphatic vessels
- Lymphatic capillary
- Thymus
- Red bone marrow
- Tonsils
- Lymph nodes (cervical)
- Lymph nodes (axillary)
- Spleen
- MALT in small intestine
- Lymph nodes (inguinal)

The lymphatic system is composed of **lymphatic vessels** that transport interstitial fluid (as lymph) back to the blood circulation, and the lymphoid organs that house lymphocytes and other cells of the body's immune defense system. **Primary lymphoid organs** are the bone marrow and thymus, where B and T lymphocytes are formed, respectively. The **secondary lymphoid organs** include the lymph nodes, MALT, and spleen.

- **Defensins**, short cationic polypeptides produced by neutrophils and various epithelial cells that kill bacteria by disrupting their cell walls;
- **Lysozyme**, an enzyme made by neutrophils and cells of epithelial barriers, which hydrolyzes bacterial cell wall components, killing the cells;
- **Complement**, a system of proteins in blood plasma, mucus, and macrophages that react with bacterial surface components to aid removal of bacteria; and
- **Interferons**, paracrine factors from leukocytes and virus-infected cells that signal NK cells to kill such cells and adjacent cells to resist viral infection.

❯❯ MEDICAL APPLICATION

Some pathogenic bacteria, such as *Haemophilus influenzae* and *Streptococcus pneumoniae*, **avoid phagocytosis** by granulocytes and macrophages of **innate immunity** by covering their cell walls with a "capsule" of polysaccharide. The capsule inhibits recognition and binding to the **phagocytes' receptors**. Eventually such bacteria can be removed by antibody-based mechanisms, including phagocytosis after **opsonization**, but in the interim of several days the cells proliferate undisturbed and establish a more dangerous infection. Elderly or immunocompromised patients, with reduced **adaptive immunity**, are particularly susceptible to infections with such bacteria.

Adaptive immune defenses, acquired gradually by exposure to microorganisms, develop more slowly and more specifically than the innate responses. The adaptive immunity involves **B** and **T lymphocytes**, described in this chapter, which become activated effector cells when "presented" with specific molecules from invasive or other pathogenic cells by **APCs**, which usually develop from monocytes. Once activated, the adaptive responses of B cells and the various functional types of T cells target specific kinds of pathogens and produce lines of B and T **memory lymphocytes**, capable of rapidly generating similar responses if the invader reappears.

❯ CYTOKINES

Within lymphoid organs and during inflammation at sites of infection or tissue injury, cells in the immune system communicate with each other primarily with **cytokines** to coordinate defensive measures. Involved in both innate and adaptive immune responses, cytokines comprise a diverse group of peptides and glycoproteins, usually with low molecular masses (between 8 and 80 kDa) and a paracrine mode of action. They coordinate cell activities in the two types of immunity. Table 14–1 lists several important cytokines. Major responses induced in target cells by such factors include the following:

- Directed cell movements, or **chemotaxis**, toward and cell accumulation at sites of inflammation, for example,

TABLE **14–1**	Examples of cytokines, grouped by their main function.
Cytokine[a]	**Main Functions**
GM-CSF, M-CSF	Growth and differentiation factors for leukocyte progenitor cells in bone marrow
TNF-α, TGF-β, IL-1	Stimulation of inflammation and fever
IL-12	Stimulation of growth in T lymphocytes and NK cells
IL-2, IL-4	Growth factors for T helper cells and B lymphocytes
IL-5	Eosinophil proliferation, differentiation, and activation
Interferon-g, IL-4	Activation of macrophages
IL-10	Inhibition of macrophages and specific adaptive immune responses
Interferon-α, interferon-β	Antiviral activity
IL-8	Chemokine for neutrophils and T lymphocytes

[a]GM-CSF, granulocyte-macrophage colony-stimulating factor; IL, Interleukin; M-CSF, macrophage colony-stimulating factor; TGF, transforming growth factor; TNF, tumor necrosis factor.

during and after diapedesis. Cytokines producing this effect are also called **chemokines**.
- Increased mitotic activity in certain leukocytes, both locally and in the bone marrow.
- Stimulation or suppression of lymphocyte activities during adaptive immunity. One large group of cytokines with such effects consists of the **interleukins**, secreted by and targeting various leukocytes primarily.
- Stimulated phagocytosis or directed cell killing by innate immune cells.

Most cytokines have multiple target cells in which they trigger multiple effects. Some are produced by and target cells besides immune cells, including endothelial cells, certain autonomic neurons, and cells of the endocrine system. The broad range of cytokine actions greatly extends the physiologic effects of infections and other stressors.

❯ ANTIGENS & ANTIBODIES

A macromolecule recognized by cells of the adaptive immune system represents an **antigen** and typically elicits a response from these cells. Antigens may consist of soluble molecules (such as proteins or polysaccharides) or molecules that are still attached as components of intact cells (bacteria, protozoa, or tumor cells). Immune cells recognize and react to small molecular domains in the antigen known as antigenic determinants or **epitopes**. The adaptive response to antigens may be **cellular**, in which lymphocytes take direct charge in the antigen's elimination; **humoral**, in which soluble antibodies play key roles in removing the antigen; or both.

All **antibodies** are glycoproteins of the **immunoglobulin** family that interact specifically with antigenic determinants. Antibodies against a specific epitope are secreted by a clone of **plasma cells** originating from a B lymphocyte triggered to proliferate when surface receptors were presented with and bound that epitope. Antibodies either accumulate in the blood plasma and the interstitial fluid of tissues or get transported across epithelia into the secretion of mucous, salivary, and mammary glands. Other antibodies exist as membrane proteins on the surface of B cells or other leukocytes. In all these situations each antibody combines with the epitope that it specifically recognizes.

Immunoglobulins of all antibody molecules have a common design, consisting of two identical light chains and two identical heavy chains with hinge regions, all held together by disulfide bonds (Figure 14–2). The isolated carboxyl-terminal tail of the heavy chains represents the **Fc region**, displaying glycosylation and relatively constant immunoglobulin domains. Fc regions of some antibodies bind surface receptors on basophils and mast cells, becoming localized to those cell surfaces only. The first 110 amino acids of the amino-terminal ends of the paired light and heavy chains differ widely from antibody to antibody and constitute an antibody's **variable Fab region**. The variable portions of one heavy and one light chain include two identical **antigen-binding sites** (Figure 14–2). DNA sequences coding for the variable regions undergo recombination and rearrangement following B lymphocyte activation against a specific antigen, so that the plasma cell progeny of the activated B cell all produce antibodies exclusively binding that antigen.

Classes of Antibodies

Table 14–2 shows five major classes of human immunoglobulins, along with their structural features, abundance in plasma, major locations, and functions. The classes are **immunoglobulin G (IgG)**, **IgA**, **IgM**, **IgE**, and **IgD**, and key aspects for each include the following:

- **IgG** represents the most abundant class, including 75%–85% of the immunoglobulin in blood. Production increases during immune responses following infections, etc. Unlike the other classes of antibodies, IgG is highly soluble, stable (half-life >3 weeks), and crosses the placental barrier into the fetal circulation. This confers **passive immunity** against certain infections until the newborn acquires their own adaptive immune system.

- **IgA** occurs in almost all exocrine secretions, produced by plasma cells in mucosae of the digestive, respiratory, and reproductive tracts. IgA has a dimeric form in which the heavy chains of two monomers are united by a short polypeptide called the **J chain**, synthesized in the plasma cell, and by another protein, the **secretory component**, furnished by the epithelial cells as the IgA dimer undergoes transcytosis. The extra modules make the structure relatively resistant to proteolysis, increasing its half-life while it deals with microorganisms in milk, saliva, tears, and mucus coating the secretory mucosae producing IgA.

- **IgM** constitutes 5%–10% of blood immunoglobulin, usually existing in a very large pentameric form with its monomers united by additional proteins. IgM originates mainly in the initial phase of an antigenic response. Bound to antigen, IgM represents the most effective antibody class for activating complement.

- **IgE**, usually a monomer, circulates with much less abundance and exists bound at its Fc region to surface receptors of mast cells and basophils. When IgE encounters the antigen that elicited its production, the antigen-antibody complexes trigger release of several biologically active substances, such as histamine, heparin, and leukotrienes, from the attached cells. This forms the basis of an **allergic reaction**, mediated by cell-bound IgE recognizing antigens (**allergens**) that stimulated the IgE synthesis initially (see Mast Cells in Chapter 5).

- **IgD**, the least abundant immunoglobulin in plasma, represents the least well-understood class of antibody. Monomers of IgD bind the surface of B lymphocytes where they (along with IgM monomers) act as antigen receptors in triggering B cell activation.

FIGURE 14–2 Basic structure of an immunoglobulin (antibody).

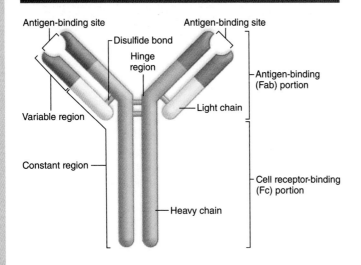

Two light chains and two heavy chains form an **antibody** molecule ("monomer"). The chains are linked by disulfide bonds. The **variable portions** (Fab) near the amino end of the light and heavy chains bind the antigen. The **constant region** (or Fc) of the molecule may bind to surface receptors of several cell types.

TABLE **14–2**	Important features of the antibody classes in humans.				
	IgG	**IgM**	**IgA**	**IgD**	**IgE**
Structure	Monomer	Pentamer	Secretory component Dimer with J chain and secretory component	Monomer	Monomer
Antibody percentage in the plasma	75%–85%	5%–10%	10%–15%	0.001%	0.002%
Presence in sites other than blood, connective tissue, and lymphoid organs	Fetal circulation in pregnant women	B lymphocyte surface (as a monomer)	Secretions (saliva, milk, tears, etc.)	Surface of B lymphocytes	Bound to the surface of mast cells and basophils
Known functions	Activates phagocytosis, neutralizes antigens	First antibody produced in initial immune response; activates complement	Protects mucosae	Antigen receptor triggering initial B cell activation	Destroys parasitic worms and participates in allergies

Actions of Antibodies

Figure 14–3a shows that antigen-binding sites of IgG and IgA antibodies bind specifically and **neutralize** certain viral particles and bacterial toxins, **agglutinate** many bacterial cells, and **precipitate** most soluble antigens. In addition the Fc portions of these and other antibodies also bind receptors for this sequence and thereby optimize three important actions of innate immunity depicted in Figure 14–3b:

- **Complement activation:** Antigen-antibody complexes containing IgG or IgM readily bind components of the **complement system**, a group of around 20 plasma proteins produced mainly in the liver, activating them through a cascade of enzymatic reactions. After activation, certain complement components bind and rupture membranes of invading cells, clump antigen-bearing bacteria or cells, and elicit the arrival of relevant leukocytes.
- **Opsonization:** This refers to the ability of receptors on macrophages, neutrophils, and eosinophils to recognize and bind the Fc portions of antibodies attached to surface antigens of microorganisms. Opsonization greatly increases the efficiency of microbial **phagocytosis** by these leukocytes at the sites of infection.
- **NK cells activation:** Primitive lymphocytes called **NK cells** recognize antibodies bound to unusual antigens of virus-infected cells, becoming activated to kill the infected cell by the release of **perforin** and various **granzymes**, which enter the cell and cause apoptosis.

› ANTIGEN PRESENTATION

Antigens recognized by lymphocytes are often bound to specialized integral membrane protein complexes on cell surfaces. These abundant antigen-presenting proteins are parts of the **major histocompatibility complex (MHC)**, which includes the two key types called MHC class I and class II. As the name implies, these proteins were first recognized by their roles in the immune rejection of grafted tissue or organs. Proteins of both classes, which on human cells are often called human leukocyte antigens (HLAs), are encoded by genes in large chromosomal loci having very high degrees of allelic variation between different individuals. T lymphocytes are specialized to recognize both classes of MHC proteins and the antigens they present. If the MHCs on cells of a tissue graft are not like those that T lymphocytes encountered during their development, the grafted cells will induce a strong immune reaction by T cells of the recipient. To these lymphocytes, the unfamiliar MHC epitopes on the graft's cells are recognized as markers of potentially tumorigenic, infected, or otherwise abnormal ("non-self") cells that they must eliminate.

Like all integral membrane protein complexes, MHC molecules are made in the rough ER and Golgi apparatus. Before leaving the ER, **MHC class I** proteins bind a wide variety of proteasome-derived peptide fragments representing the range of all proteins synthesized in that cell. All nucleated cells produce and expose on their surfaces MHC class I molecules presenting such "self-antigens," which T cells recognize as a signal to ignore those cells. By this same mechanism, some virally

FIGURE **14–3** Various specific and nonspecific functions of antibodies.

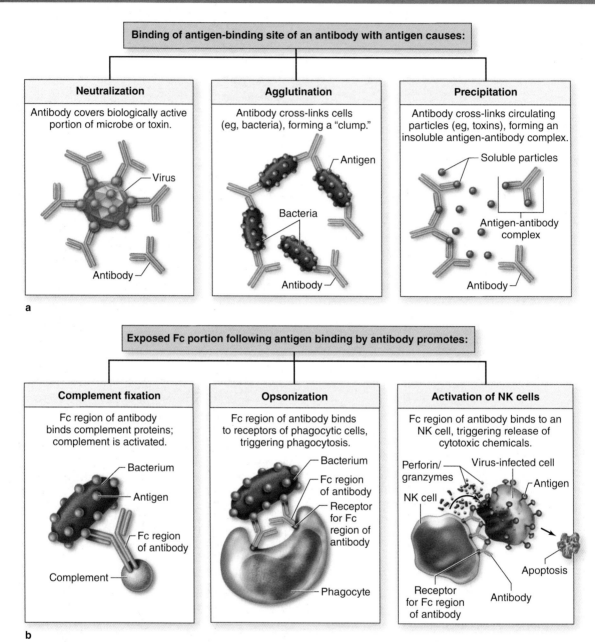

Shown here are important mechanisms by which the most common antibodies act in immunity. **(a)** Specific binding of antigens can **neutralize** or **precipitate** antigens, or cause microorganisms bearing the antigens to clump (**agglutinate**) for easier removal.

(b) Complement proteins and surface receptors on many leukocytes bind the Fc portions of antibodies attached to cell-surface antigens, producing **active complement**, more efficient phagocytosis (**opsonization**), and **NK-cell activation**.

infected cells or cells with proteins altered by gene mutation also have MHC class I proteins displaying peptides that T cells do *not* recognize as "self," helping lead to the elimination of such cells.

MHC class II proteins are synthesized and transported to the cell surface similarly but only in cells of the mononuclear phagocyte system and certain other cells under some conditions. Before joining the plasmalemma, the Golgi-derived vesicles with the MHC class II complexes first fuse with endolysosomal vesicles containing antigens ingested by receptor-mediated endocytosis, pinocytosis, or phagocytosis. This allows the class II proteins to bind fragments of whatever proteins the cells had ingested, including those from dead, infected, or abnormal cells and atypical proteins of all kinds.

At the surface of these cells, the class II complexes display the peptides from these potentially pathogenic cells, signaling T lymphocytes and activating their responses against sources of these antigens.

› CELLS OF ADAPTIVE IMMUNITY

Described in Chapter 12 with blood, lymphocytes and the monocyte-derived cells specialized for antigen presentation to lymphocytes are the major players in adaptive immune responses.

Antigen-Presenting Cells

Most specialized APCs are part of the mononuclear phagocyte system, including all types of macrophages and specialized **dendritic cells** in lymphoid organs (which are not to be confused with any cells of nervous tissue). Features common to all APCs are an active system for endocytosis and expression of MHC class II molecules for presenting peptides of exogenous antigens. Besides dendritic cells and all monocyte-derived cells, so-called "professional" APCs also include B lymphocytes and thymic epithelial cells (TECs), both discussed below.

During inflammation transient expression of MHC class II is induced by interferon-γ in certain local cells that can be considered "nonprofessional" APCs, including fibroblasts and vascular endothelial cells.

Lymphocytes

Lymphocytes both regulate and carry out adaptive immunity. In adults, stem cells for all lymphocytes are located in the red bone marrow, but cells of the major lymphoid lineages mature and become functional in two different central or **primary lymphoid organs**. Cells destined to become B lymphocytes

TABLE 14–3	Approximate percentages of B and T cells in lymphoid organs.	
Lymphoid Organ	**T Lymphocytes (%)**	**B Lymphocytes (%)**
Thymus	100	0
Bone marrow	10	90
Spleen	45	55
Lymph nodes	60	40
Blood	70	30

remain and differentiate further in the **bone marrow**. Progenitors of T lymphocytes move via the circulation into the developing **thymus**. After maturation in these primary structures, B and T cells circulate to the peripheral **secondary lymphoid organs**, which include the **MALT**, the **lymph nodes**, and the **spleen** (Figure 14–1). Lymphocytes do not stay long in the lymphoid organs; they continuously recirculate through the body in connective tissues, blood, and lymph. Because of the constant mobility of lymphocytes and APCs, the cellular locations and microscopic details of lymphoid organs differ from one day to the next. However, the relative percentages of T and B lymphocytes in these compartments are relatively steady (Table 14–3).

Lymphoid tissue is usually reticular connective tissue filled with large numbers of lymphocytes. It can be either diffuse within areas of loose connective tissue or surrounded by capsules, forming discrete (secondary) lymphoid organs. Because lymphocytes have prominent basophilic nuclei and very little cytoplasm, lymphoid tissue packed with such cells usually stains dark blue in hematoxylin and eosin (H&E)-stained sections. In all secondary lymphoid tissue, the lymphocytes are supported by a rich reticulin fiber network of type III collagen (Figure 14–4a). The fibers are produced by fibroblastic **reticular cells**, which extend numerous processes along and around the fibers (Figure 14–4b). Besides lymphocytes and reticular cells, lymphoid tissue typically contains various APCs and plasma cells.

Although most lymphocytes are morphologically indistinguishable in either the light or electron microscope, various surface proteins ("cluster of differentiation" or **CD markers**) allow them to be distinguished as B cells and subcategories of T cells by immunocytochemical methods. Key features of B and T lymphocytes also include the surface receptors involved in activating their different responses to antigens (Figure 14–5). Receptors of B cells are immunoglobulins that bind antigens directly; those on T cells react only with antigen on MHC molecules and this requires the additional cell surface proteins CD4 or CD8.

Lymphocytes in the marrow and thymus of a newborn infant not yet exposed to antigens are immunocompetent but naive and unable to recognize antigens. After circulating to the various secondary lymphoid structures, lymphocytes are exposed to antigens on APCs and become activated,

FIGURE **14–4** Reticular fibers and cells of lymphoid tissue.

(a) A three-dimensional framework of reticular fibers (collagen type III) supports the cells of most lymphoid tissues and organs (except the thymus). Areas with larger spaces between the fibers offer more mobility to cells than areas in which the fiber mesh-work is denser, such as in trabeculae (**T**) where fewer lymphocytes are aggregated and cells are generally more stationary. (×140; Silver impregnation)

(b) Cells of typical lymphoid tissue include the fibroblast-like reticular cells (**R**) producing and maintaining the trabeculae (**T**) and reticulin framework. Many cells are loosely attached to the reticulin fibers, including macrophages (**M**) and many lympho-cytes. (×240; H&E)

(*Reproduced with permission from Paulo A. Abrahamsohn, Institute of Biomedical Sciences, University of São Paulo, Brazil.*)

FIGURE **14–5** Specific receptors on T and B lymphocytes.

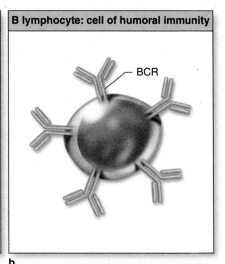

(a) All T lymphocytes have cell surface protein receptors (TCRs) with variable regions that recognize specific antigens. Cell activa-tion requires **costimulation** by the **TCR** and either **CD4 or CD8**, which characterize helper and cytotoxic T cells, respectively.

(b) B-cell receptors (BCRs) are **immunoglobulin** molecules pro-jecting from the plasmalemma.

proliferating to produce a clone of lymphocytes all able to recognize that antigen.

T Lymphocytes

T cells are long-lived lymphocytes and constitute nearly 75% of the circulating lymphocytes. They recognize antigenic epitopes via surface protein complexes termed **T-cell receptors (TCRs)**. Most TCRs include two glycoproteins called the α and β **chains**, each with variable regions produced similarly to those of immunoglobulins. Because TCRs only recognize antigenic peptides when presented as part of MHC molecules (interacting with both the MHC and the peptide it presents), T lymphocytes are said to be **MHC restricted**.

Several types of T lymphocytes exist, with various functions. Important subpopulations of T cells include the following:

- **Helper T cells** (Th cells) are characterized by **CD4**, the coreceptor with the TCR for binding MHC class II molecules and the peptides they display (Figure 14–6a). Activated by such binding, helper T cells greatly assist immune responses by producing cytokines that promote differentiation of B cells into plasma cells, activate macrophages to become phagocytic, activate cytotoxic T lymphocytes (CTLs), and induce many parts of an inflammatory reaction. Some specifically activated helper T cells persist as noncirculating or tissue-resident memory helper T cells, which allow a more rapid response if the antigen appears again later.
- **Cytotoxic T lymphocytes (CTLs)** are characteristically **CD8⁺**. Their TCRs together with the CD8 coreceptors recognize specific antigens displayed by MHC class I molecules on "foreign" cells, which include tumors cells, tissue grafts, and cells infected with virus or replicating bacteria (Figure 14–6b). In the presence of interleukin-2 (IL-2) from helper T cells, cytotoxic T cells that have recognized such antigens are activated and proliferate. Also called killer T cells, they attach to the cell sources of the antigens and remove them by releasing perforins and granzymes, which trigger apoptosis. This represents **cell-mediated immunity**, and its mechanism is broadly similar to that of NK cells. Like helper T cells, activation of cytotoxic T cells also results in a population of tissue-resident memory killer T cells.
- **Regulatory T cells** (T$_{regs}$ or suppressor T cells) are CD4⁺CD25⁺ and serve to inhibit specific immune responses. These cells, also identified by the presence of the Foxp3 transcription factor, play crucial roles in allowing immune tolerance, maintaining unresponsiveness to self-antigens and suppressing excessive immune responses. These cells produce **peripheral tolerance**, which acts to supplement the central tolerance that develops in the thymus.
- **γδ T lymphocytes** represent a smaller subpopulation whose TCRs contain γ (gamma) and δ (delta) chains instead of α and β chains. The γδ T cells migrate to the epidermis and mucosal epithelia, becoming largely intraepithelial, and do not recirculate to secondary lymphoid organs. They function in many ways like cells of innate immunity, in the front lines against invading microorganisms.

B Lymphocytes

In B lymphocytes, the surface receptors for antigens are monomers of IgM or IgD, with each B cell covered by about 150,000 such **B-cell receptors (BCRs)** (Figure 14–5b). BCRs bind an antigen, which may be free in solution, on an exposed part of an infectious agent, or already bound to antibodies, and the surface complexes then undergo endocytosis. Degraded in endosomes, peptides from the antigens are presented on MHC class II molecules of the B cell. A helper T cell then binds this B cell and activates it further by secreting IL-4, which enhances mutability in the immunoglobulin genes and stimulates several cycles of cell proliferation (Figure 14–6c).

In follicles of lymph nodes and other secondary lymphoid tissues, B lymphocytes interact with scattered **follicular dendritic cells (FDCs)**, which have long filamentous processes. Unlike other dendritic cells, FDCs are mesenchymal in origin and their function does not involve MHC class II molecules. The surfaces of these cells are covered with antibody-antigen complexes bound to receptors for complement proteins and for immunoglobulin Fc regions, causing B cells to attach, become activated, and aggregate as a small **primary lymphoid nodule** (or follicle). With the help of adjacent T cells, these B cells now form a much larger and more prominent **secondary lymphoid nodule** (Figure 14–7).

Secondary nodules are characterized by a lightly stained **germinal center** filled with large lymphoblasts (or **centroblasts**), which undergo repeated hypermutation in the genes coding for the variable regions of immunoglobulins (increasing the diversity of the antibody repertoire for recognizing and binding the initiating antigen), proliferation, and continuous quality control. Growth of activated B cells in germinal centers is very rapid, causing naive, nonproliferating B cells to be pushed aside to form the peripheral, more basophilic **follicular mantle** (Figure 14–7). After 2–3 weeks of proliferation, most cells of the germinal center and mantle are dispersed, and the structure of the secondary lymphoid nodule is gradually lost.

Most of these new, specific B lymphocytes differentiate into **plasma cells** secreting antibodies that will bind the same epitope recognized by the activated B cell. Because the

FIGURE **14–6** **Activation of lymphocytes.**

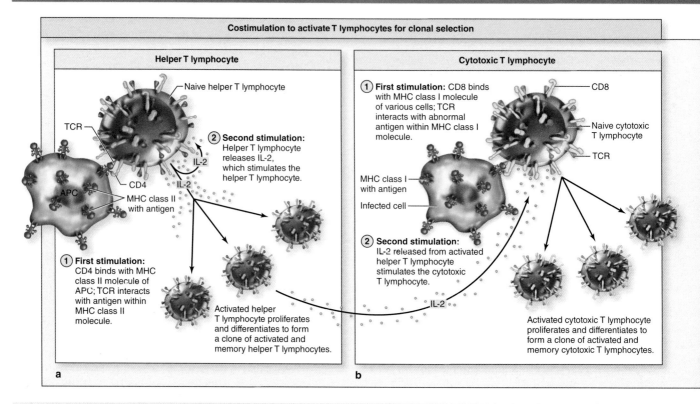

Costimulation to activate T lymphocytes for clonal selection

Helper T lymphocyte

Naive helper T lymphocyte

TCR

② **Second stimulation:**
Helper T lymphocyte
releases IL-2,
which stimulates the
helper T lymphocyte.

IL-2

CD4

IL-2

APC

MHC class II
with antigen

① **First stimulation:**
CD4 binds with MHC
class II molecule of
APC; TCR interacts
with antigen within
MHC class II
molecule.

Activated helper
T lymphocyte proliferates
and differentiates to form
a clone of activated and
memory helper T lymphocytes.

a

Cytotoxic T lymphocyte

① **First stimulation:** CD8 binds
with MHC class I molecule
of various cells; TCR
interacts with abnormal
antigen within MHC class I
molecule.

CD8

Naive cytotoxic
T lymphocyte

TCR

MHC class I
with antigen

Infected cell

② **Second stimulation:**
IL-2 released from activated
helper T lymphocyte
stimulates the cytotoxic
T lymphocyte.

IL-2

Activated cytotoxic T lymphocyte
proliferates and differentiates to
form a clone of activated and
memory cytotoxic T lymphocytes.

b

Lymphocyte activation requires costimulation of at least two receptors and causes cell proliferation that produces many effector cells and a smaller population of memory cells. In all cases, binding between cells involved in costimulation persists until lymphocyte activation is complete.

(a) The TCR and CD4 proteins of a **helper T cell** bind antigens presented on MHC class II molecules and with interleukin-2 (IL-2) stimulation, the lymphocyte is activated and proliferates.

(b) Cytotoxic T lymphocytes, or CTLs, recognize and bind abnormal or "foreign proteins" displayed on MHC class I molecules, and triggered by IL-2 from helper T cells the CTLs proliferate.

antibodies specified by B cells circulate in lymph and blood throughout the body, B cells are said to provide **humoral immunity**. Some of the newly formed B cells remain as long-lived, circulating **memory B cells**, a key feature of adaptive immunity allowing very rapid responses upon subsequent exposure to the same antigen.

❯ THYMUS

While immature B lymphocytes emerge from the bone marrow, the primary or central lymphoid organ in which T cells are produced is the **thymus**, a bilobed structure in the mediastinum (Figure 14–8). A major function of the thymus is induction of **central tolerance**, which along with regulatory T cells prevents autoimmunity. The organ originates from the embryo's third pair of pharyngeal pouches (endoderm), with precursor lymphoblasts circulating from the bone marrow to invade and proliferate in this unique thymic epithelium during its development. Fully formed and functional at birth, the thymus remains large and very active in T-cell production until puberty during which it normally undergoes **involution**, with

decreasing lymphoid tissue mass and cellularity and reduced T-cell output (Figure 14–8).

> ❯❯ **MEDICAL APPLICATION**
>
> Failure of the third (and fourth) pharyngeal pouches to develop normally in the embryo leads to **DiGeorge syndrome**, characterized by **thymic hypoplasia** (or aplasia). Lacking many or all TECs, such individuals cannot produce T lymphocytes properly and have severely depressed cell-mediated immunity.

The thymus has a vascularized connective tissue capsule that extends septa into the parenchyma, dividing the organ into many incompletely separated lobules. Each lobule has an outer darkly basophilic **cortex** surrounding a more lightly stained **medulla**. The staining differences reflect the much greater density of lymphoblasts and small lymphocytes in the cortex than the medulla (Figure 14–8b).

The thymic cortex contains an extensive population of T lymphoblasts (or **thymocytes**), some newly arrived via

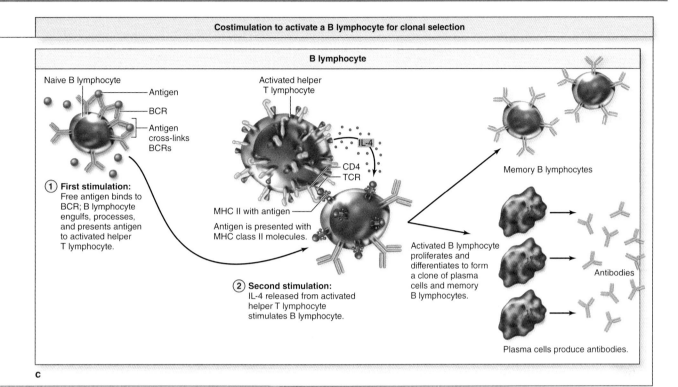

Costimulation to activate a B lymphocyte for clonal selection

B lymphocyte

Naive B lymphocyte

Antigen

BCR

Antigen cross-links BCRs

① **First stimulation:** Free antigen binds to BCR; B lymphocyte engulfs, processes, and presents antigen to activated helper T lymphocyte.

Activated helper T lymphocyte

IL-4

CD4
TCR

MHC II with antigen

Antigen is presented with MHC class II molecules.

② **Second stimulation:** IL-4 released from activated helper T lymphocyte stimulates B lymphocyte.

Memory B lymphocytes

Activated B lymphocyte proliferates and differentiates to form a clone of plasma cells and memory B lymphocytes.

Antibodies

Plasma cells produce antibodies.

c

(c) Antigen bound to the immunoglobulin receptors on B cells (BCRs) is endocytosed, processed, and presented on their MHC class II proteins to helper T cells. These then secrete IL-4 and other cytokines that stimulate gene recombination and clonal proliferation of these specific B cells. They differentiate as **plasma cells** producing antibodies against the antigen that was originally bound and processed.

venules, located among numerous macrophages and associated with the unique **thymic epithelial cells (TECs)** that have certain features of both epithelial and reticular cells. These cells usually have large euchromatic nuclei but are morphologically and functionally diverse. There are three major types of TECs in the cortex of the thymus:

- Squamous TECs form a layer, joined by desmosomes and occluding junctions, line the connective tissue of the capsule and septa and surround the microvasculature. This creates an isolated cortical compartment and, together with the vascular endothelial cells and pericytes, forms a **blood-thymus barrier** preventing unregulated exposure of thymocytes to antigens.
- Throughout this compartment another population of stellate TECs, with processes containing keratin tonofilaments joined by desmosomes, form a **cytoreticulum** to which macrophages and developing lymphocytes attach instead of to reticulin fibers (Figure 14–9). Importantly, these cells are APCs, expressing MHC class II molecules in addition to MHC class I. They also secrete numerous cytokines for T-cell development and other immune

functions, justifying this organ's inclusion among endocrine glands.

- Other squamous cortical TECs also express MHC class II molecules but form a sheetlike structure contributing to a functional **corticomedullary barrier** between these two regions of each lobule.

The more lightly stained thymic medulla contains fewer and larger, more mature lymphocytes. Three related types of medullary TECs form the following:

- A second layer of the boundary between cortex and medulla.
- A cytoreticulum that (1) supports T lymphocytes, dendritic cells, and macrophages (all less densely packed than in the cortex), and (2) expresses many specialized proteins specific to cells of other organs.
- Large aggregates of TECs, sometimes concentrically arranged, called **Hassall corpuscles** (Figure 14–10). Up to 100 μm in diameter, thymic corpuscles are unique to the medulla. Their cells secrete several cytokines that control activity of local dendritic cells, including factors promoting development of regulatory T cells for peripheral tolerance.

FIGURE **14–7** Lymphoid nodules (or follicles).

Large aggregates of B cells called lymphoid nodules or follicles transiently characterize all secondary lymphoid organs. Aggregates of uniform cell density and staining represent **primary nodules**, while those with larger, more euchromatic cells centrally are termed **secondary nodules**. Here two secondary nodules can be seen, with germinal centers (**GC**) at different stages of development. Rapid proliferation of activated B lymphoblasts in the germinal center causes smaller, naive lymphocytes to be pushed aside and crowded together peripherally as the follicular mantle (**M**).

Germinal centers represent the sites of activated B lymphoblast DNA hypermutation in genes coding for immunoglobulin variable regions, followed by rapid mitotic activity. Specific local populations of macrophages within the germinal centers clear apoptotic bodies produced by the large percentage of lymphoblasts that die after failing to receive T cell help for continued proliferation or by acquiring damaging mutations, eg mutations producing lethality or self-reactivity.

FIGURE **14–8** Thymus.

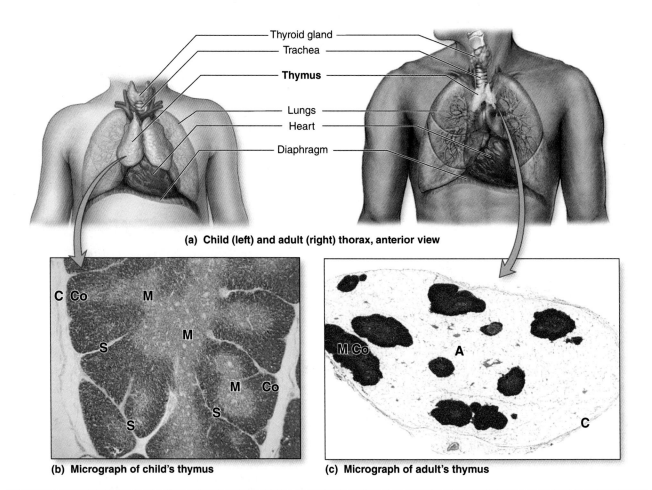

(a) Child (left) and adult (right) thorax, anterior view

(b) Micrograph of child's thymus

(c) Micrograph of adult's thymus

(a) The **thymus**, a bilobed organ located in the superior mediastinum, is most prominent and active before puberty, undergoing gradual shrinkage (involution) and loss of activity in adults.

(b) A **child's thymus**, showing connective tissue of the capsule (**C**) and septa (**S**) between thymic lobules, each having an outer cortex (**Co**) and incompletely separated medulla (**M**) of lymphoid tissue. (H&E; ×40)

(c) After **involution**, the thymus shows only small regions of lymphoid tissue, here still with cortex (**Co**) and medulla (**M**), and these are embedded in adipose tissue (**A**). Age-related thymic involution reduces production of naïve T cells and may be involved with the decline of immune function in the elderly. (H&E; ×24)

FIGURE **14–9** Cortex of the thymus.

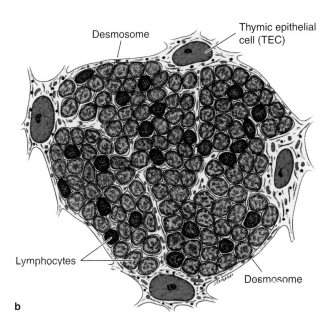

Desmosome — Thymic epithelial cell (TEC)

Lymphocytes — Desmosome

b

FIGURE **14–10** Medulla of the thymus with Hassall corpuscles.

The thymic medulla contains fewer lymphocytes than the cortex, and the epithelial cells (**E**) located here have different morphology and function. The most characteristic feature of the medulla in humans is the presence of thymic (Hassall) corpuscles (**H**). These are of variable size and contain aggregates of thymic epithelial cells releasing many cytokines important within the medullary microenvironment, especially for dendritic cell activity and for the differentiation of regulatory T cells. Dendritic cells in the medulla are difficult to discern without special staining. (×200; H&E)

(a) The cortical zone of an active thymus is packed with small, highly basophilic lymphoblasts that proliferate as well as undergo positive and negative selection in that region. The lymphoblasts are supported on a meshwork (or cytoreticulum) of unusual thymic epithelial cells (**E**). (×400; PT)

(b) The **thymic epithelial cells** throughout the cortex are APCs and extend long processes bound together by desmosomes to make a framework, the **cytoreticulum**, for the lymphoblasts. Having a cytoreticulum consisting of APC cellular processes rather than the more common network of simple reticulin fibers, allows regulated specificity of lymphocyte binding via the changing antigens on MHC proteins. Some cortical epithelial cells also secrete cytokines that promote T-cell maturation.

The microvasculature of the medulla is not surrounded by a tight layer of TECs, and mature T lymphocytes exit the thymus by passing through the walls of venules and efferent lymphatics in this region.

Role of the Thymus in T-Cell Maturation & Selection

The thymus is the site of T-lymphocyte differentiation and the selective removal of T cells reactive against self-antigens, a key part of inducing central self-tolerance.

T lymphoblasts arriving in the thymus do not yet express CD4, CD8, or a TCR. These cells populate the cortex and begin to proliferate, recombine variable regions of the TCR α and β chain

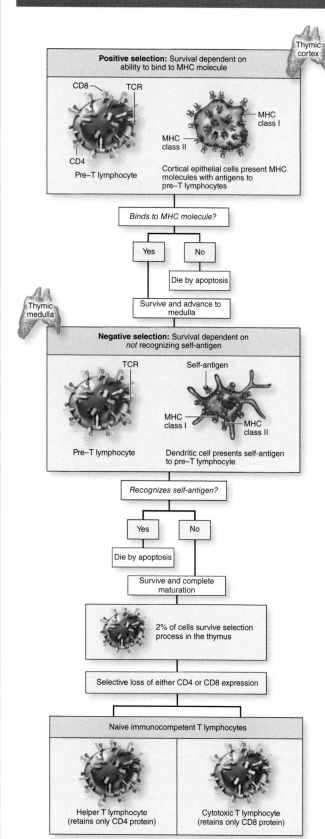

genes, and then express these TCR proteins as well as both CD4 and CD8. With these key functional components in place, thymocytes begin a stringent, **two-stage selection process** of quality control, which ensures that mature T cells have TCRs that are fully functional but do not recognize and strongly bind MHC with self-antigens. The selection process for each pre–T lymphocyte begins in the cortex, ends in the medulla, and lasts about 2 weeks. Key events are summarized in Figure 14–11, and a simplified account of how the process is currently understood is presented here.

TECs in the cytoreticulum of the cortex present the developing thymocytes with peptides on both MHC class I and class II proteins, which are important for development of CD8+ and CD4+ T cells, respectively. This interaction determines whether the newly made TCR proteins of these cells are functional. The cells are examined by **positive selection**, with a cell's survival depending on whether its TCRs can recognize and bind antigens on the MHC molecules properly. If the cell cannot pass this test, due, for example, to faulty gene recombination and expression of α and β chains, they are nonfunctional and completely useless. Such cells (as many as 80% of the total) undergo apoptosis and are removed by the macrophages. T cells with normal binding to antigens on either MHC class I or class II are positively selected and move to the medullary compartment (Figure 14–11).

In the medulla T cells with functional TCRs encounter antigens presented on both cytoreticular TECs and dendritic cells. Here the focus is on removing T cells whose TCRs strongly bind self-antigens, a process called **negative selection** because survival depends on a cell *not* binding to MHC molecules with such peptides (Figure 14–11). Among the peptides presented in this compartment are those from proteins specific for many nonthymic tissues, including those of skin, lung, liver, gut, etc. Expression of such peripheral **tissue-specific antigens** in subpopulations of medullary TECs occurs because these cells first uniquely express the nuclear protein **Aire** (*Auto*immune *re*gulator), which leads to subsequent transcription of thousands of different organ-specific genes in distinct TEC subtypes. Most of these mimetic proteins are then transferred to neighboring dendritic cells, which play the major role in presenting them to developing thymocytes.

T cells that strongly bind MHCs displaying these self-peptides undergo apoptosis, which is important because release of any such cells from the thymus would lead to a damaging autoimmune response. Only about 2% of all developing T lymphocytes pass both the positive and negative selection tests and survive to exit the thymus as immunocompetent T cells. Depending on which class of MHC they interacted with, most of these lymphocytes will have stopped expressing *either* CD8 or CD4, and become either helper T cells or cytotoxic T cells respectively (Figure 14–11).

Deletion of self-reactive helper and CTLs in the thymus is the basis for the central immunotolerance produced there.

Positive selection occurs in the cortex and allows survival only of T cells with functional TCRs recognizing MHC class I and class II molecules. **Negative selection** occurs in the medulla and allows survival only of T cells that do *not* tightly bind self-antigens presented on dendritic cells there.

Supplementing this throughout the body is the peripheral tolerance mediated by regulatory T cells, which also develop initially in the thymic medulla under the influence of cytokines from Hassall corpuscles.

MUCOSA-ASSOCIATED LYMPHOID TISSUE

Secondary lymphoid structures, where most lymphocytes are activated by antigen presentation, include the MALT, the lymph nodes, and the spleen.

The mucosa or inner lining of the digestive, respiratory, and genitourinary tracts is a common site of invasion by pathogens because their lumens open to the external environment. To protect against such invaders mucosal connective tissue of these tracts contains large and diffuse collections of lymphocytes, IgA-secreting plasma cells, APCs, and lymphoid nodules, all of which comprise the MALT. Lymphocytes are also present within the epithelial lining of such mucosae. Most of the immune cells in MALT are dispersed diffusely in the connective tissue; others are found in aggregates forming large, conspicuous structures such as the **tonsils**, the **Peyer patches** in the ileum, and the **appendix**. Collectively the MALT is one of the largest lymphoid organs, containing up to 70% of all the body's immune cells. Most of the lymphocytes here are B cells; among T cells, CD4+ helper T cells predominate.

Tonsils are large, irregular masses of lymphoid tissue in the mucosa of the posterior oral cavity and nasopharynx where their cells encounter antigens entering the mouth and nose. Named by their location these masses are the **palatine**, **lingual**, and **pharyngeal tonsils** (Figure 14–12a). In all

---

FIGURE **14–12** Tonsils.

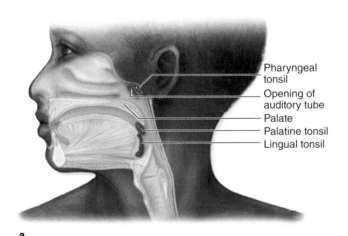

Pharyngeal tonsil
Opening of auditory tube
Palate
Palatine tonsil
Lingual tonsil

a

c

b

(a) Palatine tonsils are located in the posterior lateral walls of the oral cavity, and **lingual** tonsils are situated along the surface of the posterior third of the tongue. Both are covered with stratified squamous epithelium. The **pharyngeal tonsil** is a single medial mass situated in the posterior wall of the nasopharynx. It is usually covered by ciliated pseudostratified columnar epithelium, but areas with stratified epithelium can also be observed. Hypertrophied regions of pharyngeal tonsils resulting from chronic inflammation are called **adenoids**.

(b) A section showing several lymphoid nodules (**LN**), collectively covered by stratified squamous epithelium (**E**) on one side and a connective tissue capsule (**CT**) on the other. Some nodules show lighter staining germinal centers (**GC**). Infoldings of the mucosa in some tonsils form crypts (**C**), along which nodules are especially numerous. Lumens of crypts contain desquamated epithelial cells, live and dead lymphocytes, and bacteria. (×140; H&E)

(c) Epithelium (**E**) surrounding tonsillar crypts (**C**) often becomes infiltrated with lymphocytes and other leukocytes and can become difficult to recognize histologically. Adjacent connective tissue at the top of the photo also contains numerous lymphocytes. (×200; H&E)

(*Figure 14–12b and c, reproduced with permission from Dr Paulo A. Abrahamsohn, Institute of Biomedical Sciences, University of São Paulo, Brazil.*)

Masses of lymphoid nodules comprising tonsils are collected in three general locations in the wall of the pharynx.

tonsils, the lymphoid tissue is closely associated with the surface epithelium. Other features include the following:

- **Palatine tonsils**, located posteriorly on the soft palate, are covered by stratified squamous epithelium. The surface area of each is enlarged with 10–20 deep invaginations or **tonsillar crypts** in which the epithelial lining is densely infiltrated with lymphocytes and other leukocytes (Figure 14–12). The lymphoid tissue is filled diffusely with lymphocytes, with many secondary lymphoid nodules around the crypts. This tissue is underlain by dense connective tissue acting as a partial capsule.
- **Lingual tonsils** are situated along the base of the tongue, are also covered by stratified squamous epithelium with crypts, and have many of the same features as palatine tonsils but lack distinct capsules.
- The single **pharyngeal tonsil** is situated in the posterior wall of the nasopharynx, is covered by pseudostratified ciliated columnar epithelium, and has a thin underlying capsule. The mucosa with diffuse lymphoid tissue and lymphoid nodules is invaginated with shallow infoldings but lacks crypts.

>> MEDICAL APPLICATION

Inflammation of the tonsils, **tonsillitis**, is more common in children than adults. Chronic inflammation of the pharyngeal lymphoid tissue and tonsils of children often produces hyperplasia and enlargement of the tonsils to form "**adenoids**," which can obstruct the eustachian tube and lead to middle ear infections.

Diffuse MALT extends from the pharynx along the entire gastrointestinal tract but becomes very well developed again in the mucosa and submucosa of the ileum. Here large aggregates of lymphoid nodules comprise the **Peyer patches**, each containing dozens of nodules with no underlying connective tissue capsule (Figure 14–13a).

The simple columnar epithelium that covers the lymphoid nodules of Peyer patches includes scattered, large epithelial **M cells** with apical microfolds rather than the brush border with glycocalyx typical of the neighboring enterocytes. M cells are a unique epithelial cell type specialized for uptake of particles and intact microorganisms. The basolateral surface of each M cell is deeply invaginated to form a large "pocket" open to the underlying lymphoid tissue through a uniquely porous or sieve-like basement membrane and containing a transient population of lymphocytes and dendritic cells (Figure 14–13b). Antigens in the intestinal lumen are continuously sampled at the apical surface of these cells and transferred to the immune cells in the pockets. Lymphocytes and dendritic cells leaving the M cell pockets through the basement membrane pores interact and initiate adaptive responses to the antigens, which results in formation of the secondary lymphoid nodules. Locally produced B cells give rise to plasma cells secreting IgA, which is

transported by enterocytes into the intestinal lumen to bind and neutralize potentially harmful antigens.

Another significant collection of MALT occurs in the mucosa of the **appendix**, a short, small-diameter projection from the cecum. Typically, the mucosa of the appendix is almost completely filled with lymphoid tissue, effacing the glands otherwise found in the large intestine wall (Figure 14–14). The lumen contains the normal bacterial flora of the large intestine and may serve to retain some of these beneficial bacteria there during diarrheal illnesses.

> LYMPH NODES

Lymph nodes are bean-shaped, encapsulated structures, generally only 10 mm by 2.5 cm in size, distributed throughout the body along the lymphatic vessels (Figure 14–1). A total of 400–450 lymph nodes are present in the axillae (armpits) and groin, along the major vessels of the neck, and in the thorax and abdomen, and especially in the visceral mesenteries. The nodes constitute a series of in-line filters of lymph that defend against the spread of microorganisms and tumor cells and provide enclosed environments for antigen presentation and development of plasma cells secreting non-IgA antibodies. Before merging with the bloodstream, all lymph is filtered and has antibodies added by at least one lymph node.

Embedded in loose connective tissue, a lymph node has a convex surface where **afferent lymphatics** enter and a concave depression, the **hilum**, where an **efferent lymphatic** leaves and where an artery, vein, and nerve penetrate the organ (Figure 14–15). A dense connective tissue capsule surrounds the lymph node, extending trabeculae internally through which the blood vessels branch. Valves in the lymphatics ensure unidirectional lymph flow.

The most abundant cells of lymph nodes are lymphocytes of all types, plasma cells, dendritic cells, macrophages, and other APCs. FDCs are present within lymphoid nodules. All these cells are arranged in a stroma of reticulin fibers and reticular cells to form three major regions within each lymph node: an outer **cortex** containing the nodules; a deeper extension of cortex called the **paracortex**, which lacks nodules; and a **medulla** with prominent draining sinusoids adjacent to the hilum (Figures 14–15 and 14–16). Unlike the thymus, these regions of lymph nodes are not compartmentalized by epithelium.

The **cortex** includes the following components:

- A **subcapsular sinus**, immediately inside the capsule, receives lymph from the afferent lymphatics (Figure 14–17). From this space, **cortical sinuses** (or trabecular sinuses) branch internally among the lymphoid nodules along trabeculae. These sinuses are lined by a very thin, discontinuous endothelium penetrated by reticulin fibers and processes of dendritic cells. Lymph containing antigens, lymphocytes, and APCs passes through these sinuses and percolates easily into the surrounding lymphoid tissue.

FIGURE **14–13** Peyer patch and M cells.

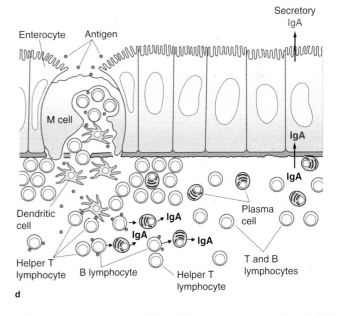

Peyer patches are very large clusters of lymphoid follicles located in the wall of the ileum, which allow close monitoring of microorganisms in the gut.

(a) A section through a Peyer patch shows a few lymphoid nodules (**N**), some with germinal centers (arrow). The mucosa of the small intestine is folded into many projecting villi (**V**). (×100; H&E)

(b) With the surface epithelial cells removed, scanning electron microscopy (SEM) shows typical basement membrane over the villi (**V**) but reveals a highly porous covering over lymphoid nodules of the Peyer patch. This sieve-like basement membrane facilitates interactions between immune cells and M cells in the epithelium over the nodules.

(c) The TEM shows that the epithelium directly over a Peyer patch lymphoid nodule has unique cells called **M (microfold) cells** with short apical folds but lacking the brush border and glycocalyx of the surrounding enterocytes. The basolateral membrane of each M cell is deeply invaginated to form a large intraepithelial pocket

containing lymphocytes (**L**) and dendritic cells (**D**) that come and go through the holes in the basement membrane (**BM**). Darker cytoplasm of adjacent enterocytes (**E**) with brush borders (**B**) is also seen. (×1000)

(d) A summary diagram showing that antigens in the gut lumen are bound by **M cells** and undergo transcytosis into their intraepithelial I pockets where **dendritic cells** take up the antigen, process it, and present it to **T helper cells**. B lymphocytes stimulated by the Th cells differentiate into **plasma cells** secreting IgA antibodies. The IgA is transported into the gut lumen where it binds its antigen on the surface of microorganisms, neutralizing potentially harmful invaders before they penetrate the mucosa.

(Figure 14–13b, Reproduced with permission from Dr Samuel G. McClugage, Department of Cell Biology and Anatomy, Louisiana State University Health Sciences Center, New Orleans, LA.)

(Figure 14–13c, Reproduced with permission from Dr Marian R. Neutra, Children's Hospital, Harvard Medical School, Boston, MA.)

FIGURE **14–14** Appendix.

A blind evagination off the cecum, the **appendix** is a significant part of the MALT with its lamina propria and submucosa filled with lymphocytes and lymphoid follicles (**L**). The small lumen contains a sample of the microbial flora of the intestine, along with undigested material. (×20; H&E)

■ **Lymphoid nodules**, with or without germinal centers, consist largely of developing B lymphocytes and occupy much of the cortex not filled with helper T lymphocytes (Figures 14–16 and 14–17). Each nodule is organized around the long, interdigitating processes of FDCs, but these are not readily seen by routine light microscopy. Macrophages in the germinal centers remove newly formed but defective B cells undergoing apoptosis.

The region between the cortex and medulla, the **paracortex** does not have precise boundaries but can be distinguished from the outer cortex by its lack of nodules (Figure 14–16). Unlike the superficial cortex, the paracortex contains lymphoid tissue rich in T cells distinguishable by immunohistochemistry (Figure 14–18).

Also located mainly in the paracortex, specialized postcapillary venules called **high endothelial venules (HEVs)**

represent an important entry point for most (90%) circulating lymphocytes into lymph nodes. Endothelial cells of these vessels become unusually enlarged or cuboidal and express specific apical surface glycoproteins that mediate the tethering and diapedesis of B and T cells from the blood into the paracortex of the lymph node (Figure 14–19). HEVs also occur in the large accumulations of MALT discussed previously but are less well characterized in those tissues.

The **medulla** of a lymph node has two major components (Figures 14–16 and 14–20):

■ **Medullary cords** are branched cordlike masses of lymphoid tissue extending from the paracortex. They contain T and B lymphocytes and many plasma cells.
■ **Medullary sinuses** are dilated spaces lined by discontinuous endothelium that separate the medullary cords. As shown in Figure 14–20, the lumens of medullary sinuses include a meshwork of processes from reticular cells, which represent a final lymph filter. These sinuses contain many macrophages and sometimes neutrophils if the lymph node is draining an infected region. They are continuous with the cortical sinuses and converge at the hilum as the efferent lymphatic vessel (Figure 14–15).

> **》》MEDICAL APPLICATION**
>
> **Metastatic cancer cells** detached from a primary tumor can enter lymphatics and are carried to nearby lymph nodes, especially the **sentinel lymph node** that is the first one downstream of the region with the tumor. Cells from well-established tumors are often immunosuppressive themselves and may continue growth as a **secondary tumor** within lymph nodes. During cancer surgery lymph nodes in the lymphatics draining the tumor area are examined by pathologists for the presence of cancer cells. The presence of such metastatic cells in lymph nodes is a key determinant in most **staging systems** for various types of cancer and an important prognostic indicator.

Role of Lymph Nodes in the Immune Response

The lymph arriving at a lymph node contains antigens free in solution or bound to antibodies or complement, still on microorganisms, or already internalized and transported by APCs. When draining from an infected or inflamed region, lymph may also contain microorganisms and cytokines. Antigens not yet phagocytosed will be internalized by APCs in the lymph nodes and presented on MHC class II molecules.

Circulating B and T lymphocytes traffic from node to node, entering via the lymph or HEVs, where B cells contact antigens on FDCs and T cells sample antigens presented on dendritic cells and other APCs. Lymphocytes whose receptors recognize such antigens will be activated. B cells will proliferate rapidly in germinal centers of follicles with the help

FIGURE **14–15** Lymph node.

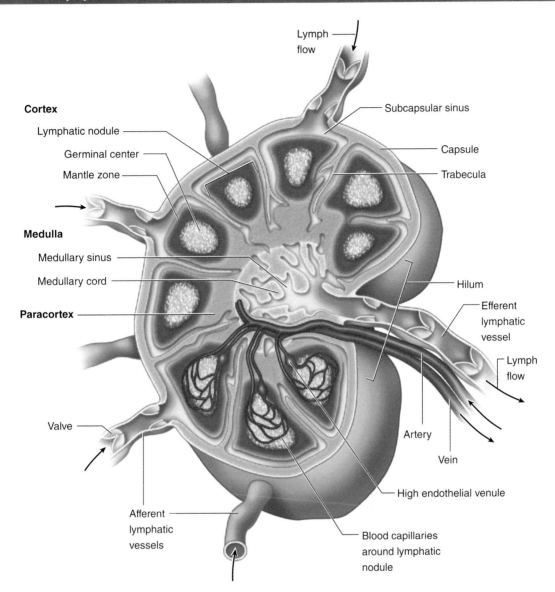

Lymph flow

Cortex
Lymphatic nodule
Germinal center
Mantle zone

Medulla
Medullary sinus
Medullary cord

Paracortex

Valve

Afferent lymphatic vessels

Subcapsular sinus
Capsule
Trabecula

Hilum
Efferent lymphatic vessel
Lymph flow

Artery
Vein
High endothelial venule

Blood capillaries around lymphatic nodule

Lymph nodes are small, encapsulated structures positioned along lymphatic vessels to filter lymph and facilitate antibody production. Valves in the lymphatic vessels ensure the one-way flow of lymph, indicated by arrows.

The three major regions of a lymph node include the outer **cortex** receiving lymph from the afferent lymphatics, an inner **paracortex** where most lymphocytes enter via HEVs, and a central **medulla** with sinuses converging at the efferent lymphatic.

of Th cells, often enlarging the entire lymph node. Activated cytotoxic T cells in the paracortex proliferate to a much lesser extent without forming follicles.

Many newly made B cells, now activated against a specific antigen, differentiate as plasma cells and move to the medulla or to downstream sites beyond the lymph node where they produce antibodies. Specific Th cells, CTLs, and T$_{regs}$ also recirculate in the efferent lymph and with the antibodies spread the immune defenses against those microorganisms throughout the body. Both B and T memory cells also move elsewhere in the body, providing long-lived protection and

proliferating more rapidly upon subsequent exposure to their specific antigen.

›› MEDICAL APPLICATION

Neoplastic proliferation of lymphocytes, producing a malignant **lymphoma**, may occur diffusely but is often located in one or more lymph nodes. Such growth can completely obliterate the normal architecture of the node and convert it to an enlarged, encapsulated structure filled with lymphocytes, a condition called **lymphadenopathy**.

FIGURE 14–16 Regions of a lymph node.

A low-magnification section of a **lymph node** shows the three functional regions: the cortex (**C**), the paracortex (**P**), and the medulla (**M**). Connective tissue of the capsule (**CT**) completely surrounds each lymph node and extends as several trabeculae (**T**) throughout the lymphoid tissue. Major spaces for lymph flow are present in this tissue under the capsule and along the trabeculae. A changing population of immune cells is suspended on reticular fibers throughout the cortex, paracortex, and medulla. Lymphoid nodules (**LN**) are normally restricted to the cortex, and the medulla is characterized by sinuses (**MS**) and cords (**MC**) of lymphoid tissue. (×40; H&E)

(Reproduced with permission from Dr Paulo A. Abrahamsohn, Institute of Biomedical Sciences, University of São Paulo, Brazil)

❯ SPLEEN

The spleen contains the largest single accumulation of lymphoid tissue in the body and is the only lymphoid organ involved in filtration of blood, making it an important organ in defense against blood-borne antigens. It is also the main site of old erythrocyte destruction. As is true of other secondary lymphoid organs, the spleen is a production site of antibodies and activated lymphocytes, which here are delivered directly into the blood.

Located high in the left upper quadrant of the abdomen and typically about 12 × 7 × 3 cm in size, the spleen's volume varies with its content of blood and tends to decrease very slowly after puberty. The organ is surrounded by a capsule of

FIGURE 14–17 Lymph node cortex.

The outer regions on the convex sides of a lymph node include the capsule (**C**), subcapsular sinuses (**S**), and a **cortex** consisting of diffuse lymphoid tissue with lymphoid nodules (**N**). Afferent lymphatic vessels (which are only rarely shown well in sections) penetrate this capsule, dumping lymph into the sinus where its contents are processed by lymphocytes and APCs. (×140; H&E)

(Reproduced with permission from Dr Paulo A. Abrahamsohn, Institute of Biomedical Sciences, University of São Paulo, Brazil)

dense connective tissue from which emerge trabeculae to penetrate the parenchyma or **splenic pulp** (Figure 14–21). Large trabeculae originate at the hilum, on the medial surface of the spleen, and carry branches of the splenic artery, vein, lymphatics, and nerves into the splenic pulp.

Functions of Splenic White & Red Pulp

The spleen is filled with reticular tissue containing reticular cells and fibers, many lymphocytes and other blood cells, macrophages, and APCs. This splenic pulp has two components: the **white pulp** (20% of the spleen) and the **red pulp** (Figure 14–21). The small masses of white pulp consist of **lymphoid nodules** and the **periarteriolar lymphoid sheaths (PALS)**, while the red pulp consists of blood-filled **sinusoids** and **splenic cords**.

As expected of an organ where the blood is monitored immunologically, the splenic microvasculature contains unique regions shown schematically in Figure 14–22. Branching from the hilum, small **trabecular arteries** leave the trabecular connective tissue and enter the parenchyma as arterioles enveloped by the PALS, which consists primarily of T cells with some macrophages, DCs, and plasma cells as part of the white pulp. Surrounded by the PALS, these vessels are known as **central arterioles** (Figure 14–23). B cells located within the PALS may be activated by a trapped antigen from the blood and form a temporary lymphoid nodule like those of other secondary lymphoid organs (Figure 14–23b). In growing nodules, the arteriole is pushed to an eccentric position

FIGURE **14–18** Lymph node cortex and paracortex.

Just deep to a lymph node's **cortex** lies the **paracortex**. Although most lymphocytes in the cortex are B cells, many located in nodules, the lymphocytes of the paracortex are largely T cells. This separation is indicated in the fluorescence micrographs here using immunohistochemistry on adjacent sections of lymph node.

(a) Antibody against a B-cell surface marker labels nearly all the lymphocytes in the cortex (**C**), as well as many cells around

an HEV (**V**) in the paracortex, but few cells in the paracortex proper (**P**).

(b) Stained with an antibody against a T-cell marker, the paracortex is heavily labeled, but only a few cells in the cortex (**C**) are stained, possibly T helper cells. (×200)

(*Reproduced with permission from I. L. Weissman, Stanford University School of Medicine, Palo Alto, CA.*)

FIGURE **14–19** High endothelial venules.

High endothelial venules or HEVs are found in the **paracortex** of lymph nodes, as shown here, as well as in tonsils and Peyer patches. Their endothelial cells are unusually shaped but generally cuboidal and facilitate rapid translocation of lymphocytes from blood into the lymphoid tissue. L-selectin on the lymphocytes recognizes sugar-rich ligands on the surfaces of these endothelial cells and, as a consequence, the lymphocytes stop there. Integrins promote adhesion between lymphocytes and the endothelial cells, and the lymphocytes cross the vessel wall into the lymph node parenchyma.

(a) HEVs can be difficult to identify in H&E-stained paraffin sections. (×400; H&E)

(b) Plastic sections more clearly reveal the HEVs (arrowheads) and the lymphocytes passing between them (arrows). (×400; PT).

(c) SEM of a sectioned HEV shows five typical lymphocytes adhering to endothelial cells (arrowheads) before migrating between them and joining other lymphocytes in the surrounding paracortex. (×500)

FIGURE **14–20** Lymph node medulla.

(a) The **medulla** of a lymph node consists mainly of the medullary sinuses (**MS**) separated by intervening medullary cords (**MC**). Lymphocytes and plasma are abundant and predominate in number over other cell types. A blood vessel within a medullary cord is also seen. (×200; H&E)

(b) Higher magnification of a medullary cord (**MC**) shows plasma cells (arrows) with spherical, eccentric nuclei and much more cytoplasm than lymphocytes. Efferent lymph is rich in newly synthesized antibodies. A medullary sinus (**MS**) with a meshwork of eosinophilic processes from surrounding reticular cells is also seen. (×400; H&E)

(*Reproduced with permission from Dr Paulo A. Abrahamsohn, Institute of Biomedical Sciences, University of São Paulo, Brazil.*)

FIGURE **14–21** Spleen.

The capsule (**C**) of the **spleen** connects to trabeculae (**T**) extending into the pulp-like interior of the organ. The red pulp (**R**) occupies most of the parenchyma, with white pulp (**W**) restricted to smaller areas, mainly around the central arterioles. Names of these splenic areas refer to their color in the fresh state: red pulp is filled with blood cells of all types, located both in cords and sinuses; white pulp is lymphoid tissue. Large blood vessels and lymphatics enter and leave the spleen at a hilum. (×20; Picro-Sirius-hematoxylin)

FIGURE **14–22** Blood flow in the spleen.

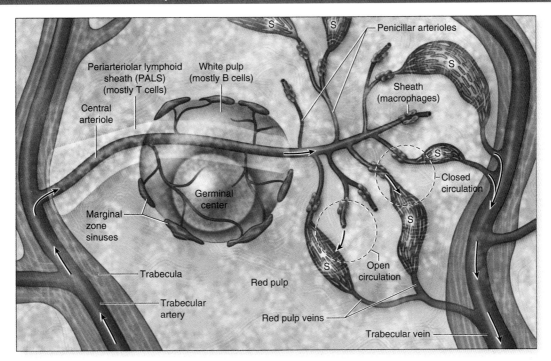

Schematic view of the blood circulation and the structure of the **spleen**, from the trabecular artery to the trabecular vein. Small branches of these arteries are called **central arterioles** and become enclosed within a sheath of lymphoid cells, the **periarteriolar lymphoid sheath (PALS)** in white pulp. B cells in these sheaths can form nodules as the largest masses of white pulp, and around these nodules are located the marginal zone sinuses.

Emerging from the white pulp, the central arteriole branches as the penicillar arterioles, which lead to sheathed capillaries. From these, blood flows into either a **closed circulation** passing directly into splenic sinuses (**S**) or an **open circulation**, being dumped from the vasculature into the lymphoid tissue of the red pulp's splenic cords. From there viable blood cells reenter the vasculature through the walls of the sinuses.

FIGURE **14–23** White pulp of the spleen.

The **splenic white pulp** consists of lymphoid tissue surrounding the central arterioles as the PALS and the nodules of proliferating B cells in this sheath.

(a) Longitudinal section of white pulp (**W**) in a PALS surrounding a central arteriole (arrowhead). Surrounding the PALS is much red pulp (**R**).

(b) A large nodule with a germinal center forms in the PALS and the central arteriole (arrowhead) is displaced to the nodule's periphery. Small vascular sinuses can be seen at the margin between white (**W**) and red (**R**) pulp. (Both ×20; H&E)

(*Reproduced with permission from Dr Paulo A. Abrahamsohn, Institute of Biomedical Sciences, University of São Paulo, Brazil.*)

but is still called the central arteriole. These arterioles send capillaries throughout the white pulp and to small sinuses in a peripheral marginal zone of developing B cells around each lymphoid nodule (Figure 14–22).

Each central arteriole eventually leaves the white pulp and enters the red pulp, losing its sheath of lymphocytes and branching as several short straight **penicillar arterioles** that continue as capillaries (Figure 14–22). Some of these capillaries are sheathed with APCs for additional immune surveillance of blood.

The red pulp is composed almost entirely of **splenic cords** (of Billroth) and **splenic sinusoids** and is the site where effete RBCs in blood are removed (Figure 14–24). The splenic cords contain a network of reticular cells and fibers filled with T and B lymphocytes, macrophages, other leukocytes, and red blood cells. The splenic cords are separated by the sinusoids (Figure 14–25). Unusual elongated endothelial cells called **stave cells** line these sinusoids, oriented parallel to the blood flow and sparsely wrapped in reticular fibers and highly discontinuous basal lamina (Figure 14–26).

Blood flow through the splenic red pulp can take either of two routes (Figure 14–22):

- In the **closed circulation**, capillaries branching from the penicillar arterioles connect directly to the sinusoids and the blood is always enclosed by endothelium.

FIGURE 14–24 Erythrocyte removal by splenic macrophages.

A micrograph showing five **macrophages** in a splenic cord engaged in phagocytosis of effete, brightly eosinophilic erythrocytes. (×400; PT)

- In the **open circulation**, capillaries from about half of the penicillar arterioles are uniquely *open-ended*, dumping blood into the stroma of the splenic cords. In this route, plasma and all the formed elements of blood must reenter the vasculature by passing through narrow slits between the stave cells into the sinusoids. These small openings present no obstacle to platelets, to the motile leukocytes, or to thin flexible erythrocytes. However stiff or effete, swollen RBCs at their normal life span of 120 days are blocked from passing between the stave cells and undergo selective removal by macrophages (Figure 14–24).

Removal of defective RBCs and recycling of their iron are major functions of the red pulp. Iron released from hemoglobin during the degradation of RBCs is stored by macrophages within complexes of ferritin proteins or bound to transferrin, returned to the circulation, and reused primarily for erythropoiesis. Iron-free heme is either bound to its transport protein, hemopexin, or is metabolized to bilirubin and excreted in the bile by liver cells. After surgical removal of the spleen (splenectomy), the number of abnormal erythrocytes in the circulation increases, although most such cells are then removed by macrophages in sinusoids of the bone marrow and liver.

From the sinusoids, blood proceeds to small red pulp veins that converge as the **trabecular veins** (Figure 14–22), which in turn form the splenic vein. The trabecular veins lack significant smooth muscle and resemble endothelium-lined channels hollowed out in the trabecular connective tissue.

Important aspects of the major lymphoid organs (thymus, MALT, lymph nodes, and spleen) are summarized and compared in Table 14–4.

›› MEDICAL APPLICATION

Enlargement of the spleen, **splenomegaly**, can occur from a variety of causes, including lymphoma or other malignant growth, infections such as mononucleosis, or sickle cell disease and other types of anemia. The splenic capsule is relatively thin, and an enlarged spleen is susceptible to traumatic rupture, a potentially life-threatening occurrence due to loss of blood into the abdominal cavity. Such rupture may require prompt surgical removal of the spleen, **splenectomy**, after which most functions of the organ are carried out by other lymphoid organs, with erythrocyte removal occurring in the liver and bone marrow.

FIGURE **14–25**   Red pulp of the spleen.

(a) The **splenic red pulp** is composed entirely of sinusoids (**S**) and splenic cords (**C**), both of which contain blood cells of all types. The cords, often called **cords of Billroth**, are reticular tissue rich in macrophages and lymphocytes. (×140; H&E)

(b) Higher magnification shows that the sinusoids (**S**) are lined by endothelial cells (arrows) with large nuclei bulging into the

sinusoidal lumens. The unusual endothelial cells are called **stave cells** and have special properties that allow separation of healthy from effete red blood cells in the splenic cords (**C**). (×200; H&E)

(*Figure 14–25a and b, reproduced with permission from Dr Paulo A. Abrahamsohn, Institute of Biomedical Sciences, University of São Paulo, Brazil.*)

TABLE **14–4**   Important histologic comparisons of the major lymphoid organs.

	Thymus	MALT	Lymph Nodes	Spleen
Cortex/medulla	Distinctly present	Absent	Present	Absent
Lymphoid nodules	Absent	Present	Present (in cortex only)	Present (in white pulp only)
Lymphatic vessels	No afferents; few efferents in septa	No afferents; efferents present	Afferents at capsule, emptying into subcapsular sinus; efferent at hilum	No afferents; efferents in trabeculae
Unique features	Hassall (thymic) corpuscles in medulla; epithelial-reticular cells in cortex and medulla	Crypts lined by surface mucosa in tonsils; epithelial M cells in mucosa over Peyer patches	Thin paracortical region between cortex and medulla, with high endothelial venules (HEV); medullary cords and sinuses	Minor white pulp component, with central arterioles; major red pulp component, with many sinusoids

FIGURE 14–26   Structure and function of splenic sinusoids.

The endothelial **stave cells** that line the sinusoids in red pulp are long cells oriented lengthwise along the sinusoids.

(a) SEM clearly shows the parallel alignment of the stave cells (**S**), as well as many macrophages (**M**) in the surrounding red pulp (**R**). (×500)

(b) A silver-stained section of spleen shows dark **reticular fibers** in the splenic cords (**C**) and wrapped around the sinusoids (**S**). The sinusoidal basement membrane is highly discontinuous and open to the passage of blood cells. (×400)

(c) Diagram showing these components of **splenic sinusoids**, with the structures resembling a loosely organized wooden barrel. In the open circulation mode of blood flow, blood cells dumped into the splenic cords move under pressure or by their own motility through the spaces between **stave cells**, reentering the vasculature and soon leaving the spleen via the splenic vein. Cells that cannot move between the stave cells, mainly effete erythrocytes, are removed by macrophages.

(Figure 14–26a, SEM photo by Yechun He and the late Prof. Emer. Tsuneo Fujita, courtesy of Prof. Tatsuo Ushiki, Niigata University, Japan.)

The Immune System & Lymphoid Organs SUMMARY OF KEY POINTS

Basic Immunology

- **Innate immunity** is present from birth and involves leukocytes (mainly granulocytes) and proteins such as defensins, complement, lysozyme, and interferons; **adaptive immunity** develops more slowly and is based on antigen presentation to **lymphocytes**.
- Immune cells communicate with one another and regulate one another's activities via polypeptide hormones called **cytokines**.
- **Antigens** are the regions of macromolecules, usually proteins, that are recognized by lymphocytes to elicit a specific immune response against them.
- **Antibodies** are immunoglobulins produced by plasma cells after a progenitor B cell is activated by a specific antigen and rearranges its immunoglobulin genes so that the antibody matches the antigen.
- Surfaces of all nucleated cells bear fragments of their constituent proteins on **MHC class I** molecules.
- Only **antigen-presenting cells (APCs)**, mostly derived from monocytes, also present fragments of endocytosed foreign proteins (usually from microorganisms) on surface **MHC class II** molecules.

Lymphocyte Origins and Differentiation

- Lymphocytes originate in the **primary lymphoid organs**: **bone marrow** for **B lymphocytes** and the **thymus** for **T lymphocytes**.
- B cells produce antibodies for **humoral immunity**; T cells function in **cell-mediated immunity**.
- T cells develop receptors (**TCRs**), usually containing α and β chains, that bind antigen along with another surface protein designated by a **CD ("cluster of differentiation") numbering system**.
- Important classes of T cells include **CD4⁺ T helper cells**; **CD8⁺ cytotoxic T cells**; **CD4⁺CD25⁺ regulatory T cells**; and γδ **T cells**, which have those TCR chains and are mainly in epithelia.
- **B-cell receptors (BCRs)** are IgM or IgD antibodies on the surfaces of B lymphocytes that bind specific antigens when they contact them.
- B and T cells are often activated, proliferate, and begin to function in the **secondary lymphoid organs**: the **lymph nodes**, all **MALT**, and the **spleen**.
- In these organs, lymphocytes are distributed within a meshwork of reticulin produced by fibroblastic **reticular cells**, and most APCs are **dendritic cells** with many processes.
- In secondary lymphoid tissues, BCRs bind antigens displayed in antibody-antigen complexes on the large surface of **follicular dendritic cells (FDCs)**.
- With cytokines from helper T cells, an FDC-activated B cell proliferates clonally to produce a large, transient **lymphoid nodule** (or follicle), which develops a pale **germinal center**.
- From lymphoid nodules, cells produced there disperse as **plasma cells**, various T cells, and **B and T memory cells** that respond and proliferate quickly if their specific antigen reappears.

Thymus

- T lymphoblasts, or **thymocytes**, attach in the **thymus** to a **cytoreticulum** composed of interconnected **thymic epithelial cells (TECs)**.
- The TECs also secrete many **cytokines**, **compartmentalize** the thymus into a **cortex** and a **medulla**, and in the cortex surround blood vessels in the **blood-thymus barrier**.
- Developing T cells with nonfunctional TCRs are detected and removed in the thymic cortex by a process of **positive selection**; cells with functional TCRs move into the thymic medulla.

- In the thymic medulla T cells whose TCRs bind strongly to "**self-proteins**," including proteins of many nonthymus cell types made by TECs expressing the *Aire* gene, undergo apoptosis there in a process of **negative selection**.
- This two-stage thymic selection leads to **central immune tolerance**, producing functional T cells that do not bind to proteins of the host.
- **Peripheral immune tolerance** occurs throughout the body when specific immune reactions are suppressed by **regulatory T cells** that also originate largely in the thymic medulla.
- Regulatory T cells form in the thymus upon interacting with dendritic cells presenting self-antigens in a process promoted by cytokines from TEC aggregates called **Hassall corpuscles**, found only in the thymic medulla.

Mucosa-Associated Lymphoid Tissue

- **MALT** is found in the mucosa of most tracts but is concentrated in the **palatine**, **lingual** and **pharyngeal tonsils**, **Peyer patches**, and the **appendix**.
- Unlike MALT, **lymph nodes** are completely **encapsulated** and occur along the lymphatic vessels; each has several **afferent lymphatics** and one **efferent lymphatic**.

Lymph Nodes

- Each lymph node **filters lymph** and **provides a site for B-cell activation** and differentiation to antibody-secreting **plasma cells**.
- A lymph node has three functional but not physically separate compartments: an outer **cortex**, a underlying **paracortex**, and an inner **medulla** adjacent to the hilum and efferent lymphatic.
- Lymphatics enter at the **cortex** of a node, where **B cells** encounter antigens, proliferate in **lymphoid nodules**, and then move into the deeper regions of the lymph node.
- Most lymphocytes enter at the **paracortex** of the lymph node via **HEVs** located there only; most lymphocytes in this region are **T helper cells**.
- The medulla has **medullary cords** containing reticular fibers with many plasma cells, macrophages, and other leukocytes; between the cords are lymph-filled **medullary sinuses** that converge at the efferent lymphatic.

Spleen

- The **spleen** is a large lymphoid organ without a cortex/medulla structure; instead, it has two intermingled but functionally different regions: **white pulp** and **red pulp**.
- **White pulp**, only 20% of the spleen, is **secondary lymphoid tissue** associated with small central arterioles that are also enclosed by **PALS** of T cells.
- **Red pulp**, which filters blood, removes defective erythrocytes, and recycles hemoglobin iron, consists of **splenic cords** with macrophages and blood cells of all kinds and **splenic sinusoids**.
- The **splenic sinusoids** are lined by unusual endothelial cells called **stave cells**, which are elongated and aligned parallel to the blood flow, with open slits between the cells.
- Blood flow in red pulp is either a **closed circulation**, moving from capillaries into the venous sinusoids, or an **open circulation**, with capillaries opening directly into the splenic cords.
- **Blood filtration** in the open circulation involves interaction with splenic cord **macrophages**, which remove old, swollen RBCs unable to slip between stave cells to reenter the venous blood flow.

The Immune System & Lymphoid Organs   ASSESS YOUR KNOWLEDGE

1. Which function is carried out by all lymphoid tissues and organs?
   a. Filtration of lymph
   b. Filtration of blood
   c. Extramedullary hemopoiesis
   d. Production of lymphocytes
   e. Destruction of old erythrocytes

2. Which structure is partly encapsulated and covered by nonkeratinized stratified squamous epithelium?
   a. Appendix
   b. Lymph node
   c. Palatine tonsil
   d. Peyer patch
   e. Thymic (Hassall) corpuscle

3. Which cell type gives rise to both memory and effector cells and is primarily associated with humoral immunity?
   a. B lymphocyte
   b. NK cell
   c. Macrophage
   d. T lymphocyte
   e. Reticular cell

4. Recycling of iron and heme, the major complex containing iron, occurs most actively in which lymphoid organ(s)/tissue(s)?
   a. Lymph nodes
   b. Peyer patches
   c. Tonsils
   d. Spleen
   e. Lymphatic vessels

5. Which description is true of all secondary (peripheral) lymphoid organs?
   a. Capable of antigen-independent lymphopoiesis
   b. Contain crypts
   c. Contain epithelial-reticular cells
   d. Lack connective tissue capsules
   e. Contain lymphoid nodules

6. Which structure would be most heavily labeled by an immunohistochemical method targeting the CD8 surface antigen?
   a. Germinal centers
   b. Paracortex
   c. Peyer patch
   d. Sheathed arterioles
   e. Splenic cords

7. A baby is born with a cleft palate and a condition called DiGeorge syndrome, which involves failure of third and fourth pharyngeal pouch derivatives to develop properly. The palate defect is corrected surgically, but regarding the pharyngeal pouch defect the parents are advised that the growing child may expect which of the following health problems?
   a. Insufficient B-cell production by lymph nodes in the head and neck
   b. Inability to secrete IgA
   c. Excessive numbers of circulating but defective erythrocytes
   d. Increased oral infections due to lack of palatine and pharyngeal tonsils
   e. Conditions related to autoimmunity

8. Many immune-related cellular activities are often impaired in aged patients. Which lymphoid organ(s) normally develop less functionality and increasing amounts of adipose tissue with age?
   a. Axillary lymph nodes
   b. Lingual tonsils
   c. Thymus
   d. Splenic white pulp
   e. Splenic red pulp

9. A 12-year-old girl of African descent presents with anemia and a large percentage of her peripheral erythrocytes appear sickle-shaped. Genetic testing reveals homozygosity for sickle cell disease. In which of the following sites will the abnormal RBCs be removed from the circulation?
   a. Thymic cortex
   b. Periarteriolar lymphoid sheaths of splenic white pulp
   c. Medullary sinuses of lymph nodes
   d. Thymic medulla
   e. Splenic cords (of Billroth)

10. A 6-year-old boy is brought to the clinic where his mother reports that he was bitten by a neighbor's dog 2 days earlier. The child's right hand is lacerated between the thumb and index finger and this area is inflamed but healing. The doctor's examination reveals small but painless swellings beneath the skin inside the right elbow and arm pit and he explains to the mother that these are active lymph nodes enlarged in response to the infection in the hand. What has produced the swelling?
    a. Increased flow of lymph through the nodes' afferent lymphatics
    b. Formation of germinal centers for B-cell proliferation in each node's cortex
    c. Arrival of antigen-presenting cells in each node's medulla
    d. Enlargement and increased activity of the nodes' high endothelial venules
    e. Increased thickness of each node's paracortex

15 Digestive Tract

The digestive system consists of the **digestive tract**—oral cavity, esophagus, stomach, small and large intestines, and anus—and its associated glands—salivary glands, liver, and pancreas (Figure 15–1). Also called the **gastrointestinal (GI) tract** or **alimentary canal**, it functions to obtain organic molecules from food that will supply the body's maintenance, growth, and energy requirements. During digestion proteins, complex carbohydrates, nucleic acids, and fats get broken down into their subunits which are absorbed in the small intestine and transferred into the microvasculature there. Most water and electrolytes undergo similar absorption in the large intestine. As introduced with the immune system, the mucosa of the digestive tract also constitutes a barrier with various defensive capabilities between ingested but not absorbed material and the body's internal tissues.

Structures within the digestive tract perform the following activities:

- **Ingestion**, or introduction of food and liquid into the oral cavity,
- **Mastication**, or chewing, which divides solid food into digestible pieces,
- **Motility**, muscular movements of materials through the tract,
- **Secretion** of lubricating and protective mucus, digestive enzymes, acidic and alkaline fluids, and bile,
- **Hormone release** for local control of motility and secretion,
- **Chemical digestion** or enzymatic degradation of large macromolecules in food to smaller molecules and their subunits,
- **Absorption** of the small molecules and water into the blood and lymph, and
- **Elimination** of indigestible, unabsorbed components of food.

› GENERAL STRUCTURE OF THE DIGESTIVE TRACT

All regions of the GI tract have certain structural features in common. A hollow tube with a variable diameter lumen, the tract's wall has four main layers: the **mucosa, submucosa, muscularis,** and **serosa**. Figure 15–2 shows a general overview of these layers; key features of each layer are summarized here.

- The **mucosa** consists of an **epithelial lining** underlaid by a **lamina propria** of loose connective tissue containing small blood vessels, lymphatics, leukocytes, and often small glands. A thin smooth muscle layer called the **muscularis mucosae** separates the mucosa from the submucosa and permits local movements of the mucosa. A frequently used synonym for "mucosa" is "**mucous membrane**," emphasizing the thinness of this layer.
- The **submucosa** contains denser connective tissue with larger blood vessels, lymphatics, and the **submucosal (Meissner) plexus** of autonomic nerves. It may also contain glands and significant lymphoid tissue.
- The thick **muscularis** (or muscularis externa) consists of smooth muscle cells organized as two or

FIGURE 15–1 The digestive system.

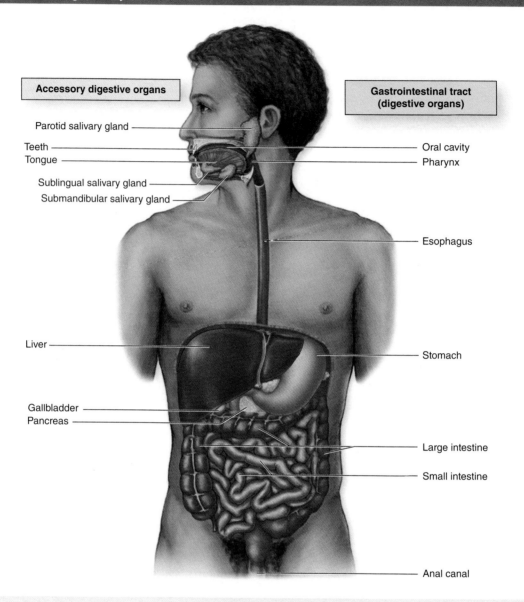

| Accessory digestive organs | | Gastrointestinal tract (digestive organs) |

Parotid salivary gland

Teeth

Tongue

Sublingual salivary gland

Submandibular salivary gland

Oral cavity

Pharynx

Esophagus

Liver

Stomach

Gallbladder

Pancreas

Large intestine

Small intestine

Anal canal

The digestive system consists of the tract from the **mouth (oral cavity)** to the **anus**, as well as the digestive glands emptying into this tract, primarily the salivary glands, liver, and pancreas. These accessory digestive glands are described in Chapter 16.

more sublayers. In the internal sublayer (closer to the lumen), the fiber orientation is generally circular; in the external sublayer it is longitudinal. The sparse connective tissue between these muscle layers holds blood and lymph vessels, as well as the **myenteric (Auerbach) nerve plexus** comprising many autonomic neurons aggregated into small ganglia and interconnected by pre- and postganglionic nerve fibers. This and the submucosal plexus together comprise the **enteric nervous system** of the digestive tract. The myenteric plexus generates and coordinates contractions of the muscularis, which mix and propel the luminal contents forward.

■ A thin cover of loose connective tissue, rich in blood vessels, lymphatics, and adipose tissue, surrounds the muscularis externa. With the stomach and intestines a simple squamous epithelium or **mesothelium** encloses this outermost layer, characterizing it here as the **serosa**. The small and large intestinal serosa continues as portions of the **mesentery**, a large fold of adipose connective tissue which suspends the intestines within the abdominal cavity and forms without interruption the **peritoneum**, or serous lining of that cavity. Digestive tract regions not suspended in the abdomen, such as the esophagus (Figure 15–1), develop directly within adjacent structures and therefore lack a serosa, having instead an outer

FIGURE 15–2 Major layers and organization of the digestive tract.

Mucosa
Epithelium
Lamina propria
Muscularis mucosae

Submucosa
Submucosal gland
Blood vessel
Submucosal nerve plexus

Muscularis
Inner circular layer
Myenteric nerve plexus
Outer longitudinal layer

Serosa

Mesentery

Vein
Artery
Lymph vessel

Lumen

Diagram showing the structure of the small intestine portion of the digestive tract, with the four main layers (**mucosa, submucosa, muscularis**, and **serosa**) and their major components listed on the left.

The stomach, small intestine, and large intestine are suspended by mesenteries, through which nerves, blood vessels, and lymphatics serve the stomach and intestines.

layer of connective tissue, the **adventitia**, continuous with that of their surroundings.

The numerous free immune cells and lymphoid nodules in the mucosa and submucosa constitute the MALT described in Chapter 14. The digestive tract normally contains thousands of microbial species, including both useful inhabitants of the gut as well as potential pathogens ingested with food and drink. The mucosa-associated immune defense system provides an essential backup to the thin physical barrier of the epithelial lining. Just below the epithelium, the lamina propria holds abundant macrophages and lymphocytes, many for production of IgA antibodies. Such antibodies undergo transcytosis into the tract's lumen bound to the secretory protein produced by the epithelial cells. This IgA complex resists

proteolysis by digestive enzymes and provides important protection against specific viral and bacterial pathogens.

›› MEDICAL APPLICATION

In diseases such as **Hirschsprung disease** (congenital aganglionic megacolon) or **Chagas disease** (**trypanosomiasis**, infection with the protozoan *Trypanosoma cruzi*), plexuses in the digestive tract's enteric nervous system are absent or severely injured, respectively. This disturbs digestive tract motility and produces dilations in some areas. The rich autonomic innervation of the enteric nervous system also provides an anatomic explanation of the well-known actions of emotional stress on the stomach and other regions of the GI tract.

» ORAL CAVITY

The **oral cavity** (Figure 15–1) lining consists of stratified squamous epithelium, which may be keratinized, partially keratinized, or nonkeratinized depending on the exact location. Epithelial differentiation, keratinization, and the interface between the epithelium and lamina propria here resemble those features in the skin and are discussed more extensively with that topic (Chapter 18). Like the keratinized surface cells of skin, the flattened superficial cells of the oral mucosa undergo continuous desquamation, or loss from the free surface. Unlike those of the epidermis, the shed cells of the nonkeratinized or partly keratinized oral epithelium retain their nuclei.

»» MEDICAL APPLICATION

Viral infections with herpes simplex 1 cause death of infected epithelial cells that can lead to vesicular or ulcerating lesions of the oral mucosa or skin near the mouth. In the oral cavity, such areas are called **canker sores**, and on the skin, they are usually called **cold sores** or **fever blisters**. Such lesions, often painful and clustered, occur when the immune defenses are weakened by emotional stress, fever, illness, or local skin damage, allowing the virus, present in the local nerves, to move into the epithelial cells.

The keratinized cell layers resist most damage from abrasion and become best developed in the **masticatory mucosa** on the gingiva (gums) and hard palate. The lamina propria in these areas rests directly on the periosteum of underlying bone. Nonkeratinized squamous epithelium predominates in the **lining mucosa** over the soft palate, cheeks, the floor of the mouth, and the oral **pharynx** (or throat), the posterior region of the oral cavity leading to the esophagus. Lining mucosa overlies a thick submucosa containing diffuse lymphoid tissue and many minor salivary glands, which secrete continuously to keep the mucosal surface wet. Throughout the oral cavity the epithelium contains transient antigen-presenting cells and rich sensory innervation.

The well-developed core of striated muscle in the **lips**, or labia (Figure 15–3) makes these structures highly mobile for ingestion, speech, and other forms of communication. Both lips have three differently covered surfaces:

- The internal mucous surfaces have lining mucosae with a thick, nonkeratinized epithelium and many minor labial salivary glands.
- The prominent red **vermilion zone** of each lip consists of very thin keratinized stratified squamous epithelium and represents the transition from oral mucosa to skin. Moistened with saliva by the tongue, this lip region lacks salivary and sweat glands. The underlying connective tissue is very rich in both sensory innervation and capillaries, which impart the pink color to the surface here.
- The more peripheral outer surface has thin skin, consisting of epidermal and dermal layers, sweat glands, and many hair follicles with sebaceous glands.

FIGURE 15–3 Lip.

Low-magnification micrograph of a **lip** section showing one side covered by typical oral mucosa (**OM**), the opposite side covered by skin (**S**) containing hair follicles (**F**), and associated glands. The area between the lip's oral mucosa and normal skin represents the vermilion zone (**V**), where epidermis remains very thin, lightly keratinized, and transparent to blood in the rich microvasculature of the underlying connective tissue.

Because this region lacks the glands for oil and sweat, it is prone to excessive dryness and chapping in cold, dry weather. Internally, the lips contain much striated muscle (**M**) and many minor salivary glands (**G**). (×10; H&E)

Tongue

The **tongue** forms as a mass of striated muscle covered by mucosa, which can manipulate ingested material during mastication and swallowing. Fascicles of muscle fibers develop in all directions, allowing a high level of mobility. Connective tissue from the lamina propria penetrates between these small fascicles, making the mucous membrane strongly adherent to the muscular core. The lower surface of the tongue shows typical lining mucosa. The irregular dorsal surface has hundreds of small protruding **papillae** of various types on its anterior two-thirds and the massed lingual tonsils on the posterior third, or root of the tongue (Figure 15–4). A V-shaped groove, the **sulcus terminalis**, demarcates the papillary and tonsillar areas of the tongue's dorsal surface.

The lingual papillae represent elevations of the mucous membrane that assume various forms and functions. There are four main types (Figure 15–4):

- **Filiform papillae** (Figure 15–5) have elongated conical shapes and are very numerous and heavily keratinized,

FIGURE 15–4 Tongue, lingual papillae, and taste buds.

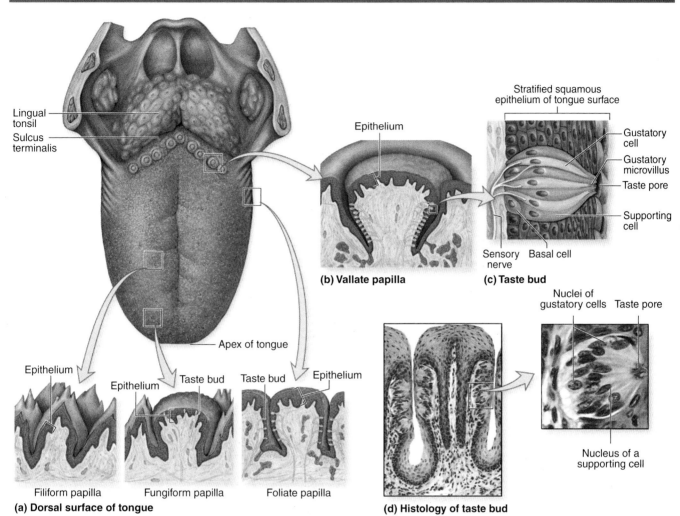

(a) Dorsal surface of tongue

(b) Vallate papilla

(c) Taste bud

(d) Histology of taste bud

(a) On its dorsal surface the posterior third of the tongue produces the **lingual tonsils** and the anterior portion bears numerous **lingual papillae** of four types. Pointed **filiform papillae** provide friction to help move food during chewing. Ridge-like **foliate papillae** on the sides of the tongue are best developed in young children. **Fungiform papillae** occur scattered across the dorsal surface

(b) 8–12 large **vallate papillae** form a V-shaped line near the terminal sulcus. **Taste buds** develop on fungiform and foliate papillae but become much more abundant on the vallate papillae.

(c) Diagram of a single taste bud shows the **gustatory (taste) cells**, the **supporting cells** whose function remains poorly understood, and the basal **stem cells**. Microvilli at the ends of the gustatory cells project through an opening in the epithelium, the **taste pore**. Afferent sensory axons enter the basal end of taste buds and synapse with the gustatory cells.

(d) In the stratified squamous epithelium of the tongue surface, taste buds form as distinct clusters of cells recognizable histologically even at low magnification. At higher power the taste pore may be visible, as shown here, as well as the elongated nuclei of gustatory and supporting cells. (×140 and ×500; H&E)

which can give this lingual surface a whitish appearance. They provide a rough surface that facilitates movement of food during chewing.

- **Fungiform papillae** (Figure 15–5) are much less numerous, interspersed among the filiform papillae, and lightly keratinized. Bulbous or mushroom-shaped, these have well-vascularized and innervated cores of lamina propria.
- **Foliate papillae** consist of several parallel ridges on each side of the tongue, anterior to the sulcus

terminalis, but are rudimentary in humans, especially older individuals.

- **Vallate** (or **circumvallate**) **papillae** (Figure 15–5) are the largest papillae, lightly keratinized with diameters of 1–3 mm. Eight to 12 vallate papillae normally become aligned just in front of the terminal sulcus. Ducts of several small, serous **salivary (von Ebner) glands** empty into the deep, moat-like groove that surrounds each vallate papilla.

FIGURE **15–5** Lingual papillae.

(a) Section of the dorsal surface of tongue showing both filiform (**FI**) and fungiform papillae (**F**). Both types are elevations of the connective tissue (**CT**) covered by stratified squamous epithelium (**SSE**), but the filiform type becomes pointed and heavily keratinized while the fungiform type is mushroom-shaped, lightly keratinized, with scattered taste buds.

(b) Micrograph shows a single very large **vallate papilla** with two distinctive features: many taste buds (**TB**) around the sides and several small salivary glands (**GL**) emptying into the cleft or moat formed by the elevated mucosa surrounding the papilla. These glands continuously flush the cleft, renewing the fluid in contact with the taste buds. (Both ×20; H&E)

These glands provide a continuous watery flow over the abundant taste buds on the sides of the less keratinized papillae, washing away food particles so that the taste buds can receive and process new gustatory stimuli. Secretions from these and other minor salivary glands associated with taste buds contain a lipase preventing formation of a hydrophobic film on these structures that would interfere with gustation.

All **taste buds** develop as ovoid structures within the stratified epithelium on the tongue's surface, and continuously sample the general composition of ingested material (Figures 15–4 and 15–5). Approximately 250 taste buds occur on the lateral surface of each vallate papilla, with many others present on fungiform and foliate (but not the keratinized filiform) papillae. Taste buds are not restricted to lingual papillae and appear scattered much more sparsely elsewhere on the dorsal and lateral surfaces of the tongue and oral mucosa, where they are also continuously flushed by numerous minor salivary glands.

A taste bud has 50–100 cells, about half of which consist of elongated **gustatory (taste) cells**, which turn over with a 7- to 10-day life span. Other cell types in the structure represent slender **supportive cells**, differentiating cells, and slowly dividing basal **stem cells** that give rise to the other cell types. The base of each bud rests on the basal lamina which allows afferent sensory axons to enter and form synapses with the gustatory cells. At the apical ends of the gustatory cells, microvilli project toward a 2-μm-wide opening in the structure called the **taste pore**. Molecules (or tastants) dissolved in saliva contact the microvilli through the pore and interact with cell surface taste receptors (Figure 15–4).

Taste buds detect at least five broad categories of tastants: sodium ions (salty); hydrogen ions from acids (sour); sugars and related compounds (sweet); alkaloids and certain toxins (bitter); and amino acids such as glutamate and aspartate (umami; Jap. *umami*, savory). Salt and sour tastes arise from the actions of ion channel receptors; the other three taste categories involve G-protein-coupled receptors. In all cases, receptor binding produces depolarization of the gustatory cells, stimulating the sensory nerve fibers to send impulses to the brain. Conscious perception of tastes in food requires olfactory and other sensations in addition to taste bud activity.

Teeth

In the adult human normally 32 **permanent teeth** occur in two bilaterally symmetric arches in the maxillary and mandibular bones (Figure 15–6a). Each quadrant has eight teeth: two incisors, one canine, two premolars, and three permanent

FIGURE **15–6** Teeth.

Central incisor (7–8 y)
Lateral incisor (8–9 y)
Canine (11–12 y)
1st premolar (10–11 y)
2nd premolar (10–12 y)
1st molar (6–7 y)
2nd molar (12–13 y)
3rd molar (17–25 y)

Upper teeth

Hard palate

3rd molar (17–25 y)
2nd molar (11–13 y)
1st molar (6–7 y)
2nd premolar (11–12 y)
1st premolar (10–12 y)
Canine (9–10 y)
Lateral incisor (7–8 y)
Central incisor (6–7 y)

Lower teeth

(a) Permanent teeth

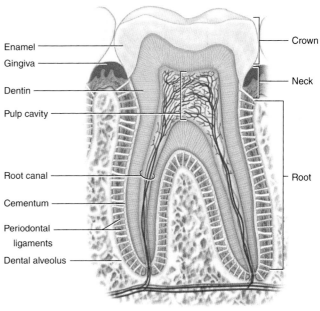

Enamel
Gingiva
Dentin
Pulp cavity
Root canal
Cementum
Periodontal ligaments
Dental alveolus

Crown
Neck
Root

(b) Molar

All teeth are similar embryologically and histologically.

(a) The drawing shows dentition of the permanent teeth, along with the approximate age each tooth erupts.

(b) Diagram of a molar's internal structure, which is like that of all teeth, with an enamel-covered **crown**, cementum-covered **roots** anchoring the tooth to alveolar bone of the jaw, and a slightly

constricted **neck** where the **enamel** and **cementum** coverings meet at the gingiva. Most of the roots and neck consists of **dentin**. Extending into the neck, a **pulp cavity** contains well-vascularized, well-innervated mesenchymal connective tissue. Blood vessels and nerves enter the tooth through apical foramina at the root tips. **Periodontal ligaments** hold the tooth to bone of the jaw.

molars. Twenty of the permanent teeth are preceded by **primary teeth** (deciduous or milk teeth) that undergo loss; the others represent permanent molars with no deciduous precursors. Each tooth has a **crown** exposed above the gingiva, a constricted **neck** at the gum, and one or more **roots** that fit firmly into bony sockets called **dental alveoli** (Figure 15–6b).

Very hard, acellular **enamel** covers the crown and a bone-like tissue called **cementum** surrounds the roots. These two casings meet at the neck of the tooth. The bulk of a tooth consists of another calcified material, **dentin**, which surrounds an internal **pulp cavity** (Figure 15–6b). The cavity contains **dental pulp**, highly vascular, well-innervated, and composed largely of loose, mesenchymal connective tissue with much ground substance, thin collagen fibers, fibroblasts, and mesenchymal stem cells. The pulp cavity narrows in each root as the **root canal** and opens as an **apical foramen** at the root's tip for passage of the blood vessels, lymphatics, and nerves serving the pulp cavity. With roots **periodontal ligaments** develop as dense bundles of collagen fibers inserted into both the cementum and the alveolar bone holding the tooth firmly in place.

Dentin

Dentin is a calcified tissue harder than bone, consisting of 70% hydroxyapatite. Its organic matrix contains type I collagen and proteoglycans secreted from the apical ends of **odontoblasts**, tall cells derived from the cranial neural crest, which form a lining of the pulp cavity (Figure 15–7a). Mineralization of the **predentin** matrix secreted by odontoblasts involves matrix vesicles in a process like that which occurs in osteoid during bone formation (see Chapter 8).

Long apical **odontoblast processes** extend from the odontoblasts within **dentinal tubules** (Figure 15–7b), which penetrate the full thickness of the dentin and gradually become longer as dentin becomes thicker. Along their length, these processes extend fine branches into smaller lateral branches of the tubules (Figure 15–7c). The odontoblast processes maintain dentin matrix, and odontoblasts slowly continue predentin production into adult life, gradually reducing the size of the pulp cavity, and remain capable of repairing damaged dentin.

FIGURE **15–7** Dentin and odontoblasts.

(a) Odontoblasts (**O**) mature as long polarized cells derived from undifferentiated cells in the developing pulp cavity (**PC**) and become specialized for collagen and GAG synthesis. They are bound together by junctional complexes as a layer, with no basal lamina, and secrete a collagen-rich matrix called predentin (**P**) only from their apical ends at the dentinal surface. Within approximately 1 day of secretion, predentin mineralizes to become dentin (**D**) as hydroxyapatite crystals form in a process like that occurring in osteoid of developing bones (see Chapter 8). In this process, the collagen is engulfed, and calcified matrix becomes much more acidophilic and stains quite differently than that of predentin. When predentin secretion begins, an apical extension from each cell, the odontoblast process (**OP**), forms and becomes surrounded by new matrix. As the dentin-predentin layer thickens, these processes lengthen. When tooth formation is complete, odontoblasts persist

and their processes reside in canals called **dentinal tubules**, which run through the full thickness of the dentin. (×400; Mallory trichrome)

(b) Silver staining can reveal odontoblast processes sharply, along with their branching near the junction of dentin with enamel (**E**) and along their length closer to their source (**c**). The lateral branches occupy smaller canaliculi within dentin. (Both ×400; Silver)

(d) A trichrome stain reveals the odontoblast processes' (**OP**) connections to the odontoblasts (**O**), shown with stained nuclei, which allow for maintenance of dentin in adult teeth. (×400; Mallory trichrome)

(Figure 15–7b, c, and d, reproduced with permission from M. F. Santos, Department of Histology and Embryology, Institute of Biomedical Sciences, University of São Paulo, Brazil.)

FIGURE **15–8** Ultrastructure of dentinal tubule.

(a) TEM shows the calcification of dentin (**D**) at its border with not-yet calcified predentin (**P**). An odontoblast process (**OP**) with microtubules and a few secretory vesicles is shown in the fluid-filled space (**S**) in the dentinal tubule. A process extends from each odontoblast, and the tubules continue completely across the dentin layer. (×32,000)

(b) TEM cross section of an odontoblast process (**OP**) near predentin (**P**) shows its close association with an unmyelinated nerve fiber (**N**) extending there from fibers in the pulp cavity. These nerves respond to various stimuli, such as cold temperatures, reaching the nerve fibers through the dentinal tubules. (×61,000)

Teeth are sensitive to stimuli such as cold, heat, and acidic pH, all of which can be perceived as pain. This sensitivity involves the highly innervated pulp and originates in unmyelinated nerve fibers that extend into the dentinal tubules along with odontoblast processes (Figure 15–8) when such stimuli affect fluid inside the dentinal tubules, stimulating these nerve fibers.

> ### ❯❯ MEDICAL APPLICATION
>
> Immune defenses in the oral cavity cannot protect against all infections. **Pharyngitis** and **tonsillitis** are often due to the bacterium *Streptococcus pyogenes*. White excrescences or **leukoplakia** on the sides of the tongue can be caused by Epstein-Barr virus. **Oral thrush**, a white exudate on the tongue's dorsal surface, is due to a yeast (*Candida albicans*) infection and usually affects neonates or immunocompromised patients.

Enamel

Enamel, the hardest component of the human body, contains 96% calcium hydroxyapatite and only 2%–3% organic material, including very few proteins and no collagen. Other ions, such as fluoride, can be incorporated or adsorbed by the hydroxyapatite crystals; enamel containing fluorapatite more effectively resists acidic dissolution caused by microorganisms, leading to the addition of fluoride to toothpaste and water supplies.

Enamel consists of uniform, interlocking columns called **enamel rods** (or prisms), each about 5 μm in diameter and

surrounded by a thinner layer of other enamel. Each rod extends through the entire thickness of the enamel layer, which averages 2 mm. The precise, interlocked arrangement of the enamel rods is crucial for enamel's hardness and resistance to great pressures during mastication.

In a developing tooth bud, the unmineralized matrix for the enamel rods is secreted by tall, polarized cells called **ameloblasts** (Figure 15–9a), which comprise a specialized epithelium within the tooth bud called the **enamel organ**. The apical ends of the ameloblasts face those of the odontoblasts producing predentin (Figure 15–10). An apical extension from each ameloblast, the **ameloblast (or Tomes) process**, contains numerous secretory granules with the proteins of the enamel matrix. The secreted matrix undergoes very rapid mineralization. A small (20 kDa) protein called **amelogenin**, the main structural protein of developing enamel, initiates and guides growth of hydroxyapatite crystals within elongating enamel rods.

Ameloblasts develop from the ectodermal lining of the embryonic oral cavity, while odontoblasts and most tissues of the pulp cavity differentiate from neural crest cells and mesoderm, respectively. Together, these tissues produce a series of 52 tooth buds in the developing oral cavity, 20 for the primary teeth and 32 for the secondary or permanent teeth. Primary teeth complete development and begin to erupt about 6 months after birth. Secondary tooth bud development occurs slowly through the "bell stage" shown in Figure 15–10a, until about 6 years of age, when these teeth begin to erupt and the primary teeth loosen and are shed.

FIGURE **15–9** Ameloblasts and enamel.

(a) In a section of embryonic **tooth bud**, ameloblasts (**A**) are tall, polarized cells whose apical ends initially contact dentin (**D**). Ameloblasts join to form a cell layer surrounded basally by connective tissue (**CT**). After odontoblasts begin to secrete predentin, ameloblasts secrete a matrix lacking collagen but rich in the protein amelogenin that quickly initiates calcium hydroxyapatite formation to make enamel (**E**), the hardest material in the body. Enamel forms a layer but consists of enamel rods or prisms, solidly fused together by more enamel. Each enamel rod represents the product of one ameloblast. No cellular processes occur in enamel, and the layer of ameloblasts surrounding the developing crown disappears during tooth eruption. Teeth that have been decalcified for histologic sectioning typically lose their enamel layer completely. (×400; H&E)

(b) Micrograph of a thin preparation of a tooth prepared by grinding. Fine, long tubules can be observed in the dentin (**D**), and rods aligned the same way can be very faintly observed (arrows) in the enamel (**E**). The more prominent lines that cross enamel diagonally represent incremental growth lines produced as the enamel matrix develops with cyclic secretion by the ameloblast layer. (×400; Unstained)

>> MEDICAL APPLICATION

Periodontal diseases include **gingivitis**, inflammation of the gums, and **periodontitis**, which involves inflammation at deeper sites, both of which are caused most commonly by bacterial infections with poor oral hygiene. Chronic periodontitis weakens the periodontal ligament and can lead to loosening of the teeth. The depth of the gingival sulcus, measured during clinical dental examinations, is an important indicator of potential periodontal disease.

Periodontium

The **periodontium** comprises the structures responsible for maintaining the teeth in the maxillary and mandibular bones, and includes the **cementum**, the **periodontal ligament**, and the **alveolar bone** with the associated **gingiva** (Figures 15–6b and 15–11a).

Cementum covers the dentin of the root and resembles bone, but is avascular. It is thickest around the root tips where **cementocytes** reside in lacunae with processes in canaliculi, especially near the cementum surface. Although less labile than bone, cementocytes maintain their surrounding matrix and react to stresses by gradual matrix remodeling.

The **periodontal ligament** represents connective tissue with short bundles of collagen fibers (Sharpey fibers) binding the cementum and the alveolar bone (Figure 15–11b). Unlike typical ligaments, it is highly cellular and supplied with blood vessels and nerves, giving the periodontal ligament sensory and nutritive functions in addition to its role in supporting the tooth. It permits very limited movement of the tooth within the alveolus and helps protect the alveolus from the recurrent pressure exerted during mastication. Its thickness (150–350 μm) remains uniform along the root but decreases with age.

The **alveolar bone** lacks the typical lamellar pattern of adult bone but has osteoblasts and osteocytes engaging in continuous remodeling of the bony matrix. Surrounding cementum of the roots, the periodontal ligament serves as the periosteum for alveolar bone, bound to it by the collagen fiber bundles which also penetrate the cementum (Figure 15–11c).

At the neck of each tooth the keratinized **gingival mucosa** becomes firmly bound to typical periosteum of the maxillary and mandibular bones (Figure 15–11a). Just above the most narrow part of the neck, a specialized portion of gingival epithelium forms a thick basal lamina which adheres strongly to the enamel (or the cementum of

FIGURE **15–10** Tooth formation.

Tooth formation begins in the embryo when ectodermal epithelium lining the oral cavity grows into the underlying mesenchyme of the developing jaws. At a series of sites corresponding to each future tooth, these epithelial cells proliferate extensively and become organized as **enamel organs**, each shaped like a wine glass with its stem initially still attached to the oral lining. **Ameloblasts** form from the innermost layer of cells in the enamel organ. Mesenchymal cells inside the concave portion of the enamel organ include neural crest cells that differentiate as the layer of **odontoblasts**.

(a) A section of a developing tooth in which production of dentin and enamel has begun. The ameloblast layer (**A**) is separated from the outer enamel epithelium (**OEE**) by a thick intervening region rich in GAGs but with few, widely separated cells. Surrounding the enamel organ is mesenchyme, some parts of which begin to undergo intramembranous bone formation (**B**). Inside the cavity of each enamel organ, mesenchymal cells comprise the dental papilla (**DP**), in which the outermost cells comprise the layer of odontoblasts (**O**) facing the ameloblasts. These two cell layers

begin to move apart as the odontoblasts begin to produce the layer of predentin (**PD**). Contact with dentin induces each ameloblast to begin secretion of an enamel rod. More slowly, calcifying interprismatic enamel fuses all the enamel rods into a very strong, solid mass. (×20; H&E)

(b) Detail of an enamel organ showing the layers of predentin (**PD**) and dentin (**D**) and a layer of enamel (**E**), along with the organized cell layers that produced this material. Odontoblasts (**O**) contact at their basal ends the mesenchyme of the dental papilla (**DP**) that will become the pulp cavity. Ameloblasts (**A**) are prominent in the now much thinner enamel organ, which is very close to developing bone (**B**). Enamel formation continues until shortly before tooth eruption; formation of dentin continues until the tooth develops fully. Odontoblasts persist surrounding the pulp cavity, with processes penetrating the dental layer, producing factors to help maintain dentin. Mesenchymal cells immediately around the enamel organ differentiate into the cells of cementum and other periodontal tissues. (×120; H&E)

older teeth) and to which the epithelial cells attach by numerous hemidesmosomes.

› ESOPHAGUS

The **esophagus** develops as a muscular tube, about 25 cm long in adults, which transports swallowed material from the pharynx to the stomach. The four layers of the GI tract (Figure 15–12) become well-established and clearly seen in the esophagus. The esophageal mucosa has nonkeratinized stratified squamous epithelium, and the submucosa contains small mucus-secreting glands, the **esophageal glands**, which lubricate and protect the mucosa (Figure 15–13a). Near the stomach the mucosa also contains other groups of glands, the **esophageal cardiac glands**, which secrete additional mucus.

›› MEDICAL APPLICATION

The lubricating mucus produced in the esophagus offers little protection against acid that may move there from the stomach. Such movement can produce **heartburn** or **reflux esophagitis**. An incompetent inferior esophageal sphincter may result in chronic heartburn, which can lead to erosion of the esophageal mucosa or **gastroesophageal reflux disease (GERD)**. Untreated GERD can produce metaplastic changes in the stratified squamous epithelium of the esophageal mucosa, a condition called **Barrett esophagus**.

Swallowing begins with voluntary muscle action but finishes with involuntary peristalsis. In approximately the upper one-third of the esophagus, the muscularis consists exclusively

FIGURE **15–11** Periodontium.

The periodontium of each tooth consists of the **cementum**, **periodontal ligament**, **alveolar bone**, and **gingiva**.

(a) Micrograph of a decalcified tooth showing the **periodontium**. The free gingiva (**FG**) overlies dentin (**D**) here since most enamel was removed. Compare this photo to the same region in the diagram of Figure 15–6b. Gingiva has stratified squamous epithelium over connective tissue of the lamina propria (**LP**), which is continuous with that of the periosteum (**P**) of the alveolar bone (**B**) and with the periodontal ligament (**PL**). (×10; H&E)

(b) Micrograph shows the periodontal ligament (**L**) with its many blood vessels (**V**) and insertions into the alveolar bone (**B**). This ligament serves as the periosteum of the alveolar bone in the tooth sockets and continues into the developing layer of cementum (**C**) that covers the dentin. Cementum forms a thin layer of bone-like material secreted by large, elongated surface cells called **cementoblasts**. (×100; H&E)

(c) Polarizing light micrograph shows the continuity of collagen in alveolar bone (**B**) periosteum with the bundled collagen in the periodontal ligament (**L**). (×200; Picrosirius in polarized light)

FIGURE **15–12** Esophagus.

Mucosa

Submucosa

Muscularis

Adventitia

(a) In an **esophagus** cross section, the four major layers of the GI tract are clearly seen. The esophageal mucosa is folded longitudinally, with the lumen largely closed. (×10; H&E)

(b) Higher magnification of the esophageal **mucosa** shows the thick stratified squamous epithelium (**E**), the lamina propria (**LP**) with scattered lymphocytes, and strands of smooth muscle in the muscularis mucosae (**MM**). (×65; H&E)

FIGURE **15–13** Esophagus.

(a) Longitudinal section of esophagus shows **mucosa** consisting of nonkeratinized stratified squamous epithelium (**SSE**), lamina propria (**LP**), and smooth muscles of the muscularis mucosae (**MM**). Beneath the mucosa lies the **submucosa** containing esophageal mucous glands (**GL**) that empty via ducts (**D**) onto the luminal surface. (×40; H&E)

(b) Transverse section showing the **muscularis** halfway along the esophagus reveals a combination of large skeletal or striated muscle fibers (**St**) and smooth muscle fibers (**Sm**) in the outer layer, cut transversely here. This transition from muscles under voluntary control to the type controlled autonomically is important in the swallowing mechanism. (×200; H&E)

of skeletal muscle like that of the tongue. The middle portion of the esophagus contains a combination of skeletal and smooth muscle fibers (Figure 15–13b), and the lower third the muscularis has exclusively smooth muscle. Only the distal 1–2 cm of the esophagus extends into the peritoneal cavity and has a serosa cover; the rest is enclosed by the loose connective tissue of the adventitia, which blends into the surrounding tissue.

❯ STOMACH

The **stomach** is a greatly dilated segment of the digestive tract whose main functions are:

- To continue the digestion of carbohydrates initiated by the amylase of saliva,
- To add an acidic fluid to the ingested food and mixing its contents into a viscous mass called **chyme** by the churning action of the muscularis,
- To begin digestion of triglycerides by a secreted lipase, and
- To promote the initial digestion of proteins with the enzyme **pepsin**.

❯❯ MEDICAL APPLICATION

For various reasons, including autoimmunity, parietal cells may be damaged to the extent that insufficient quantities of intrinsic factor are secreted and **vitamin B$_{12}$** is not absorbed adequately. This vitamin is a cofactor required for DNA synthesis; low levels of vitamin B$_{12}$ can reduce proliferation of erythroblasts, producing **pernicious anemia**.

Four major regions make up the stomach: the cardia, fundus, body, and pylorus (Figure 15–14a). The **cardia** makes up a narrow transitional zone, 1.5-3 cm wide, just beyond the esophagus; the **pylorus** denotes the funnel-shaped region opening into the small intestine. Both these regions have mucous glands primarily and are histologically similar. The much larger **fundus** and **body** regions (Figure 15–14a) have similar microscopic structures and contain gastric glands releasing acidic gastric juice. The mucosa and submucosa of the empty stomach form large, longitudinally directed folds called **rugae**, which flatten when the stomach fills with food. As Figures 15–14 and 15–15 show, the stomach wall in all its regions consists of the four major layers.

❯❯ MEDICAL APPLICATION

Gastric and duodenal ulcers are painful erosive lesions of the mucosa that may extend to deeper layers. Such ulcers can occur anywhere between the lower esophagus and the jejunum, and their causes include bacterial infections with *Helicobacter pylori*, effects of nonsteroidal anti-inflammatory drugs, overproduction of HCl or pepsin, and lowered production or secretion of mucus or bicarbonate.

Mucosa

Changing abruptly at the esophagogastric junction (Figure 15–14b), the mucosal surface of the stomach is a simple columnar epithelium that invaginates deeply into the lamina propria. The invaginations form millions of **gastric pits**, each opening to the stomach lumen (Figures 15–14 and 15–16).

FIGURE **15–14** Stomach.

(a) Stomach regions, anterior view

- Esophagus
- **Fundus**
- **Cardia**
- Pyloric orifice
- Pyloric sphincter
- Lesser curvature
- Duodenum
- Longitudinal layer
- Circular layer — Muscularis
- Oblique layer
- **Body**
- Greater curvature
- **Pylorus**
- Gastric folds

b — SCE, SSE, LP, MM, ECG

(c) Stomach wall, sectional view

- Gastric pit
- Stomach lumen
- Simple columnar epithelium
- Lamina propria — **Mucosa**
- Muscularis mucosae
- **Submucosa**
- Oblique layer
- Circular layer — **Muscularis**
- Longitudinal layer
- **Serosa**
- Blood vessel
- Lymph vessel
- Artery
- Vein
- Submucosal nerve plexus
- Myenteric nerve plexus

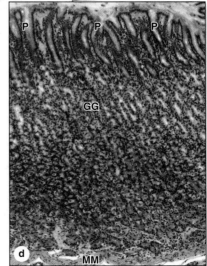

The **stomach** develops as a muscular, more dilated part of the digestive tract where mechanical and chemical digestion occurs.

(a) The major stomach regions are the **cardia**, **fundus**, **body**, and **pylorus**, all with longitudinal gastric folds, or rugae. The muscularis has three layers here.

(b) At the **esophagogastric junction**, stratified squamous epithelium (**SSE**) lining the esophagus abruptly gives away to the simple columnar epithelium (**SCE**) of the stomach. Also seen here are the mucous esophageal cardiac glands (**ECG**) beneath the lamina propria (**LP**) and muscularis mucosae (**MM**). (×60; H&E)

(c) The **mucosa** of the stomach wall contains invaginations called **gastric pits** that lead into **gastric glands**. These structures are lined by simple columnar epithelium containing five functional cell types.

(d) A histologic section of the gastric **mucosa** shows the gastric pits (**P**) and glands (**GG**) surrounded by cells of the lamina propria. The thin underlying muscularis mucosae (**MM**) is also shown. (×60; H&E)

FIGURE **15–15** Wall of the stomach with rugae.

A low-magnification micrograph of the **stomach wall** at the fundus shows the relative thickness of the four major layers: the mucosa (**M**), the submucosa (**SM**), the muscularis externa (**ME**), and the serosa (**S**). Two rugae (folds) cut transversely and consisting of mucosa and submucosa are included.

The mucosa is filled with branched tubular glands penetrating the full thickness of the lamina propria so that this sublayer cannot be distinguished at this magnification. The **muscularis mucosae** (arrows), immediately beneath the basal ends of the gastric glands, is shown. The submucosa consists largely of loose connective tissue, with blood vessels (**V**) and lymphatics. (×12; H&E)

FIGURE **15–16** Gastric pits and glands.

(a) SEM of the **stomach lining** cleared of its mucous layer reveals closely placed gastric pits (**P**) surrounded by polygonal apical ends of surface mucous cells. (×600)

(b) A section of the same lining shows that these surface mucous cells are part of a simple columnar epithelium continuous with the lining of the pits (**P**). Each pit extends into the sparse lamina propria and then branches into several tubular glands. These glands coil and fill most of the mucosa. Barely visible around the various cells of the closely packed gastric glands are cells, capillaries, and small lymphatics of the connective tissue lamina propria. (×200; H&E)

The **surface mucous cells** that line the lumen and gastric pits secrete a thick, highly viscous, and adherent mucous layer, which is rich in bicarbonate ions and protects the mucosa from both the abrasive effects of food and the corrosive effects of stomach acid.

Each gastric pit leads to a long, branched, tubular gland extending through the full thickness of the lamina propria. **Stem cells** for the epithelium lining the glands, pits, and stomach lumen become localized in a narrow neck or isthmus segment between each gastric pit and the deeper gland. The pluripotent stem cells divide asymmetrically, producing progenitor cells for all the other epithelial cells. Some of these move upward to replace the pit lining and surface mucous cells, which have a turnover time of 4–7 days. Other progenitor cells migrate more deeply and differentiate into the secretory cells of the glands which turn over much more slowly than the surface mucous cells.

The vascularized **lamina propria** surrounds and becomes crowded with the gastric pits and glands but includes the usual scattered smooth muscle fibers, lymphoid cells, capillaries, and lymphatics. A thin layer of smooth muscle, the **muscularis mucosae**, separates the mucosa from the underlying submucosa (Figure 15–15).

In the fundus and body, the **gastric glands** themselves fill most of the mucosa, with several such glands formed by branching at the neck of each gastric pit. Secretory epithelial cells of the gastric glands get distributed unevenly and release products that produce and regulate the stomach's functions. Four major secretory cell types occur in the gastric glands:

- **Mucous neck cells** are present mainly as clusters but also singly among the other cells in the necks of gastric glands and include many progenitor and immature surface mucous cells (Figure 15–17). Less columnar than the surface mucous cells and those lining the gastric pits, mucous neck cells often appear distorted by neighboring cells, but have round nuclei and apical secretory granules. Their mucus secretion is less alkaline than that of the surface mucous cells.

FIGURE 15–17   Gastric glands.

Throughout the **fundus** and **body** regions of the stomach, the gastric pits lead to **gastric glands** with various cell types.

(a) The long, coiled gastric glands penetrate the complete thickness of the mucosa, from the gastric pits (**GP**) to the muscularis mucosae (**MM**).

(b) In the neck of a gastric gland, below the surface mucous cells (**SM**) lining the gastric pit, are small mucous neck cells (**MN**), scattered individually or clustered among parietal cells (**P**) and stem cells that give rise to all epithelial cells of the glands. The numerous parietal cells (**P**) are large distinctive cells often bulging from the tubules, with central nuclei surrounded by intensely eosinophilic cytoplasm with unusual ultrastructure. These cells produce HCl, and the numerous mitochondria required for this process

cause the eosinophilia. Chief cells (**C**) begin to appear in the neck region. Around these tubular glands are various cells and microvasculature of the connective tissue.

(c) Near the muscularis mucosae (**MM**), the bases of these glands contain fewer parietal cells (**P**) but many more zymogenic chief cells (**C**). Chief cells occur in clusters, with basal nuclei and basophilic cytoplasm. From their apical ends chief cells secrete pepsinogen, the zymogen precursor for the major protease pepsin. Zymogen granules are often removed or stain poorly in routine preparations. (Both ×200; H&E)

(d) Diagram showing general morphology and functions of the five major cell types comprising gastric glands.

■ **Parietal** (oxyntic) **cells** produce hydrochloric acid (HCl) and occur scattered among the mucous neck cells and throughout deeper parts of the gland. They are large cells, usually appearing rounded or pyramidal, each with one (sometimes two) central round nucleus. Their intensely eosinophilic cytoplasm includes a high density of mitochondria (Figure 15–17).

A striking and unique ultrastructural feature of an active parietal cell is a deep, circular invagination of the apical plasma membrane to form an **intracellular canaliculus** with a large surface area produced by thousands of microvilli (Figure 15–18). As shown in Figure 15–19, parietal cell **carbonic anhydrase**

FIGURE **15–18** Ultrastructure of parietal cells.

(a) A TEM of an active **parietal cell** shows abundant microvilli (**MV**) protruding into the **intracellular canaliculi**, near the lumen and deeper in the cell. The cytoplasm surrounding these canaliculi contains numerous mitochondria (**M**). (×10,200)

(b) Composite diagram of a **parietal cell** showing the ultrastructural differences between a **resting cell (left)** and an **active cell (right)**. In the resting cell tubular vesicles (**TV**) occur apically (left), but the cell has few microvilli and only short intracellular canaliculi

(**IC**) among the mitochondria (**M**) and Golgi vesicles (**G**). When activated to produce HCl (right), the tubular vesicles fuse with the cell membrane to form large intracellular canaliculi (**IC**) with many microvilli (**MV**), thus providing a generous increase in the surface of the cell membrane for diffusion and ion pumps. Prolonged activity may produce more mitochondria.

(Figure 15–18a, reproduced with permission from Dr Susumu Ito, Department of Cell Biology, Harvard Medical School, Boston, MA.)

FIGURE **15–19** Synthesis of HCl by parietal cells.

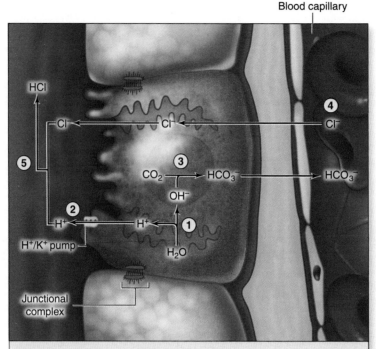

Blood capillary

(1) Water (H_2O) within the parietal cell is split into a hydrogen ion (H^+) and a hydroxide ion (OH^-).

(2) H^+ is pumped into the lumen of the gastric gland by an H^+/K^+ pump.

(3) OH^- bonds with carbon dioxide (CO_2) to form bicarbonate ion (HCO_3^-).

(4) An exchange occurs as HCO_3^- is transported out of the parietal cell (HCO_3^- then enters the blood), while chloride ion (Cl^-) is transported into the parietal cell; Cl^- then enters the lumen of the gastric gland.

(5) Within the lumen of the gastric gland, Cl^- combines with H^+ to form hydrochloric acid (HCl).

A diagram indicating the main steps of HCl synthesis in parietal cells. Conversion of H_2O and CO_2 to HCO_3^- (**bicarbonate ion)** and H^+ (**a proton**) is catalyzed by the enzyme carbonic anhydrase. Active transport is used to pump H^+ into canaliculi in exchange for K^+ and to discharge HCO_3^- by an antiport at the basal cell domain in exchange for Cl^-. The Cl^- ions diffuse into the canaliculi, leave the cell, and combine with the protons in the lumen of the gastric gland to form HCl.

Basally released bicarbonate ions enter the local interstitial fluid and microvasculature, helping to maintain the neutral pH of the mucosa. Other HCO_3^- is taken up by surface mucous cells and used to raise the pH of mucus.

catalyzes the conversion of cytoplasmic water and CO_2 into HCO_3^- and H^+. The HCO_3^- is transported from the basal end of the cell and H^+ is pumped from the cell apically, along with Cl^-. In the canalicular lumens, the H^+ and Cl^- ions combine to form HCl. While the gastric secretion becomes highly acidic, the mucosa itself remains at a more neutral pH partly because of the bicarbonate released into the lamina propria. The abundant mitochondria provide energy primarily for operating the cells' many ion pumps.

Parietal cells also secrete **intrinsic factor**, a glycoprotein required for uptake of vitamin B_{12} in the small intestine.

Control of parietal cell secretory activity occurs both by local parasympathetic innervation and by paracrine release of histamine and the polypeptide **gastrin** from enteroendocrine cells.

■ **Chief (zymogenic) cells** predominate in the deeper regions of gastric glands (Figure 15–17) and have all the characteristics of active protein-secreting cells. Ultrastructurally chief cells show abundant RER and

FIGURE **15–20** Ultrastructure of parietal, chief, and enteroendocrine cells.

TEM of a transversely sectioned gastric gland shows the ultrastructure of three major cell types. Parietal cells (**P**) contain abundant mitochondria and intracellular canaliculi (**IC**). Also shown are chief cells (**C**), which have extensive rough ER and apical secretory granules near the lumen (**L**).

An enteroendocrine cell (**E**) shows dense basal secretory granules and represents a closed-type enteroendocrine cell, it lacks contact with the gland's lumen and secretes product basally in an endocrine/paracrine manner. (×1200)

numerous apical secretory granules (Figure 15–20). The granules contain inactive enzyme **pepsinogens**, precursors converted into active **pepsins** (Gr. *peptein*, to digest) in the acid environment of the stomach. Pepsins represent broadly specific endoproteinases, with maximal activity at a pH between 1.8 and 3.5, that initiate hydrolysis of ingested protein in the stomach. Chief cells also produce **gastric lipase**, which digests many lipids.

■ **Enteroendocrine cells**, scattered among the epithelial cells deep in gastric glands, sense signals in the lumen of the gut and secrete factors with endocrine or paracrine functions. In the fundus, small enteroendocrine cells secreting **serotonin** (5-hydroxytryptamine) become localized at the basal lamina of the gastric glands (Figure 15–20). In the pylorus other enteroendocrine cells appear in contact with the glandular lumens, including **G cells** producing the peptide **gastrin**.

Table 15–1 lists the locations, products, and major actions of the stomach's enteroendocrine cells, along with those occurring in the intestinal mucosa which secrete different hormones, all of which have major importance for digestive function. Seldom seen by routine light microscopy, these cells can be visualized by processing the tissue with chromium

or silver salts. This method provided the alternative names **enterochromaffin (EC) cells** and **argentaffin cells**, respectively. Now usually visualized immunohistochemically using antibodies against their product, they are commonly named with the initial letter of their major hormone product (Table 15–1). Most of these cells process amines and are also collectively called **APUD cells** for their "amine precursor uptake and decarboxylation" activity. More generally all such cells make up parts of the **diffuse neuroendocrine system (DNES)**, a subject discussed further in Chapter 20.

>> **MEDICAL APPLICATION**

Tumors called **carcinoids**, which arise from enteroendocrine EC cells, are responsible for the clinical symptoms caused by overproduction of serotonin. Serotonin increases gut motility, and chronic high levels of this hormone/neurotransmitter can produce mucosal vasoconstriction and tissue damage.

Upon stimulation, these cells release their hormone products that then exert paracrine (local) or endocrine (systemic) effects via the vasculature. Cells of the digestive tract DNES fall into two classes: a "closed" type, in which the cellular apex

TABLE 15–1	Principal enteroendocrine cells in the gastrointestinal tract.			
			Major Action	
Cell Type	**Major Location**	**Hormone Produced**	**Promotes**	**Inhibits**
D cells	Pylorus, duodenum, and pancreatic islets	Somatostatin		Secretion from other DNES cells nearby
EC cells	Stomach, small and large intestines	Serotonin and substance P	Increased gut motility	
G cells	Pylorus	Gastrin	Gastric acid secretion	
I cells	Small intestine	Cholecystokinin (CCK)	Pancreatic enzyme secretion, gallbladder contraction	Gastric acid secretion
K cells	Duodenum and jejunum	Gastric inhibitory polypeptide (GIP)		Gastric acid secretion
L cells	Ileum and colon	Glucagon-like peptide (GLP-1)	Insulin secretion	Gastric acid secretion Sense of hunger
L cells	Ileum and colon	Peptide YY	H_2O and electrolyte absorption in large intestine	Gastric acid secretion
Mo cells	Small intestine	Motilin	Increased gut motility	
N cells	Ileum	Neurotensin		Gastric acid secretion
S cells	Small intestine	Secretin	Pancreatic and biliary bicarbonate and water secretion	Gastric acid secretion Stomach emptying

lies beneath neighboring epithelial cells (Figure 15–20), and an "open" type, in which the constricted apical end of the cell contacts the lumen and bears chemoreceptors that sample the lumen's contents. Effects of the hormones include regulation of peristalsis and tract motility; secretion of digestive enzymes, water, and electrolytes; and the sense of being satiated after eating.

In the cardia and pylorus regions of the stomach, the mucosa also contains tubular glands, with long pits, branching into coiled secretory portions, called **cardiac glands** and **pyloric glands**, respectively (Figure 15–21). Importantly, these glands lack both parietal and chief cells, primarily secreting abundant mucus that helps protect the adjacent digestive tract regions from stomach acid.

Other Layers

Figures 15–14 and 15–15 summarize the other major layers of the stomach wall. In all stomach regions the **submucosa** consists of connective tissue with large blood and lymph vessels and many lymphoid cells, macrophages, and mast cells. The **muscularis** has three poorly defined layers of smooth muscle: an outer longitudinal layer, a middle circular layer, and an innermost oblique layer. Rhythmic contractions of the muscularis thoroughly mix ingested food and chyme with mucus, HCl, and digestive enzymes from the gastric mucosa. At the pylorus the circular muscle layer thickens greatly to form the **pyloric sphincter**. A thin **serosa** covers the entire stomach.

› SMALL INTESTINE

In the **small intestine** digestive processes are completed and the products of digestion (nutrients) are absorbed by cells of the epithelial lining. Approximately 5 m long, the small intestine consists of three segments: the **duodenum**, **jejunum**, and **ileum**. These segments have most histologic features in common and are discussed together.

›› MEDICAL APPLICATION

Leiomyomas, benign tumors of smooth muscle cells, represent the most common type of tumor in the stomach and small intestine and may become large. Autopsy records suggest that the muscularis of the stomach may include leiomyomas in up to 50% of the population older than 50 years.

Mucosa

Viewed macroscopically the lining of the small intestine shows a series of permanent circular or semilunar folds, the **plicae circulares**, involving both mucosa and submucosa (Figures 15–22a and 15–23), and best developed in the jejunum. Short (0.5-1.5 mm) mucosal outgrowths called **villi** projecting into the lumen densely cover the entire mucosa of the small intestine (Figure 15–22). These finger- or leaflike projections

FIGURE **15–21** Pyloric glands.

The pyloric region of the stomach has deep gastric pits (**P**) leading to short, coiled pyloric glands (**G**) in the lamina propria (**LP**). Cardiac glands are rather similar histologically and functionally. Cells of these glands secrete mucus and lysozyme primarily, with a few enteroendocrine G cells also present.

The glands and pits are surrounded by cells of the lamina propria connective tissue containing capillaries, lymphatics, and MALT. Beneath the glands a few smooth muscle fibers of the muscularis mucosae can also be detected. (×140; H&E)

consist of a simple columnar epithelium of absorptive cells called **enterocytes**, with many interspersed **goblet cells**, that surrounds a core of loose connective tissue extending from the lamina propria and containing fibroblasts, smooth muscle fibers, lymphocytes and plasma cells, fenestrated capillaries, and a central lymphatic called a **lacteal**.

Celiac disease (celiac sprue) is a disorder of the small intestine mucosa that causes **malabsorption** and can lead to damage or destruction of the villi. The cause of celiac disease includes an immune reaction against gluten or other proteins in wheat and certain other types of grain. The resulting inflammation affects the enterocytes, leading to reduced nutrient absorption.

Openings of short tubular glands called **intestinal glands** or **crypts** (or **crypts of Lieberkühn**) occur between the villi, with the epithelium lining each crypt continuous with that covering the villi (Figure 15–22c). The epithelium of the intestinal glands includes differentiating cells and pluripotent stem cells for all the cell types of the small intestinal epithelium. These include the following:

- **Enterocytes**, the tall absorptive cells, have basal nuclei and the apical end of each displays a prominent ordered region called the **striated (or brush) border**, seen ultrastructurally as an area of densely packed **microvilli** covered by **glycocalyx** (Figures 15–22e and 15–24c). As discussed in Chapter 4, each microvillus is a cylindrical protrusion of apical cytoplasm approximately 1 μm tall and 0.1 μm in diameter containing actin filaments enclosed by the cell membrane. Each enterocyte displays an average of 3000 microvilli and each 1 mm² of mucosal surface contains about 200 million of these structures, through which nutrients undergo absorption by the cells. Microvilli, villi, and the plicae circulares all greatly increase the mucosal surface area in contact with nutrients in the lumen and represent important feature in an organ specialized for nutrient absorption. It is estimated that plicae increase the intestinal surface area 3-fold, the villi increase it 10-fold, and the microvilli increase it another 20-fold, resulting in a total absorptive surface area of over 200 m² in the small intestine.

Enterocytes' mechanism of absorption varies with the different molecular products of digestion. Disaccharidases and peptidases secreted by the enterocytes and located within the glycocalyx hydrolyze disaccharides and dipeptides into monosaccharides and amino acids which undergo rapid active transport, transcytosis and release basally for uptake by the capillaries. Digestion of fats by gastric and pancreatic lipases produces lipid subunits, including glycerol, monoglycerides, and fatty acids, which bile salts emulsify into small (2 nm) micelles that allow lipid entry into enterocytes by passive diffusion and membrane transporters. In enterocytes these lipids are re-esterified into triglycerides in smooth ER and complexed with apoproteins in the Golgi apparatus, producing **chylomicrons** that are discharged from the cell's basolateral surface for uptake by the lacteal. Figure 15–25 summarizes basic aspects of lipid absorption.

- **Goblet** cells, described in Chapter 4, occur scattered among the absorptive enterocytes (Figures 15–22d and

FIGURE 15–22   Absorptive surface of the small intestine.

(a) Layers

Mucosa
Submucosa
Muscularis
Inner circular layer
Outer longitudinal layer
Serosa

Circular folds

Circular fold

(b) Section of small intestine

Intestinal villi
Submucosa
Serosa
Inner circular layer
Outer longitudinal layer
Muscularis

(c) Intestinal villus

Enterocyte
(absorbs nutrients)

Capillary network
Goblet cells
(produce mucin)
Lacteal

Paneth cells
(innate immunity)

Intestinal gland
Lymphatic nodule

Muscularis mucosae
Venule
Lymph vessel
Arteriole

(d) Intestinal villi

Intestinal lumen
Villi
Simple columnar
epithelium
Lamina propria
Goblet cells

(e) Microvilli

Microvilli
Intestinal
lumen

(a) The **mucosa** and **submucosa** are the inner two of the gut's four concentric layers and include its absorptive components.

(b) The mucosa and submucosa together form circular folds or **plicae circulares** covered by a dense covering of fingerlike projections called **villi**, which increase the absorptive area.

(c) An intestinal villus bears a surface epithelium which consists goblet cells and more numerous **enterocytes**. This epithelium continues downward into the lamina propria to form the short

intestinal glands, or **crypts**, with stem cells and **Paneth cells** below each villus. Internally each villus contains lamina propria connective tissue with microvasculature and lymphatics called **lacteals**.

(d) A micrograph of villi featuring the simple columnar epithelium composed of absorptive enterocytes and goblet cells. (×70; H&E)

(e) A TEM showing the dense brush of **microvilli** at the apical end of each enterocyte, which serve to increase greatly the absorptive surface of the cell. (×18,000; TEM)

FIGURE **15–23** Circular folds (plicae circulares) of the jejunum.

The mucosa and submucosa (**SM**) of the small intestine form distinct projecting folds called plicae (**P**), which encircle or spiral around the inner circumference and develop most fully in the jejunum. On each fold the mucosa forms a dense covering of projecting **villi** (**V**). In this longitudinal section, the two layers of the muscularis (**M**) are clearly distinguished. The inner layer has smooth muscle encircling the submucosa; the outer layer runs lengthwise just inside the serosa (**S**), the gut's outer layer. This arrangement of smooth muscle provides for strong peristaltic movement of the gut's contents. (×12; Masson trichrome)

15–24a, b). They secrete specific antibacterial peptides and glycoprotein mucins, which undergo hydration to form a mucus layer that functions to protect and lubricate the lining of the intestine.

- **Paneth cells**, located in the basal portion of the intestinal crypts below the stem cells, develop as exocrine cells with large, eosinophilic secretory granules in their apical cytoplasm (Figure 15–26). Paneth cell granules release lysozyme, phospholipase A_2, and hydrophobic peptides called **defensins**, all of which serve to protect the crypts by binding and breaking down bacterial cell walls. Paneth cells make up another example of innate immunity and have important roles in regulating the microenvironment of the intestinal crypts.

- **Enteroendocrine cells** occur in varying numbers throughout the length of the small intestine, secreting various peptide hormones (Table 15–1). Many of these exemplify the "open" type of enteroendocrine cells, in which the apical end of the cell contacts the intestinal lumen with chemoreceptors resembling those of taste buds, to sample levels of certain nutrients such as sugars that regulate specific hormone release from their basal ends (Figure 15–27).

- **M (microfold) cells** develop as unique cells specialized for transepithelial transport of particles and microorganisms, located mainly in the ileum's mucosa overlying the lymphoid follicles of Peyer patches. As discussed in Chapter 14, each M cell has a large pocket formed by deep invagination of the basolateral membrane and containing lymphocytes and macrophages (see Figure 14–13c, d). Continuous sampling of intestinal microorganisms by the M cells and the immune cells within and below the M cells make up an important part of the defense provided by mucosal immunity.

Other Layers

Along the entire small intestine loose connective tissue of the mucosal lamina propria contains extensive blood and lymph microvasculature, nerve fibers, smooth muscle cells, and diffuse lymphoid tissue. Lamina propria penetrates the core of

FIGURE **15–24** Cells covering the villi.

(a) The columnar epithelium that covers intestinal villi consists mainly of the tall absorptive enterocytes (**E**). The apical ends of these cells are joined and covered by a **brush border** of microvilli. Covered by a coating of glycoproteins, the brush border, along with the mucus-secreting goblet cells (**G**), stains with carbohydrate staining methods. Other cells of the epithelium are scattered enteroendocrine cells, which are difficult to identify in routine preparations, and various immune cells such as intraepithelial lymphocytes. The small spherical nuclei of such lymphocytes can be seen here between the enterocytes. (X250; PAS-hematoxylin)

(b) At higher magnification individual **microvilli** of enterocytes (**E**) are better seen and the striated appearance of the brush border is apparent. The secretory goblet cells (**G**) lack the well-developed brush border. (×500)

(c) TEM shows microvilli and densely packed mitochondria of enterocytes (**E**). An enteroendocrine cell (**EC**) of the closed type with basal secretory granules can be distinguished along the basal lamina. (×2500)

each villus, bringing with it microvasculature, lymphatics, and nerves (Figures 15–22c and 15–28). Smooth muscle fibers extending from the muscularis mucosae produce rhythmic movements of the villi that increase the absorption efficiency. Fibers of the muscularis mucosae also produce local movements of plicae circulares that help propel lymph from the lacteals into submucosal and mesenteric lymphatics.

The submucosa has larger blood and lymph vessels and the diffuse, interconnected neurons of the **submucosal (Meissner) nerve plexus**, which produce coordinated local movements of the plicae circulares and villi. The proximal part of the duodenum includes in its submucosa and mucosa large clusters of branched tubular mucous glands, the **duodenal (or Brunner) glands**, with small excretory ducts opening among the intestinal crypts (Figure 15–29). Mucus from these

glands is distinctly alkaline (pH 8.1–9.3), which neutralizes chyme entering the duodenum from the pylorus, protecting the mucous membrane, and bringing the intestinal contents to the optimum pH for pancreatic enzyme action. In the ileum, both the lamina propria and submucosa contain well-developed mucosa-associated lymphoid tissue (MALT), consisting of the large lymphoid nodule aggregates known as **Peyer patches** that underlie the epithelial M cells.

The muscularis becomes well developed in the small intestine, consisting of an internal circular layer, an external longitudinal layer, with the neurons of the **myenteric (Auerbach) nerve plexus** between them producing their contractions for peristalsis (Figure 15–30). Neurons of both the submucosal and myenteric plexuses are largely autonomic and collectively make up the large enteric nervous system. A thin

FIGURE **15–25** Lipid absorption and processing by enterocytes.

(a) TEM shows that enterocytes involved in lipid absorption accumulate many small lipid droplets in vesicles of the smooth ER (**SER**). These vesicles fuse near the nucleus, forming larger globules that are moved laterally and cross the cell membrane to the extracellular space (**arrows**) for eventual uptake by lymphatic capillaries (lacteals) in the lamina propria. (×3000)

(b) (1) Simplified diagram showing lipid processing by enterocytes. Ingested fats are emulsified by **bile acids** to form a suspension of lipid droplets from which lipids are digested by **lipases** to produce glycerol, fatty acids, and monoglycerides. **(2)** The products of hydrolysis diffuse passively across the microvilli membranes and are collected in the cisternae of the smooth ER, where they are resynthesized as **triglycerides**. **(3)** Processed through the RER and Golgi, these triglycerides become surrounded by a thin layer of proteins and packaged in vesicles containing **chylomicrons** (0.2–1 μm in diameter) of lipid complexed with protein. **(4)** Chylomicrons are transferred to the lateral cell membrane, secreted by exocytosis, and flow into the extracellular space in the direction of the lamina propria, where most enter the lymph in **lacteals**.

Absorbed cholesterol and fatty acids not used in chylomicron formation may be released from the enterocytes basally, along with amino acids and monosaccharides, for uptake by local blood capillaries. As discussed in the next chapter, venous blood from the small intestine is carried by the hepatic portal vein directly to the liver, which absorbs and processes these dietary nutrients released from enterocytes.

Chylomicrons are too large to pass through the fenestrae of blood capillaries but enter the lacteals through the larger openings between the lymphatic endothelial cells (see Figure 11–24) and are carried with lymph to the thoracic duct, from which they enter the blood circulation and are distributed systemically. As a result, most triglycerides and other factors bound within chylomicrons such as fat-soluble vitamins from the diet are carried by blood capillaries for use by cells throughout the body or for storage in adipocytes without passing initially through the hepatic portal vein and liver.

(Figure 15–25a, reproduced with permission from Dr Robert R. Cardell, Jr, Department of Cancer and Cell Biology, University of Cincinnati College of Medicine, Cincinnati, OH.)

FIGURE **15–26** Intestinal crypts or glands, with Paneth cells.

(a) Between villi (**V**) throughout the small intestine, the covering epithelium invaginates into the lamina propria (**LP**) to form short tubular glands called intestinal glands or intestinal crypts (**IC**). The lining near the openings of the crypts contains a population of stem cells for the entire epithelial lining of the small intestine. Daughter cells slowly move with the growing epithelium out of the crypts, differentiating as **goblet cells, enterocytes,** and **enteroendocrine cells**. These cells continue to move up each villus and within a week are shed at the tip, with billions shed throughout the small intestine each day. At the base of the crypts are many Paneth cells (**P**) with an innate immune function. The submucosa (**S**) has many lymphatics draining lacteals. (×200; Mallory trichrome)

(b) Higher magnification at the base of an intestinal gland shows the typical eosinophilic granules of Paneth cells (**P**), along with an "open" type enteroendocrine cell (**EC**) and a differentiating goblet cell (**G**). (×400; H&E)

serosa with mesothelium continuous with that of mesenteries covers the small intestine (Figure 15–22a).

❯❯ MEDICAL APPLICATION

Crohn disease is a chronic inflammatory bowel disease that occurs most commonly in the ileum or colon, resulting from a poorly understood combination of immune, environmental, and genetic factors. Excessive lymphocytic activity and inflammation occur in any or all layers of the tract wall, producing pain, localized bleeding, malabsorption, and diarrhea.

❯ LARGE INTESTINE

The **large intestine** or bowel, which absorbs water and electrolytes and forms indigestible material into feces, includes the following regions: the short **cecum**, with the **ileocecal valve** and the **appendix**; the ascending, transverse, descending, and sigmoid **colon**; and the **rectum**, containing feces prior to evacuation (Figure 15–31). The large bowel mucosa lacks villi and except in the rectum has no major folds. Less than one-third the length of the small intestine, the large intestine has a greater diameter (6–7 cm). The wall of the colon is puckered by muscularis action into a series of large outpocketings called **haustra** (L. sing. *haustrum*, bucket, scoop).

Tubular **intestinal glands** penetrate the mucosa of the large bowel along its entire length. These small glands and the intestinal lumen are lined by absorptive and goblet cells, with a small number of enteroendocrine cells (Figures 15–32 and 15–33). The columnar absorptive cells or **colonocytes** have irregular microvilli and dilated intercellular spaces indicating active fluid absorption (Figure 15–33d). Goblet cells producing lubricating mucus become more numerous along the length of the colon and in the rectum. Epithelial stem cells become localized in the bottom third of each gland.

FIGURE **15–27** Enteroendocrine cell.

TEM of an "open" **enteroendocrine cell** in the epithelium of the duodenum shows microvilli at its apical end in contact with the lumen. The microvilli have components of nutrient-sensing and signal transduction systems similar in some components to those of taste bud gustatory cells.

Activation of these cells by nutrients triggers the release at the basolateral membranes of peptide factors, including satiation peptides, which diffuse through extracellular fluid to enter capillaries (endocrine) or to bind receptors on nearby nerve terminals, smooth muscle fibers, or other cells (paracrine).

Hormones from the various enteroendocrine cells act in a coordinated manner to control gut motility; regulate secretion of enzymes, HCl, bile, and other components for digestion; and produce the sense of satiety in the brain. (×4500)

(Reproduced with permission from AGE Pearse, Department of Histochemistry, Royal Postgraduate Medical School, London, UK.)

FIGURE **15–28** Microvasculature, lymphatics, and muscle in villi.

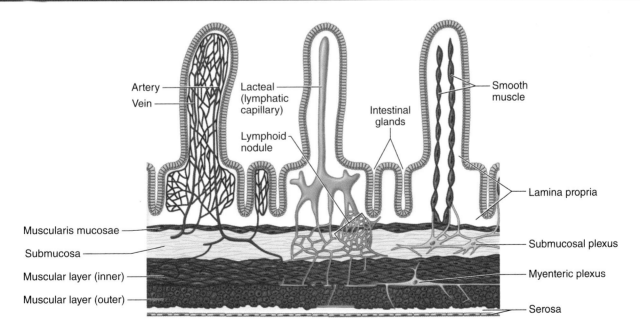

Diagrammatic representations of the small intestine villi **blood microvasculature (left)**, lymphatic capillaries called **lacteals (center)**, and both **innervation and smooth muscle fibers (right)**.

FIGURE 15–29 Duodenal (Brunner) glands.

Concentrated in the upper duodenum are large masses of compound tubular **mucous glands**, the duodenal glands (**DG**), with many lobules that occupy much of the submucosa and may extend above the muscularis mucosae (**MM**) into the mucosa. Many small excretory ducts (**D**) extend from these lobules through the lamina propria and empty into the lumen among the small intestinal crypts.

Alkaline mucus from duodenal glands neutralizes the pH of material entering the duodenum and supplements the mucus from goblet cells in lubricating and protecting the lining of the small intestine. (×100; H&E)

FIGURE 15–30 Small intestine muscularis and myenteric plexus.

(a) Transverse sections of the **small intestinal wall** show the orientation of the internal (**IM**) and external (**EM**) smooth muscle layers. The inner layer is predominantly circular, while the outer layer runs longitudinally. The serosa (**S**) is a thin connective tissue covered here by a mesothelium of cuboidal or squamous cells. (×200; PT)

(b) Between the internal and external layers of muscularis (**IM** and **EM**) are ganglia of pale-staining neurons and other cells of the myenteric plexus (**MP**). (×100; H&E)

The lamina propria here has many lymphoid cells and lymphoid nodules that frequently extend into the submucosa (Figure 15–32). The richness in MALT relates directly to the large bacterial population of the large intestine. The appendix at the cecum has little or no absorptive function but constitutes a significant component of MALT (see Chapter 14).

The muscularis of the colon has longitudinal and circular layers but its organization differs from that of the small intestine, with fibers of the outer layer gathered into three separate longitudinal bands called **teniae coli** (L., ribbons of the colon)

FIGURE **15–31** Large intestine.

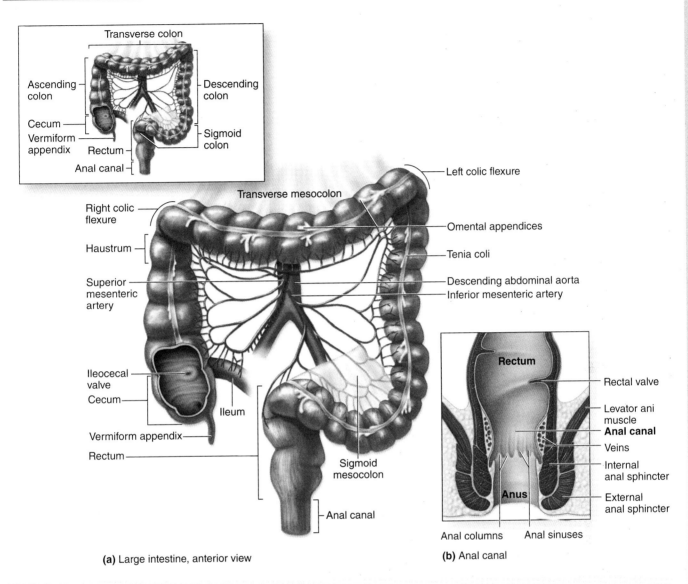

(a) Large intestine, anterior view

(b) Anal canal

As shown at the top, the **large intestine** consists of the **cecum**; the ascending, transverse, descending, and sigmoid regions of the **colon**; and the rectum, which leads to the anal canal.

(a) Anterior view of the large intestine with the proximal end exposed shows the **ileocecal valve** at its attachment to the ileum, along with the sac called the **cecum** and its extension, the **appendix**. The mucosa has only shallow plicae and no villi.

The muscularis has two layers, but the outer longitudinal layer consists mainly of three distinct bundles of muscle fibers called **teniae coli** that produce the bulging haustra in the colon wall. The serosa of the colon is continuous with that of the supporting

mesenteries and displays a series of suspended masses of adipose tissue called **omental appendages**.

(b) At the distal end of the rectum, the anal canal, the mucosa, and submucosa are highly vascularized, with venous sinuses, and are folded as a series of longitudinal folds called **anal columns** (of Morgagni) with intervening **anal sinuses**.

Fecal material accumulating in the rectum is eliminated by muscular contraction, including action of an **internal anal sphincter** continuous with the circular layer of the muscularis and an **external sphincter** of striated (voluntary) muscle.

FIGURE **15–32** Wall of the large intestine.

(a) Large intestine tunics

(b) Large intestine mucosa and submucosa

(a) Diagram shows the wall of the large intestine composed of the four typical layers. The **submucosa** is well-vascularized. The **muscularis** has a typical inner circular layer, but the outer longitudinal muscle occurs as three equally spaced bands, the **teniae coli**.

(b) Light micrographs show that the large intestinal **mucosa** is occupied mostly by tubular **intestinal glands** lined mainly by goblet cells and extending as deep as the muscularis mucosae. The lamina propria contains abundant MALT. (×80; H&E)

(Figure 15–32a), in which local contractions produce the haustra mentioned above. Intraperitoneal portions of the colon have a covering serosa characterized by small, pendulous protuberances of adipose tissue.

❯❯ MEDICAL APPLICATION

Colorectal cancer represents an **adenocarcinoma** that develops initially from benign **adenomatous polyps** in the mucosal epithelium. Such polyps usually occur in epithelium of the rectum, sigmoid colon, or distal descending colon and are more common in individuals with low-fiber diets, which reduce the bulk of fecal material, and this in turn prolongs contact of the mucosa with toxins in feces. Screens for colorectal cancer include **sigmoidoscopy** or **colonoscopy** to see polyps and tests for **fecal occult blood** resulting from mucosal bleeding as an adenocarcinoma invades more deeply into the mucosa.

❯❯ MEDICAL APPLICATION

Swollen blood vessels in the mucosa or submucosa of the anal canal can cause a painful disorder called **hemorrhoids**. This common condition typically results from a low-fiber diet, **constipation**, prolonged sitting, or straining at defecation, conditions that produce increased pressure on these blood vessels.

Continuous medially with the sigmoid colon, the **rectum** lacks haustra. Here the teniae coli merge along its 10-12 cm length as a tube of longitudinally arrayed muscle. The **anal canal**, 3-4 cm long makes up the posterior end of the rectum. At the **rectoanal junction**, the simple columnar mucosal lining of the rectum transitions to stratified squamous epithelium (Figure 15–34). The mucosa and submucosa of the anal canal form several longitudinal folds, the **anal columns** (Figure 15–31b), in which the lamina propria and submucosa include

FIGURE **15–33** Colon mucosa.

(a) Transverse section of the colon shows the muscularis externa (**ME**), including a **tenia coli** cut transversely in the lower part of the figure, the submucosa (**S**), the mucosa (**M**) filled with **tubular intestinal glands**. Some of these glands are cut longitudinally, but most seen here are cut transversely. (×14; H&E)

(b) Transversely cut glands are seen to consist of simple columnar epithelium surrounded by a tubular lumen (**L**) and embedded in lamina propria (**LP**) with many free lymphocytes. Lymphocytes can also be seen penetrating the epithelium (**arrow**). (×200; H&E)

(c) Longitudinal section of one intestinal gland stained for glycoproteins shows **mucus** in the lumen and two major cell types in the epithelium: goblet cells (**G**) and the neighboring columnar cells specialized for water absorption. (×400; PAS)

(d) TEM of the absorptive cells, or **colonocytes**, reveals short **microvilli** at their apical ends and dilated **intercellular spaces** with interdigitating leaflets of cell membrane (**L**), a sign of active water transport. The absorption of water is passive, following the active transport of sodium from the basolateral surfaces of the epithelial cells. (×2500)

FIGURE **15–34** Mucosa of the rectoanal junction.

The simple columnar epithelium of goblet cells comprising the tubular **intestinal glands** in the **rectum** (left side of photo) changes abruptly to stratified squamous epithelium of **skin** in the **anal canal** (right side of photo), as seen in this longitudinal section. The connective tissue of the lamina propria contains many free lymphocytes. (×40; H&E)

TABLE 15–2	Summary of distinguishing digestive tract features, by region and layers.			
Region and Subdivisions	Mucosa (Epithelium, Lamina Propria, Muscularis Mucosae)	Submucosa (With Submucosal Plexuses)	Muscularis (Inner Circular and Outer Longitudinal Layers, With Myenteric Plexuses Between Them)	Adventitia/Serosa
Esophagus (upper, middle, lower)	Nonkeratinized **stratified squamous epithelium**; **cardiac glands** at lower end	Small **esophageal glands** (mainly mucous)	Both layers **striated muscle** in upper region; both layers **smooth muscle** in lower region; **smooth and striated muscle** fascicles mingled in middle region	Adventitia, except at lower end with serosa
Stomach (cardia, fundus, body, pylorus)	**Surface mucous cells** and **gastric pits** leading to **gastric glands** with **parietal and chief cells,** (in the fundus and body) or to mucous **cardiac glands** and **pyloric glands**	No distinguishing features	**Three indistinct layers** of smooth muscle (inner oblique, middle circular, and outer longitudinal)	Serosa
Small intestine (duodenum, jejunum, ileum)	**Plicae circulares; villi,** with **enterocytes** and **goblet cells,** and **crypts/glands** with **Paneth cells** and **stem cells; Peyer patches** in ileum	**Duodenal (Brunner) glands** (entirely mucous); possible extensions of Peyer patches in ileum	No distinguishing features	Mainly serosa
Large intestine (cecum, colon, rectum)	**Intestinal glands** with **goblet cells** and **absorptive cells**	No distinguishing features	Outer longitudinal layer separated into three bands, the **teniae coli**	Mainly serosa, with adventitia at rectum
Anal canal	**Stratified squamous epithelium;** longitudinal **anal columns**	Venous sinuses	Inner circular layer thickened as **internal sphincter**	Adventitia

sinuses of the rectal venous plexus. Near the anus, the rectum's muscularis changes to a thick circular layer, the **internal anal sphincter**. Defecation involves its coordinated contraction together with that of voluntary, striated muscle comprising the **external anal sphincter** (Figure 15–31b).

Table 15–2 summarizes all the major histologic features distinguishing each region of the digestive tract.

❯❯ MEDICAL APPLICATION

Herniation or outpocketing of the mucosa and submucosa of the colon can occur between the teniae coli, forming bulges (diverticula) and a condition called **diverticulosis**. This disorder can result from structural defects in the colon wall or from high intraluminal pressure or **constipation**. Fecal material can become immobilized in the diverticula and cause localized inflammation or **diverticulitis**.

Digestive Tract SUMMARY OF KEY POINTS

Oral Cavity

- The **oral cavity** lining or **mucosa** primarily has **nonkeratinized stratified squamous epithelium**, with **keratinized stratified squamous epithelium** on the **hard palate** and **gingiva**.
- The dorsal surface mucosa of the tongue has projecting **lingual papillae** of four types: **filiform** papillae with keratinized epithelium and nonkeratinized **foliate, fungiform,** and large **vallate** papillae.

- All lingual papillae, except the filiform type, have epithelial **taste buds** on their sides, with chemosensory **gustatory cells** with synapses to basal sensory innervation, **support cells**, and an apical **taste pore**.
- Each tooth has **enamel** covering its **crown** and **neck** and a vascularized, innervated central **pulp cavity** within the **dentin** that makes up the **roots** and extends into the neck.

- Enamel calcifies as parallel **enamel rods** in a process guided by the protein **amelogenin** after secretion from columnar epithelial cells called **ameloblasts** in the **enamel organ** of the embryonic **tooth bud**.
- **Predentin** is secreted as elongated **dentinal tubules** from tall **odontoblasts**, which line the pulp cavity and persist in the fully formed tooth, with apical **odontoblast processes** extending between the tubules.
- The **periodontium** of each tooth consists of a thin layer of bone-like **cementum** surrounding dentin of the roots and the **periodontal ligament** binding the cementum to **alveolar bone** on the jaw socket.

Layers of the Digestive Tract

- From the esophagus to the rectum, the digestive tract has **four major layers**: a lining **mucosa**, a **submucosa**, a **muscularis**, and an outermost **adventitia** or mesothelium-covered **serosa**.
- The **mucosa** varies regionally along the tract but always consists of a lining **epithelium** on a **lamina propria** of loose connective tissue and smooth muscle fibers extending from a **muscularis mucosae** layer.

Esophagus

- The mucosa of the **esophagus** has **nonkeratinized stratified squamous epithelium**; its muscularis is striated at its superior end with smooth muscle at its inferior end, with mixed fiber types in the middle.
- Along almost all of its length the outer layer of the esophagus is **adventitia**, merging with other tissues of the mediastinum.
- At the **esophagogastric junction**, stratified squamous epithelium changes abruptly to **simple columnar epithelium** invaginating into the lamina propria as branched tubular glands and a serosa replaces the adventitia.

Stomach

- The **stomach** has four major regions: the superior **cardia** and inferior **pylorus**, which resemble each other histologically, and the intervening **fundus** and **body**, which are also similar.
- The mucosa of the stomach fundus and body shows innumerable penetrating **gastric pits**, which are lined like the stomach lumen with **surface mucous cells** and which lead into branching **gastric glands**.
- The surface mucous cells secrete a thick layer of **viscous mucus with bicarbonate ions**, which protects these cells and the underlying lamina propria.
- Four **major cell types** comprise the epithelium lining the **gastric glands**, along with their pluripotent **stem cells** located in the narrow neck regions of these glands:
  - **Mucous neck cells** include immature precursors of the surface mucous cells but produce less alkaline mucus while migrating up into the gastric pits.
  - **Parietal cells** are large cells with many mitochondria and **large intracellular canaliculi** for production of **HCl** in the gastric secretion; they also secrete **intrinsic factor** for vitamin B$_{12}$ uptake.
  - **Chief (zymogenic) cells**, clustered mainly in the lower half of the gastric glands, secrete the protein **pepsinogen** which undergoes activation in the low pH of the lumen to form the major protease **pepsin**.

- **Enteroendocrine cells** are scattered epithelial cells of the **diffuse neuroendocrine system**, which release **peptide hormones** to regulate activities of neighboring tissues during food digestion.
- The mucosa of the stomach cardiac and pyloric regions has branching **cardiac and pyloric glands**, which consist almost entirely of columnar **mucous cells**, lacking parietal and chief cells.

Small Intestine

- The **small intestine** has three regions: the **duodenum** with large mucous glands in the submucosa called **duodenal glands**; the **jejunum**; and the **ileum** with large mucosal and submucosal **Peyer patches**.
- In all regions of small intestine, the mucosa has millions of projecting **villi**, with simple columnar epithelium over cores of lamina propria, and intervening simple tubular **intestinal glands** (or crypts).
- Stem cells in these glands produce the columnar epithelial cells of villi, mainly **enterocytes** for nutrient absorption and **goblet cells**, as well as defensin-producing **Paneth cells** deep in the glands.
- **Sugars** and **amino acids** produced by final steps of digesting carbohydrates and polypeptides in the **glycocalyx** undergo transcytosis through **enterocytes** for uptake by **capillaries**.
- Products of **lipid** digestion associate with bile salts, are taken up by enterocytes, and are converted to **triglycerides** and **lipoproteins** for release as **chylomicrons** and uptake by a lymphatic called a **lacteal** in the core of each villus.
- Smooth muscle of the **lamina propria** and **muscularis mucosae**, under the control of the autonomic **submucosal (Meissner) plexus**, moves the villi and helps propel lymph through the lacteals.
- Smooth muscle in the **inner circular layer** and the **outer longitudinal layer** of the muscularis, under the control of the autonomic **myenteric (Auerbach) plexus**, produces strong **peristalsis**.

Large Intestine

- The **large intestine** has three major regions: the short **cecum**, with the appendix; the long **colon**, with its ascending, transverse, descending, and sigmoid portions; and the **rectum**.
- Along its entire length the mucosa of the large intestine has millions of short simple tubular **intestinal glands**, lined by lubricant **goblet cells** and absorptive cells called **colonocytes** for the uptake of water and electrolytes.
- The **muscularis** of the colon has its outer longitudinal layer subdivided into three bands of smooth muscle called **teniae coli**, which act in the peristaltic movement of feces to the rectum.

Anal Canal

- At the **anal canal** the simple columnar epithelium lining the rectum shifts abruptly to **stratified squamous epithelium** of the skin at the **anus**.
- Near the anus, the circular layer of the rectum's muscularis forms the **internal anal sphincter**, with further control exerted by **striated muscle** of the **external anal sphincter**.

Digestive Tract ASSESS YOUR KNOWLEDGE

1. In which of the following structures of the oral cavity would taste buds be localized in the highest concentration?
   a. Fungiform papillae
   b. Gingiva
   c. Filiform papillae
   d. Ventral surface of the tongue
   e. Vallate papillae

2. Certain antibiotic therapies slow the replacement of the cells lining the small intestine. This may cause the loss of what tissue type?
   a. Ciliated pseudostratified columnar epithelium
   b. Simple cuboidal epithelium
   c. Simple columnar epithelium
   d. Pseudostratified columnar epithelium with stereocilia
   e. Stratified squamous, nonkeratinized epithelium

3. The teniae coli of the large intestine represent an organ-specific specialization of which layer of the intestinal tract wall?
   a. Epithelium
   b. Lamina propria
   c. Muscularis mucosa
   d. Muscularis externa
   e. Serosa

4. Which of the following would most likely result from a reduction in the number of Paneth cells?
   a. Thinning of the glycocalyx
   b. Reduced breakdown of fats
   c. Elevated levels of undigested proteins
   d. Decreased mucus in the intestine
   e. Increased number of intestinal bacteria

5. A medical student on a rotation in the pathology laboratory is given an unlabeled microscope slide with tissue provided by a gastroenterologist from a cancer patient she is attending. The mucosa and submucosa are poorly preserved, with only the thick muscularis well-stained, showing striated fibers. The slide most likely shows a biopsy of which region of the GI tract?
   a. Pyloric sphincter
   b. Esophagus
   c. Colon
   d. Corpus of the stomach
   e. Ileum

6. Diarrhea may result if which of the following organs fails to carry out its role in absorbing water from the feces?
   a. Anal canal
   b. Cecum
   c. Colon
   d. Jejunum
   e. Duodenum

7. Which of the following is true of the absorptive cells of the small intestine?
   a. Also called enteroendocrine cells
   b. Have many microvilli covering their basal surfaces
   c. Absorb lipids by active transport
   d. Synthesize triglycerides from absorbed lipids
   e. Undergo mitosis at tips of villi and are sloughed off into crypts

8. A 52-year-old man is diagnosed with a carcinoid after an appendectomy. The enteroendocrine cells producing this disorder differ from goblet cells in which of the following?
   a. The direction of release of secretion
   b. The use of exocytosis for release of secretory product
   c. Their presence in the small and large intestines
   d. The origin from a crypt stem cell
   e. Their location in a simple columnar epithelium

9. A 14-month-old girl is brought to the pediatric dentistry clinic because her erupted deciduous teeth are opalescent with fractured and chipped surfaces. X-rays reveal bulb-shaped crowns, thin roots, and enlarged central cavities. Tissue immediately surrounding one tooth's central cavity is biopsied and prepared for histology, which reveals irregular, widely spaced tubules. Which of the following applies to this irregular tissue layer?
   a. It has a composition similar to that of bone and is produced by cells similar in appearance to osteocytes.
   b. It is formed on a noncollagenous matrix that is resorbed after mineralization by the same cells that secreted it.
   c. It contains abundant nerves, microvasculature, and loose connective tissue.
   d. It consists of mineralized collagen secreted by cells derived from the neural crest.
   e. It is the site of inflammation in diabetic patients and is sensitive to vitamin C deficiency.

10. A 39-year-old woman presents with dyspnea, fatigue, pallor, tachycardia, anosmia, and diarrhea. Laboratory results are: hematocrit 32% (normal 36.1%–44.3%), MCV 102 fL (normal 78–98 fL), 0.3% reticulocytes (normal 0.5%–2.0%), 95 pg/mL vitamin B_{12} (normal 200–900 pg/mL), and an abnormal stage I of the Schilling test. Autoantibodies are detected against a cell type located in one region of the GI tract. In which regions would those cells be found?
    a. Esophagus
    b. Body of the stomach
    c. Pyloric region of the stomach
    d. Cardiac region of the stomach
    e. Duodenum

16 Organs Associated with the Digestive Tract

The organs associated with the digestive tract include the major salivary glands, pancreas, liver, and gallbladder. Products of these organs facilitate movement and digestion of food within the gastrointestinal tract. The main functions of the **salivary glands** include moistening and lubricating ingested food and the oral mucosa, beginning digestion of carbohydrates and lipids with amylase and lipase, and secreting innate immune components such as lysozyme and lactoferrin.

The **pancreas** secretes digestive enzymes that act in the small intestine and hormones important for the metabolism of the absorbed nutrients. Bile, whose components are necessary for digestion and absorption of fats, makes up the exocrine secretion of the **liver** but is stored and concentrated in the **gallbladder** for later delivery to the duodenum. The liver also plays a major role in carbohydrate and protein metabolism, inactivates many toxic substances and drugs, and synthesizes most plasma proteins and factors necessary for blood coagulation.

❯ SALIVARY GLANDS

Exocrine glands in the oral mucosa produce saliva, which has digestive, lubricating, and protective functions. With a normal pH near neutrality saliva has an important buffering function in addition to its varied hydrolytic, mucous, and immune components. The large salivary glands occur as three pairs: the **parotid**, **submandibular**, and **sublingual glands** (Figure 16–1). Numerous minor or intrinsic salivary glands located throughout most of the oral mucosa secrete about 10% of the total saliva volume.

❯❯ MEDICAL APPLICATION

Inadequate saliva production, leading to **dry mouth** or **xerostomia**, can occur with various factors affecting the major salivary glands, such as **mumps** viral infection, radiation of the glands, or the normal side effect of drugs such as **antihistamines**.

A connective tissue capsule surrounds each major salivary gland. The parenchyma of each consists of secretory units on a branching duct system arranged in lobules, separated by septa of connective tissue. Each gland produces a largely serous, seromucous, or mucous secretion, depending on its content of the glycoprotein mucin. The parotid glands release a serous, watery saliva. The submandibular and sublingual glands produce a seromucous secretion, while that of the minor glands is mostly mucous. Cells of the duct system draining the glands' secretory units modify saliva, reabsorbing and adding various electrolytes.

Three epithelial cell types comprise the salivary secretory units:

- **Serous cells** are polarized protein-secreting cells, usually pyramidal in shape, with round nuclei, well-stained RER, and apical secretory granules (Figures 16–2 through 16–4). Joined apically by tight and adherent junctions, serous cells usually comprise a somewhat spherical unit called an **acinus** (L. berry), with a small central lumen (Figure 16–2), which may also have mucous cells. Serous cells secrete enzymes and other proteins.
- **Mucous cells** are more columnar, showing compressed basal nuclei (Figures 16–2 and 16–4). Mucous cells contain apical granules with hydrophilic mucins which after secretion provide lubricating properties in saliva but cause poor cellular staining in routine preparations (Figure 16–5). Mucous cells occur in mixed seromucous acini or become organized as short **tubules** rather than acini. Mixed salivary glands have seromucous acini and tubuloacinar secretory units for both serous and mucous secretion (see Table 4–4).
- **Myoepithelial cells**, described in Chapter 4, occur inside the basal lamina surrounding acini or tubules and the proximal ends of the duct system (Figures 16–2 and 16–4).

FIGURE **16–1** Major salivary glands.

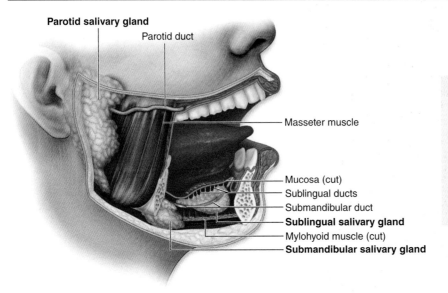

Parotid salivary gland
Parotid duct
Masseter muscle
Mucosa (cut)
Sublingual ducts
Submandibular duct
Sublingual salivary gland
Mylohyoid muscle (cut)
Submandibular salivary gland

Three large bilateral pairs of major salivary glands develop in the oral cavity, the **parotid**, **submandibular**, and **sublingual glands**, which together produce about 90% of saliva. The figure indicates their locations, relative sizes, and excretory ducts. These glands plus microscopic minor salivary glands scattered throughout the oral mucosa produce 0.75–1.50 L of saliva daily.

FIGURE **16–2** Epithelial components of a submandibular gland lobule.

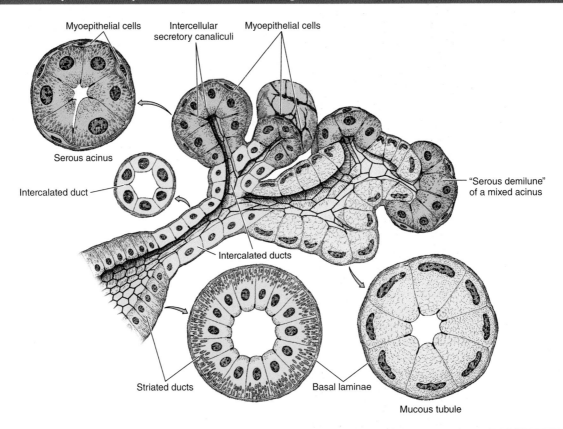

Myoepithelial cells
Intercellular secretory canaliculi
Myoepithelial cells
Serous acinus
Intercalated duct
"Serous demilune" of a mixed acinus
Intercalated ducts
Striated ducts
Basal laminae
Mucous tubule

The **submandibular gland's** secretory portions consist of pyramidal serous (violet) and mucous (tan) cells. **Serous acini** have typical protein-secreting cells with rounded nuclei, basal accumulation of RER, and apical ends filled with secretory granules. The cells of **mucous tubules** have flattened, basal nuclei with condensed chromatin. Mixed tubuloacinar secretory units also occur, combining short mucous tubules with distal clusters of serous cells called "**serous demilunes**." The short **intercalated ducts** are lined with low cuboidal epithelium. The **striated ducts** consist of columnar cells with characteristics of ion-transporting cells: basal membrane invaginations with mitochondrial accumulations. **Myoepithelial cell** processes surround the serous acini.

FIGURE **16–3** Parotid gland.

The large **parotid gland** consists entirely of serous acini with cells producing amylase and other proteins for storage in secretory granules.

(a) Micrograph of a parotid gland shows densely packed serous acini (**A**) with ducts. Secretory granules of serous cells are clearly shown in this plastic section, as well as an intercalated duct (**ID**) and striated duct (**SD**), both cut transversely. (×400; PT)

(b) Faint striations of a duct (**SD**) are better seen here, along with a septum (**CT**) and numerous serous acini (**A**). The connective tissue often includes adipocytes. (×200; H&E)

These small, flattened cells extend several contractile processes around the associated secretory unit or duct and their activity is important for moving secretory products into and through the ducts.

❯❯ MEDICAL APPLICATION

Excessive saliva production, or **sialorrhea**, is associated with the autonomic activity of **nausea**, inflammation within the oral cavity, and **rabies** viral infection.

In the **intralobular duct system**, secretory acini and tubules empty into short **intercalated ducts**, lined by cuboidal epithelial cells, and several of these ducts join to form a **striated duct** (Figure 16–2). The more columnar striated duct cells develop many infoldings of their basolateral membrane, all aligned with numerous mitochondria that, by light microscopy, appear as faint basal striations radiating toward the nuclei (Figure 16–6). Striated ducts reabsorb Na^+ and Cl^- from the initial secretion and add HCO_3^-, with their folded cell membranes providing a large surface area with ion transporters, facilitating rapid ion transcytosis and making the secretion slightly hypotonic.

Plasma cells in the connective tissue surrounding the small intralobular ducts release **IgA**, which forms a complex with the secretory component synthesized by the epithelial cells of the serous acini and intralobular ducts. Transferred into the saliva, the IgA complex provides defense against specific pathogens in the oral cavity.

Ducts from each lobule converge and drain into interlobular **excretory ducts** with increasing size and thicker

TEM of a mixed acinus from a submandibular gland shows both **serous and mucous cells** surrounding the small lumen (**L**). Mucous cells (**M**) have large, hydrophilic granules like those of goblet cells, while serous cells (**S**) have small, dense granules. Small myoepithelial cells (**My**) extend contractile processes around each acinus. (×2500)

(Reproduced with permission from Dr John D. Harrison, King's College London Dental Institute, London, UK.)

copious watery secretion with relatively little organic content. Sympathetic stimulation inhibits such secretion and produces the potential for dry mouth often associated with anxiety.

Features specific to each pair of major salivary glands include the following:

- **Parotid glands**, located in each cheek near the ear, comprise large branched acinar glands with exclusively serous acini (Figure 16–3). Serous cells of parotid glands secrete abundant **α-amylase**, which initiates hydrolysis of carbohydrates, and proline-rich proteins with antimicrobial and other protective properties.
- **Submandibular glands** produce two-thirds of all saliva and represent the mixed type of gland, developing as branched tubuloacinar glands having many mixed secretory units but serous acini primarily (Figures 16–4 and 16–5a). Within the mixed units, most serous cells occur distally on short mucous tubules, often assuming "serous demilune" (Fr., half-moon) arrangements (Figure 16–5a). In addition to α-amylase and proline-rich proteins, serous cells of the submandibular gland secrete **lysozyme** which hydrolyses bacterial walls.
- **Sublingual glands**, the smallest of the major glands, also consist of branched tubuloacinar units, having a few serous acini but mostly short tubules of mucous cells, with mucus as their main product (Figure 16–5b). The serous cells there add amylase and lysozyme to the secretion.

As described in Chapter 15 small, nonencapsulated salivary glands also occur distributed throughout the oral mucosa and submucosa with short ducts to the oral cavity. These minor salivary glands are usually mucous, except for the small serous (von Ebner) glands at the bases of circumvallate papillae. Plasma cells releasing IgA also commonly appear within the minor salivary glands.

› PANCREAS

The **pancreas** develops as a mixed exocrine-endocrine gland producing both digestive enzymes and hormones. It is an elongated retroperitoneal organ, with a large head portion near the duodenum and more narrow body and tail regions extending away to the left (Figure 16–7). The pancreas has a very thin capsule of connective tissue, from which septa extend to cover the larger vessels and ducts and to separate the parenchyma into lobules (Figure 16–8). Each secretory acinus is covered by a basal lamina surrounded only by a delicate sheath of reticular fibers, forming a sparse stroma but with a rich capillary network. Endocrine function of the pancreas involves primarily smaller cells resembling enteroendocrine cells and occurring in variously sized clusters called the **pancreatic islets** (islets of Langerhans). These are described with the endocrine organs in Chapter 20.

connective tissue layers. The unusual lining of these ducts appears to combine various epithelial types, including simple cuboidal or columnar, stratified cuboidal or columnar, and pseudostratified epithelia, distributed in no apparent pattern. These atypical epithelia may reflect their composition of cells with many diverse functions, including cells for ion reabsorption, cells for secretion of mucin and other proteins, enteroendocrine cells, and basal stem cells, all in highly branched ducts of small diameter. Before emptying into the oral cavity, the main duct of each gland becomes lined with nonkeratinized stratified squamous epithelium.

Vessels and nerves enter the large salivary glands at a hilum and gradually branch into the lobules, forming a rich vascular and nerve plexus surrounding the secretory and duct components. The capillaries surrounding the secretory units provide fluid important for saliva production, stimulated by the autonomic nervous system. Parasympathetic stimulation, usually elicited through the smell or taste of food, provokes a

FIGURE **16–5** Submandibular gland and sublingual gland.

(a) The **submandibular gland** is a mixed serous and mucous gland, with serous cells predominating, and shows well-stained serous acini (**A**) and "serous demilunes" (**S**) and pale-staining mucous cells (**M**) grouped as tubules in this tubuloacinar gland. (The crescent-shaped "serous demilunes" appear to arise at least in part artifactually, due to disproportionate swelling of the adjacent

mucous cells during tissue processing.) Small intralobular ducts (**ID**) drain each lobule. (×340; H&E)

(b) The **sublingual gland** is a mixed but largely mucous gland with a tubuloacinar arrangement of poorly stained mucous cells (**M**). Small intralobular ducts (**ID**) are seen in connective tissue, as well as small fascicles of lingual striated muscle (**SM**). (×140; H&E)

❯❯ MEDICAL APPLICATION

Pancreatic cancer, usually a carcinoma of pancreatic duct cells, can arise anywhere in the gland but occurs most often in the head of the organ near the duodenum. The disorder usually remains asymptomatic until growth and metastasis are well advanced, leading to the low rate of early detection and subsequent high rate of mortality. Metastasis may be facilitated by the relatively sparse connective tissue around the ducts and vasculature of the pancreas.

The digestive enzymes are produced by cells of serous acini in the larger exocrine portion of the pancreas (Figure 16–9a). With well-stained acinar cells and little stroma,

pancreatic acinar tissue somewhat resembles the parotid gland histologically, except that pancreas lacks striated ducts and the parotid glands lack islets of endocrine cells. Each pancreatic acinus consists of several serous cells surrounding a very small lumen, without myoepithelial cells (Figure 16–9). The acinar cells are pyramidal and polarized, with round basal nuclei and numerous apical zymogen granules, typical features of protein-secreting cells (Figures 16–9 and 16–10).

Each acinus is drained by a short **intercalated duct** of simple squamous or low cuboidal epithelium. The initial cells of these small ducts extend into the lumen of the acinus as small pale-staining **centroacinar cells** that are unique to the pancreas. Cells of the intercalated ducts secrete a large volume of fluid, rich in HCO_3^- (bicarbonate ions), which alkalinizes

FIGURE **16–6** Striated ducts.

(a) A striated duct (**SD**) shows faint striations in the basal half of the columnar cells, which represent mitochondria located in the folds of the lateral cell membrane. (×200; H&E)

(b) SEM indicates that the apical ends of the cells are joined together near the small lumen (**L**), with interdigitating folds of cell membrane best developed at the basal end (**B**). (×4000)

(c) SEM shows the bases (**B**) of several such cells with the basal lamina removed, revealing the interlocking of folded membrane between neighboring cells. Mitochondria within the folds supply energy for rapid ion uptake from saliva. (×4000)

and transports hydrolytic enzymes also produced in the acini. The intercalated ducts merge with **intralobular ducts** and larger **interlobular ducts**, which have increasingly columnar epithelia before joining the main pancreatic duct that runs the length of the gland.

The exocrine pancreas secretes approximately 1.5 L of alkaline pancreatic juice per day and delivers it directly into the duodenum where the HCO_3^- ions neutralize the acidic chyme entering there from the stomach and establish the pH for optimal activity of the pancreatic enzymes. These digestive enzymes include several **proteases**, **α-amylase**, **lipases**, and **nucleases** (**DNAase** and **RNAase**). The proteases are secreted as inactive zymogens (**trypsinogen**, **chymotrypsinogen**, proelastase, kallikreinogen, and procarboxipeptidases). Trypsinogen is cleaved and activated by enteropeptidases in the duodenum, generating trypsin that activates the other proteases in a cascade. Pancreatic tissue itself is protected against autodigestion by the following features:

- Restricting protease activation to the duodenum;
- Trypsin inhibitor, which is packaged in the secretory granules along with trypsinogen; and

- The high pH in the acini and duct system due to HCO_3^- secreted by the centroacinar and intercalated duct cells, which helps keep all the enzymes inactive.

›› MEDICAL APPLICATION

In **acute pancreatitis**, the proenzymes may be activated and digest pancreatic tissues, leading to very serious complications. Possible causes include infection, gallstones, alcoholism, drugs, and trauma. **Chronic pancreatitis** can produce progressive fibrosis and loss of pancreatic function.

Regulation of exocrine secretion in the pancreas happens mainly through two polypeptide hormones produced by enteroendocrine cells of the small intestine:

- **Cholecystokinin (CCK)**, which stimulates enzyme secretion by the acinar cells, and
- **Secretin**, which promotes water and HCO_3^- secretion by the duct cells.

Autonomic (parasympathetic) nerve fibers also stimulate secretion from both acinar and duct cells.

FIGURE **16–7** Pancreas and duodenum.

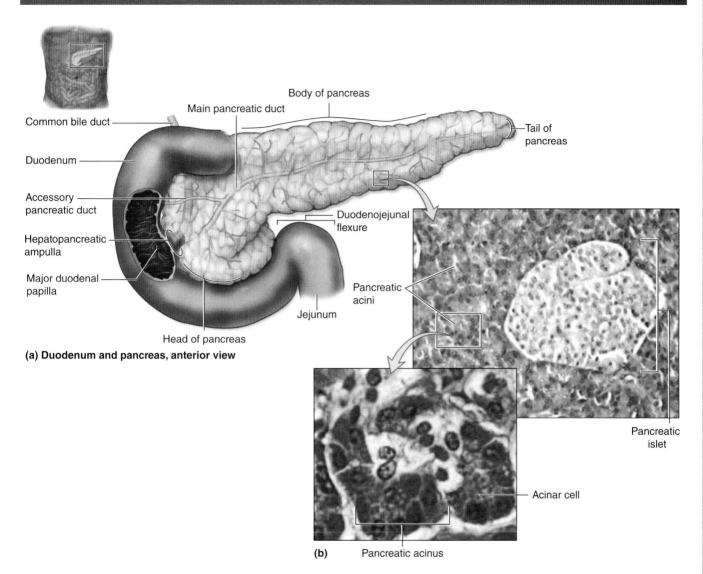

(a) Duodenum and pancreas, anterior view

- Common bile duct
- Duodenum
- Accessory pancreatic duct
- Hepatopancreatic ampulla
- Major duodenal papilla
- Head of pancreas
- Main pancreatic duct
- Body of pancreas
- Tail of pancreas
- Duodenojejunal flexure
- Jejunum
- Pancreatic acini
- Pancreatic islet
- Acinar cell

(b) Pancreatic acinus

(a) The main regions of the **pancreas** are shown in relation to the two **pancreatic ducts** and the **duodenum**.

(b) Micrographs showing a **pancreatic islet** and two **pancreatic acini**. (×75 and ×200; H&E)

›› MEDICAL APPLICATION

In the normal liver dense connective tissue occurs mostly in the portal areas, surrounding the blood vessels and bile ductule. In liver **cirrhosis**, which occurs late in **chronic liver disease**, fibrosis and proliferation of fibroblasts and hepatic stellate cells occur beyond the portal areas. The excessive connective tissue may disrupt the normal hepatic architecture and interfere with liver function.

› LIVER

The **liver** is the largest internal organ, in adults averaging about 1.5 kg or 2% of the body weight, and is supported by ligaments in the right upper quadrant of the abdomen just below the diaphragm (see Figure 15–1). The liver has two major lobes, left and right, with the latter much larger and comprising two other smaller inferior lobes. Deep fissures incompletely separate these four hepatic lobes, each enclosed by a thin layer of fibrous connective tissue called Glisson's capsule. The serous mesothelium of the visceral peritoneum covers most of this capsule, except where the liver maintains contact with the diaphragm or other organs. The capsule thickens as loose connective tissue at the hilum (or porta hepatis) on the inferior side, where the **dual blood supply** from the **hepatic portal vein** and **hepatic artery** enters the organ and where lymphatics and the left and right hepatic (bile) ducts exit.

The main digestive function of the liver is production of **bile**, a complex substance required for the emulsification, hydrolysis, and uptake of fats in the duodenum. As the organ

FIGURE **16–8** Pancreas.

Low-power view of **pancreas** includes several islets (**I**) surrounded by many smaller serous acini (**A**). The larger intra-lobular ducts (**D**) are lined by simple columnar epithelium. The ducts and blood vessels (**V**) are embedded in con-nective tissue, which also provides a thin capsule to the entire gland and thin septa separating the lobules of secretory acini. (×20; H&E)

FIGURE **16–9** Pancreatic acini.

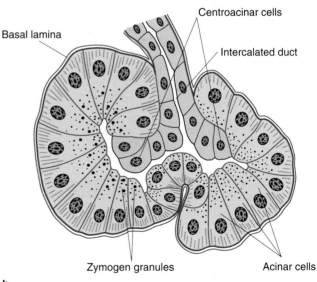

Centroacinar cells

Basal lamina

Intercalated duct

Zymogen granules

Acinar cells

(a) Micrograph of **exocrine pancreas** shows the serous, enzyme-producing cells arranged in small acini (**A**) with very small lumens. Acini are surrounded by only small amounts of connective tissue with fibroblasts (**F**). Each acinus drains into an intercalated duct with its initial cells, the centroacinar cells (**arrow**), inserted into the acinar lumen. (×200; H&E)

(b) The diagram shows the arrangement of cells more clearly. Under the influence of secretin, the **centroacinar** and **interca-lated duct cells** secrete a copious HCO_3^--rich fluid that hydrates, flushes, and alkalinizes the enzymatic secretion of the acini.

FIGURE **16–10** Pancreatic acinar cell ultrastructure.

TEM of a pancreatic acinar cell shows its pyramidal shape and the round, basal nucleus (**N**) surrounded by cytoplasm packed with cisternae of rough ER (**RER**). The Golgi apparatus (**G**) is situated at the apical side of the nucleus and is associated with condensing vacuoles (**C**) and numerous secretory granules (**S**) with zymogen.

The small lumen (**L**) of the acinus contains proteins recently released from the cell by exocytosis. Exocytosis of digestive enzymes from secretory granules is promoted by CCK, released by enteroendocrine cells of the duodenum when food enters that region from the stomach. (×8000)

in which nutrients absorbed in the small intestine undergo processing before distribution throughout the body, the liver also serves as the major interface between the digestive and circulatory systems. About 75% of the blood entering the liver is nutrient-rich (but O_2-poor) blood from the portal vein arising from the stomach, intestines, and spleen; the other 25% comes from the hepatic artery and supplies the organ with O_2.

Hepatocytes (Gr. *hepar*, liver), the key cells of this organ, are among the most functionally diverse cells of the body. In addition to an exocrine function in the secretion of bile components, hepatocytes and other liver cells process the contents of blood through many specific activities:

■ Synthesis and endocrine secretion into the blood of the major **plasma proteins**, including albumins, fibrinogen, apolipoproteins, transferrin, and many others;

■ Conversion of amino acids into glucose (**gluconeogenesis**);

■ Breakdown (**detoxification**) and conjugation of ingested toxins, including many drugs;

■ Amino acid **deamination**, producing **urea** removed from blood in kidneys;

■ **Storage of glucose** in glycogen granules and **triglycerides** in small lipid droplets;

■ **Storage of vitamin A** and other fat-soluble vitamins in **hepatic stellate cells**;

- Removal of effete erythrocytes by specialized macrophages called **Kupffer cells**; and
- **Storage of iron** in complexes with the protein **ferritin**.

Hepatocytes & Hepatic Lobules

The liver's unique histologic organization and microvasculature allow hepatocytes to perform their diverse metabolic, exocrine, and endocrine functions. Hepatocytes are large cuboidal or polyhedral epithelial cells, with big, round central nuclei and eosinophilic cytoplasm rich in mitochondria. The cells are frequently binucleated and about 50% of them are polyploid, with two to eight times the normal chromosome number.

The liver parenchyma becomes organized as thousands of small (~0.7 × 2 mm) **hepatic lobules** in which hepatocytes form hundreds of irregular plates arranged radially around a small **central vein** (Figures 16–11 through 16–13). The hepatocyte plates are supported by a delicate stroma of reticulin fibers (Figure 16–13b). Peripherally each lobule has three to six portal areas with more fibrous connective tissue, each containing three interlobular structures that make up the **portal triad** (Figures 16–11 and 16–13d):

FIGURE 16–11 Liver.

(a) Hepatic lobules

Hepatic sinusoid
Hepatocytes
Hepatic lobule
Central vein
Bile canaliculi

To inferior vena cava
To hepatic veins
Central vein
Mixing of arterial and venous blood

(b) Hepatocytes and sinusoids

Bile canaliculi
Reticuloendothelial cell
Hepatic sinusoid
Hepatocyte
Portal triad
Bile ductule
Branch of hepatic portal vein
Branch of hepatic artery
Oxygenated blood from aorta
Deoxygenated but nutrient-rich blood from digestive organs

(c) Portal triad and hepatic lobule

C   PV   H   L   B   HA

The **liver**, a large organ in the upper right quadrant of the abdomen, immediately below the diaphragm, consists of thousands of polygonal structures called **hepatic lobules**, which are the basic functional units of the organ.

(a) Diagram showing a small **central vein** in the center of a hepatic lobule and several sets of blood vessels at its periphery. The peripheral vessels are grouped in connective tissue of the **portal tracts** and include a branch of the portal vein, a branch of the hepatic artery, and a branch of the bile duct (the **portal triad**).

(b) This diagram indicates the flow of arterial (red) and venous (blue) blood from two vessels in the portal tract, and how this blood mixes in the **hepatic sinusoids**. Both blood vessels branch and join sinusoids which run between plates of **hepatocytes** and drain into the central vein. Flow of bile to a bile ductule is also shown here (green).

(c) Micrograph of a **lobule** shows the central vein (**C**), plates of hepatocytes (**H**), and in an adjacent portal area a small lymphatic (**L**) and components of the **portal triad**: a portal venule (**PV**), hepatic arteriole (**HA**), and bile ductule (**B**). (×220; H&E)

FIGURE **16–12** Hepatic lobule.

Cut transversely, **hepatic lobules** appear as polygonal units with numerous irregular plates of **hepatocytes** converging on a central venule (**C**).

(a) Hepatic lobules in some mammalian livers, such as the pig liver shown here, are very well delimited by connective tissue (arrows) on all sides.

(b) In humans, these lobules have much less connective tissue and their boundaries are more difficult to distinguish. In both cases, peripheral connective tissue of portal areas contains the portal triad: small bile ductules (**D**), venule (**V**) branches of the portal vein, and arteriole (**A**) branches of the hepatic artery. (Both ×150; H&E)

- A **venule** branch of the portal vein, with blood rich in nutrients but low in O₂,
- An **arteriole** branch of the hepatic artery, which supplies O₂, and
- One or two small **bile ductules** of cuboidal epithelium, branches of the bile conducting system.

Most of the peripheral portal areas also contain lymphatics and nerve fibers and, in some species (eg, pigs), extend thicker sheets of fibrous connective tissue completely around the lobules, making individual lobules easier to distinguish than in human liver sections. (Figure 16–12b).

Between all the anastomosing plates of hepatocytes of a hepatic lobule are important vascular **sinusoids**, which emerge from the peripheral branches of the portal triad's portal vein and hepatic artery and converge on the lobule's **central vein** (Figures 16–11 through 16–13c). Mixing of venous and arterial blood, from those two vascular components of the portal triad, occurs in these irregular hepatic sinusoids. The anastomosing sinusoids have thin, discontinuous linings of fenestrated endothelial cells surrounded by sparse basal lamina and reticular fibers. The endothelial discontinuities and fenestrations allow plasma to fill a narrow **perisinusoidal space** (or **space of Disse**) and directly bathe the many

irregular microvilli that project from the hepatocytes into this space (Figure 16–14). This direct contact between hepatocytes and plasma facilitates most key hepatocyte functions involving uptake and release of potential toxins, proteins, and nutrients.

Two other functionally important cells occur along the sinusoids of hepatic lobules:

- Numerous specialized **stellate macrophages**, usually called **Kupffer cells**, are localized within the sinusoid lining (Figure 16–15). These monocyte-derived cells recognize and phagocytose aged erythrocytes, freeing heme and iron for local reuse or storage in ferritin complexes. Kupffer cells are also antigen-presenting cells and remove bacteria or debris present in the portal blood.
- Occurring in the perisinusoidal space, **hepatic stellate cells** (or **Ito cells**) contain small lipid droplets, which store vitamin A and other fat-soluble vitamins (Figure 16–15b). These mesenchymal cells, which are difficult to see in routine preparations, also produce extracellular matrix (ECM) components (becoming myofibroblasts after liver injury) and cytokines that help regulate Kupffer cell activity.

The endothelium of the central vein in the middle of each hepatic lobule supports a very thin layer of fibrous connective tissue (Figure 16–13c). Central venules from each lobule

FIGURE **16–13** Hepatic lobule microvasculature.

(a) Hepatocytes (**H**) are polygonal epithelial cells, which form branching, irregular plates separated by venous sinusoids (**S**). (H&E ×400)

(b) Reticulin (collagen type III) fibers (**R**) running along the plates of hepatocytes (**H**), supporting these and the intervening sinusoids. Most connective tissue in the liver is found in the septa and portal tracts. (×400; Silver)

(c) With plates of hepatocytes (**H**) converging on it, the central vein (**C**) of the lobule has more collagen than the smaller sinusoids (**S**) that drain into it from all directions (arrows). (×200; Mallory trichrome)

(d) Peripheral portal areas contain most of the connective tissue and each houses a **portal triad**: a portal venule (**PV**), an arteriole branching off the hepatic artery (**HA**), and one or two bile ductules (**BD**). (×200; H&E)

converge into larger veins, which eventually form three major and several minor **hepatic veins**, all of which empty into the inferior vena cava.

Blood flows unidirectionally in each hepatic lobule, from the peripheral triads to the center. Consequently, oxygen and metabolites, along with toxic substances absorbed in the intestines, reach the lobule's peripheral cells first and then the more central cells. Reflecting this structure, the properties and functions of the periportal hepatocytes differ from those of the cells near the central venule. Hepatocytes near the portal areas can rely on aerobic metabolism and display more active protein synthesis, while the more central cells exist with lower concentrations of nutrients and oxygen and become more specialized for detoxification and glycogen metabolism.

While the sinusoidal (basolateral) domains of hepatocytes process nutrients and other blood components and secrete

FIGURE **16–14** Ultrastructure of hepatocytes, perisinusoidal space, and bile canaliculi.

(a) TEM of **hepatocytes** shows small bile canaliculi (**BC**) between tight junctions (**TJ**) joining two cells. A hepatocyte nucleus (**H**) is in the lower right corner, surrounded by small tubular vesicles of smooth ER (**SER**), much rough ER (**RER**), many mitochondria (**M**), small electron-dense glycogen granules, and Golgi complexes (**G**). Between the hepatocytes and the fenestrated endothelial cell (**E**) of the sinusoid (**S**) is the very small perisinusoidal space (**PS**) almost filled with **microvilli**. (×9500)

(b) SEM of the luminal surface of the endothelium lining a hepatic sinusoid shows grouped fenestrations (**F**). At the border are seen cut edges of endothelial cells (**E**) in this discontinuous sinusoid and hepatocytes (**H**). Between these two cells is the narrow perisinusoidal space (**PS**), into which project **microvilli** from the hepatocytes surface. (×6500)

(c) SEM of hepatocytes (**H**) broken apart from one another reveals the length of a bile canaliculus (**BC**) along the cell's surface. Such canaliculi run between the cells of the hepatocyte plates in the hepatic lobules and carry bile toward the portal areas where the canaliculi join cuboidal bile ductules. (×8000)

(Figure 16–14a, reproduced with permission from Douglas L. Schmucker, Department of Anatomy, University of California, San Francisco, CA. Figure 16–14b, reproduced with permission from Eddie Wisse, Electron Microscopy Unit, Department of Pathology, University of Maastricht, Maastricht, the Netherlands.)

plasma proteins, the smaller apical surfaces of the hepatocytes form **bile canaliculi** for exocrine secretion of bile (Figures 16–14 and 16–16). Within the hepatic plates, hepatocytes adhere together firmly with desmosomes and junctional complexes. At specific locations, however, the apical surfaces of two adherent hepatocytes become grooved and juxtaposed to form the canaliculus, sealed by tight junctions, into which bile

components are secreted (Figure 16–14). Running between hepatocytes these canaliculi represent elongated spaces (total length >1 km!) with lumens only 0.5–1 μm in diameter but large surface areas due to the many short microvilli projecting from the constituent hepatocytes (Figures 16–14 and 16–16).

The bile canaliculi form a complex anastomosing network of channels through the hepatocyte plates that end near

FIGURE **16–15** Hepatic sinusoids.

In the endothelial lining of the **hepatic sinusoids** are numerous specialized stellate macrophages or **Kupffer cells**, which detect and phagocytose effete erythrocytes.

(a) Kupffer cells (**K**) appear here as black cells in a liver lobule from a rat injected with particulate India ink. (×200; H&E)

(b) In a plastic section, Kupffer cells (**K**) are seen in the sinusoid (**S**) between two groups of hepatocytes (**H**) and larger than the

flattened endothelial cells (**E**). Between the endothelium and the hepatocytes is a very narrow space called the perisinusoidal space (**PS**) of Disse, in which are located small hepatic stellate cells (**HS**), or Ito cells, which maintain the sparse ECM of this compartment and also store vitamin A in small lipid droplets. These cells are numerous but are difficult to demonstrate in routine histologic preparations. (×750; PT)

the portal tracts (Figures 16–11b and 16–17). The bile flow progresses in a direction opposite to that of the blood, that is, from the center of the lobule to its periphery. Bile canaliculi are the smallest branches of the biliary tree or bile conducting system. At the portal tract they empty into bile **canals of Hering** (Figure 16–17) composed of cuboidal epithelial cells called **cholangiocytes**. These short bile canals quickly merge in the portal areas with the **bile ductules** lined by cuboidal or columnar cholangiocytes and distinctly sheathed by connective tissue. Bile ductules gradually merge, enlarge, and form the right and left **hepatic ducts** leaving the liver.

Into the canaliculi hepatocytes continuously secrete bile, a mixture of **bile acids** (organic acids such as cholic acid), **bile salts** (the deprotonated forms of bile acids), electrolytes, fatty acids, phospholipids, cholesterol, and **bilirubin**. Some bile components are synthesized in hepatocyte SER, but most are taken up from the perisinusoidal space; all are quickly secreted into the bile canaliculi (Figure 16–16). Bile acids/salts have an important function in emulsifying the lipids in the duodenum, promoting their digestion and absorption.

Bilirubin represents a pigmented breakdown product of heme released primarily from splenic macrophages and carried to hepatocytes bound to albumen, but also from Kupffer cells. Released into the duodenum with bile, bilirubin is converted by intestinal bacteria into other pigmented products, some of which are absorbed in the intestinal mucosa to be

processed and excreted again in the liver or excreted into urine by the kidneys. These bilirubin-related compounds give feces and urine their characteristic colors.

> **≫ MEDICAL APPLICATION**
>
> The **fibrosis** characteristic of **cirrhosis** produces connective tissue that can fill the perisinusoidal space and interfere with metabolic exchange between the hepatocytes and the sinusoids. Blockage of hepatocyte secretion into the blood can result in **clotting disorders**, **hypoalbuminemia**, and other medical problems.

Hepatocytes & Liver Functions

As mentioned previously, hepatocytes are highly versatile cells with diverse functions reflected in their cytoplasmic contents (Figure 16–16). Abundant **rough ER** produces mainly plasma proteins and causes cytoplasmic basophilia, more pronounced in hepatocytes near the portal areas (Figure 16–12). As discussed more fully below, hepatocytes deeper in the lobules have more **smooth ER**, the site of enzyme systems for the biotransformation or detoxification of substances removed from blood in the sinusoids, processed, and then usually excreted with bile. These enzymes include those responsible for oxidation, methylation, and conjugation of steroids, barbiturates,

FIGURE **16–16** Hepatocyte ultrastructure and major functions.

A diagram of hepatocyte cytoplasmic organization, with locations of its major functions.

(**1**) RER is primarily engaged in synthesis of **plasma proteins** for release into the perisinusoidal space.

(**2**) Potentially toxic compounds bilirubin (bound to albumin) and bile acids are taken up from the perisinusoidal space, processed by enzymes in the tubulovesicular system of the SER, and secreted into the **bile canaliculi**.

(**3**) Glucose is taken up from the perisinusoidal space and stored in **glycogen granules**, with the process reversed when glucose is needed.

antihistamines, anticonvulsants, and other drugs. Under some conditions prolonged presence of drugs can lead to increased amounts of SER in hepatocytes, thus enhancing the liver's detoxification capacity. Other SER enzymes (glucuronosyl transferases) conjugate bilirubin to glucuronate, rendering it more soluble and facilitating its excretion in bile.

Glycogen granules and small **lipid droplets** in hepatocytes, and very small electron-dense **ferritin complexes** (hemosiderin) primarily in the Kupffer cells, respectively mediate temporary storage of glucose, triglycerides, and iron.

Hepatocyte **peroxisomes** are also abundant and important for oxidation of excess fatty acids, catalase-mediated breakdown of hydrogen peroxide generated by fatty acid oxidation (by catalase activity), and conversion of excess purines to uric acid. Many **Golgi complexes** are also present, involved in synthesis of both plasma proteins and bile components. The numerous mitochondria provide energy for all these activities (Figure 16–16).

❯❯ MEDICAL APPLICATION

Fatty liver disease develops as a reversible condition in which large lipid droplets containing triglycerides accumulate abnormally in hepatocytes via the process called **steatosis**. This disorder has multiple causes, but it occurs most commonly in individuals with **alcoholism** or **obesity**. Accumulation of fat in hepatocytes may produce a progressive inflammation of the liver, or **hepatitis**, in this case called **steatohepatitis**.

FIGURE **16–17** Bile ductules.

Near the periphery of each hepatic lobule, many **bile canaliculi** join with the larger **bile canals** of Hering, which are lined by cuboidal epithelial cells called **cholangiocytes**. These canals soon join the **bile ductules** in the portal areas and drain into the biliary tree.

The different categories of hepatocyte functions—including secretion of proteins into blood, the exocrine secretion of bile, and the removal of diverse small compounds from blood—have led to three ways of considering liver lobule structure, as summarized in Figure 16–18.

■ The classic **hepatic lobule** (Figure 16–18a), with blood flowing past hepatocytes from the portal areas to the central venule, emphasizes the endocrine function of the structure producing factors for uptake by the blood.

■ The concept of **portal lobules** of hepatocytes is more useful when considering the exocrine function of these cells, bile secretion. The roughly triangular portal area has a bile ductule as its central feature (Figure 16–18b), into which bile drains along many canaliculi between hepatocytes in two or more classic hepatic lobules. In

this structure the central venules of the classic lobules occur peripherally, as shown diagrammatically in Figure 16–18b which depicts one portal lobule with the central veins of three classic lobules at its corners.

■ The **hepatic acinus**, a third way of viewing liver cells, highlights the dual nature of their blood supply and the oxygen gradient from the hepatic artery branch to the central vein. In a liver acinus, hepatocytes make up an irregular oval or diamond-shaped area extending from two portal triads to the two closest central veins (Figure 16–18c). Periportal hepatocytes, nearest the hepatic arteriole, comprise zone I in the acinus, get the most oxygen and nutrients and can most readily carry out functions requiring oxidative metabolism, such as protein synthesis. Hepatocytes in zone III, near the central vein, get the least oxygen and nutrients. These cells make up

FIGURE 16–18 Concepts of structure-function relationships in liver.

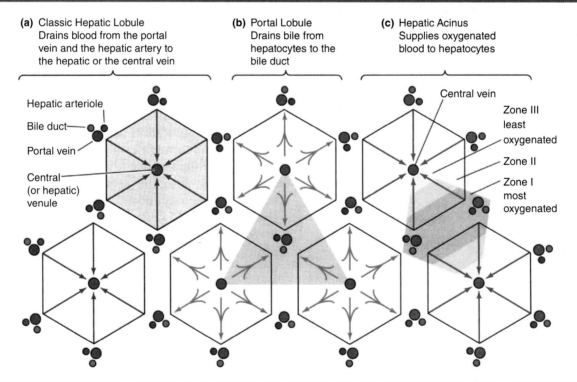

(a) Classic Hepatic Lobule
Drains blood from the portal vein and the hepatic artery to the hepatic or the central vein

(b) Portal Lobule
Drains bile from hepatocytes to the bile duct

(c) Hepatic Acinus
Supplies oxygenated blood to hepatocytes

Hepatic arteriole
Bile duct
Portal vein
Central (or hepatic) venule

Central vein
Zone III least oxygenated
Zone II
Zone I most oxygenated

Studies of liver microanatomy, physiology, and pathology have given rise to three related ways to view the liver's organization, which emphasize different aspects of hepatocyte activity.

(a) The **classic lobule** concept offers a basic understanding of the structure-function relationship in liver organization and emphasizes the endocrine function of hepatocytes as blood flows past them toward the central vein.

(b) The **portal lobule** emphasizes the hepatocytes' exocrine function and the flow of bile from regions of three classic lobules toward the bile duct in the portal triad at the center here. The area drained by each bile duct is roughly triangular.

(c) The **hepatic acinus** concept emphasizes the different oxygen and nutrient contents of sinusoidal blood at different distances from the portal tract, with microvasculature from each portal area supplying sinusoids and cells in two or more classic lobules. Major activities of each hepatocyte are determined by its location along the oxygen/nutrient gradient from the portal tract to the central venule: periportal cells of zone I get the most oxygen and nutrients and show metabolic activity generally different from the pericentral hepatocytes of zone III, exposed to the lowest oxygen and nutrient concentrations. Many pathologic changes in the liver are best understood from the point of view of liver acini.

the preferential sites for glycolysis, lipid formation, and drug biotransformations and are the first hepatocytes to undergo fatty accumulation and ischemic necrosis. Hepatocytes in the transitional zone II have a range of metabolic functions intermediate between those in zones I and III. The major activities in any given hepatocyte result from the cell adapting to the microenvironment produced by the contents of the blood to which it is exposed.

›› MEDICAL APPLICATION

An important function of hepatocyte SER is the conjugation of hydrophobic (water-insoluble), yellow bilirubin by glucuronosyl transferases to form water-soluble, nontoxic bilirubin glucuronide, which is excreted into the bile canaliculi. When bilirubin glucuronide is not formed or excreted properly, various diseases characterized by jaundice can result.

A frequent cause of jaundice in newborns is an underdeveloped state of the hepatocyte SER (neonatal hyperbilirubinemia). A treatment in these cases is exposure to blue light from ordinary fluorescent tubes, which transforms unconjugated bilirubin into a water-soluble photoisomer that can be excreted by the kidneys.

Unlike the salivary glands and pancreas, the liver has a strong capacity for **regeneration** despite its normal slow rate of cell renewal. Hepatocyte loss from the action of toxic substances triggers mitosis in the remaining healthy hepatocytes in a process of **compensatory hyperplasia** that maintains the original tissue mass. Surgically removing a portion of the liver produces a similar response in the hepatocytes of the remaining lobe(s). The regenerated liver tissue is usually well organized, with the typical lobular architecture, and replaces the functions of the destroyed or missing tissue. This regenerative capacity has clinical importance because a major liver lobe can often be donated by a living relative for surgical transplantation, with full liver function eventually restored in both donor and recipient.

Besides proliferation of existing hepatocytes, a role for **liver stem cells** in regeneration has been shown in some experimental models. Such cells, often called **oval cells**, are present among cholangiocytes of the bile canals near portal areas and produce progenitor cells for both hepatocytes and cholangiocytes.

›› MEDICAL APPLICATION

Most malignant tumors of the liver derive from hepatocytes or cholangiocytes of the hepatic ducts. The pathogenesis of **liver carcinoma** is associated with a variety of acquired disorders, such as **chronic viral hepatitis** (B or C) and cirrhosis.

› BILIARY TRACT & GALLBLADDER

As already discussed, bile produced by the hepatocytes flows through the **bile canaliculi**, **bile ductules**, and **bile ducts**. As shown in Figure 16–19 these structures gradually merge in a network that ultimately forms the **common hepatic duct**, which branches as the **cystic duct** to the gallbladder and continues to the duodenum as the **common bile duct**.

The hepatic, cystic, and common bile ducts are all lined by mucous membranes having simple columnar epithelia of cholangiocytes. The lamina propria and submucosa are relatively thin, with mucous glands in some areas of the cystic duct, and surrounded by a thin muscularis. This muscle layer becomes thicker near the duodenum and finally, in the duodenal papilla, forms a sphincter that regulates bile flow into the small intestine.

The gallbladder develops as a hollow, pear-shaped organ (Figure 16–19) attached to the lower surface of the liver, capable of storing 30–50 mL of bile that is concentrated during storage. The wall of the gallbladder consists of a mucosa composed of simple columnar epithelium and lamina propria, a thin muscularis with bundles of muscle fibers oriented in several directions, and an external adventitia or serosa (Figure 16–20a). The mucosa has numerous folds that are particularly evident when the gallbladder is empty.

The tall cholangiocytes lining the gallbladder have prominent mitochondria, microvilli, and distinct intercellular spaces, all indicative of cells actively transporting water, in this case for concentrating bile (Figure 16–20b). The mechanism for this includes activity of Na^+ pumps in the basolateral membranes, followed by passive movement of water from the bile. To move stored bile into the duodenum, contraction of the gallbladder muscularis is induced by cholecystokinin (CCK) from enteroendocrine cells of the small intestine. Release of CCK occurs when those endocrine cells detect the presence of ingested fats. Gallbladder removal due to obstruction or chronic inflammation leads to the direct flow of bile from liver to gut, with few major consequences on digestion.

›› MEDICAL APPLICATION

Reabsorption of water from bile in the gallbladder is involved in the formation of **gallstones** in the lumen of the gallbladder or biliary ducts, a condition called **cholelithiasis**.

This disorder usually originates with bile that already contains excessive amounts of normal bile components. Supersaturation of cholesterol in bile can lead to the formation of **cholesterol stones**, the most common form. Brown or black **pigment stones** can form when bile contains excessive amounts of unconjugated bilirubin, which can result from chronic hemolysis associated with disorders such as sickle cell anemia. Gallstones can lead to biliary obstruction or more commonly to inflammation in **acute or chronic cholecystitis**.

FIGURE **16–19** Biliary tract and gallbladder.

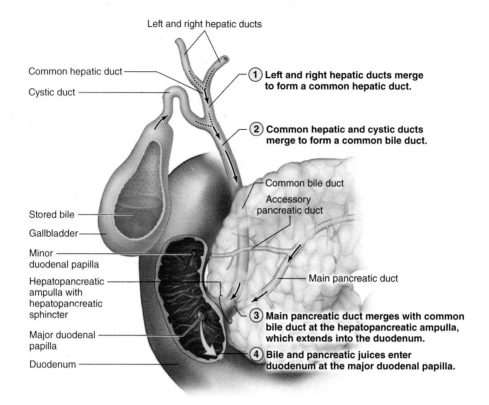

Left and right hepatic ducts

Common hepatic duct

Cystic duct

1 Left and right hepatic ducts merge to form a common hepatic duct.

2 Common hepatic and cystic ducts merge to form a common bile duct.

Common bile duct

Accessory pancreatic duct

Stored bile

Gallbladder

Minor duodenal papilla

Main pancreatic duct

Hepatopancreatic ampulla with hepatopancreatic sphincter

Major duodenal papilla

Duodenum

3 Main pancreatic duct merges with common bile duct at the hepatopancreatic ampulla, which extends into the duodenum.

4 Bile and pancreatic juices enter duodenum at the major duodenal papilla.

Bile leaves the liver in the left and right hepatic ducts (1), which merge to form the common hepatic duct, which connects to the cystic duct serving the gallbladder. The latter two ducts merge to form a common bile duct (2). All these ducts are lined by cuboidal or low columnar cells called **cholangiocytes**, similar to those of the small bile ductules in the liver.

The main pancreatic duct merges with the common bile duct at the hepatopancreatic ampulla, which enters the wall of the duodenum at a major papilla (of Vater) (3). The accessory pancreatic duct enters the duodenum at a minor papilla. Bile and pancreatic juice mix before their release into the duodenum at the major papilla (4).

Organs Associated with the Digestive Tract SUMMARY OF KEY POINTS

Salivary Glands

- **Salivary glands** have secretory units of either **protein-secreting serous cells**, usually organized in round or oval **acini**, or of **mucin-secreting mucous cells** in elongated **tubules**.
- **Parotid glands** have only serous acini; **sublingual glands** are mixed but have primarily mucous tubules, some with **serous demilunes**; **submandibular glands** are also mixed but have mainly serous acini.
- With help from **myoepithelial cells**, salivary secretory units drain into simple cuboidal **intercalated ducts**, which merge as simple columnar **striated ducts**, which merge further as the larger interlobular or **excretory ducts**.
- Cells of **striated ducts** have mitochondria-lined, basolateral membrane folds specialized for electrolyte reabsorption from the secretion; **excretory ducts** are unusual in having **stratified cuboidal or columnar** cells.

Pancreas

- **Pancreatic islets** of endocrine cells are embedded in exocrine **serous acinar tissue**, which comprises most of the pancreas and in which the cells secrete hydrolytic **digestive enzymes** for delivery to the duodenum.
- Each pancreatic **acinar cell** is pyramidal, with **secretory (zymogen) granules** in the narrow apical end and Golgi complexes, much rough ER, and a large nucleus at the basal end.
- **Intercalated ducts** draining pancreatic acini, including their initial **centroacinar cells** inserted into the acinar lumen, **secrete bicarbonate** ions (HCO_3^-) to neutralize chyme entering the duodenum from the stomach.

Liver

- Liver **hepatocytes** are large epithelial cells with large central nuclei (polyploid and often binucleated), much smooth and rough ER, and many small Golgi complexes.

FIGURE **16–20** Gallbladder.

The **gallbladder** consists of a saclike structure that stores and concentrates bile, and releases it into the duodenum after a meal.

(a) Its wall consists largely of a highly folded mucosa, with a simple columnar epithelium (arrows) overlying a typical lamina propria (**LP**); a muscularis (**M**) with bundles of muscle fibers oriented in all directions to facilitate emptying of the organ; and an external adventitia (**A**) where it is against the liver and a serosa where it is exposed. (×60; H&E)

(b) TEM of the epithelium shows cells specialized for water uptake across apical microvilli (**MV**) and release into the intercellular spaces (**arrows**) along the folded basolateral cell membranes. From these spaces, water is quickly removed by capillaries in the lamina propria. Abundant mitochondria provide the energy for this pumping process. Scattered apical secretory granules (**G**) contain mucus. (×5600)

- **Hepatocytes** have many functions, including endocrine (**plasma protein**) secretion, exocrine (**bile**) secretion, glucose storage (**glycogen granules**), and **detoxification** (using SER and peroxisomes).
- In the liver, **hepatocytes** develop within irregular plates of cells to form polygonal **hepatic lobules** in which the hepatocyte plates radiate toward a small **central vein**.
- Each hepatic lobule is surrounded by very sparse connective tissue that becomes more abundant in the **portal areas** at the lobule corners.
- **Portal areas** or tracts contain a small lymphatic and the **portal triad**: a **portal venule** branch from the portal vein, a **hepatic arteriole** branch of the hepatic artery, and a **bile ductule** branch of the biliary tree.
- In the lobules the portal venule and hepatic arteriole both branch into irregular **sinusoids** between the hepatic plates where the nutrient-rich and O$_2$-rich blood mixes, flows past hepatocytes, and drains to the central vein.

- The endothelium of the hepatic **sinusoids** is **discontinuous and fenestrated**; between it and the hepatocytes is the **perisinusoidal space (of Disse)** where exchange occurs between the hepatocytes and blood plasma.
- The sinusoidal endothelium includes many specialized **stellate macrophages** or **Kupffer cells**, which recognize and remove effete erythrocytes, **releasing iron and bilirubin** for uptake by hepatocytes.
- Also present in the perisinusoidal spaces are **hepatic stellate cells** (or Ito cells) containing many small lipid droplets for **storage of vitamin A** and other fat-soluble vitamins.
- Between adherent hepatocytes in the hepatic plates are grooves forming **bile canaliculi**, sealed by tight junctions, into which hepatocytes secrete water and **bile components**, including **bilirubin** and **bile acids**.
- In each hepatic lobule, all bile canaliculi converge on the **bile canals (of Hering)**, which join the **bile ductules** in the portal areas and eventually all merge to form the left and right **hepatic ducts**.

Biliary Tract and Gallbladder

- All bile-conducting structures after the bile canaliculi have an epithelial lining of simple cuboidal or columnar cells called **cholangiocytes**.
- The common hepatic duct leads to the cystic duct, which carries bile to the **gallbladder** for temporary **bile storage** and concentration.

- The mucosa of the **gallbladder** has many **folds** conferring a large surface area, a well-vascularized lamina propria, and a lining of **columnar cholangiocytes** specialized for water uptake from bile.
- Contraction of the gallbladder **muscularis** sends bile to the duodenum via the **common bile duct** and is induced by **cholecystokinin (CCK)** from enteroendocrine cells in the duodenum when food is present.

Organs Associated with the Digestive Tract ASSESS YOUR KNOWLEDGE

1. In a liver biopsy from a long-time drug user which of the following hepatocyte organelles would be expected to be more extensive than normal?
   a. Rough endoplasmic reticulum
   b. Golgi apparatus
   c. Lysosomes
   d. Peroxisomes
   e. Smooth endoplasmic reticulum

2. Which description is true of pancreatic zymogens?
   a. Are packaged for secretion in the SER
   b. Are synthesized on free ribosomes
   c. Are inactive until they reach the duodenal lumen
   d. Are stored in the basal cytoplasm of acinar cells
   e. Are produced by cuboidal cells lining the pancreatic duct

3. Which process increases in response to parasympathetic stimulation of the salivary glands?
   a. Volume of secretion
   b. Cell division in secretory acini
   c. Mucus content of saliva
   d. Inorganic salts content of saliva
   e. Cell division in interlobular ducts

4. Which feature is unique to the exocrine pancreas?
   a. Insulin-secreting β cells
   b. Centroacinar cells
   c. Predominately serous secretory cells
   d. Striated interlobular ducts
   e. Striated intralobular ducts

5. Which description is true of the bile canaliculi?
   a. Are bordered directly by endothelial cells.
   b. Are part of the portal triad.
   c. Are surrounded by the hepatic sinusoids.
   d. Lumens are entirely sealed by junctional complexes.
   e. Normally contain some blood plasma.

6. Which description is true of the gallbladder?
   a. Dilutes bile
   b. Absorbs bile
   c. Secretes mucus
   d. Has a thick submucosa
   e. Is covered entirely by serosa

7. Which description is true for the hepatic space of Disse?
   a. Is surrounded by the hepatic sinusoid.
   b. Contents flow toward the central vein.
   c. Is directly contacted by hepatocytes.
   d. Lumen sealed by junctional complexes.
   e. Contents empty into canals of Hering lined by cholangiocytes.

8. A 50-year-old woman presents to the family medicine clinic. She admits to drinking a six-pack of beer each day with a little more intake on weekends. Laboratory tests show elevated alanine aminotransferase/serum glutamic oxaloacetic transaminase (AST/SGOT). Her sclerae appear jaundiced and her serum bilirubin is 2.5 mg/dL (normal 0.3–1.9 mg/dL). A biopsy shows hepatic fibrosis with significant loss of normal lobular structure. Jaundice is most likely to result when the proper location or orientation of what hepatic structures is disrupted?
   a. Central veins
   b. Spaces of Disse
   c. Kupffer cells
   d. Hepatocytes
   e. Merging sinusoids

9. A 48-year-old woman is referred to an allergy and rheumatology specialist with itching eyes, dryness of the mouth, difficulty swallowing, loss of the sense of taste, hoarseness, fatigue, and swollen parotid glands. She reports increasing joint pain over the past 2 years. She complains of frequent mouth sores. Laboratory tests show a positive antinuclear antibody (ANA) and rheumatoid factor (RF) levels of 70 U/mL (normal <60 U/mL) by the nephelometric method. A parotid gland biopsy shows inflammatory infiltrates in the interlobular connective tissue with damage to the acinar cells and striated ducts. In this case, resorption of which of the following will be most altered by destruction of those ducts?
   a. Na^+
   b. H_2O
   c. HCO_3^-
   d. Cl^-
   e. Ca^{2+}

10. A young child presents with hepatomegaly and renomegaly, failure to thrive, stunted growth, and hypoglycemia. A deficiency in glucose-6-phosphatase is identified and the diagnosis of von Gierke disease is made. What cellular structures would be expected to accumulate in hepatocytes during progression of this disorder?
    a. Chylomicrons
    b. Glycogen granules
    c. Mitochondria
    d. Zymogen granules
    e. Ribosomes

17 The Respiratory System

The respiratory system provides for exchange of O_2 and CO_2 to and from the blood. Respiratory organs include the **lungs** and a branching system of bronchial tubes connecting the sites of gas exchange with the external environment. Air moves through the lungs by a ventilating mechanism that involves the thoracic cage, intercostal muscles, diaphragm, and elastic components of the lung tissue. As shown in Figure 17–1 anatomically the system consists of the upper and lower respiratory tracts. Functionally the system has two descriptive components:

- The **conducting portion**, which consists of the nasal cavities, pharynx, larynx, trachea, bronchi (Gr. *bronchos*, windpipe), bronchioles, and terminal bronchioles.
- The **respiratory portion**, where the system's main function of gas exchange occurs, consisting of respiratory bronchioles, alveolar ducts, and alveoli (Figure 17–1).

Alveoli, the cellular sites for the exchange of O_2 and CO_2 between inspired air and blood, are small, air-filled, saclike structures, which make up most of the lung structure.

The conducting portion cleans and humidifies inspired air and provides the conduits for air movement to and from alveoli. To ensure an uninterrupted supply of air, a combination of cartilage, collagen and elastic fibers, and smooth muscle provides the conducting portion with both rigid structural support and the necessary flexibility and extensibility.

❯ NASAL CAVITIES

The left and right nasal cavities each have two components: the external, dilated **vestibule** and the internal **nasal cavity**. Skin of the nose enters the **nares** (nostrils) partway into the vestibule and includes sweat glands, sebaceous glands, and coarse, moist **vibrissae** (hairs), which filter out particulate material from inspired air. Within the vestibule, the epithelium loses its keratinized nature and undergoes a transition to typical pseudostratified columnar epithelium which lines the nasal cavities.

The nasal cavities lie within the skull as two cavernous chambers separated by the bony **nasal septum**. Three curving projections called **conchae** (*L. concha*, seashell) or turbinate bones, extend from each side of the septum, forming partially separate passages that create turbulence in the air passing along them. The highly vascular mucosa covering the conchae and other parts of the nasal cavities conditions inhaled air. Loops of capillaries very near the epithelial surface carry blood in a general direction against the flow of inspired air, releasing heat that warms the air while water secreted from small seromucous glands humidifies it. A thin layer of surface mucus produced by these glands and goblet cells traps and removes small inhaled particles and microorganisms, with the latter also bound and inactivated by immunoglobulin A (IgA) from plasma cells in the lamina propria.

Respiratory epithelium covers the middle and inferior conchae; specialized olfactory epithelium spreads over the superior conchae along with the roof of the nasal cavities.

Respiratory Epithelium

The mucosa lining most regions of the nasal cavities and conducting portion of the respiratory system bears ciliated pseudostratified columnar epithelium, described with epithelia in Chapter 4 and commonly known as **respiratory epithelium**

FIGURE **17–1** Anatomy of the respiratory system.

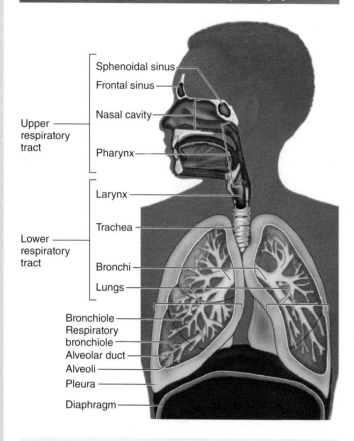

Sphenoidal sinus
Frontal sinus
Nasal cavity

Upper respiratory tract

Pharynx

Larynx

Trachea

Lower respiratory tract

Bronchi

Lungs

Bronchiole
Respiratory bronchiole
Alveolar duct
Alveoli
Pleura
Diaphragm

Anatomically, the respiratory tract has **upper** and **lower parts**. Histologically and functionally, the respiratory system has a **conducting portion**, which consists of all the components that condition air and bring it into the lungs, and a **respiratory portion**, where gas exchange actually occurs, consisting of respiratory bronchioles, alveolar ducts, and alveoli in the lungs. Portions of two sets of paranasal sinuses are also shown here.

(Figure 17–2). This epithelium consists of five major cell types, all of which contact an unusually thick basement membrane:

- **Ciliated columnar cells** are the most abundant, each with 250–300 cilia on its apical surface (Figure 17–2).
- **Goblet cells**, also numerous and predominant in some areas (Figure 17–2), have basal nuclei and apical domains filled with granules containing mucin glycoproteins.
- **Brush cells** represent a much less numerous, columnar cell type, in which the small apical surfaces bear sparse, blunt microvilli (Figure 17–2c). Brush cells are **chemosensory receptors** resembling gustatory cells, with similar signal transduction components and synaptic contact with afferent nerve endings on their basal surfaces.
- **Small granule cells** (or Kulchitsky cells) are difficult to distinguish in routine preparations but possess numerous dense core granules 100–300 nm in diameter. Like enteroendocrine cells of the gut, they are part of the **diffuse neuroendocrine system (DNES)** (see Chapter 20).

Like brush cells, they represent only about 3% of the cells in respiratory epithelium.
- **Basal cells** denote mitotically active stem and progenitor cells that give rise to the other epithelial cell types.

❯❯ MEDICAL APPLICATION

The chronic presence or accumulation of toxins that occur with heavy cigarette smoking or industrial air pollution affects the respiratory epithelium beginning in the nasal cavities. Immobilization of the cilia causes failure to clear mucus containing filtered material and exacerbates the problem, leading eventually to the likelihood of **squamous metaplasia** of the epithelium. A change from pseudostratified ciliated columnar to stratified squamous epithelium can occur, particularly in the mucosa of bronchi. This can produce precancerous **cell dysplasia** in this tissue.

Olfactory Epithelium

The olfactory chemoreceptors needed for the sense of smell develop within the **olfactory epithelium**, a specialized region of the mucous membrane covering the superior conchae and roof of the nasal cavity. In adult humans it is about 10 cm² in area and up to 100 μm thick. This pseudostratified columnar epithelium has three major cell types (Figure 17–3):

- **Olfactory neurons** are bipolar neurons present throughout this epithelium. Their nuclei form an irregular row near the middle of the thick epithelium. The apical (luminal) pole of each olfactory cell forms a dendritic process, the tip of which projects into the overlying layer of watery mucus and expands as a knoblike structure. About 20 very long, nonmotile cilia emerge radially from basal bodies in this knob and collectively provide a large surface with transmembrane receptors for inhaled odorant molecules solubilized in the mucus. Receptor binding, either directly to odorant molecules or by recognizing small odorant-binding proteins that solubilize and carry hydrophobic odorants, triggers an action potential along the axons extending from these neurons basally. The axons leave the olfactory epithelium, uniting in the lamina propria as very small nerves that then pass to the brain through foramina in the **cribriform plate** of the ethmoid bone (Figure 17–3). From there they form the olfactory nerve (cranial nerve I) and eventually synapse with neurons in the olfactory bulb, part of the brain's elaborate decoding system for the sense of smell.
- **Supporting cells** or sustentacular cells are also columnar, have narrow bases and broad apexes containing the nuclei and extending microvilli into the fluid layer. Well-developed apical junctional complexes bind supporting cells to the olfactory cells, stabilizing the apical surface. Understanding of their complete repertoire remains poor, but some sustentacular cells ensheath olfactory cells and their axons, regulating the microenvironments

FIGURE 17–2 Respiratory epithelium.

Respiratory epithelium is the classic example of **pseudostratified ciliated columnar epithelium**.

(a) Details of this epithelium's structure vary in different regions of the respiratory tract, but it usually rests on a very thick basement membrane (**BM**), stained blue here with a trichrome stain, and has several cell types, some columnar, some basal, and all contacting the basement membrane.

Ciliated columnar cells are most abundant, with hundreds of long robust cilia (**C**) on each of their bulging apical ends that provide a lush cover of cilia on the luminal surface.

Most of the small, rounded cells at the basement membrane are stem cells and their differentiating progeny, which together make up about 30% of the epithelium.

Mucus-secreting goblet cells (**G**) and intraepithelial lymphocytes and dendritic cells are also present in respiratory epithelium. The lamina propria is well-vascularized (**V**). (×400; Mallory trichrome)

(b) Scanning electron microscopy (SEM) shows the luminal surface of goblet cells (**G**) among the numerous ciliated cells.

(c) SEM of another region shows that goblet cells (**G**) predominate in some areas, with subsurface accumulations of mucus evident in some (**arrows**). The film of mucus traps most airborne dust particles and microorganisms, and the ciliary movements continuously propel the sheet of mucus toward the pharynx for elimination. Other columnar cells, representing only about 3% of the cells in respiratory epithelium, are brush cells (**B**) with small apical surfaces bearing a tuft of short, blunt microvilli. (Both ×3000)

in some respects like astrocytes or nonmyelinating Schwann cells.

- **Basal cells** represent small, spherical, or cone-shaped cells near the basal lamina comprising the stem cells for the other two types, replacing the olfactory neurons every 1–2 months and support cells less frequently.

The lamina propria of the olfactory epithelium possesses tubuloacinar serous glands, the **olfactory glands** (of Bowman), secreting into the surface mucus a watery fluid containing lysozyme and other innate immune factors, IgA, together with some of the odorant-binding proteins important for olfactory neuron function.

Paranasal Sinuses

The **paranasal sinuses** develop as bilateral cavities in the frontal, maxillary, ethmoid, and sphenoid bones of the

skull (Figure 17–1), lined with thin respiratory epithelium with goblet cells. The lamina propria, continuous with the underlying periosteum, contains only a few small glands. The paranasal sinuses communicate with the nasal cavities through small openings; mucus produced there moves into the nasal cavities by the activity of the ciliated epithelial cells.

›› MEDICAL APPLICATION

Sinusitis is an inflammatory process of the sinuses that may persist for long periods of time, mainly because of obstruction of drainage orifices. Chronic sinusitis and **bronchitis** are components of **primary ciliary dyskinesia**, or Kartagener syndrome, an inherited genetic disorder characterized by defective ciliary action.

FIGURE **17–3** Olfactory mucosa.

(a) The **olfactory mucosa** covers the superior conchae bilaterally and sends axons from throughout its entire 10 cm² area to the brain via small openings in the cribriform plate of the ethmoid bone. It is a **pseudostratified epithelium**, containing basal stem cells and columnar support cells in addition to the **bipolar olfactory neurons**. The dendrites of these neurons expand at the mucosal surface and have long nonmotile cilia specialized with many membrane receptors for odor molecules. Binding such ligands causes depolarization which passes along axons to the olfactory bulb of the brain.

Head trauma causing damage to the ethmoid bone can produce loss or reduction of the sense of smell, **anosmia** or **hyposmia**, respectively, by severing olfactory nerve axons in the cribriform plate. Similar loss can occur with damage to the olfactory epithelium caused by intranasal drug use.

(b) Only a thin basement membrane separates the olfactory basal cells (**B**) from the underlying lamina propria (**LP**). Nuclei of the bipolar olfactory neurons (**ON**) lie in the middle of the pseudostratified olfactory epithelium, with a zone of supporting cell (**S**) nuclei above it. At the apical end of the cells are the nonmotile cilia (**C**), or olfactory hairs, and a layer of mucus (**M**). (×200; H&E)

The olfactory neurons are the best-known example of neurons capable of regular replacement due to **regenerative activity** of the epithelial stem cells from which they arise. For this reason, loss of the olfactory sense due to toxic fumes or physical injury to the olfactory mucosa itself is often temporary.

❯ PHARYNX

The left and right nasal cavities open posteriorly into the nasopharynx, the first part of the **pharynx** (Figure 17–1). The nasopharynx is lined by respiratory mucosa which contains the medial pharyngeal tonsil as well as the openings of the two auditory tubes from each middle ear cavity. It is continuous caudally with the posterior part of the oral cavity, the oropharynx (throat), the mucosa of which has nonkeratinized stratified squamous epithelium and includes the palatine and lingual tonsils. The oropharynx leads to a short, narrow region with similar lining, the laryngopharynx, continuous at its inferior end with both the larynx and the esophagus (Figure 17–1).

❯ LARYNX

The **larynx** is a short (4 cm × 4 cm) passage for air between the pharynx and the trachea (Figure 17–1). Its rigid wall is reinforced by hyaline cartilage (in the thyroid, cricoid, and the inferior arytenoid cartilages) and smaller elastic cartilages (in the epiglottis, cuneiform, corniculate, and the superior arytenoid cartilages), all of which are connected by ligaments. In addition to maintaining an open airway, movements of these cartilages by skeletal muscles participate in sound production during phonation.

The **epiglottis**, a flattened structure projecting from the upper rim of the larynx, serves to prevent swallowed food or fluid from entering that passage. Its upper, or lingual, surface has stratified squamous epithelium; at variable points on its laryngeal surface, this epithelium undergoes a transition to ciliated pseudostratified columnar (respiratory) epithelium. Mixed mucous and serous glands are found in the lamina propria beneath the epithelium.

Below the epiglottis and vestibule of the larynx, the mucosa projects bilaterally into the lumen with two pairs of folds separated by a narrow space or ventricle (Figure 17–4). The upper pair, the immovable **vestibular folds**, is partly covered with typical respiratory epithelium overlying numerous seromucous glands and occasional lymphoid nodules. The

FIGURE **17–4** Larynx.

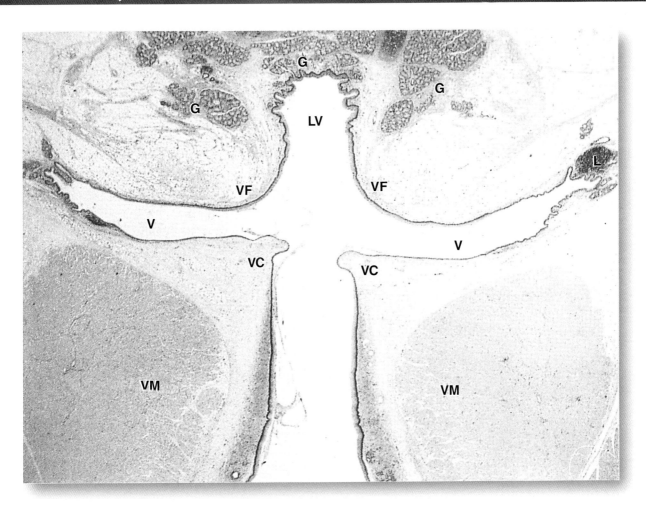

The **larynx** is a short air passage between the pharynx and trachea. Its wall contains skeletal muscles and pieces of cartilage, all of which make the larynx specialized for sound production, or phonation. This low-power micrograph shows the laryngeal vestibule (**LV**), which is surrounded by seromucous glands (**G**). The lateral walls of this region bulge as a pair of vestibular folds (**VF**). These also contain seromucous glands and areolar tissue with MALT, often with lymphoid nodules (**L**), and are largely covered by respiratory epithelium, with regions near the epiglottis having stratified squamous epithelium.

Below each large vestibular fold is a narrow space or ventricle (**V**), below which is another pair of lateral folds, the vocal folds or cords (**VC**). These are covered by stratified squamous epithelium and project more sharply into the lumen. Each contains a large striated vocalis muscle (**VM**) and nearer the surface a small ligament, which is cut transversely, and therefore difficult to see here. Variable tension of these ligaments caused by the muscles produces different sounds as air is expelled across the vocal cords. All the structures and spaces above these folds add resonance to the sounds, assisting phonation. (×15; H&E)

lower pair of folds, the **vocal folds** (or cords), have features important for phonation or sound production:

- Each vocal fold is covered with nonkeratinized stratified squamous epithelium that protects the mucosa from abrasion and desiccation from rapid air movement.
- A dense regular bundle of elastic connective tissue, the vocal ligament, supports the free edge of each vocal fold.
- Deep to the mucosa are large bundles of striated fibers comprising the **vocalis muscle** that allow each vocal fold to be moved.

During phonation muscles of the larynx draw the paired vocal folds together (adduction), which narrows the opening between them, the **rima glottidis**, and air expelled from the lungs causes the adducted vocal folds (cords) to vibrate and produce sound.

The pitch and other qualities of the sound are altered by changing the tension on the vocal folds, the width of the rima glottidis, the volume of air expelled, etc. The vestibular folds and ventricles, along with other structures and spaces higher in the respiratory tract, contribute to the resonance of sound produced in the larynx. Speech is produced when sounds made in the larynx are modified by movements of the pharynx, tongue, and lips. The larynx is larger and the vocal folds longer in males than in females after puberty, causing men's voices typically to have a deeper range than women's voices.

> ❯❯ **MEDICAL APPLICATION**
>
> Inflammation of the larynx, or **laryngitis**, is typically due to viral infection and is usually accompanied by **edema** or swelling of the organ's lamina propria. This changes the shape of the vocal folds or other parts of the larynx, producing **hoarseness** or complete **loss of voice**. Croup is a similar syndrome in young children in which edema of the laryngeal mucosa is accompanied by both hoarseness and **coughs** that typically are loud and harsh. Benign reactive polyps, called **singer's nodules**, are frequent in the stratified squamous epithelium of the true vocal cords, affecting the voice.

❯ TRACHEA

The **trachea**, 10–12 cm long in adults, is lined with typical respiratory mucosa in which the lamina propria contains numerous seromucous glands producing watery mucus (Figure 17–5). A series with about a dozen C-shaped rings of hyaline cartilage between the submucosa and adventitia reinforces the wall and keeps the tracheal lumen open (Figure 17–6). The open ends of the cartilage rings are on the posterior surface, against the esophagus, and are bridged by a bundle of smooth muscle called the **trachealis muscle** and a sheet of fibroelastic tissue attached to the perichondrium.

The trachealis muscle relaxes during swallowing to facilitate the passage of food by allowing the esophagus to bulge into the lumen of the trachea, with the elastic layer preventing excessive distention of the lumen. The muscle strongly contracts in the cough reflex to narrow the tracheal lumen and provide for increased velocity of the expelled air and better loosening of material in the air passage.

Table 17–1 summarizes the major features of all the upper respiratory tract structures.

> ❯❯ **MEDICAL APPLICATION**
>
> **Coughing** is a reflex action produced most often by viral infection or other irritation of the trachea or other region of the respiratory tract. A persistent **dry cough**, in which no mucus (phlegm) is produced, can be treated by **cough suppressants** that act on the brainstem and vagus nerve, while **productive coughs** are often treated with **expectorants** that help loosen mucus covering the respiratory mucosa.

FIGURE **17–5** Tracheal wall.

The **trachea** is lined by typical respiratory epithelium (**RE**) underlain by connective tissue of the lamina propria (**LP**) and seromucous glands (**G**) in the lamina propria and submucosa. Adjacent to the submucosa are the C-shaped rings of hyaline cartilage (**C**) covered by perichondrium (**P**). (×50; H&E)

FIGURE **17–6** Bronchial tree.

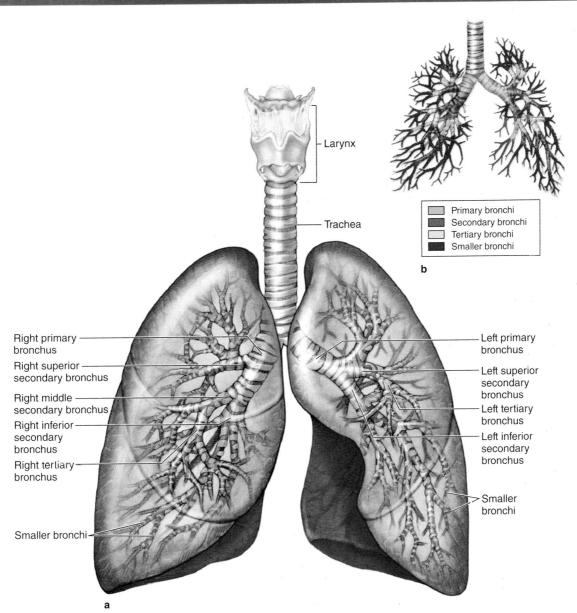

Larynx

Trachea

Primary bronchi
Secondary bronchi
Tertiary bronchi
Smaller bronchi

b

Right primary bronchus

Right superior secondary bronchus

Right middle secondary bronchus

Right inferior secondary bronchus

Right tertiary bronchus

Smaller bronchi

Left primary bronchus

Left superior secondary bronchus

Left tertiary bronchus

Left inferior secondary bronchus

Smaller bronchi

a

The **trachea** bifurcates as right and left **primary bronchi** that enter the hilum on the posterior side of each **lung** along with the pulmonary vessels, lymphatics, and nerves.

(a) Within each lung, bronchi subdivide further to form the **bronchial tree**, the last component of the air conducting system.

(b) The small diagram shows the color-coded major branches of the bronchial tree.

The vast surface area of the lungs, including the bronchial trees and the many million alveoli they support, makes the lung highly susceptible to inhaled pathogens escaping the defenses in the upper respiratory tract. Such pathogens include a variety of common bacteria and viruses capable of causing bronchitis, pneumonia, influenza, and other respiratory diseases.

❯ BRONCHIAL TREE & LUNG

The trachea divides into two **primary bronchi** that enter each lung at the hilum, along with arteries, veins, and lymphatic vessels. After entering the lungs, the primary bronchi course downward and outward, giving rise to three **secondary (lobar) bronchi** in the right lung and two in the left lung (Figure 17–6),

each of which supplies a pulmonary lobe. These lobar bronchi again divide, forming **tertiary (segmental) bronchi**. Each of the tertiary bronchi, together with the smaller branches it supplies, constitutes a **bronchopulmonary segment**—approximately 10%–12% of each lung with its own connective tissue capsule and blood supply. The existence of such lung

TABLE 17–1	Histologic features of the upper respiratory tract, larynx, and trachea.			
Region	**Epithelium**	**Glands**	**Musculoskeletal Support**	**Other Features and Major Functions**
Vestibules of nasal cavities	Stratified squamous, keratinized to nonkeratinized	Sebaceous and sweat glands	Hyaline cartilage	Vibrissae (stiff hairs) and moisture both filter and humidify air
Most areas of nasal cavities	Respiratory	Seromucous glands	Bone and hyaline cartilage	Rich vasculature and glands warm, humidify, and clean air
Superior areas of nasal cavities	Olfactory, with bipolar neurons	Serous (Bowman) glands	Bone (ethmoid)	Solubilize and detect odorant molecules in air
Nasopharynx and posterior oropharynx	Respiratory and stratified squamous	Seromucous glands	Bone and skeletal muscle	Conduct air to larynx; pharyngeal and palatine tonsils
Larynx	Respiratory and stratified squamous	Mucous glands, smaller seromucous glands	Elastic and hyaline cartilage, ligaments, skeletal muscle	Site for phonation; epiglottis closes while swallowing
Trachea	Respiratory	Mainly mucous glands, some serous or mixed glands	C-shaped rings of hyaline cartilage, with smooth (trachealis) muscle in posterior opening of each	Conduct air to primary bronchi entering lungs; some MALT

segments facilitates the specific surgical resection of diseased lung tissue without affecting nearby healthy tissue.

The tertiary bronchi give rise to smaller and smaller bronchi, whose terminal branches are called **bronchioles**. Each bronchiole enters a pulmonary lobule, where it branches to form five to seven **terminal bronchioles**. The pulmonary lobules are each pyramid-shaped, with the apex aimed at the pulmonary hilum, and each is delineated by a thin layer of connective tissue, which in adults is frequently incomplete. Moving through the smaller bronchi and bronchioles toward the respiratory portion, the histological organization of both the epithelium and the underlying lamina propria gradually becomes more simplified (Table 17–2).

Bronchi

Each primary bronchus branches repeatedly, with each branch becoming progressively smaller until it reaches a diameter of 1–2 mm. The mucosa of the larger bronchi is structurally similar to the tracheal mucosa except for the organization of cartilage and smooth muscle (Figure 17–7). In the primary bronchi, most cartilage rings completely encircle the lumen, but as the bronchial diameter decreases, cartilage rings are gradually replaced with smaller isolated plates of hyaline cartilage. Small mucous and serous glands are abundant, with ducts opening into the bronchial lumen. The lamina propria also contains crisscrossing bundles of spirally arranged smooth muscle and elastic fibers (Figures 17–7 and 17–8), which become more

TABLE 17–2	Features of airways within the lungs.		
Region of Airway	**Epithelium**	**Muscle and Skeletal Support**	**Other Features and Major Functions**
Bronchi	Respiratory	Prominent spiral bands of smooth muscle; irregular hyaline cartilage plates	Repeated branching; conduct air deeper into lungs
Bronchioles	Simple ciliated cuboidal to columnar, with exocrine club cells	Prominent circular layer of smooth muscle; no cartilage	Conduct air; important in bronchoconstriction and bronchodilation
Terminal bronchioles	Simple cuboidal, ciliated cells and club cells	Thin, incomplete circular layer of smooth muscle; no cartilage	Conduct air to respiratory portions of lungs; exocrine club cells with several protective and surfactant functions
Respiratory bronchioles	Simple cuboidal, ciliated cells and club cells, with scattered alveoli	Fewer smooth muscle fibers, mostly around alveolar openings	Conduct air deeper, with some gas exchange, and protective and surfactant functions of club cells
Alveolar ducts and sacs	Simple cuboidal between many alveoli	Bands of smooth muscle around alveolar openings	Conduct air, with much gas exchange
Alveoli	Types I and II alveolar cells (pneumocytes)	None (but with network of elastic and reticular fibers)	Sites of all gas exchange; surfactant from type II pneumocytes; dust cells

FIGURE **17–7** Tertiary (segmental) bronchus.

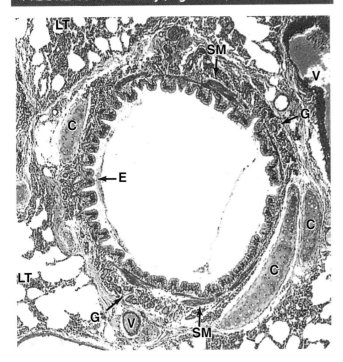

In a cross section of a tertiary bronchus, the lining of respiratory epithelium (**E**) and the mucosa are folded due to contraction of its smooth muscle (**SM**). At this stage in the bronchial tree, the wall is also surrounded by many pieces of hyaline cartilage (**C**) and contains many seromucous glands (**G**) in the submucosa which drain into the lumen. In the connective tissue surrounding the bronchi can be seen arteries and veins (**V**), which are also branching as smaller and smaller vessels in the approach to the respiratory bronchioles. All bronchi are surrounded by distinctive lung tissue (**LT**) showing the many empty spaces of pulmonary alveoli. (×56; H&E)

prominent in the smaller bronchial branches. Contraction of this muscle layer is responsible for the folded appearance of the bronchial mucosa observed histologically in cross sections.

Numerous lymphocytes are found both within the lamina propria and among the epithelial cells. Lymphatic nodules are present, especially at the branching points of the bronchial tree. Like the smooth muscle and elastic fibers, mucosa-associated lymphoid tissue (MALT) also becomes relatively more abundant as bronchi become smaller and the cartilage and other connective tissue are reduced.

Bronchioles

Bronchioles are the intralobular airways with diameters of 1 mm or less, formed after about the tenth generation of branching; they lack both mucosal glands and cartilage, although dense connective tissue is associated with the smooth muscle (Figure 17–9). In the larger bronchioles, the epithelium is still ciliated pseudostratified columnar, but this decreases in height and complexity to become ciliated simple columnar or

simple cuboidal epithelium in the smallest **terminal bronchioles**, which are the last parts of the air conducting system. The ciliated epithelial lining of bronchioles begins the **mucociliary apparatus** or escalator, important in clearing debris and mucus by moving it upward along the bronchial tree and trachea.

›› MEDICAL APPLICATION

Bronchioles constitute the air passages affected most often, especially in young children, by the **measles virus** or **adenovirus**, both of which can cause **bronchiolitis**. If persistent, the inflammation produced by either infection can lead to **obliterative bronchiolitis**, complete or partial closure of the airway lumen due to fibrosis in the wall. Most types of **lung cancer** are **carcinomas** involving epithelial cells lining the larger segments of bronchi, not bronchioles.

The cuboidal epithelium of terminal bronchioles consists largely of **club cells** or bronchiolar exocrine cells (previously called Clara cells), with nonciliated, dome-shaped apical ends containing secretory granules (Figure 17–10). These exocrine cells have various functions, including the following:

- **Secretion of surfactant** lipoproteins and mucins in the fluid layer on the epithelial surface,
- **Detoxification** of inhaled xenobiotic compounds by enzymes of the SER, and
- Secretion of **antimicrobial peptides** and cytokines for local immune defense.

Also present in the terminal bronchiole epithelium are chemosensory **brush cells** and **DNES small granule cells** like those of the epithelium higher in the respiratory system. A small population of stem cells provides for replacement of the other bronchiolar cell types.

The bronchiolar lamina propria still contains elastic fibers and smooth muscle, producing folds in the mucosa. Muscular contraction in both the bronchi and the bronchioles is controlled primarily by nerves of the autonomic nervous system.

›› MEDICAL APPLICATION

Asthma is a common condition produced by chronic inflammation within the bronchial tree of the lungs. The disorder is characterized by sudden constrictions of the smooth muscle in bronchioles called **bronchospasms**, or bronchial spasms. Constriction is caused by mast cell degranulation triggered by the presence of specific antigens. The resulting difficulty in breathing can be very mild to severe. **Epinephrine** and other sympathomimetic drugs relax the muscle and increase the bronchiole diameter by stimulating the sympathetic nervous system, and they are administered during asthma attacks. When the thickness of the bronchial walls is compared with that of the bronchiolar walls, the bronchiolar muscle layer is seen to be proportionately greater.

FIGURE **17–8** Bronchial wall.

(a) The epithelial lining (**E**) of bronchi is mainly pseudostratified cili-ated columnar cells with a few goblet cells. The lamina propria (**LP**) contains the distinct layer of smooth muscle (**SM**) surrounding the entire bronchus. The submucosa is the site of the supporting cartilage (**C**) and the adventitia includes blood vessels (**V**) and nerves (**N**). Lung tissue (**LT**) directly surrounds the adventitia of bronchi. (×140; H&E)

(b) In the smaller bronchi the epithelium is primarily of columnar cells with cilia (arrows), with fewer goblet cells. The lamina propria has both smooth muscle (**SM**) and small serous glands (**G**) near cartilage (**C**). (×400; H&E)

Respiratory Bronchioles

Each terminal bronchiole subdivides into two or more **respiratory bronchioles**, which always include saclike **alveoli** and represent, therefore, the first part of this system's respiratory region (Figure 17–11). The respiratory bronchiolar mucosa resembles that of the terminal bronchioles, except for having a few openings to alveoli where gas exchange occurs. Smooth muscle and elastic connective tissue comprise the lamina propria and the epithelium consists of club cells, with simple squamous cells at the alveolar openings and extending into the alveolus. Proceeding distally along the respiratory

bronchioles, alveoli become more numerous and closer together.

>> **MEDICAL APPLICATION**

Obstruction of the air supply in bronchi due to excess mucus or to aspirated material can lead to collapse of pulmonary lobules as circulating blood absorbs gases from the affected alveoli. This condition, called **atelectasis**, is normally revers-ible when the blockage is relieved but, if persistent, can cause fibrosis and loss of respiratory function.

FIGURE **17–9** Bronchioles.

The smallest branches of the bronchial tree are the **bronchioles**, which lack supporting cartilage and glands.

(a) A large bronchiole has the characteristically folded respiratory epithelium (**E**) and prominent smooth muscle (arrows), but it is supported only by fibrous connective tissue (**CT**). (×140; H&E)

(b) Staining for elastic fibers reveals the high elastic content of the smooth muscle (**arrowhead**) associated with the muscle of a smaller bronchiole in which the epithelium is simple columnar

but still ciliated. Darkly stained elastic fibers are also present in the tunica media of a large arteriole (**A**) nearby and to a lesser extent in the accompanying venule (**V**). The connective tissue includes many lymphocytes (**L**) of diffuse MALT and lymphoid nodules. (×180; Aldehyde fuchsin)

(c) In very small bronchioles the epithelium (**E**) is reduced to simple cuboidal cells with cilia. Several layers of smooth muscle cells (**arrows**) comprise a high proportion of the wall. (×300; H&E)

Alveolar Ducts

The distal ends of respiratory bronchioles branch into tubes called **alveolar ducts**, which are completely lined by the openings of alveoli (Figures 17–11 and 17–12). Both the alveolar ducts and the alveoli themselves are lined with extremely attenuated squamous cells. In the thin lamina propria, a strand of smooth muscle cells surrounds each alveolar opening, and a network of elastic and collagen fibers supports both the duct and its alveoli.

Larger clusters of alveoli called **alveolar sacs** form the ends of alveolar ducts distally and occur occasionally along their length (Figures 17–11 and 17–12). The lamina propria is now extremely thin, consisting essentially of a web of **elastic** and **reticular fibers** that encircles the alveolar openings and closely surrounds each alveolus. Prominent in this sparse connective tissue, a network of **capillaries** also surrounds each alveolus.

FIGURE **17–10** Terminal bronchiole and exocrine bronchiolar cells.

The last parts of the air conducting system before the sites of gas exchange appear are called the **terminal bronchioles**.

(a) A terminal bronchiole has a mucosa with nonciliated cuboidal or low columnar epithelium (**E**), surrounded by only one or two layers of smooth muscle (**SM**) embedded in connective tissue (**CT**). Alveoli (**A**) are seen in the surrounding lung tissue. (×300; PT)

(b) Most of the epithelium here consists of exocrine bronchiolar cells, or **club cells** (**C**), with bulging domes of apical cytoplasm contain granules, as shown here in a plastic section. These cells have several important functions. They secrete components of surfactant which reduces surface tension and helps prevent collapse of the bronchioles. The P450 enzyme system of their smooth ER detoxifies potentially harmful compounds in air. In other defensive functions, the cells also produce the secretory component for the transfer of IgA into the bronchiolar lumen; lysozyme and other enzymes active against bacteria and viruses; and several cytokines regulating local inflammatory responses. Also included among the cuboidal cells are stem cells that give rise to all of the cells within the bronchiolar epithelium. (×500; PT)

❯❯ MEDICAL APPLICATION

Diffuse alveolar damage or **acute respiratory distress syndrome** can be produced by various types of injuries to the alveolar epithelial and the capillary endothelial cells. Common causes of such injuries include viral and bacterial respiratory tract infections and inhalation of toxic gases, chemicals, or air with excessive oxygen. With removal of the initiating factors, normal alveolar wall components can often be repaired and at least partial function restored.

FIGURE 17–11 Pulmonary circulation, terminal and respiratory bronchioles, and alveoli.

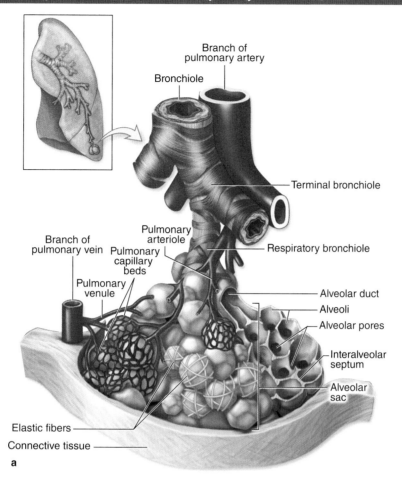

Branch of pulmonary artery

Bronchiole

Terminal bronchiole

Pulmonary arteriole

Respiratory bronchiole

Branch of pulmonary vein

Pulmonary capillary beds

Pulmonary venule

Alveolar duct

Alveoli

Alveolar pores

Interalveolar septum

Alveolar sac

Elastic fibers

Connective tissue

a

b

c

Terminal bronchioles branch into **respiratory bronchioles**, which then branch further into **alveolar ducts** and individual **alveoli**. Respiratory bronchioles are similar in most respects to terminal bronchioles except for the presence of scattered alveoli along their length.

(a) The diagram shows this branching relationship, as well as the **pulmonary blood vessels**, which parallel the bronchioles, and the dense layer of branching **capillaries** and **elastic fibers** surrounding each alveolus.

(b) The micrograph shows the branching nature of the air passages in two dimensions: respiratory bronchioles (**RB**), which open to alveolar ducts (**AD**), alveolar sacs (**AS**), and individual alveoli (**A**). (×60; H&E)

(c) SEM reveals better the three-dimensional, interconnected relationship of a terminal bronchiole (**TB**), respiratory bronchiole (**RB**), alveolar duct (**AD**), alveolar sacs (**AS**), and individual alveoli (**A**). (×180)

FIGURE **17–12** Respiratory bronchioles, alveolar ducts, and alveoli.

Lung tissue has a spongy structure because of the abundant air passages and pockets called alveoli.

(a) Typical section of lung tissue includes many bronchioles, some of which are respiratory bronchioles (**RB**) cut lengthwise, and shows the branching continuity with alveolar ducts (**AD**) and sacs (**AS**). Respiratory bronchioles still have a layer of smooth muscle and some regions of cuboidal epithelium, but alveolar ducts consist of a linear series of alveoli, each with smooth muscle fibers around the opening. Individual alveoli (**A**) all open to the sacs or ducts. The respiratory bronchiole runs along a

thin-walled branch of the pulmonary artery (**PA**), while branches of the pulmonary vein (**V**) course elsewhere in the parenchyma. (×14; H&E)

(b) Higher magnification shows the relationship of the many rounded, thin-walled alveoli (**A**) to alveolar ducts (**AD**). Alveolar ducts end in two or more clusters of alveoli called alveolar sacs (**AS**). Smooth muscle around the alveolar openings appears as eosinophilic "knobs" between adjacent alveoli. The alveoli here that do not show openings to the ducts or the sacs have their connections in planes of adjacent sections. (×140; H&E)

Alveoli

Alveoli are saclike evaginations, each about 200 μm in diameter, from the respiratory bronchioles, alveolar ducts, and alveolar sacs. Along with the airways, alveoli are responsible for the spongy structure of the lungs (Figures 17–11 and 17–12). Each adult lung has approximately 200 million alveoli with a total internal surface area of 75 m². Each alveolus resembles a small, rounded pouch open on one side to an alveolar duct or alveolar sac. Air in these structures exchanges O_2 and CO_2 with the blood in surrounding capillaries, through thin specialized alveolar walls that enhance diffusion between the external and internal environments.

Between neighboring alveoli lie thin **interalveolar septa** consisting of scattered fibroblasts and sparse extracellular matrix (ECM), notably elastic and reticular fibers, of connective tissue. The arrangement of elastic fibers enables alveoli to expand with inspiration and contract passively with expiration; reticular fibers prevent both collapse and excessive distention of alveoli. The interalveolar septa are vascularized with the richest capillary networks in the body (Figure 17–11).

The densely anastomosing pulmonary capillaries within the interalveolar septa are supported by the meshwork of reticular and elastic fibers in the alveolar walls. Air in the alveoli is separated from capillary blood by three components collectively referred to as the respiratory membrane or **blood-air barrier** (Figures 17–13 through 17–15):

- Two or three highly attenuated, thin cells lining the alveolus,
- The fused basal laminae of these cells and the endothelial cells of capillaries, and
- The thin capillary endothelial cells.

The total thickness of these layers varies from 0.1 to 1.5 μm. Macrophages and other leukocytes can also be found within the septa (Figures 17–13 and 17–14). **Alveolar pores** (of Kohn), ranging 10–15 μm in diameter, penetrate the interalveolar septa (Figure 17–13) and connect neighboring alveoli that open to different bronchioles. Such pores equalize air pressure in these alveoli and permit collateral circulation of air if a bronchiole becomes obstructed.

O_2 from the alveolar air diffuses through the blood-air barrier into the capillary blood and binds **hemoglobin** in erythrocytes; CO_2 diffuses into the alveolar air from the pulmonary blood. Most CO_2 arrives in the lungs as part of H_2CO_3 inside erythrocytes and is liberated through the action of carbonic anhydrase.

Capillary endothelial cells of alveolar walls are very thin, but continuous (not fenestrated) (Figure 17–15). Perinuclear clustering of most organelles allows the rest of the cell to become very thin and demonstrate highly efficient gas exchange. Ultrastructurally, the most prominent features in the flattened portions of the cell are numerous pinocytotic vesicles.

FIGURE **17–13** Alveoli and the blood-air barrier.

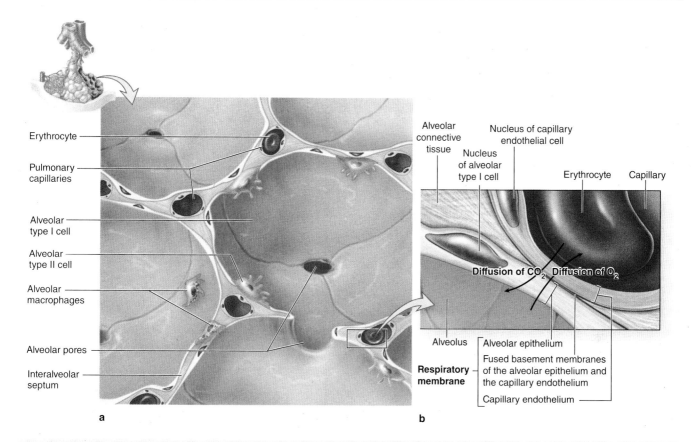

Erythrocyte

Pulmonary capillaries

Alveolar type I cell

Alveolar type II cell

Alveolar macrophages

Alveolar pores

Interalveolar septum

a

Alveolar connective tissue

Nucleus of capillary endothelial cell

Nucleus of alveolar type I cell

Erythrocyte   Capillary

Diffusion of CO_2 Diffusion of O_2

Alveolus

Respiratory membrane

Alveolar epithelium

Fused basement membranes of the alveolar epithelium and the capillary endothelium

Capillary endothelium

b

Gas exchange between air and blood occurs at a membranous barrier between each **alveolus** and the **capillaries** surrounding it.

(a) This diagram shows the relationship between capillaries in the **interalveolar septa** and the saclike **alveoli**. The **alveolar pores** (of Kohn) allow air pressure to equilibrate and air to circulate between alveoli on different ducts or sacs if the local airway becomes blocked.

(b) The **air-blood barrier** consists of an alveolar type I cell, a capillary endothelial cell, and their fused basement membranes. Oxygen diffuses through this barrier from alveolar air into capillary blood and carbon dioxide moves in the opposite direction. The inner lining of alveoli is covered by a layer of surfactant (not shown), which lowers fluid surface tension and helps prevent collapse of alveoli.

Type I alveolar cells (or **type I pneumocytes**) are also extremely attenuated cells lining the alveolar surfaces. Type I cells constitute the alveolar side of the blood-air barrier and make up about 95% of the alveolar lining; type II alveolar cells (described as follows) make up the remainder. Type I cells are so thin that the TEM was needed to demonstrate that all alveoli have such linings (Figure 17–15). Organelles here are also grouped around the nucleus, reducing the thickness of the remaining cytoplasm at the blood-air barrier to as little as 25 nm. Pinocytotic vesicles in the attenuated cytoplasm may play a role in the turnover of surfactant and the removal of small particulate contaminants from the outer surface. In addition to desmosomes, all type I epithelial cells have tight junctions that prevent the leakage of tissue fluid into the alveolar air space (Figure 17–16).

Type II alveolar cells (type II pneumocytes or septal cells) are cuboidal cells bulging into the air space, interspersed among the type I alveolar cells, and bound to them with tight junctions and desmosomes (Figure 17–16). Type II cells often occur in groups of two or three at points where two or more alveolar walls unite. These epithelial cells rest on the same basal lamina and have the same origin as the type I cells that line most of the alveolus. Type II cell nuclei are rounded and may have nucleoli, and their cytoplasm is typically lightly stained with many vesicles.

Many vesicles of type II alveolar cells are structures termed **lamellar bodies**, which TEM reveals to be membrane-bound granules 100–400 nm in diameter containing closely stacked parallel membrane lamellae (Figures 17–16 and 17–17). Lamellar bodies contain a variety of lipids, phospholipids, and proteins, which are continuously synthesized and released at the apical cell surface. The secreted material acts as **pulmonary surfactant** by spreading over the entire inner alveolar surface as a complex film of phospholipids and lipoproteins

FIGURE **17–14** Alveolar walls.

The septa between alveoli (**A**) contain several cell types. As seen here, the capillaries (**C**) include erythrocytes and leukocytes. The alveoli are lined mainly by squamous type I alveolar cells (**I**), which line almost the entire alveolus surface and across which gas exchange occurs. Type II alveolar cells line a bit of each alveolus and are large, rounded cells, often bulging into the alveolus (**II**). These type II cells have many functions of club cells, including production of surfactant. Also present are alveolar macrophages (**M**), sometimes called **dust cells**, which may be in the alveoli or in the interalveolar septa. (×450; H&E)

over a thin aqueous phase at the cell membranes. The surfactant film lowers surface tension at the air-epithelium interface, which helps prevent alveolar collapse at exhalation and allows alveoli to be inflated with less inspiratory force, easing the work of breathing.

Critical components of the surfactant layer produced by type II alveolar cells include the phospholipid **dipalmitoylphosphatidylcholine (DPPC)**, cholesterol, and four surfactant proteins (Figure 17–17). Surfactant protein A (SP-A), an abundant hydrophilic glycoprotein, and SP-D are important for innate immune protection within alveoli. SP-B and SP-C are hydrophobic membrane proteins required for the proper orientation of DPPC in the surfactant film lining the alveolus.

The surfactant layer turns over constantly, being gradually removed by pinocytosis in both types of alveolar cells and by macrophages. In fetal development, surfactant appears in the last weeks of gestation as type II cells differentiate and form lamellar bodies. Lack of adequate surfactant is a major cause of respiratory distress in premature neonates.

>> **MEDICAL APPLICATION**

Type II pneumocytes are the major target cell in lungs for the **severe acute respiratory syndrome coronavirus clade 2**, which causes **COVID-19**. The virus docks with a receptor, angiotensin-converting enzyme 2 (ACE2), an integral membrane protein that balances the activity of ACE on pulmonary capillaries by catalyzing hydrolysis of the vasoconstrictor peptide angiotensin II, thus helping to maintain blood pressure (see Chapter 19). Spike proteins on the coronavirus bind ACE2 on the type II cells, inducing endocytosis and translocation of the virus-enzyme complex into the cell's endosomal system, where the virus' coat is disassembled, and its RNA genome replicated and transcribed to begin new virus production. Infected cells reduce surfactant production, leading to alveolar collapse, reduced O_2-CO_2 exchange, and variable levels of hypoxia. Subsequent pathological changes locally include cell loss, fluid accumulation in alveoli and bronchioles, fibrin exudate from local capillaries, and edema.

FIGURE **17–15** Ultrastructure of the blood-air barrier.

TEM of a capillary (**C**) in an interalveolar septum shows areas for gas exchange between blood and air in three alveoli (**A**). The capillary endothelium is continuous but extremely thin, and its basal lamina (**B**) fuses with that of the type I alveolar cells (**I**) and type II cells. A fibroblast (**F**) can be seen in the septum, and the thickened nuclear regions of two endothelial cells (**E**) are also included. The nucleus at the bottom belongs to an endothelial cell or a circulating leukocyte. (×17,000)

Alveolar macrophages, also called **dust cells**, are found in alveoli and in the interalveolar septum (Figures 17–13 and 17–14). Millions of monocytes migrate daily from the microvasculature into the lung tissue, where they phagocytose excess surfactant, erythrocytes lost from damaged capillaries, and airborne particulate matter that has penetrated as far as alveoli. Active alveolar macrophages can often be distinguished from type II pneumocytes because they are slightly darker due to their content of dust and carbon from air and complexed iron (hemosiderin) from erythrocytes (Figure 17–14). Filled macrophages have various fates: most migrate into bronchioles where they move up the mucociliary apparatus for removal

into the esophagus; others exit the lungs in the lymphatic drainage; and some remain in the interalveolar septa connective tissue for years.

Alveolar lining fluids are also removed via the conducting passages as a result of the ciliary activity. As the secretions pass up through the airways, they combine with bronchial mucus to form **bronchoalveolar fluid**, which helps remove particulate components from inspired air. The bronchoalveolar fluid is bacteriostatic, containing lysozyme and other protective agents produced by club cells, type II alveolar cells, and alveolar macrophages.

Table 17–2 summarizes important histologic features and major functions at each level of the airways in lungs.

FIGURE **17–16** Ultrastructure of type II alveolar cells.

TEM of a **type II alveolar cell** protruding into the alveolar lumen shows unusual lamellar bodies (**L**), which contain newly synthesized pulmonary surfactant after processing of its components in rough ER (**RER**) and the Golgi apparatus (**G**). Smaller multivesicular bodies (**MVB**) with intraluminal vesicles are also present. Short microvilli (**M**) cover the apical cell surface at the alveolus (**A**)

lumen. The type II cell is attached via junctional complexes (**JC**) to the neighboring type I cell (**I**). Reticular fibers (**RF**) are prominent in the ECM. (×30,000)

(Reproduced with permission from Dr Mary C. Williams, Pulmonary Center Boston University School of Medicine, MA.)

❯❯ MEDICAL APPLICATION

In congestive heart failure, the lungs become congested with blood, and erythrocytes pass into the alveoli, where they are phagocytized by alveolar macrophages. In such cases, these macrophages are called **heart failure cells** when present in the lung and sputum; they are identified by a positive histochemical reaction for iron pigment (hemosiderin).

Regeneration in the Alveolar Lining

Inhalation of toxic gases or similar materials can kill type I and II cells lining pulmonary alveoli. Death of alveolar cells stimulates mitotic activity in the remaining type II cells, the progeny of which become progenitors for both cell types. The normal turnover rate of type II cells is estimated to be 1% per day and results in a continuous renewal of both

FIGURE **17-17** Type II alveolar cell function.

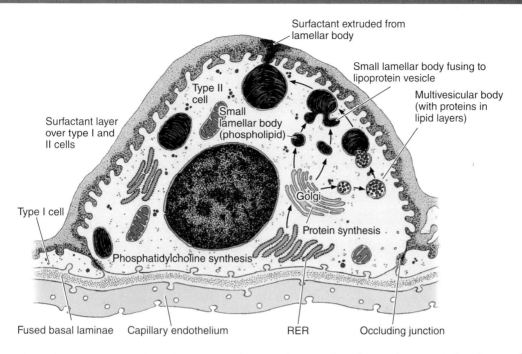

The diagram illustrates **surfactant production** by a **type II alveolar cell**. Surfactant contains protein-lipid complexes synthesized initially in the ER and Golgi apparatus, with further processing and storage in **lipoprotein vesicles** that fuse into large organelles called **lamellar bodies**.

Also present are smaller **multivesicular bodies**, which form when membrane components of an early endosome are sorted, invaginate, and pinch off into smaller vesicles inside the endosome's lumen. In surfactant-producing cells, the vesicles in multivesicular bodies are added to the lamellar bodies. Surfactant is secreted continuously by exocytosis and forms an oily film containing phospholipids and surfactant proteins.

Incomplete differentiation of type II alveolar cells is the leading cause of infant respiratory distress syndrome in premature babies, in whom the resulting deficit of surfactant leads to difficulty in expanding the alveoli for efficient respiratory exchange with breathing. Treatment involves insertion of an endotracheal tube to provide both continuous positive airway pressure (CPAP) and synthetic exogenous surfactant.

alveolar cells. With increased toxic stress, stem cells are also stimulated to divide and give rise to new alveolar cell progenitors.

❯ LUNG VASCULATURE & NERVES

Blood circulation in the lungs includes both the **pulmonary circulation**, carrying O_2-depleted blood for gas exchange, and **bronchial circulation**, carrying O_2-rich blood. The pulmonary arteries and veins are both relatively thin walled as a result of the low pressures (25 mm Hg systolic, 5 mm Hg diastolic) within the pulmonary circuit. Entering the lung at the hilum, the pulmonary artery branches and accompanies the bronchial tree (Figures 17–11 and 17–12), with its branches sharing the connective tissue of the bronchi and bronchioles. Beginning at the level of the respiratory bronchioles, branches of this artery give rise to dense capillary networks that surround each alveolus in the interalveolar septa.

❯❯ MEDICAL APPLICATION

Emphysema, a chronic lung disease most commonly caused by cigarette smoking, involves dilation and permanent enlargement of the bronchioles leading to pulmonary acini. Emphysema is accompanied by loss of cells in the alveoli and other parts of the airway walls, leading to an irreversible loss of respiratory function. Any type of infection in the respiratory regions of the lung produces the local inflammatory condition called **pneumonia**.

Venules arising from the capillary networks are found singly in the lung parenchyma, somewhat removed from the airways (Figures 17–11 and 17–12), supported by a thin covering of connective tissue. After small pulmonary veins leave a lobule, they follow the bronchial tree toward the hilum.

Bronchial arteries also enter the lung hilum and branch along with the bronchial tree, distributing blood to most of the lung down to the level of the respiratory bronchioles, at which point they anastomose with small branches of the pulmonary artery and mix their blood with that entering the capillary networks drained by pulmonary venules.

The lymphatic vessels originate in the connective tissue of bronchioles. They follow the bronchioles, bronchi, and pulmonary vessels and all drain into lymph nodes in the region of the hilum. This deep network of lymphatics parallels a superficial network draining areas near the lung surfaces located in the visceral pleura. Lymphatic vessels are not found in the terminal portions of the bronchial tree beyond the alveolar ducts.

Both parasympathetic and sympathetic autonomic fibers innervate the lungs and control reflexes regulating smooth muscle contractions which determine the diameters of the airways. General visceral afferent fibers, carrying poorly localized pain sensations, are also present. The nerves are found primarily in the connective tissue surrounding the larger elements of the bronchial tree and exit the lung at the hilum.

› PLEURAL MEMBRANES

The lung's outer surface and the internal wall of the thoracic cavity are covered by a serous membrane called the **pleura** (Figure 17–18). The membrane attached to lung tissue is called the **visceral pleura** and the membrane lining the thoracic walls is the **parietal pleura**. The two layers are continuous at the hilum and are both composed of simple squamous mesothelial cells on a thin connective tissue layer containing collagen and elastic fibers. The elastic fibers of the visceral pleura are continuous with those of the pulmonary parenchyma.

Between the parietal and visceral layers, the narrow **pleural cavity** (Figure 17–18) is entirely lined with the mesothelial cells producing a thin film of serous fluid, which acts as a lubricant, facilitating the smooth sliding of one surface over the other during respiratory movements.

In certain pathologic states, the pleural cavity may contain liquid or air. Like the walls of the peritoneal and pericardial cavities, the serosa of the pleural cavity is water-permeable, and fluid exuded from blood plasma commonly accumulates (as a pleural effusion) in this cavity during inflammation and other abnormal conditions.

›› MEDICAL APPLICATION

The condition **pneumothorax** is a partially or completely **collapsed lung** caused by air trapped in the pleural cavity, typically resulting from blunt or penetrating trauma to the chest and producing shortness of breath and hypoxia. Inflammation of the pleura, a condition called either **pleuritis** or **pleurisy**, is most commonly caused by an acute viral infection or pneumonia. **Pleural effusion** or fluid buildup in the pleural cavity produces shortness of breath and can be one result of inflamed pleura.

FIGURE 17–18 Pleura.

The **pleura** are serous membranes (serosa) associated with each lung and thoracic cavity. **(a)** The diagram shows the **parietal pleura** lining the inner surface of the thoracic cavity and the **visceral pleura** covering the outer surface of the lung. Between these layers is the narrow space of the pleural cavity.

(b) Both layers are similar histologically and consist of a simple squamous mesothelium (**M**) on a thin layer of connective tissue, as shown here for visceral pleura covering alveoli (**A**). The connective tissue is rich in both collagen and elastic fibers and contains both blood vessels (**V**) and lymphatics (**L**). (×140; H&E)

❯ RESPIRATORY MOVEMENTS

During inhalation, contraction of the external intercostal muscles elevates the ribs, and contraction of the diaphragm lowers the bottom of the thoracic cavity, increasing its diameter and resulting in pulmonary expansion. The bronchi and bronchioles increase in diameter and length during inhalation. The respiratory portion also enlarges, mainly as a result of expansion of the alveolar ducts. Individual alveoli enlarge only slightly. The elastic fibers of the pulmonary parenchyma are stretched by this expansion. During exhalation, the lungs retract passively because of muscle relaxation, and the elastic fibers' return to the unstretched condition.

❯❯ MEDICAL APPLICATION

Lung cancer is one of the most common forms of this disease. **Squamous cell carcinoma**, which is closely correlated with a history of smoking, arises most often from epithelial cells of segmental bronchi. **Adenocarcinoma**, the most common lung cancer in nonsmokers, usually arises from epithelial cells more peripherally, in bronchioles and alveoli. **Small cell carcinoma**, a less common but highly malignant form of lung cancer, develops after neoplastic transformation of small granule Kulchitsky cells in bronchial respiratory epithelium.

The Respiratory System SUMMARY OF KEY POINTS

- The function of the respiratory system is to provide **oxygen to the blood**, with a secondary function of sound production in the larynx.
- The respiratory system consists of an air **conducting region** (the upper respiratory tract in the head, as well as the larynx, trachea, bronchi, and most bronchioles) and a **respiratory region** with **alveoli**.

Nasal Cavities

- The left and right **nasal cavities** of the upper respiratory tract have **vestibules** where air enters and three projections called **conchae** from their medial walls, which create turbulence in inspired air.
- Moist **vibrissae** in the vestibular openings, the **nares** or nostrils, filter some material from inspired air.
- Deeper areas of the vestibules and the floor, lateral walls, and most of the conchae of the nasal cavities themselves are lined by **respiratory epithelium: pseudostratified ciliated columnar epithelium**.
- **Respiratory epithelium** includes **goblet cells** secreting mucus, **ciliated columnar cells** sweeping the mucus along the surface, chemosensory **brush cells**, scattered **endocrine cells**, and basal **stem cells**.
- The roof and part of the superior concha in each nasal cavity are covered by **olfactory epithelium**, which is pseudostratified epithelium containing bipolar **olfactory neurons**, **support cells**, and **stem cells**.
- The mucosa of the **nasal cavities** and **nasopharynx** also contains a rich vasculature and many **seromucous glands**, which help warm, humidify, and clean inspired air.

Larynx, Trachea, and Bronchial Tree

- Within the lumen of the **larynx**, bilateral projecting **vocal folds** (or cords) can be placed under variable tension by the underlying **vocalis muscles** and caused to vibrate by expelled air, producing sounds.
- The **trachea** is completely lined by **respiratory epithelium** and is supported by C-shaped rings of **hyaline cartilage**, with smooth **trachealis muscles** in the posterior opening of the rings.
- Left and right **primary bronchi** enter the two lungs and bifurcate repeatedly as **secondary**, **tertiary**, and **smaller segmental bronchi** with the lung tissue as the **bronchial tree**.

- **Bronchi** and their branches are lined by **respiratory mucosa**, with prominent spiraling bands of **smooth muscle**, **elastic fibers**, and increasingly smaller pieces of **hyaline cartilage**.
- Branches of the bronchial tree with diameters of 1 mm or less are generally called **bronchioles**, which are lined by **simple columnar** or **cuboidal ciliated cells**, with circular smooth muscle and elastic fibers, but **no cartilage**.
- **Terminal bronchioles** are the last branches to lack alveoli and are lined by **simple cuboidal epithelium** consisting mainly of **club cells**, which have **innate immune** and **surfactant secretory functions**.

Respiratory Region

- Terminal bronchioles subdivide into two or three **respiratory bronchioles**, lined by simple cuboidal epithelium and interrupted by scattered squamous evaginations called **alveoli**, the sites of gas exchange.
- A respiratory bronchiole leads to an **alveolar duct**, which is lined by a continuous series of alveoli, and which ends in a cluster of alveoli called the **alveolar sac**.
- All alveoli are surrounded by sparse connective tissue in **interalveolar septa** consisting primarily of **elastic and reticular fibers** and a dense **capillary network**.
- The wall of each alveolus consists of **alveolar cells**, or **pneumocytes**, of two types: extremely **thin type I alveolar cells** and cuboidal **type II alveolar cells** with **surfactant** secreting and **innate immune** properties.
- **Type II alveolar cells** are characterized ultrastructurally by unique cytoplasmic **lamellar bodies**, large granules with closely stacked layers of membrane involved in **surfactant synthesis**.
- The **blood-air barrier** allowing gas exchange at each alveolus consists of the **thin type I alveolar cell**, the **thin capillary endothelial cells**, and the **fused basal laminae** of these two cells.
- The **surfactant material** secreted by exocrine club cells and type II alveolar cells is an oily mixture of cholesterol, **phospholipids**, and **surfactant proteins**, which forms a film and **lowers surface tension** in alveoli.
- Each lung is covered by **visceral pleura**, a layer of thin connective tissue and mesothelium, and is continuous with **parietal pleura**, a similar tissue layer that lines the pleural cavity.

The Respiratory System ASSESS YOUR KNOWLEDGE

1. Which of the following components increase(s) as a proportion of the respiratory tract wall from trachea to alveoli?
   a. Cilia
   b. Elastic fibers
   c. Smooth muscle
   d. Cartilage
   e. Goblet cells

2. Air moving rapidly across the vocal cords and causing them to vibrate and produce sound is contacting what type of epithelium?
   a. Pseudostratified ciliated
   b. Stratified squamous keratinized
   c. Stratified squamous nonkeratinized
   d. Simple squamous
   e. Simple cuboidal

3. Which structural feature distinguishes between terminal and respiratory bronchioles?
   a. Alveoli
   b. Cilia
   c. Exocrine bronchiolar cells
   d. Mucous glands in lamina propria
   e. Smooth muscle

4. Which of the following features distinguishes a bronchus within a lung from the primary bronchi?
   a. Glands in the submucosa
   b. Pseudostratified ciliated columnar epithelium
   c. Smooth muscle in the wall
   d. Irregular plates of cartilage
   e. Goblet cells in the epithelium

5. Which feature involved in protection of the respiratory tract is absent from the digestive tract?
   a. Goblet cells
   b. Cilia
   c. Lymphoid nodules
   d. Secretory IgA
   e. Tight junctions

6. Which of the following is true of pulmonary surfactant?
   a. Secreted by type I pneumocytes
   b. Forms layer rich in phospholipid overlying a thin aqueous phase
   c. Prevents alveolar collapse by increasing surface tension
   d. Does not affect bacterial survival
   e. Is secreted by goblet cells

7. The pulmonary (functional) and bronchial (nutritive) arterial systems enter the lungs separately at the hilus but anastomose into a single system at which level?
   a. Bronchi
   b. Larynx
   c. Terminal bronchioles
   d. Segmental bronchioles
   e. Respiratory bronchioles

8. After 35 weeks of gestation, a 5-lb 5-oz girl is born to a 30-year-old gravid 2, para 2 (G2P2) woman. The infant has rapid and labored breathing, which is viewed as transient tachypnea of the newborn. The infant's 1- and 5-min APGAR scores are 8 and 9, respectively. She has respiratory distress, with a normal pulse and no heart murmurs. She is transported to the neonatal intensive care unit with worsening tachypnea. In this infant which of the following is likely to be involved?
   a. Failure of the type I pneumocytes to form complete blood-air barriers
   b. Absence of elastic fibers from the bronchiolar walls and interalveolar septa
   c. Failure of type II pneumocytes to complete differentiation and become fully functional
   d. Failure of type II pneumocyte progenitors to proliferate adequately during gestation
   e. Inadequate development of the parietal and visceral pleura

9. A teenage girl presents at the hospital emergency department with paroxysms of dyspnea, cough, and wheezing. Her parents indicate that she had these "attacks" during the past winter and that they have worsened and become more frequent during the spring. Which of the following cell types and their location is correctly matched to a function it may perform in this patient's disorder?
   a. Cilia in alveolar ducts, enhanced mucociliary transport
   b. Plasma cells in bronchus-associated lymphoid tissue (BALT), bronchoconstriction
   c. Eosinophils in BALT, bronchodilation
   d. Goblet cells in bronchioles, hyposecretion
   e. Mast cells in BALT, bronchoconstriction, and edema

10. A 28-year-old man is diagnosed with a testicular germ cell tumor. The tumor is surgically removed, and he begins chemotherapy with cisplatin, etoposide, and bleomycin. Bleomycin chemotherapy is known to affect the lung blood-air barrier. Which of the following best describes the structural site of those effects?
   a. Fused basal laminae of epithelial and endothelial cells
   b. Alveolar pores of Kohn
   c. Alveolar macrophages in interalveolar septa
   d. Type II pneumocytes linked by junctional complexes
   e. Smooth muscle cells of the pulmonary and bronchial arteries

Answers: 1b, 2c, 3a, 4d, 5b, 6b, 7e, 8c, 9e, 10a

18 Skin

As the largest single organ of the body, the skin typically accounts for 15%–20% of total body weight and, in adults, presents 1.5–2 m² of surface to the external environment. Also known as the **integument** (L. *integumentum*, covering) or **cutaneous layer**, the skin consists of the **epidermis**, an epithelial layer of ectodermal origin, and the **dermis**, a layer of mesodermal connective tissue (Figure 18–1). At the irregular junction between the dermis and epidermis, projections called **dermal papillae** interdigitate with invaginating **epidermal ridges** to strengthen adhesion of the two layers. Epidermal derivatives include hairs, nails, and sebaceous and sweat glands. Beneath the dermis lies the **subcutaneous tissue** or **hypodermis** (Gr. *hypo*, under + *derma*, skin), a loose connective tissue layer usually containing pads of adipocytes. The subcutaneous tissue binds the skin loosely to the underlying tissues and corresponds to the superficial fascia of gross anatomy.

The specific functions of the skin fall into several broad categories.

- **Protective:** It provides a physical barrier against thermal and mechanical insults, such as friction, and against most potential pathogens and other material. Microorganisms that do penetrate skin alert resident lymphocytes and antigen-presenting cells (APCs) in skin to trigger an immune response. The dark pigment melanin in the epidermis protects cell nuclei from ultraviolet (UV) radiation. Skin also forms a permeability barrier against excessive loss or uptake of water, which has allowed for terrestrial life. Fortuitously, skin's selective permeability allows some lipophilic drugs, such as certain steroid hormones and medications, to be administered via skin patches.

- **Sensory:** Many types of sensory receptors allow skin to constantly monitor the environment, and various skin mechanoreceptors help regulate the body's interactions with physical objects.

- **Thermoregulatory:** A constant body temperature is normally easily maintained, thanks to the skin's insulating components (eg, the fatty layer and hair on the head) and its mechanisms for accelerating heat loss (sweat production and a dense superficial microvasculature).

- **Metabolic:** Cells of skin synthesize vitamin D₃, needed in calcium metabolism and proper bone formation, through the local action of UV light on the vitamin's precursor. Sweating helps remove excess electrolytes, and the subcutaneous layer stores a significant amount of energy in the form of fat.

- **Sexual signaling:** Many features of skin, such as pigmentation and hair, serve as visual indicators of health involved in attraction between the sexes in all vertebrate species, including humans. The effects of sex pheromones produced by the apocrine sweat glands and other skin glands also factor into this attraction.

The dermal-epidermal interdigitations are of the peg-and-socket variety in most skin (Figure 18–1), but they occur as well-formed ridges and grooves in the thick skin of the palms and soles, sites to the most intense friction. These ridges and the intervening sulci form distinctive patterns unique for everyone, appearing as combinations of loops, arches, and whorls, called dermatoglyphs, also known as fingerprints and footprints. Skin is elastic and can expand rapidly to cover swollen areas and, like the gut lining, is self-renewing throughout life. In healthy individuals, injured skin undergoes rapid repair. The molecular basis of skin healing is increasingly well

FIGURE **18–1**   **Layers and appendages of skin.**

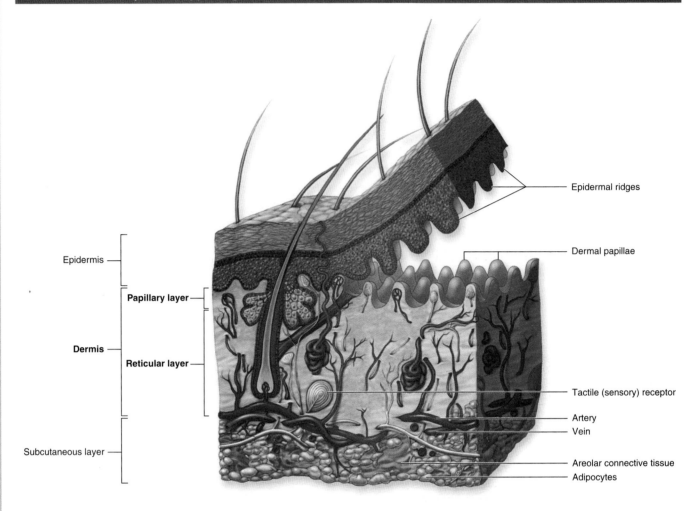

Epidermis

Dermis

Papillary layer

Reticular layer

Subcutaneous layer

Epidermal ridges

Dermal papillae

Tactile (sensory) receptor

Artery

Vein

Areolar connective tissue

Adipocytes

Diagrammatic overview of **skin**, showing the three **major layers** and **epidermal appendages** (hair follicles, sweat, and sebaceous glands), the **vasculature**, and the major **sensory receptors**.

understood and provides a basis for better understanding of repair and regeneration in other organs.

〉 EPIDERMIS

The **epidermis** consists mainly of a stratified squamous keratinized epithelium composed of cells called **keratino-cytes**. Three much less abundant epidermal cell types also occur: pigment-producing **melanocytes**, antigen-presenting **Langerhans cells**, and tactile epithelial cells called **Merkel cells** Figure 18–2.

The epidermis forms the major distinction between **thick skin** (Figure 18–2a), found on the palms and soles, and **thin skin** (Figure 18–3) found everywhere else on the body. The depth of the epidermal layer alone varies from 75 to 150 μm for thin skin and from 400 to 600 μm (0.6 mm) for thick skin. Total skin thickness (epidermis plus dermis) also differs

according to the site. For example, full skin on the back is about 4 mm thick, whereas that of the scalp is about 1.5 mm thick. Like all epithelia, the stratified squamous epidermis lacks microvasculature, its cells receiving nutrients and O_2 by diffusion from the dermis.

From the dermis, the epidermis consists of four layers of keratinocytes (or five layers in thick skin, Figure 18–2):

■ The **basal layer** (stratum basale) comprises a single layer of basophilic cuboidal or columnar cells on the basement membrane at the dermal-epidermal junction (Figures 18–2 and 18–3). Hemidesmosomes in the basal cell membranes attach these cells to the basal lamina, and desmosomes connect the cells of this layer together in their lateral and upper surfaces. Intense mitotic activity characterizes the basal layer, especially among pro-genitor cells for keratinocytes located here and in the deepest part of the next layer. In addition to the basal

FIGURE **18–2** Layers or strata of epidermis in thick skin.

(a) Micrograph showing the sequence of the **epidermal layers** in thick skin, with the layers' traditional but still widely used Latin names. Coarse bundles of collagen occur in the dermis and on the far left, the duct from a sweat gland enters the epidermis from a dermal papilla and coils through a surface pore. (×100; H&E)

(b) Diagram illustrating the sequence of the epidermal layers also indicates the normal locations of three important nonkeratinocyte cells in the epidermis: **melanocytes**, a **Langerhans cell**, and a **tactile Merkel cell**.

stem cells for keratinocytes found here, a niche for such cells also occurs in the hair follicle sheaths continuous with the epidermis. The human epidermis turns over about every 15–30 days, depending on age, the region of the body, and other factors. Activation of genes for cytoskeletal **keratins** to form intermediate filaments about 10 nm in diameter constitutes an important feature of keratinocytes in the basal layer. During maturation the cells move upward, and the amount and types of keratin filaments increase until they represent half the total protein in the superficial keratinocytes.

❯❯ MEDICAL APPLICATION

Friction blisters represent lymph-filled spaces created between the epidermis and dermis of thick skin by excessive rubbing, as with ill-fitting shoes or hard use of the hands. If continued, such activity produces protective thickening and hardening of the outer cornified epidermal layers, seen as **corns** and **calluses**.

■ The **spinous layer** (stratum spinosum) develops as maturing basal cells move up to form a thick layer of cells, especially in the epidermal ridges (Figures 18–2 and 18–3). Cells here have generally polyhedral shapes,

central nuclei, nucleoli, and cytoplasm actively synthesizing keratins. Just above the basal layer, some progenitor cells of this layer still divide. Keratin filaments assemble here into microscopically visible bundles called **tonofibrils**, which converge and terminate at the numerous desmosomes holding the layered cells together. The cells extend slightly around the tonofibrils on both sides of each desmosome (and the extensions elongate if the cells shrink at all during histologic processing), leading to the appearance of many short "spines" or prickles at the cell surfaces (Figure 18–4). The epidermis of thick skin subject to continuous friction and pressure has a thicker spinous layer, with more abundant tonofibrils and desmosomes.

❯❯ MEDICAL APPLICATION

In adults, one-third of all cancers originate in the skin. Most of these derive from cells of the basal or spinous layers, producing, respectively, basal cell carcinomas and squamous cell carcinomas. Fortunately, both types of tumors can be diagnosed and excised early and consequently are rarely lethal. Skin cancer shows an increased incidence in fair-skinned individuals residing in regions with high amounts of solar radiation.

FIGURE **18–3** Layers of epidermis in thin skin.

The interface between dermis and **epidermis** in thin skin is held together firmly by interlocking epidermal protrusions or pegs (**EP**) and dermal papillae (**DP**). The dermis (**D**) of thin skin is both more cellular and vascularized than that of thick skin, with elastin and less coarse bundles of collagen. The epidermis usually shows only four layers in thin skin: the one-cell-thick basal layer (**B**) containing most mitotic cells; the spinous layer (**S**) where synthesis of much keratin and other proteins takes place; the granular layer (**G**); and the cornified layer (**C**), consisting of dead squames composed mostly of keratin. (×240; H&E)

■ The **granular layer (stratum granulosum)** consists of three to five layers of flattened cells, now undergoing the terminal differentiation process of **keratinization**. Their cytoplasm has become filled with intensely basophilic masses (Figures 18–2, 18–3, and 18–5) called **keratohyaline granules**. These represent dense, non-membrane-bound masses of **filaggrin** and other proteins associated with the keratins of tonofibrils, linking them further into large cytoplasmic structures.

Characteristic features in cells of the granular layer also include Golgi-derived **lamellar granules**, small ovoid (100 × 300 nm) structures with many lamellae containing lipids and glycolipids. Among the last activities of the keratinocytes, the lamellar granules undergo exocytosis to produce a lipid-rich, impermeable layer around the cells. This material forms a major part of the skin's barrier against water loss. Formation of this barrier, which appeared first in ancestral reptiles, evolved as a key process that permitted animals to develop on land. Together, keratinization and production of the lipid-rich layer also have a crucial sealing effect in skin, forming the barrier to penetration by most foreign materials.

■ A clear layer, the stratum lucidum occurs only in thick palmar and plantar skin and consists of a thin, optically refractile sheet of flattened acidophilic keratinocytes held together by desmosomes (Figures 18–2 and 18–5). Nuclei and organelles have disappeared and the cytoplasm consists almost exclusively of packed keratin filaments embedded in an electron-dense matrix.

■ The **cornified layer (stratum corneum)** (Figures 18–2 and 18–3) comprises 15–20 layers of squamous, keratinized cells filled with filamentous keratins. Keratin filaments

FIGURE **18–4** Keratinocytes of the spinous layer.

(a) A section of the epidermal spinous layer of thick skin, showing **keratinocytes** with numerous short cytoplasmic projections (**arrow**). (×400; PT)

(b) TEM of a single spinous **keratinocyte** with surface projections (**arrows**). (×8400)

(c) Detail of the desmosomes joining two **keratinocytes** showing intermediate filaments associated with desmosomes. The desmosomes occur on the tips of the cytoplasmic projections or "spines" seen by light microscopy. (×40,000)

FIGURE **18–5** Granular and clear layers: thick skin.

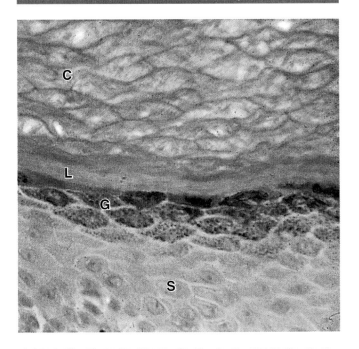

In keratinocytes moving upward from the spinous layer (**S**), differentiation proceeds with the cells becoming filled with large, amorphous protein masses called **keratohyaline granules**.

Cells with these basophilic granules make up the granular layer (**G**), where keratin filaments become cross-linked with filaggrin and other proteins from these granules to produce tight bundles filling the cytoplasm and flattening the cells. Smaller organelles called **lamellar granules** undergo exocytosis in this layer, secreting a lipid-rich layer around the cells which makes the epidermis impermeable to water. Together, the lipid envelope and the keratin-filled cells determine most of the physical properties of the epidermis.

The cells leaving the granular layer, still bound together by desmosomes, undergo terminal differentiation and in **thick skin** form a dense, thin layer called the clear layer, or **stratum lucidum** (**L**). Here proteins are dispersed through the tonofibril bundles, giving this layer a regular, "clear" appearance. In the most superficial cornified layer (**C**), most cells have lost nuclei and cytoplasm, consisting only of flattened, keratinized structures called **squames** bound by hydrophobic, lipid-rich intercellular cement. At the surface, they get worn away (thick skin) or flake off (thin skin). (×560; H&E)

contain at least six different polypeptides with molecular masses ranging from 40 to 70 kDa, synthesized during cell differentiation in the immature layers. As they form, keratin tonofibrils become heavily massed with filaggrin and other proteins in keratohyaline granules. By the end of keratinization, the cells contain only amorphous, fibrillar proteins with their plasma membranes surrounded by the lipid-rich layer. These fully keratinized or cornified cells, called **squames**, undergo continuous disintegration or shedding at the epidermal surface as the desmosomes and lipid-rich cell envelopes break down. Table 18–1 summarizes the important features of all the epidermal layers.

In the chronic skin condition called **psoriasis**, keratocytes are typically produced and differentiate at accelerated rates, causing at least slight thickening of the epidermal layers and increased keratinization and desquamation. Caused by overactive T lymphocytes triggering an autoimmune reaction in the skin, psoriasis can also lead to inflammation with redness, irritation, itching, and scaling, with a defective skin barrier.

Melanocytes

Skin color results from several factors, including the presence of carotene along with the amount and kind of **melanin** in the keratinocytes, recent prolonged exposure to sunlight, and the microvascular density in the dermis.

Melanocytes (Figures 18–6 and 18–7), a specialized epidermal cell type found among the basal keratinocytes of skin and hair follicles, synthesize brown-black pigments called **eumelanin**. **Pheomelanin** (Gr. *phaios*, dusky) is a similar red-yellow pigment. Melanocytes develop from neural crest cells migrating into the embryonic epidermis' basal layer, where eventually one melanocyte accumulates for every five or six keratinocytes (600–1200/mm² of thin skin). They are approximately four times more numerous and active in thin skin than in thick palmar and plantar skin.

Melanocytes have pale-staining, rounded cell bodies attached by hemidesmosomes to the basal lamina but lack attachments to the neighboring keratinocytes. Several long irregular cytoplasmic extensions from each melanocyte cell body course among the cells of the basal and spinous layers and terminate within invaginations of 10–30 keratinocytes. Ultrastructurally, a melanocyte has numerous small mitochondria, short cisternae of RER, and a well-developed Golgi apparatus (Figure 18–6).

As indicated in Figure 18–7 **tyrosinase**, a transmembrane enzyme in Golgi-derived vesicles, catalyzes the first step in melanin synthesis. Tyrosinase activity converts tyrosine into **3,4-dihydroxyphenylalanine (DOPA)**, which then undergoes further transformations and polymerizes into the different forms of melanin. Melanin pigment becomes linked to a matrix of structural proteins and accumulates in the Golgi vesicles, which develop and mature into elliptical granules called **melanosomes** (Figure 18–7).

Melanosomes then move via kinesin to the tips of the melanocyte's cytoplasmic extensions. The neighboring keratinocytes engulf the tips of these processes, take in the melanosomes, and transport them via dynein toward their nuclei. The melanosomes accumulate within keratinocytes as a supranuclear cap which prior to keratinization absorbs and scatters sunlight, protecting DNA of the living cells from the ionizing, mutagenic effects of UV radiation.

Although melanocytes produce melanosomes, the keratinocytes comprise the melanin depots and contain more of this pigment than the cells that make it. One melanocyte plus the keratinocytes into which it transfers melanosomes make up an **epidermal-melanin unit**. Similar densities of such units exist

TABLE **18–1**	Summary of skin and subcutaneous layers.	
Layer	**Specific Layer**	**Description**
Epidermis 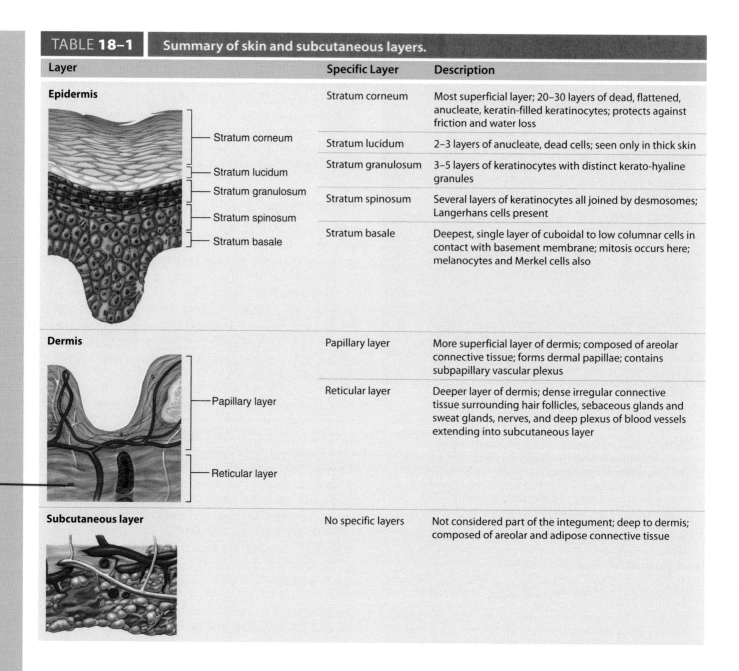	Stratum corneum	Most superficial layer; 20–30 layers of dead, flattened, anucleate, keratin-filled keratinocytes; protects against friction and water loss
	Stratum lucidum	2–3 layers of anucleate, dead cells; seen only in thick skin
	Stratum granulosum	3–5 layers of keratinocytes with distinct kerato-hyaline granules
	Stratum spinosum	Several layers of keratinocytes all joined by desmosomes; Langerhans cells present
	Stratum basale	Deepest, single layer of cuboidal to low columnar cells in contact with basement membrane; mitosis occurs here; melanocytes and Merkel cells also
Dermis	Papillary layer	More superficial layer of dermis; composed of areolar connective tissue; forms dermal papillae; contains subpapillary vascular plexus
	Reticular layer	Deeper layer of dermis; dense irregular connective tissue surrounding hair follicles, sebaceous glands and sweat glands, nerves, and deep plexus of blood vessels extending into subcutaneous layer
Subcutaneous layer	No specific layers	Not considered part of the integument; deep to dermis; composed of areolar and adipose connective tissue

Diagram labels (Epidermis): Stratum corneum, Stratum lucidum, Stratum granulosum, Stratum spinosum, Stratum basale

Diagram labels (Dermis): Papillary layer, Reticular layer

in the skin of all individuals; melanocytes of people with ancestral origins near the equator, where the maximal need for protection against the sun occurs, produce melanin granules more rapidly and accumulate them in keratinocytes more abundantly.

›› MEDICAL APPLICATION

Albinism represents a congenital disorder producing skin **hypopigmentation** due to a defect in tyrosinase or some other component of the melanin-producing pathway. An acquired condition called **vitiligo** involves skin **depigmentation**, often only in affected patches, due to the loss or decreased activity of melanocytes. The causes of melanocyte loss are not clear, but they may include environmental, genetic, or autoimmune conditions.

In regions with much less sunlight, such as Northern Europe, the small amount of UV radiation penetrating dark skin barely sustains adequate vitamin D_3 synthesis. Individuals with ancestry in these regions have one or more genetic polymorphisms that affect steps in melanin formation and result in more lightly pigmented keratinocytes, which allow increased UV penetration and vitamin D_3 synthesis.

Darkening of the skin, or tanning, after exposure to solar radiation at wavelengths of 290–320 nm involves two processes. A physicochemical reaction quickly darkens pre-existing melanin, and at the same time, paracrine factors secreted by keratinocytes experiencing increased UV radiation accelerate melanin synthesis and its accumulation in the epidermis.

FIGURE **18–6** Melanocytes.

Vesicle filled with melanin
Melanin pigment in keratinocyte
Melanin pigment
Melanocyte
Basement membrane

Melanocytes occur in the epidermal basal layer, synthesizing **melanin granules** and transferring them into the nearest **keratinocytes**. Transfer occurs through many long, branching melanocyte processes that extend into the spinous layer but are not routinely seen by light microscopy.

(a) In light microscopy melanocytes (**M**) typically appear as rounded, pale-staining cells just above the dermis (**D**). Melanocytes are difficult to distinguish from Merkel cells by routine microscopy. Langerhans cells are also rounded, poorly stained cells but are typically located more superficially than melanocytes, in the spinous layer. (×400; H&E)

(b) Diagram of a **melanocyte** in its niche showing the irregular cytoplasmic processes between neighboring keratinocytes for transfer of melanin to those cells, a process described with Figure 18–7.

(c) This TEM shows the large nucleus of a melanocyte (**M**) on the basal lamina (**BL**). Large Golgi complexes (**G**) produce vesicles called **melanosomes**, containing matrix proteins and enzymes for melanin synthesis. These vesicles gradually transform into dark melanin-containing granules (**MG**), which mature and accumulate at the tips of the dendritic cytoplasmic extensions (**CE**) before transfer to keratinocytes (**K**). (×14,000)

›› MEDICAL APPLICATION

Melanocytes can normally proliferate in skin to produce **moles**, or **benign melanocytic nevi** of various types. Changes in the size or appearance of moles are sometimes indicative of dysplasia that can progress further to **malignant melanoma**. Dividing rapidly, malignantly transformed melanocytes often penetrate the basal lamina, enter the dermis, and metastasize by invading blood and lymphatic vessels.

Langerhans Cells

APCs called **Langerhans cells**, derived from monocytes, represent a more variable population of cells in epidermis, averaging 2%–8% with more in thin skin than thick. These dendritic cells usually appear most clearly in the spinous layer, but their cytoplasmic processes extend between keratinocytes of all the layers, forming a dense network in the epidermis (Figure 18–8).

Langerhans cells bind, process, and present antigens to T lymphocytes in the same manner as immune dendritic cells in other organs (see Chapter 14). Microorganisms cannot penetrate the epidermis without alerting these dendritic cells and triggering an immune response. Langerhans cells, along with more scattered epidermal lymphocytes and other APCs in the dermis, comprise a major component of the skin's adaptive immunity.

Because of its location, the skin is continuously in close contact with many antigenic molecules. Various epidermal features participate in both innate and adaptive immunity (Chapter 14), providing an important immunologic component to the skin's overall protective function.

Merkel Cells

Merkel cells, or **epithelial tactile cells**, develop as low-threshold mechanoreceptors in the basal epidermal layer and

FIGURE 18–7 Melanosome formation.

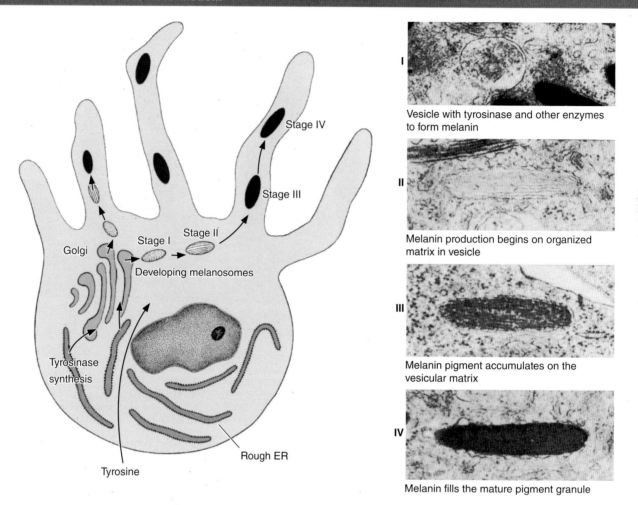

I

Vesicle with tyrosinase and other enzymes to form melanin

II

Melanin production begins on organized matrix in vesicle

III

Melanin pigment accumulates on the vesicular matrix

IV

Melanin fills the mature pigment granule

The diagram of a **melanocyte** shows the main features of **melanin formation**. The granules containing melanin mature through four stages that are characterized ultrastructurally, as shown on the right. **Tyrosinase** is synthesized in the rough ER, processed through the Golgi apparatus, and accumulates in vesicles that also have a fine granular matrix of other proteins (**stage I** melanosomes). Melanin synthesis begins in the ovoid **stage II** melanosomes, in which the matrix has been organized into parallel filaments on which polymerized melanin is deposited and accumulates in **stage III**. A mature melanin granule (**stage IV**)

has lost enzymatic activities and has the internal matrix filled with melanin. The mature granules are ellipsoid, approximately 0.5 by 1 μm in size, and visible by light microscopy.

Melanin granules are transported to the tips of the processes of melanocyte and are then transferred to the neighboring keratinocytes of the basal and spinous layers. In keratinocytes, the melanin granules undergo transport to a region near the nucleus, where they accumulate as a supranuclear cap shading the DNA against the harmful effects of UV radiation.

are essential for sensing gentle touch, becoming abundant in highly sensitive skin like that of fingertips and at the bases of some hair follicles. Originating from the embryonic neural crest, Merkel cells become localized in both thin and thick skin, achieving a higher cell percentage in the latter. They resemble the surrounding keratinocytes by light microscopy but contain few if any melanosomes. Their ultrastructural characteristics include small, Golgi-derived dense-core granules concentrated in areas near the basolateral surface where the cells form synaptic contacts with the expanded terminal discs of unmyelinated afferent fibers penetrating the basal lamina (Figure 18–9). Light touch to the skin initiates release of neurotransmitters and tactile sensation from that location.

❯❯ MEDICAL APPLICATION

Merkel cells have clinical importance because Merkel cell carcinomas, though uncommon, are very aggressive and difficult to treat. Merkel cell carcinoma is 40 times less common than malignant melanoma but has twice the mortality of that disease.

FIGURE **18–8** Langerhans cells.

Langerhans cells are dendritic APCs of the epidermis where they comprise an important defense against pathogens and environmental toxins. Like other APCs, they develop in the bone marrow, move into the blood circulation, and finally migrate into the stratified squamous epithelia where they are difficult to identify in routinely stained sections.

(a) Section of immunostained skin shows **Langerhans cells** (yellow) abundant in hair follicles (**F**), where many microorganisms live, and throughout the superficial layers of epidermis (**E**). Keratin

of the epidermis and follicles is stained green. (×40) Antibodies against langerin/CD207 and keratin.

(b) Face-on view of an epidermal sheet stained using the same antibody conjugated to a red fluor. A network of interdigitating **Langerhans cells** acts as an alarm system to detect any invading microorganisms. After sampling the invaders' antigens, the triggering Langerhans cells leave the epidermis and travel to the nearest lymph node to elicit lymphocytes that can mount a collective immune response. (×200; Anti-langerin/CD207)

FIGURE **18–9** Merkel or tactile cell.

Derived embryonically from the neural crest, **Merkel cells** develop in the epidermis' basal layer and function as highly sensitive mechanoreceptors, especially abundant in skin of the fingertips and external genitalia. This TEM of a Merkel cell shows a mass of Golgi-derived dense-core cytoplasmic granules (**G**) near the basolateral cell membrane, which is in direct synaptic contact with the expanded, disc-like ending of an unmyelinated sensory nerve fiber (**N**) that has penetrated the epidermis. (×14,000)

Inset: Granules are similar in morphology and content to the granules of many other neuroendocrine cells. Here the vesicles contain both classic neurotransmitters like serotonin and a variety of neuropeptides. When slight mechanical displacement of the epidermis activates calcium-channels in the Merkel cell membrane, neurotransmitters undergo exocytosis and initiate a neural impulse producing the sensation of touch. (×61,500)

❯ DERMIS

The **dermis** represents the layer of connective tissue (Figures 18–1 and 18–2) that supports the epidermis and binds it to the subcutaneous tissue (hypodermis). The thickness of the dermis varies with the region of the body and reaches its maximum of 4 mm on the back. The surface of the dermis is very irregular and has many projections (dermal papillae) that interdigitate with projections (epidermal pegs or ridges) of the epidermis (Figure 18–1), especially in skin subject to frequent pressure, where they reinforce the dermal-epidermal junction.

A **basement membrane** always occurs between the basal epidermal layer and the dermis and follows the contour of the interdigitations between these layers. Nutrients for keratinocytes diffuse into the avascular epidermis from the dermal vasculature through the basement membrane.

> ❯❯ **MEDICAL APPLICATION**
>
> Abnormalities of the dermal-epidermal junction can lead to one type of blistering disorder (bullous pemphigoid). Another type of blistering disorder (pemphigus) is caused by autoimmune damage to intercellular junctions between keratinocytes.

As indicated in Table 18–1 and Figure 18–1, the dermis contains two sublayers with indistinct boundaries:

- The thin **papillary layer**, which includes the dermal papillae, consists of loose connective tissue, with types I and III collagen fibers, fibroblasts and scattered mast cells, dendritic cells, and leukocytes. From this layer, anchoring fibrils of type VII collagen insert into the basal lamina, helping to bind the dermis to the epidermis.
- The underlying **reticular layer** becomes much thicker and consists of dense irregular connective tissue (mainly bundles of type I collagen), with more fibers and fewer cells than the papillary layer. A network of elastic fibers also develops (Figure 18–10), providing elasticity to the skin. Proteoglycans rich in dermatan sulfate occur abundantly among the collagen and elastic fibers.

> ❯❯ **MEDICAL APPLICATION**
>
> With age changes in the dermal ECM are normal: thickening of collagen fibers, less collagen synthesis, and loss of hyaluronan and other GAGs. In old age, extensive cross-linking of collagen fibers and the loss of elastic fibers, especially after excessive exposure to the sun (solar elastosis), cause the skin to become more fragile, lose its suppleness, and develop wrinkles. The epidermis also normally thins and becomes more transparent during aging. In several disorders, such as cutis laxa and Ehlers-Danlos syndromes, there is a considerable increase in skin and ligament extensibility caused by defective collagen fibril processing.

FIGURE 18–10   Elastic fibers of dermis.

A section of thin skin stained for **elastic fibers** shows the extensive distribution of these darkly stained fibers among the eosinophilic **collagen bundles**. In the dermal papillary layer, the diameter of fibers decreases as they approach the epidermis and insert into the basement membrane. (×100; Weigert elastic stain)

Both dermal regions contain a rich network of blood and lymphatic vessels. The nutritive vessels form two major plexuses (Table 18–1):

- Between the papillary and reticular dermal layers lies the microvascular **subpapillary plexus**, from which capillary branches extend into the dermal papillae and form a rich, nutritive capillary network just below the epidermis.
- A deep plexus with larger blood and lymphatic vessels lies near the interface of the dermis and the subcutaneous layer.

In addition to the nutritive function, dermal vasculature has a thermoregulatory function, which involves numerous **arteriovenous anastomoses** or shunts (see Chapter 11) located between the two major plexuses. The shunts decrease blood flow in the papillary layer to minimize heat loss in cold conditions and increase this flow to facilitate heat loss in

FIGURE **18–11** Tactile sensory receptors.

Tactile disc

Epidermis

Dermis

Subcutaneous layer

Free nerve ending

Tactile corpuscle

Krause bulb

Ruffini corpuscle

Root hair plexus

Lamellated corpuscle

Skin contains several types of **sensory receptors**, with or without capsules of connective tissue and modified Schwann cells. Most are difficult to see in routine preparations. In the epidermis are **free nerve endings** and tactile discs of nerve fibers associated with **Merkel cells** (shown in light blue) within the basal epidermal layer. Both involve unencapsulated nerve fibers, as does the **root hair plexus** around the bases of hair follicles in the dermis, which detects light touch or hair movements. Epidermal free nerve endings also detect pain (nociception), temperature extremes, and mechanical movements of the skin.

More complex, encapsulated tactile receptors occur in the dermis and hypodermis, and include **Meissner corpuscles** for light touch, **lamellated (Pacinian) corpuscles** detecting pressure and high-frequency vibration, **Krause end bulbs** for detection of low-frequency vibrations/movements, and **Ruffini corpuscles** detecting tissue distortion. The latter two receptors are much less widely distributed in skin and less commonly seen.

warm environments, thus helping maintain a constant body temperature. Lymphatic vessels begin in the dermal papillae and converge to form two plexuses located with the blood vessels.

The dermis also has a rich nerve supply. Sensory afferent nerve fibers form a network in the papillary dermis and around hair follicles, ending at the epithelial and dermal receptors shown in Figure 18–11. Autonomic effector nerves to dermal sweat glands and smooth muscle fibers in the skin of some areas are postganglionic fibers of sympathetic ganglia; no parasympathetic innervation is present.

❯ SUBCUTANEOUS TISSUE

The subcutaneous layer (Figure 18–1) consists of loose connective tissue that binds the skin loosely to the subjacent organs, making it possible for the skin to slide over them. This layer, also called the **hypodermis** or **superficial fascia**, contains adipocytes that vary in number in different body regions and vary in size according to nutritional state. Besides storing fat, this adipose tissue allows the hypodermis to serve as both insulation and cushion to protect deeper structures. The extensive vascular supply at this layer promotes rapid uptake of insulin or drugs injected into this tissue.

❯ SENSORY RECEPTORS

With its large surface and external location, the skin functions as an extensive receiver for diverse environmental stimuli. A variety of sensory receptors develop in skin, including both simple nerve endings with no Schwann cell or collagenous coverings and more complex structures with sensory fibers enclosed by glia and delicate connective tissue capsules (Figure 18–11). The unencapsulated receptors include the following:

- Tactile (or **Merkel cells**) mentioned above, each associated with a disc or expanded axonal ending (Figure 18–9), which function as tonic receptors for sustained light touch and for sensing an object's texture.
- **Free nerve endings** in the papillary dermis and extending into lower epidermal layers, which respond primarily

to high and low temperatures (thermoreception), pain (nociception), and itching (pruritus), but also function as important tactile receptors.

- **Root hair plexuses**, a web of sensory fibers surrounding the bases of hair follicles in the reticular dermis that detects movements of the hairs.

The encapsulated receptors all represent phasic mechanoreceptors, responding rapidly to stimuli on the skin. Four of these occur in human skin, although only the first two listed here appear in routine slide preparations:

- **Meissner corpuscles** develop in dermal papillae as elliptical structures, 30–75 μm by 50–150 μm, consisting of sensory axons winding among flattened Schwann cells arranged perpendicular to the long axis (Figure 18–12a). These sensory receptors initiate impulses when light-touch

---

FIGURE 18–12 Meissner and lamellated (Pacinian) corpuscles.

Micrographs show the two most common encapsulated sensory receptors of skin: **Meissner** and **Pacinian corpuscles**.

(a) Meissner tactile corpuscles (**TC**) are specialized to detect light touch and are usually seen in dermal papillae (**DP**), partially surrounded by epidermis (**E**). They are elliptical, approximately 150-μm long, with an outer capsule (from the perineurium) and thin, stacked inner layers of modified Schwann cells, around which course nerve fibers. (×400; H&E)

(b) Lamellated (Pacinian) corpuscles (**PC**) detect coarse touch or pressure and develop as large oval structures, frequently 1 mm in length, found among adipose tissue (**A**) deep in the reticular dermis or in the subcutaneous tissue. Here the outer connective tissue capsule surrounds 15–50 thin, concentric layers of modified Schwann cells, each separated by slightly viscous interstitial fluid. Several axons enter one end of the corpuscle and lie in the cylindrical, inner core of the structure. Movement or pressure of this corpuscle from any direction displaces the inner core, leading to a nerve impulse. (×40; H&E)

or low-frequency stimuli against the skin temporarily deform their shape. They are numerous in the fingertips, palms, and soles but decline slowly in number during aging.

- **Lamellated (Pacinian) corpuscles** represent much larger, oval structures, approximately 0.5 mm by 1 mm, found deep in the reticular dermis and hypodermis, with an outer capsule and 15–50 thin, concentric lamellae of flattened Schwann cells and collagen surrounding a highly branched, unmyelinated axon (Figure 18–12b). Lamellated corpuscles specialize in sensing coarse touch, pressure (sustained touch), and vibrations, with distortion of the capsule amplifying a mechanical stimulus to the axonal core where an impulse is initiated. Pacinian corpuscles also occur in connective tissue of organs located deep in the body, including the walls of the rectum and urinary bladder, where they also produce the sensation of pressure when the surrounding tissue undergoes stretching.
- **Krause end bulbs** exist as simpler encapsulated, ovoid structures, with extremely thin, collagenous capsules penetrated by a sensory fiber. They are found primarily in the skin of the penis and clitoris where they sense low-frequency vibrations.
- **Ruffini corpuscles** have collagenous, fusiform capsules anchored firmly to the surrounding connective tissue, with sensory axons stimulated by stretch (tension) or twisting (torque) in the skin.

> HAIR

Hairs consist of elongated keratinized structures that form within epidermal invaginations, the **hair follicles** (Figure 18–13). The color, size, shape, and texture of hairs vary according to age, genetic background, and region of the body. All skin has at least minimal hair except the glabrous skin of the palms, soles, lips, glans penis, clitoris, and labia minora. The face has about 600 hairs/cm² and the remainder of the body has about 60/cm². Hairs grow discontinuously, with alternating periods of growth and rest, and this growth does not occur synchronously in all regions of the body or even in the same area.

The growing hair follicle has a terminal dilation called a **hair bulb** (Figure 18–13a). A single **dermal papilla** inserts into the base of the hair bulb, bringing a capillary network required to sustain the hair follicle. Keratinocytes continuous with those of the basal epidermis cover the hair bulb and dermal papilla. These cells give rise to the matrix of the elongating **hair root**; the part of a hair extending beyond the skin surface makes up the **hair shaft**.

The keratinocytes of the hair bulb generally resemble those in the basal and spinous layers of epidermis. They divide rapidly in a matrix region immediately around the dermal papilla and then undergo keratinization, melanin accumulation, and terminal differentiation. As described above with epidermis, melanocytes among the hair bulb epithelial cells transfer melanosomes into the keratinocytes that will later move into the matrix and differentiate to form the hair. Unlike the epidermis in which all keratinocytes contribute to the cornified layer, cells in the hair root matrix differentiate with variable amounts and types of keratin. The keratin of hair has properties making it harder and more compact than that of the outer epidermal layer, maintaining its structure as the hair shaft much longer.

In most thick hairs large, vacuolated, and moderately keratinized cells form a central **medulla** of the hair root (Figures 18–13b and 18–14). Heavily keratinized, densely packed cells make up the **cortex** around the medulla. The most peripheral cells of the hair root comprise the **cuticle**, a thin layer of heavily keratinized, squamous cells covering the cortex (Figures 18–13c and 18–14).

The outermost cells of the hair bulb develop in continuity with the epithelial root sheath, which has two parts. The **internal root sheath** surrounds the deep part of the hair root but degenerates above the level of the attached sebaceous glands. The **external root sheath** covers the internal sheath and extends all the way to the epidermis, where it merges with the basal and spinous layers. This sheath's thickened basement membrane, called the **glassy membrane**, separates the hair follicle from the dermis (Figure 18–14b). The surrounding dermis forms a connective tissue sheath.

The **arrector pili muscle**, a small bundle of smooth muscle cells, extends from the midpoint of the fibrous sheath to the dermal papillary layer (Figure 18–13a). Contraction of these muscles pulls the hair shafts to a more erect position, usually under cold conditions, to trap a layer of warm air near the skin. In skin regions with short thin hair, contraction of arrector pili muscles produces tiny bumps on the skin surface ("goose bumps") where each contracting muscle distorts the attached dermis.

As mentioned earlier hairs grow asynchronously, cyclically, and at different rates in different regions of the body. The hair growth cycle has three major phases:

- A generally long period of mitotic activity and growth (**anagen**),
- A brief period of arrested growth and regression of the hair bulb (**catagen**), and
- A final long period of inactivity (**telogen**) during which the hair may be shed.

FIGURE **18–13** Hair.

a

b

c

All types of body **hair** have a similar composition and form in hair follicles derived from the epidermis but extending deep into the dermis.

(a) The diagram shows major parts of a **hair** and its **follicle**, including the vascularized, nutritive hair dermal **papilla** and the **arrector pili muscle** that pulls the hair erect.

(b) A longitudinal section of a hair root and bulb shows the **matrix**, **medulla**, and **cortex** in the root and the surrounding

epithelial and connective tissue sheaths. Cells of the hair bulb matrix proliferate, take up melanosomes, and undergo keratinization to differentiate as the three concentric layers of the hair. (×70; H&E)

(c) The thin **cuticle** forms the outermost layer of the hair, composed of shingle-like cells, shown in this SEM of a hair shaft emerging from the epidermis. (×260)

At the beginning of the next anagen phase, epidermal stem cells located in a small bulge of the external root sheath near the arrector pili muscle produce progenitor cells for the matrix of a new hair bulb. Hair growth on the face and pubis responds strongly to the influence of sex hormones, especially androgens, and begins at puberty.

❯❯ MEDICAL APPLICATION

Loss of hair to produce **baldness** or **alopecia** results from a complex combination of genetic and hormonal factors that is not well understood. Arresting mitotic activity in the hair

matrix during cancer **chemotherapy** disrupts both the function and the structural integrity of hair follicles and usually leads to rapid, reversible alopecia.

❯ NAILS

A similar process of keratinization also produces the **nails**, consisting of hard plates of keratin on the dorsal surface of each distal phalanx (Figure 18–15). The proximal part of the nail, the **nail root**, lies beneath a fold of skin, from which the epidermal cornified layer extends as the **cuticle**, or

FIGURE **18–14** Layers of a hair and its follicle.

(a) The base of a **hair follicle** sectioned obliquely shows the vascularized dermal papilla (**DP**) continuous with the surrounding connective tissue sheath (**CTS**). The papilla is enclosed by the deepest part of the epithelial sheath, which is continuous with the internal root sheath (**IRS**) and external root sheath (**ERS**), both of which have continuity with the stratified epidermis. Just outside the ERS is the glassy membrane (**G**) that is continuous with the basement membrane of the epidermis. The epithelial cells (keratinocytes) around the papilla proliferate and differentiate as the root of the hair itself. Above the papilla, only the cortex (**CO**) of the hair is clearly seen in this section. (×140; H&E)

(b) A **hair root** sectioned more transversely shows the same layers of the follicular sheath, but the layers of the hair root are now seen to include the medulla (**M**), cortex (**CO**), and cuticle (**CU**). Other labels are like those of part (a). (×140; H&E)

(c) A rat whisker **follicle** sectioned longitudinally and stained indirectly with fluorescent antibodies against **laminin** in basal laminae is used here to emphasize both structural and developmental features of hair follicles. The abundant laminin staining in the mesenchymal dermal papilla (**DP**) reveals the high density of capillaries in that tissue.

In contrast, the cortex (**CO**) of the growing hair and the internal and external root sheaths (**RS**) almost completely lack laminin, like the epidermis with which the outer sheath is continuous. Only the prominent basement membrane supporting the basal keratinocytes around the dermal papilla and continuing as the thick "glassy membrane" (**G**) between the external root sheath and surrounding connective tissue stains positively for laminin, along with variously sized blood vessels in the adjacent connective tissue. (×150)

eponychium. The **nail plate** is bound to a floor of epidermis, the **nail bed**, containing only the basal and spinous epidermal layers.

The nail root develops from the **nail matrix** in which the epithelial cells (here completely devoid of melanocytes) divide, move distally, and become keratinized in a process somewhat like hair formation but without keratohyaline granules. The nail root matures and hardens as the nail plate (Figure 18–15). Continuous growth in the matrix pushes the nail plate forward over the nail bed (which makes no contribution to the plate) at a rate of about 3 mm/mo for fingernails and 1 mm/mo for toenails. The distal end of the plate becomes free of the nail bed at the epidermal fold called the **hyponychium**. The nearly transparent nail plate and the thin epithelium of the nail bed provide a useful window on the amount of oxygen in the blood by showing the color of blood in the dermal vessels.

❯ SKIN GLANDS

Sebaceous Glands

Sebaceous glands are embedded in the dermis over most of the body, except in the thick, glabrous skin of the palms and soles. Thin skin averages about 100 such glands per square centimeter, but the frequency increases to 400–900/cm² on the face and scalp. Sebaceous glands develop as branched acinar glands with several acini converging at a short duct that usually empties into the upper portion of a hair follicle (Figure 18–16). A hair follicle and its associated sebaceous glands make up a **pilosebaceous unit**. The stem cell niche of the hair follicle's bulge region gives rise to progenitor cells for the associated sebaceous glands, in addition to keratinocytes and melanocytes. In certain hairless regions, such as the penis,

FIGURE **18–15** Nails.

a

- Free edge
- Nail groove
- Nail fold
- Lunula
- Nail body
- Eponychium (cuticle)

b

- Phalanx (finger bone)
- Nail matrix
- Nail root
- Nail bed
- Hyponychium
- Nail plate
- Dermis
- Epidermis

c

PNF · DNM · E · NR · VNM · NB · NP · D

Nails are hard, keratinized derivatives formed in a process resembling that of both the epidermal cornified layer and hair.

(a) Surface view of a finger shows the nail's major regions, including the crescent-shaped white area called the **lunula**, which derives its color from the opaque nail matrix and immature nail plate below it.

(b) A diagrammatic sagittal section includes major internal details of the growing **nail** and the hyponychium where the free end of the nail plate is bound to epidermis.

(c) A sagittal section from a finger shows the proximal nail fold (**PNF**) and its epidermal extension, the eponychium (**E**) or cuticle. The nail root (**NR**), the most proximal region of the nail plate (**NP**), is formed like the hair root by a matrix of proliferating, differentiating keratinocytes. These cells make up the dorsal nail matrix (**DNM**) and ventral nail matrix (**VNM**), which contribute keratinized cells to the nail root. The mature nail plate remains attached to the nail bed (**NB**), which consists of basal and spinous epidermal layers over dermis (**D**) but moves forward on this bed due to continuous growth in the nail matrix. (×100; Mallory trichrome)

FIGURE **18–16** Glands of skin.

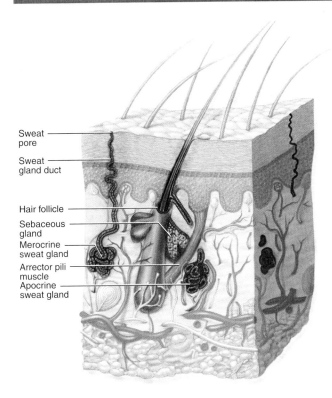

Skin includes three major types of **exocrine glands**.

Sebaceous glands usually comprise one or more parts of a pilosebaceous unit with a hair follicle and secrete oily sebum into the space around the hair root. Thermoregulatory **eccrine sweat glands** empty their secretion onto the skin surface via sweat pores.

Apocrine sweat glands secrete a more protein-rich sweat into the hair follicles of axillary and perineal skin.

(Labels on figure:) Sweat pore; Sweat gland duct; Hair follicle; Sebaceous gland; Merocrine sweat gland; Arrector pili muscle; Apocrine sweat gland

Acne vulgaris is an inflammatory disorder of the pilosebaceous unit, which can be expected to occur during adolescence. It involves excessive keratinization within this unit and excess sebum production, both of which contribute to the blockage of ducts in the follicle. Anaerobic bacteria, typically *Propionibacterium acnes*, grow in the accumulated sebum, leading to localized inflammation and neutrophil infiltration. The resulting enlarged follicle is called a **comedone**.

Sweat Glands

Sweat glands form as long epidermal invaginations embedded in the dermis (Figure 18–1). Two types of sweat glands develop, eccrine and apocrine, with distinct functions, distributions, and structural details.

Eccrine sweat glands (Figures 18–16 and 18–18) make up the most effective means of temperature regulation in humans. They have wide distribution in skin of all body regions, but become most numerous on the soles of the feet (620/cm²). The average person's 3 million eccrine sweat glands collectively approximate the mass of a kidney and can produce sweat at a rate of 10 L/d, a secretory rate far exceeding that of other exocrine glands. Sweating increases as a physiologic response to raised body temperature during physical exercise or thermal stress and during periods of anxiety.

Both the secretory components and ducts of eccrine sweat glands develop coils and small lumens. The **secretory part** generally stains more poorly than the ducts and consists of an unusual stratified cuboidal epithelium with three cell types (Figure 18–18b):

- Pale-staining **clear cells** located on the basal lamina produce the sweat, having abundant mitochondria and large surface areas provided by basolateral surface infoldings. Interstitial fluid from the capillary-rich dermis surrounding the gland undergoes transcytosis through clear cells, either directly into the gland's lumen or into intercellular canaliculi opening to the lumen.
- **Dark cells** filled with strongly eosinophilic granules line most of the lumen and do not contact the basal lamina (Figure 18–18). The granules undergo merocrine secretion to release a poorly understood mixture of glycoproteins with bactericidal activity.
- **Myoepithelial cells** on the basal lamina (Figure 18–18b) contract to move the watery secretion and glycoproteins into the duct.

The **ducts** of eccrine sweat glands have two layers of more acidophilic cells filled with mitochondria and cell membranes rich in Na⁺, K⁺-ATPase. These duct cells absorb Na⁺ ions from the secreted water to prevent excessive loss of this electrolyte. Typically independent of hair follicles, each duct merges with the epidermal basal layer and sweat flow continues in a spiraling channel through the epidermal strata to an excretory **sweat pore** at the skin surface (Figures 18–2a and 18–16).

clitoris, eyelids, and nipples, sebaceous ducts open directly onto the epidermal surface.

The acini of sebaceous glands represent the classic example of holocrine secretion. On the basal lamina is a layer of low-cuboidal epithelial cells, which proliferate and become displaced centrally, undergoing terminal differentiation as large, lipid-producing **sebocytes** filled with small fat droplets (Figure 18–17). Their nuclei shrink and undergo autophagy along with other organelles, and near the duct the cells disintegrate, releasing the lipids as the main secretory product. This product, called **sebum**, gradually covers the surfaces of both the epidermis and hair shafts.

Sebum contains a complex mixture of lipids, including wax esters, squalene, cholesterol, and triglycerides that undergo hydrolysis by bacterial enzymes after secretion. Secretion from sebaceous glands increases greatly at puberty, stimulated primarily by testosterone in men and by ovarian and adrenal androgens in women. Sebum helps maintain the stratum corneum and hair shafts and exerts weak antibacterial and antifungal properties.

FIGURE **18–17** Sebaceous glands.

Sebaceous glands secrete a complex, oily mixture of lipids called **sebum** into short ducts, which in most areas open into hair follicles. Sebum production is the classic example of holocrine secretion, in which the entire cell dies and contributes to the secretory product.

(a) A section of a **pilosebaceous unit** shows acini composed of large sebocytes (**S**), which undergo terminal differentiation by

filling with small lipid droplets and then disintegrating near the ducts (**D**) opening at the hair (**H**) shaft. (×122; H&E)

(b) A section of **sebaceous gland** showing the gland's capsule (**C**) and differentiating sebocytes (**S**) at higher magnification. Proliferation and enlargement of the progenitor cells just inside the capsule continuously forces terminally differentiated sebocytes as sebum into the ducts; myoepithelial cells are not involved. (×400; H&E)

Sweat quickly evaporates upon release, cooling the skin and the blood present there. Eccrine sweat glands also function as auxiliary excretory organs, eliminating small amounts of nitrogenous waste and excess salts.

Apocrine sweat glands occur almost exclusively in skin of the axillary and perineal regions. Their development depends on sex hormones and becomes complete and functional only after puberty. The secretory components of apocrine glands, with much larger lumens than those of eccrine sweat glands (Figure 18–19), have both myoepithelial cells and a single, eosinophilic cell type in a simple epithelium. Many of these cells show apical blebs, suggesting a pinching-off secretory process, as well as features typical of apical granule exocytosis. Thus, the gland's name is controversial since its cells apparently utilize both merocrine and apocrine secretion.

The ducts of apocrine glands resemble those of eccrine glands, but usually open into axillary or other hair follicles (Figure 18–16), thus resulting in a protein-rich product mixed with sebum. The slightly viscous secretion is initially odorless but may acquire a distinctive odor because of bacterial activity. The production of sex-related pheromones by apocrine glands is well established in many mammals, and likely occurs at least vestigially in humans. Apocrine sweat glands are innervated

by adrenergic nerve endings, whereas eccrine sweat glands receive cholinergic fibers.

> **›› MEDICAL APPLICATION**
>
> The sweat of infants with cystic fibrosis (CF) is often salty and is commonly taken as indicative of this genetic disease. CF patients have defects in a transmembrane conductance regulator (CFTR) of epithelial cells that lead to disruptive accumulations of thick mucus in the respiratory and digestive tracts. Failure to remove salt from sweat is related to the same genetic defect.

› SKIN REPAIR

Skin has a good capacity for **repair**, an important attribute in this exposed and easily damaged organ. The process of **cutaneous wound healing**, whether initiated surgically or accidentally, involves several overlapping stages that vary in duration with the size of the wound (Figure 18–20). In the first phase blood from cut vessels clots in the wound, releasing polypeptide growth factors and chemokines from the

FIGURE **18–18** Eccrine sweat glands.

a

b

(a) Histologically **eccrine glands** have small lumens in the secretory components (**S**) and ducts (**D**), both of which have an irregular stratified cuboidal appearance. Both clear and acidophilic cells occur in the stratified cuboidal epithelium of the secretory units. The box indicates an area with such cells shown ultrastructurally in part (b). (×200; Mallory trichrome)

(b) TEM of these important thermoregulatory structures reveals three cell types in their secretory portions. Myoepithelial cells (**M**)

are present at the basal lamina (**BL**) to propel sweat into the duct. Irregular pyramidal cells called dark cells (**D**) border the lumen (**L**) and are filled with electron-dense, eosinophilic secretory granules that release bactericidal peptides and other components of innate immunity. Columnar or cuboidal clear cells (**C**) on the basal lamina rapidly transport water from interstitial fluid in the capillary-rich dermis directly into the lumen or into intercellular canaliculi (**IC**) continuous with the lumen. Na^+ ions are recovered from this fluid through the action of cells in the ducts. (×6500)

FIGURE **18–19** Apocrine sweat glands.

The secretory portions (**S**) of **apocrine sweat glands** have lumens much larger than those of eccrine sweat glands. The ducts (**D**) of apocrine glands also differ from those of eccrine glands in opening into hair follicles (**H**) rather than to the epidermal surface. (×200; Mallory trichrome)

FIGURE 18–20　Major stages of cutaneous wound healing.

① Cut blood vessels bleed into the wound.

② Blood clot forms, and leukocytes clean wound.

③ Blood vessels regrow, and granulation tissue forms.

④ Epithelium regenerates, and connective tissue fibrosis occurs.

Skin repair occurs in overlapping stages shown here schematically.

The process begins with blood quickly **clotting** at the wound site, releasing **platelet-derived growth factors** and other substances (**1**).

Macrophages and **neutrophils** enter the wound as **inflammation** begins, and **keratinocytes** from the cut edges of the epidermal basal layer begin to migrate beneath and through the blood clot (**2**).

Under the influence of growth factors and hydrolytic enzymes released in part from macrophages, **fibroblasts proliferate** and produce much new collagen to form "**granulation tissue**" containing many new, growing capillaries (**3**).

The epidermis gradually reestablishes continuity over the wound site, but **excessive collagen** usually remains in the dermis as **scar tissue** (**4**).

disintegrating platelets. Neutrophils and macrophages undergo diapedesis locally and remove bacteria and debris from the wound. These comprise major events of **inflammation** that typically lasts 2–3 days.

Before completion of this phase, **epithelialization** begins as cells of the epidermal basal layer remove their desmosomes and hemidesmosomes and migrate laterally beneath the blood clot, which becomes an increasingly desiccated eschar, or scab. If much epidermis has been lost, new cells may migrate from the bulge region of surviving hair follicles. Epidermal cell and fibroblast proliferation is stimulated by several different growth factors released from macrophages and other cells and from binding sites in ECM proteoglycans. Matrix metalloproteinases and other proteases from the migrating cells and macrophages facilitate cell migration.

New fibroblasts and newly sprouted capillaries produce another collagen-rich, well-vascularized tissue in the dermis called **granulation tissue**, which gradually replaces the blood clot (Figure 18–20). In the final stage, the epidermis reestablishes continuity but typically lacks the ability to form new hair or glands. The granulation tissue undergoes **remodeling,** and a more normal vasculature reappears. Collagen bundles and fibroblasts in this new connective tissue are at least initially much more abundant and disorganized than in uninjured skin, forming **scar tissue** at the wound site.

Skin SUMMARY OF KEY POINTS

- Skin consists mainly of a superficial stratified squamous epithelium, the **epidermis**, and a thicker layer of connective tissue, the **dermis**, which overlies a **subcutaneous hypodermis**.

Epidermis

- The epidermis consists of **keratinocytes** that undergo a terminal differentiation process called **keratinization** in a series of steps that form distinct epidermal layers or strata.
- The **basal layer** is a single sheet of mitotically active cuboidal cells attached by **hemidesmosomes** and integrins to the basement membrane and to each other by **desmosomes**.
- The **spinous layer** has several tiers of polyhedral cells attached to each other by desmosomes at the tips of short projections containing **bundled keratin**, or **tonofibrils**.
- The **granular layer** is a thinner layer of keratinocytes, now flattened and filled densely with lipid-rich **lamellar granules** and **keratohyaline granules** containing **filaggrin** and other proteins binding the tonofibrils.
- The superficial **cornified layer** protects against water loss, friction, and microbial invasion, and consists of flattened, terminally differentiated cells, or **squames**, which slowly disintegrate.
- The epidermis-dermis interface is enlarged and strengthened by interdigitating **epidermal ridges** or **pegs** and **dermal papillae** in which microvasculature also supplies nutrients and O$_2$ for the epidermis.
- **Melanocytes** in the basal epidermis synthesize dark melanin pigment in **melanosomes** and transport these to adjacent keratinocytes, which accumulate them to protect nuclear DNA from UV damage.
- Antigen-presenting cells called **Langerhans cells** form a network through the epidermis, intercepting and sampling microbial invaders before moving to lymph nodes in an adaptive immune response.

Dermis

- The **dermis** has two major layers: a superficial **papillary layer** or loose connective tissue with a microvascular plexus, and a thicker dense irregular **reticular layer** containing larger blood vessels.

Cutaneous Sensory Receptors

- Sensory receptors in the epidermis include **free nerve endings**, which detect pain and temperature extremes, and basal **tactile or Merkel cells**, light-touch receptors associated with sensory nerve fibers.
- Other cutaneous sensory structures include **Meissner corpuscles**, encapsulated elliptical mechanoreceptors that surround sensory axons and detect light touch.
- Deeper in the dermis and subcutaneous layer are **lamellated** or **Pacinian corpuscles**, which are ovoid and much larger than Meissner corpuscles, for detection of pressure or firm touch.

Epidermal Appendages

- **Hairs** form in **hair follicles**, in which keratinocytes comprising the matrix of the deep **hair bulb** proliferate rapidly and undergo keratinization to form the medulla, cortex, and cuticle of a **hair root**.
- A large dermal **hair papilla** penetrates the base of the hair bulb, and its vasculature supplies nutrients and O$_2$ for proliferating and differentiating cells.
- The growing **hair root** is surrounded by **internal and external root sheaths** continuous with the epidermis, a **glassy membrane** formed in part by the basal lamina, and a **connective tissue sheath**.
- **Nails** are formed in a manner similar to hairs: keratinocytes proliferate in the matrix of the **nail root** and differentiate with the formation of **hard keratin** as a growing **nail plate** with edges covered by skin folds.
- **Sebaceous glands** produce **sebum** by terminal differentiation of **sebocytes**, the classic example of **holocrine secretion**, secreting this oily substance onto hair in the follicles or **pilosebaceous units**.
- **Eccrine sweat glands** in the dermis produce sweat that is mostly water onto the skin surface, where its evaporation provides an important mechanism for cooling the body.
- **Apocrine sweat glands,** restricted to skin of the axillae and perineum, have much wider lumens than eccrine glands, develop after puberty, and secrete protein-rich sweat onto the hair of hair follicles.

Skin ASSESS YOUR KNOWLEDGE

1. Which of the following components of the epidermis provides sealant between adjacent cells, blocking water loss from skin?
   a. Keratohyaline granules
   b. Glycolipids and lipids
   c. Melanin
   d. Desmosomes
   e. Adherent junctions

2. Which cells derive from precursors originating in the bone marrow and function as antigen-presenting cells in skin?
   a. Keratinocytes
   b. Langerhans cells
   c. Melanocytes
   d. Merkel cell
   e. Arrector pili

3. Cells responsible for producing the pigment for dark hair are located in which of the following?
   a. The cortex of the hair shaft
   b. Throughout the hair shaft
   c. The internal root sheath of the hair
   d. The dermal papilla of the hair bulb
   e. The hair matrix (zone of dividing and differentiating cells) of the hair bulb

4. Which of the following separates the hair follicle from the connective tissue of the dermis?
   a. External root sheath
   b. Internal root sheath
   c. Glassy membrane
   d. Hair cuticle
   e. Medulla

5. Which structure typifies reticular dermis but not papillary dermis?
   a. Capillaries
   b. Dense irregular connective tissue
   c. Meissner tactile corpuscles
   d. Sweat gland ducts
   e. Type I collagen fibers

6. Which of the following best characterizes sebaceous glands?
   a. Its duct drains onto the skin surface.
   b. It releases its contents via holocrine secretion.
   c. It primarily secretes water and salts.
   d. Its secretory units are supplied by adrenergic stimulation.
   e. It is located typically in the reticular dermis.

7. Myoepithelial cells aid in the secretory process of which of the following?
   a. Melanocytes
   b. Sebaceous glands
   c. Keratinocytes of the granular layer
   d. Eccrine sweat glands
   e. Apocrine sweat glands

8. A 52-year-old woman presents with severe blistering over her buttocks. Analysis of her serum demonstrates the presence of antibodies which by immunohistochemical techniques stain material located at the basement membrane of the epidermis in a biopsy of her skin. The underlying biological mechanism of her skin disorder involves an abnormality in which of the following structures?
   a. Macula adherens
   b. Gap junctions
   c. Hemidesmosomes
   d. Zonula occludens (tight junctions)
   e. Zonula adherens

9. A 64-year-old woman, who has always been proud of her suntanned, healthy look, is referred to a dermatologist with a blue-violet, painless, 1.5-cm lump in the skin of her left shoulder. The lump is firm and cannot be moved, and has grown very rapidly over the past few weeks. The mass is removed surgically and the pathologist diagnoses it as a Merkel cell carcinoma. If the UV radiation to which her skin was exposed affected the Merkel cells, what other cell type sharing the same specific epidermal layer might also be affected?
   a. Fibroblasts of the papillary layer
   b. Keratinocytes of the stratum granulosum
   c. Cells of tactile (Meissner) corpuscles
   d. Keratinized epithelial cells
   e. Basal stem cells for keratinocytes

10. A 37-year-old woman presents with a suspected Schwannoma. The radiology report indicates "a soft tissue mass to the right of L1 at the level of the L1 to L2 neural foramen." The neurologist presses the base of a vibrating 128 cps tuning fork to the skin of the patient's right and left thighs and asks her to describe the sensation. She asks the patient to close her eyes and then to tell her whether the tuning fork is vibrating or not. With that instrument, the doctor is primarily testing the function of which of the following sensory receptors?
    a. Lamellated (Pacinian) corpuscles
    b. Kraus end bulbs
    c. Meissner corpuscles
    d. Merkel cells
    e. Free nerve endings

19 The Urinary System

The urinary system consists of the paired kidneys and ureters, the bladder, and the urethra. This system's most important function ensures optimal properties of the blood, which the kidneys continuously monitor and adjust. This general role of the kidneys involves a complex combination of renal tasks:

- Regulation of the balance between water and electrolytes (inorganic ions), in addition to the acid-base balance;
- Excretion of metabolic wastes along with excess water and electrolytes in **urine**, the kidneys' excretory product which passes through the ureters for temporary storage in the bladder before its release to the exterior by the urethra;
- Excretion of many bioactive substances, including many drugs;
- Secretion of **renin**, a protease important for regulation of blood pressure by cleaving circulating angiotensinogen to angiotensin I;
- Secretion of **erythropoietin**, a glycoprotein growth factor that stimulates erythrocyte production in red marrow when the blood O_2 level is low;
- Conversion of the steroid prohormone vitamin D, initially produced in the skin, to the active form (**1,25-dihydroxyvitamin D$_3$** or calcitriol); and
- Gluconeogenesis during starvation or periods of prolonged fasting, making glucose from amino acids to supplement this process in the liver.

› KIDNEYS

Approximately 12 cm long, 6 cm wide, and 2.5 cm thick in adults, each **kidney** has a concave medial border, the **hilum**—where nerves enter, the ureter exits, lymphatics exit, and blood vessels do both—and a convex lateral surface,

both covered by a thin fibrous capsule (Figure 19–1). Inside the hilum, the upper end of the ureter expands as the **renal pelvis** and divides into two or three **major calyces**. Smaller branches, the minor calyces, arise from each major calyx. The area surrounding the renal pelvis and calyces contains adipose tissue.

The parenchyma of each kidney has an outer **renal cortex**, a darker stained region with many round corpuscles and tubule cross sections, and an inner **renal medulla** consisting mostly of aligned linear tubules and ducts (Figure 19–1). The renal medulla in humans consists of 8–15 conical structures called **renal pyramids**, all with their bases meeting the cortex (at the corticomedullary junction) and separated from each other by extensions of the cortex called renal columns. Each pyramid plus the cortical tissue at its base and extending along its sides constitutes a **renal lobe**. Parallel ducts and tubules extending from the medulla into the cortex comprise the medullary rays; these plus their associated cortical tissue are considered renal lobules. The tip of each pyramid, called the **renal papilla**, projects into a minor calyx that collects urine formed by tubules in one renal lobe (Figure 19–1).

Each kidney contains roughly 1.25 million functional units called **nephrons** (Figure 19–2). Each nephron consists of a corpuscle attached to a long, simple epithelial renal tubule with three different regions along its length. The major parts of nephron include the following:

- **Renal corpuscle**, an initial dilated part enclosing a tuft of capillary loops and the site of blood filtration, always located in the cortex;
- **Proximal tubule**, a long, very convoluted part, located entirely in the cortex, with a shorter straight part entering the medulla;
- **Loop of Henle** (or nephron loop), in the medulla, with a **thin descending** and a **thin ascending** limb;

FIGURE **19–1** Kidney.

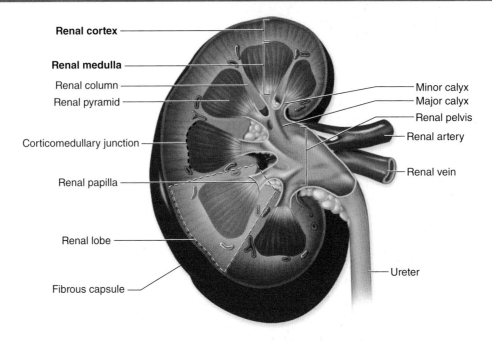

Each **kidney** is bean-shaped, with a concave **hilum** where the ureter and the renal artery and vein enter. The ureter divides and subdivides into several **major and minor calyces**, around which is located the renal sinus containing adipose tissue.

Attached to each minor calyx is a **renal pyramid**, a conical region of medulla delimited by extensions of **cortex**. The cortex and hilum are covered with a fibrous capsule.

- **Distal tubule**, consisting of a thick straight part ascending from the loop of Henle back into the cortex and a convoluted part completely in the cortex; and a
- **Connecting tubule**, a short minor part linking the nephron to collecting ducts.

Connecting tubules from several nephrons merge to form **collecting tubules** that then merge as larger **collecting ducts**. These converge in the renal papilla, where they deliver urine to a minor calyx. **Cortical nephrons** are those located almost completely in the cortex while **juxtamedullary nephrons** (about one-seventh of the total) lie closer to the medulla and have longer loops of Henle extending deeper into the medulla.

⟩⟩ MEDICAL APPLICATION

Polycystic kidney disease represents an inherited disorder in which normal cortical organization of both kidneys is lost due to the formation of multiple, large, fluid-filled cysts. The cysts may arise from any epithelial cells of the nephron and can lead to gross kidney enlargement and loss of renal function.

⟩ BLOOD CIRCULATION

As expected for an organ specialized to process the blood, the kidney vasculature is large, well-organized, and closely associated with all components of the nephron. As Figure 19–3 indicates, the names of blood vessels in kidneys come from their locations or contours.

Each kidney's **renal artery** divides into two or more segmental arteries at the hilum. Around the renal pelvis, these arteries branch further as the **interlobar arteries**, which extend between the renal pyramids toward the corticomedullary junction (Figure 19–3). Here the interlobar arteries divide again to form the **arcuate arteries**, which run in an arc along this junction at the base of each renal pyramid. Smaller **interlobular arteries** (or cortical radial arteries) radiate from the arcuate arteries, extending deeply into the cortex.

From the interlobular arteries arise the microvascular **afferent arterioles**, which divide to form a plexus of looping fenestrated capillaries called the **glomerulus**, each of which develops within a renal corpuscle specialized for filtering blood (Figures 19–3 and 19–4). Blood drains from these glomerular capillaries, not via venules, but via **efferent arterioles**, which at once branch again to form a second capillary network, mostly **peritubular capillaries** profusely distributed throughout the cortex. Efferent arterioles leaving the juxtaglomerular corpuscles near the medulla do not form peritubular capillaries, but instead branch repeatedly as parallel tassel-like bundles of capillary loops called the **vasa recta** (L. *recta*, straight), which penetrate deep into the medulla in association with the loops of Henle and collecting ducts. Collectively, the cortex receives over 10 times more blood than the medulla.

FIGURE **19–2** A nephron and its parts.

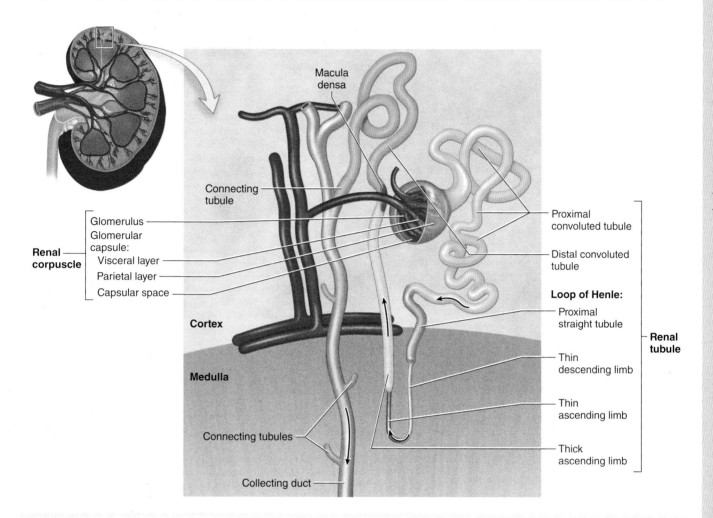

Each kidney contains about 1.25 million functional units called **nephrons**. Each nephron originates in the cortex, at the **renal corpuscle** surrounding a small tuft of glomerular capillaries. Extending from the corpuscle is the long **PCT** which leads to the short **proximal straight tubule** that enters the outer medulla. This tubule continues as the **thin descending limb** and the **thin ascending limb** of the nephron's loop of Henle in the medulla.

The loop of Henle ends with a **thick ascending limb**, a straight tubule that reenters the cortex and ends at its thickened **macula densa** area where it contacts the arterioles entering the glomerulus. Beyond the macula densa this tubule is the **distal convoluted tubule**, the end of which is the short **connecting tubule**. Connecting tubules from many nephrons merge into cortical collecting tubules and a **collecting duct** that transports urine to the calyx.

Blood leaves the kidney in veins that follow the same courses as the arteries and have the same names (Figure 19–3). The outermost peritubular capillaries and capillaries in the kidney capsule converge into small stellate veins that empty into the interlobular veins.

›› MEDICAL APPLICATION

There are many different **glomerular diseases** involving the renal corpuscles, with different causes calling for different treatments. Accurate diagnoses of such disorders by pathologists require sampling of the cortex and may involve examination of the renal corpuscles by immunofluorescence light microscopy or even by TEM.

› RENAL FUNCTION: FILTRATION, SECRETION, & REABSORPTION

Specialized epithelial cells of the nephrons and collecting systems perform the major functions of the kidneys in producing urine: the removal of metabolic wastes as well as excess water and electrolytes from blood. Urine formation involves the following specific activities:

- **Filtration**, by which water and solutes in the blood leave the vascular space and enter the lumen of the nephron;
- Tubular **secretion**, by which substances move from epithelial cells of the tubules into the lumens, usually after

FIGURE **19–3** Blood supply to the kidneys.

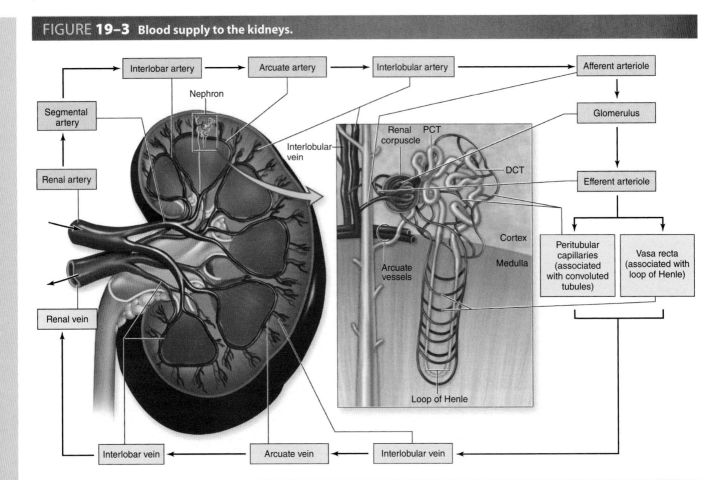

A coronal view of a **kidney** (left) shows the major **blood vessels**, with their names.

An expanded diagram (right) includes the **microvascular components** extending into the cortex and medulla from the interlobular vessels.

Pink boxes indicate vessels with arterial blood and light blue indicates the venous return. The intervening lavender boxes and vessels indicate capillaries where specific reabsorbed substances reenter the blood.

uptake from the surrounding interstitium and capillaries; and

- Tubular **reabsorption**, by which substances move from the tubular lumen across the epithelium into the interstitium and surrounding capillaries.

Along the length of the nephron and collecting system the filtrate receives various secreted molecules and has others reabsorbed, before it enters the minor calyces as **urine** and undergoes **excretion**.

The number of nephrons decreases substantially in older adults, a process accelerated by high blood pressure. Removal of a kidney from a transplant donor (unilateral nephrectomy) causes the remaining kidney to undergo compensatory growth with cellular hypertrophy in the proximal parts of the nephron tubules and an increased rate of filtration, which allow renal function to continue within normal levels.

›› MEDICAL APPLICATION

Inflammation within the glomeruli, or **glomerulonephritis**, which can range from acute or chronic, usually stems from humoral immune reactions. Varieties of this condition involve the deposition of circulating antibody-antigen complexes within glomeruli or circulating antibodies binding to either glomerular antigens or extraneous antigens deposited in the glomeruli. Regardless of the source, the accumulating immune complexes can then elicit a local inflammatory response.

Renal Corpuscles & Blood Filtration

Each nephron begins in a renal corpuscle, about 200 μm in diameter and containing a tuft of glomerular capillaries, surrounded by a double-walled epithelial capsule called the **glomerular (Bowman) capsule** (Figure 19–2). As depicted

FIGURE **19–4** Microvasculature of the renal cortex.

Cortical vasculature is revealed in a section of the kidney with the renal artery injected with carmine dye before fixation. Small interlobular arteries (**I**) branch from the arcuate arteries and radiate out through the cortex giving off the afferent arterioles (**A**) that bring blood to the glomerular capillaries. Each glomerulus (**G**) contains a mass of capillary loops that drain into an efferent arteriole. These then branch as a large, diffuse network of peritubular capillaries (**PT**) throughout the cortex. (×125)

and the visceral layer. Each renal corpuscle has a **vascular pole**, where the afferent arteriole enters and the efferent arteriole leaves, and a **tubular pole**, where the proximal convoluted tubule (PCT) begins (Figure 19–5).

The outer parietal layer of a glomerular capsule consists of a simple squamous epithelium supported externally by a basal lamina. At the tubular pole this epithelium changes to the simple cuboidal epithelium that continues and forms the proximal tubule (Figure 19–5).

The visceral layer of a renal corpuscle consists of unique stellate epithelial cells called **podocytes** (Figures 19–5c and 19–5d), which together with the capillary endothelial cells comprise the apparatus for renal filtration. From the cell body of each podocyte, several **primary processes** extend and curve along and around a length of glomerular capillary. Each primary process gives rise to much more numerous parallel, interdigitating secondary processes or **pedicels** (L. *pedicellus*, little foot; Figures 19–5c and 19–5d). The pedicels cover much of the capillary surfaces, in direct contact with the basal laminae (Figures 19–5c, 19–5d, and 19–6).

Between the interdigitating pedicels are elongated spaces, or filtration **slit pores**, each 25–30 nm wide (Figures 19–5c and 19–6). Electron microscopy reveals that zipper-like **slit diaphragms** bridge these slit pores of adjacent pedicels (Figure 19–6). Slit diaphragms are modified and specialized occluding junctions formed by P-cadherin, **nephrins**, and most abundantly the polyanionic glycoprotein **podocalyxin**. Projecting from cell membrane on each side of the filtration slit, the glycoproteins interact to form a negatively charged molecular mesh within the slit diaphragm which repels organic anions and some polypeptides in the capillary.

The thick (300–360 nm) **glomerular basement membrane** (GBM) occurs between the fenestrated capillary endothelial cells and the covering podocytes (Figure 19–6). The GBM forms the thickest and most substantial part of the filtration barrier separating blood from the capsular space and develops by fusion of the capillary's and the podocyte's basal laminae. Laminin and fibronectin in this blended basement membrane bind integrins in both the podocyte and endothelial cell membranes, and the meshwork of cross-linked type IV collagen and proteoglycans further restricts passage of proteins larger than about 70 kDa, which includes the most abundant proteins in plasma. Small proteins that do make it through the filtration barrier undergo endocytosis within the proximal tubule. The abundant polyanionic GAGs in the glomerular membrane, like the negatively charged components of the slit diaphragms, tend to restrict filtration of organic anions.

Filtration, therefore, occurs through a structure with three parts:

- The fenestrations of the capillary endothelium, which blocks blood cells and platelets;
- The thick, combined basal laminae, or GBM, which restricts large plasma proteins and some organic anions; and
- The filtration slit diaphragms between pedicels, which restrict some small proteins and organic anions.

in Figure 19–5 the capsule's internal or **visceral layer** closely envelops portions of the glomerular capillaries, the walls of which have abundant fenestrations or pores. The outer **parietal layer** forms the external surface of the capsule. Between these two capsular layers is the **capsular** (or **urinary**) **space**, which receives the fluid filtered through the capillary walls

FIGURE **19–5** Renal corpuscles.

(a) Renal corpuscle

Visceral layer of glomerular capsule

(c) Filtration membrane

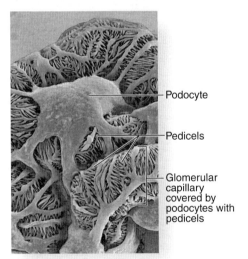

(b) Histology of renal corpuscle

(d) Podocytes

(a) The **renal corpuscle** consists of a small mass of capillaries called the **glomerulus**, housed within a bulbous glomerular capsule. The visceral layer of the capsule is composed of complex epithelial cells called **podocytes**, which cover each capillary, forming slit-like spaces between interdigitating processes called **pedicels**. Blood enters and leaves the glomerulus through the afferent and efferent arterioles, respectively.

(b) The micrograph shows the major histologic features of a **renal corpuscle**. The glomerulus (**G**) of capillaries is surrounded by the capsular space (**CS**) covered by the simple squamous parietal layer (**PL**) of Bowman capsule. Near the corpuscle is that nephron's

macula densa (**MD**) and sections of proximal convoluted tubules (**PCT**) and distal convoluted tubules (**DCT**). (H&E; ×300)

(c) This diagram shows that filtration is produced in the corpuscle when blood plasma in the glomerular capillaries is forced under pressure through the **capillary fenestrations**, across the filtration **membrane** or GBM surrounding the capillary, and through the **filtration slit** diaphragms located between the podocyte pedicels.

(d) The scanning electron microscopy (SEM) shows the distinctive appearance of **podocytes** and their **pedicel** processes that cover **glomerular capillaries**. (×800)

FIGURE 19–6 Glomerular filtration barrier.

The **glomerular filtration barrier** consists of three layered components: the fenestrated **capillary endothelium**, the **GBM**, and **filtration slit** diaphragms between pedicels. The major component of the filter is formed by fusion of the basal laminae of a podocyte and a capillary endothelial cell.

(a) TEM shows cell bodies of two podocytes (**PC**) and the series of pedicels on the capillary (**C**) basement membrane separated by the filtration slit diaphragms. Around the capillaries and podocytes is the capsular space (**CS**) into which the filtrate enters. The enclosed area is shown in part (**b**). (×10,000)

(b) At higher magnification, both the fenestrations (**F**) in the endothelium (**E**) of the capillary (**C**) and the filtration slits (**FS**) separating the pedicels (**P**) are clearly seen on the two sides of the thick, fused basement membrane (**BM**). Thin slit diaphragms (**SD**) bridge the slits between pedicels. (×45,750)

(c) Diagram shows the three major parts of the **glomerular filter** and their major functions.

Glomerular filter
- **Fenestrated capillary endothelium**
- **Glomerular basement membrane** (blocks large proteins)
- **Filtration slit diaphragms** between pedicels (Regulate passage of many small proteins)

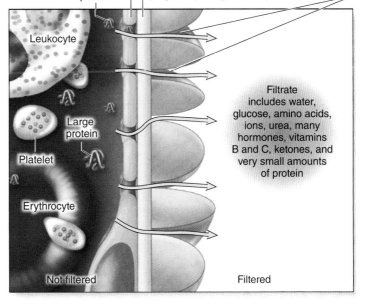

(c) Substances filtered by filtration membrane

Normally about 20% of the blood plasma entering a glomerulus filters into the capsular space. The initial glomerular filtrate has a chemical composition like that of plasma except for its very low protein content. The glomerular filter blocks filtration of most plasma proteins, but smaller proteins, including most polypeptide hormones, pass into the filtrate.

Unlike the shifting pressures affecting most capillary beds which drain into a venule (see Figure 5–18), the glomerular capillaries (each totaling approximately 1 cm in length) are uniquely situated between the two arterioles, afferent and efferent. Importantly, contractile activity of these arterioles causes hydrostatic pressure in the glomerular capillaries to remain higher than the osmotic pressure exerted by their contents, resulting in the constant filtration of plasma by the glomerular filter along its total length, with no reabsorption of the filtrate. Regulation of the glomerular filtration rate (GFR) occurs continuously by neural and hormonal inputs that affect the degree of constriction in the two arterioles. The total glomerular filtration area of an adult has been estimated at 500 cm^2 and the average GFR at 125 mL/min or 180 L/d. Because the total amount of circulating blood plasma averages 3 L, it follows that the kidneys typically filter the entire blood volume 60 times every day.

In addition to capillary endothelial cells and podocytes, renal corpuscles also contain **mesangial cells** (Gr. *mesos*, in the midst + *angion*, vessel), most of which resemble vascular pericytes in having contractile properties and producing components of an external lamina. Mesangial cells are difficult to distinguish from podocytes in routine sections, but often stain more darkly. They and their surrounding matrix comprise the mesangium (Figure 19–7), which fills interstices between capillaries that lack podocytes. Functions of the mesangium include the following:

- Physical support of capillaries within the glomerulus;
- Adjusted contractions in response to blood pressure changes, which help maintain an optimal filtration rate;
- Phagocytosis of protein aggregates adhering to the glomerular filtration barrier, including antibody-antigen complexes abundant in many pathological conditions; and
- Secretion of several cytokines, prostaglandins, and other factors important for immune defense and repair in the glomerulus.

FIGURE **19–7** Mesangium.

(a) Diagram shows that **mesangial cells** in renal corpuscles are located between capillaries and cover those capillary surfaces not covered by **podocyte processes**.

(b) The TEM shows one mesangial cell (**MC**) and the surrounding mesangial matrix (**MM**). This matrix appears similar to and in many places continuous with basement membrane (**BM**) and supports capillaries where podocytes are lacking. Mesangial cells extend contractile processes (arrows) along capillaries that help regulate blood flow in the glomerulus. Some mesangial processes appear to pass between endothelial cells (**EC**) into the capillary lumen (asterisks) where they may help remove or endocytose adherent protein aggregates. The capillary at the left contains an erythrocyte (**E**) and a lymphocyte (**L**). Podocytes (**P**) and their pedicels (**PD**) open to the urinary space (**US**) and associate with the capillary surfaces not covered by mesangial cells. (×3500)

Proximal Convoluted Tubule

Cells in many parts of the nephron tubule and collecting system reabsorb water and electrolytes, but other activities occur primarily in specific tubular regions. Table 19–1 summarizes the functionally specialized regions/cells of nephron tubules and collecting ducts, along with their histologic features, their location in the kidney, and the functions performed there.

TABLE 19–1	Histologic features and major functions of regions within renal tubules.		
Region of Tubule	**Histologic Features**	**Locations**	**Major Functions**
PCT	Simple cuboidal epithelium; cells well-stained, with numerous mitochondria, prominent basal folds and lateral interdigitations; long microvilli, lumens often occluded	Cortex	Reabsorption of all organic nutrients, all proteins, most water, and electrolytes; secretion of organic anions and cations, H$^+$, and NH$_4^+$
Loop of Henle			
Thin limbs	Simple squamous epithelium; few mitochondria	Medulla	Passive reabsorption of Na$^+$ and Cl$^-$
TAL	Simple cuboidal epithelium; no microvilli, but many mitochondria	Medulla and medullary rays	Active reabsorption of various electrolytes
DCT	Simple cuboidal epithelium; cells smaller than in PCT, short microvilli and basolateral folds, more empty lumens	Cortex	Reabsorption of electrolytes
Collecting system			
Principal cells	Most abundant, cuboidal to columnar; pale-staining, distinct cell membranes	Medullary rays and medulla	Regulated reabsorption of water & electrolytes; regulated secretion of K$^+$
Intercalated cells	Few and scattered; slightly darker staining	Medullary rays	Reabsorption of K$^+$ (low-K$^+$ diet); help maintain acid-base balance

DCT, distal convoluted tubule; PCT, proximal convoluted tubule; TAL, thick ascending limb.

At the tubular pole of the renal corpuscle, the simple squamous epithelium of the capsule's parietal layer transforms smoothly into the simple cuboidal epithelium of the **proximal convoluted tubule (PCT)** (Figures 19–8 and 19–9). These long, tortuously winding tubules fill most of the cortex, with their cells specialized for both absorption and secretion. The PCT normally reabsorbs two-thirds of the water and electrolytes, and all the organic nutrients (glucose, amino acids, vitamins, etc.), filtered from plasma in the corpuscle. These reabsorbed molecules all undergo transfer directly across the tubular wall for immediate uptake back into the blood plasma of the adjacent peritubular capillaries.

The cells of the PCTs have central nuclei and very acidophilic cytoplasm (Figures 19–8 and 19–9) because of the abundant mitochondria. The cell apex displays numerous long microvilli that form a prominent **brush border** in the lumen that facilitates reabsorption from the filtrate (Figures 19–8 through 19–10). Because of the large cell size each transverse section of a PCT typically contains only three to five nuclei. In routine histologic preparations, the long brush border appears disorganized and often gives the lumens a fuzz-filled appearance. Peritubular capillaries occur abundantly in the sparse surrounding connective tissue interstitium, which fills only about 10% of the cortex (Figure 19–8).

Ultrastructurally the apical cytoplasm of PCT cells shows numerous pits and **vesicles** near the bases of the microvilli, indicating active endocytosis and pinocytosis (Figure 19–10).

These vesicles contain the small, reabsorbed proteins that will be degraded in lysosomes, with the amino acids released to the circulation. Proximal tubular cells also have many long basal **membrane invaginations** and lateral interdigitations with neighboring cells (Figure 19–10). Both the brush border and the basolateral folds contain many types of transmembrane proteins that mediate tubular reabsorption and secretion. Long mitochondria concentrated along the basal invaginations (Figure 19–10) supply ATP locally for the membrane proteins involved in active transport. Because of the extensive interdigitations of the lateral membranes, routine light microscopy can seldom resolve discrete boundaries between cells of the PCT epithelium.

Transcellular **reabsorption** here involves both active and passive mechanisms, with the cells of the PCT having a large variety of aquaporin channels, transmembrane ion pumps, ion channels, transporters, enzymes, and carrier proteins. Water and certain solutes can also move passively between the cells (paracellular transport) along osmotic gradients through leaky apical tight junctions.

Small proteins in the filtrate either undergo receptor-mediated endocytosis and proteolysis in the cuboidal cells or get degraded by peptidases on the luminal surface. In both cases the resulting amino acids are released at the basolateral cell surfaces for uptake by nearby peritubular capillaries.

Conversely, organic anions and cations not filtered in the renal corpuscle (because of the polyanions in the filter

FIGURE **19–8** **Renal cortex: proximal and distal convoluted tubules.**

(a) The micrograph shows the continuity at a renal corpuscle's tubular pole (**TP**) between the simple cuboidal epithelium of a proximal convoluted tubule (**P**) and the simple squamous epithelium of the capsule's parietal layer. The urinary space (**U**) between the parietal layer and the glomerulus (**G**) drains into the lumen of the proximal tubule. The lumens of the proximal tubules appear filled, because of the long microvilli of the brush border

and aggregates of small plasma proteins bound to this structure. By contrast, the lumens of distal convoluted tubules (**D**) appear empty, lacking a brush border and protein.

(b) Here the abundant peritubular capillaries and draining venules (arrows) surrounding the proximal (**P**) and distal (**D**) convoluted tubules are clearly seen. (Both ×400; H&E)

or by binding to plasma proteins) may be released from the peritubular capillaries, taken up by the cells of the proximal tubules and undergo **secretion** back into the filtrate by active transport (Table 19–1). Organic anion and cation transporters in the PCT allow kidneys to dispose of such substances at a higher rate than by glomerular filtration alone. Because these molecules include important substances (such as bile salts and creatinine) and many antibiotics and other drugs, this process of tubular secretion has great pharmacologic importance as a key mechanism of drug clearance.

Besides their major roles in reabsorption and secretion, cells of the proximal tubule also perform hydroxylation of vitamin D and release it to the capillaries. Moreover,

fibroblastic interstitial cells in cortical areas near the proximal tubules produce erythropoietin, the erythroblast growth factor secreted in response to a prolonged decrease in local oxygen concentration.

〉〉 MEDICAL APPLICATION

Diabetic glomerulosclerosis, the thickening and loss of function in the GBM produced as part of the systemic microvascular sclerosis in diabetes mellitus, is the leading cause of (irreversible) **end-stage kidney disease** in the United States. Treatment requires either a **kidney transplant** or regular **artificial hemodialysis**.

FIGURE 19–9 Convoluted tubules, nephron loops, and collecting ducts.

(a) Nephron components

Efferent arteriole

Connecting tubule

Afferent arteriole

Collecting duct

Distal convoluted atubule

Renal corpuscle

Proximal convoluted tubule

Nephron loop

(b) Renal cortex

RC

DCT

PCT

(c) Convoluted tubule epithelia

Tall microvilli

Short, sparse microvilli

Nucleus
Mitochondria
Basement membrane

Proximal convoluted tubule

Distal convoluted tubule

(d) Cross section of renal medulla

T

A

T

CD

CD

A

(a) Diagram of a **nephron** shows levels of the sections in the photos.

(b) A section of cortical tissue shows two renal corpuscles (**RC**), the eosinophilic proximal convoluted tubules (**PCT**) with lumens containing microvilli and small proteins, and the less abundant, less well-stained distal convoluted tubules (**DCT**) with empty lumens. (×120; H&E)

(c) Diagram shows the major structural differences between the cuboidal cells of **proximal and distal tubules**. Cells of both tubules have basal membrane invaginations associated with mitochondria.

(d) A cross section through a **medullary renal pyramid** shows the simple squamous epithelium of the thin descending and ascending limbs of loops of Henle (**T**) and its thick ascending limbs (**A**), as well as the pale columnar cells of collecting ducts (**CD**). Note also the homogeneous **interstitium** with capillaries smaller than the thin limbs. (×160; Mallory trichrome)

Loop of Henle (or Nephron Loop)

Near the medulla the PCT continues with a much shorter portion, less specialized for reabsorption, called the proximal straight tubule, which enters the medulla and continues as the nephron's **loop of Henle** (Figure 19–2). This is a U-shaped structure with a **thin descending limb** into the medulla and a **thin ascending limb** back to the cortex, with both limbs composed of simple squamous epithelia. The straight part of

TEM reveals important features of the cuboidal cells of the **proximal convoluted epithelium**: the long, dense apical microvilli (**MV**), the abundant endocytotic pits and vesicles (**V**) in the apical regions near lysosomes (**L**). Small proteins brought into the cells nonspecifically by pinocytosis are degraded in lysosomes and the amino acids released basally.

Apical ends of adjacent cells are sealed with zonula occludens, but the basolateral sides are characterized by long invaginating folds of membrane along which many long mitochondria (**M**) are situated. Water and the small molecules released from the PCTs are taken up immediately by the adjacent peritubular capillaries (**C**). Between the basement membranes of the tubule and the capillary shown here is an extension of a fibroblast (**F**). (×10,500)

the proximal tubule has an outer diameter of about 60 μm, but it narrows abruptly to about 30 μm in the thin limbs of the loop. The squamous cells comprising the wall of the thin segments contain few organelles, indicating a primarily passive role in transcellular transport, and the lumen is prominent (Figures 19–9 and 19–11). Near the cortex the thin ascending limb of the loop becomes the **thick ascending limb (TAL)**, with simple cuboidal epithelium and many mitochondria again, and extends as far as the macula densa near the nephron's glomerulus (Figure 19–2).

Further important adjustments to the salt content of the filtrate involve the loops of Henle and the surrounding interstitial connective tissue. Cuboidal cells of the loops' thick ascending limbs transport Na$^+$ actively and other ions passively out of the tubule against a concentration gradient into the hyaluronate-rich interstitium, making that compartment hyperosmotic. This causes water to diffuse from the thin descending part of the loop, concentrating the filtrate. The countercurrent flow of filtrate (descending, then immediately ascending) in the two parallel limbs of the nephron loop establishes a gradient of osmolarity in the interstitium of the renal pyramids, an effect "multiplied" at deeper levels in the medulla by the activity of many additional loops from juxtamedullary nephrons penetrating deeper into the medullary pyramids. As mentioned earlier and shown diagrammatically in Figure 19–3, fenestrated capillaries of the **vasa recta** develop in very close association with all parts of the nephron loop (Figure 19–11). Countercurrent blood flow in the looping vasa recta capillaries helps maintain the hyperosmotic interstitium, allowing the interstitial osmolarity to become maximal near the apex of the medullary pyramid. The mechanism of the **countercurrent exchange system** established by the loops of Henle and vasa recta is an important topic in renal physiology.

> **›› MEDICAL APPLICATION**
>
> **Sickle cell nephropathy**, one of the most common problems caused by sickle cell disease, occurs when the affected erythrocytes sickle in the vasa recta because of the low oxygen tension there. The nephropathy results from **renal infarcts**, usually within the renal papillae or pyramids.

Distal Convoluted Tubule & Juxtaglomerular Apparatus

The ascending limb of the nephron is straight as it enters the cortex and forms the macula densa, and then becomes tortuous as the **distal convoluted tubule (DCT)** (Figure 19–2). Much less tubular reabsorption occurs here than in the proximal tubule. The simple cuboidal cells of the distal tubules differ from those of the proximal tubules in being smaller and having no brush border and more empty lumens (Figure 19–9). Because distal tubule cells are flatter and smaller than those of the proximal tubule, more nuclei are typically seen in sections of distal tubules than in those of proximal tubules (Figure 19–8). Cells of the DCT also have fewer mitochondria than cells of proximal tubules, making them less acidophilic (Figure 19–9). The rate of Na$^+$ absorption here is regulated by **aldosterone** from the adrenal glands.

Where the initial, straight part of the distal tubule contacts the arterioles at the vascular pole of the renal corpuscle of its parent nephron, its cells become more columnar and closely packed, forming the **macula densa** (L. thicker spot). This is part of a specialized sensory structure, the **juxtaglomerular apparatus (JGA)** that utilizes feedback mechanisms to regulate glomerular blood flow and keep the rate of glomerular filtration relatively constant. The JGA is shown in Figures 19–5 and 19–12. Cells of the macula densa typically have apical nuclei, basal Golgi complexes, and a more elaborate and varied system

FIGURE **19–11** Renal medulla: nephron loops and collecting ducts.

(a) A micrograph of a **medullary renal pyramid** cut transversely shows closely packed cross sections of the many nephron loops' thin descending and ascending limbs (**T**) and thick ascending limbs (**A**), intermingled with parallel vasa recta capillaries containing blood (**C**) and collecting ducts (**CD**). All these structures are embedded in the interstitium (**I**), which contains sparse myofibroblast-like cells in a matrix very rich in hydrophilic hyaluronate.

The specialized nature of the interstitial tissue helps maintain the osmolarity gradient established by differential salt and water transport across the wall of the nephron loop, which is required to concentrate urine and conserve body water. (×400; Mallory trichrome)

(b) The TEM reveals the slightly fibrous nature of the interstitium (**I**) and shows that the simple squamous epithelium of the thin limbs (**T**) is slightly thicker than that of the nearby vasa recta capillaries (**C**). (×3300)

(Figure 19–11b, reproduced with permission from Dr Johannes Rhodin, Department of Cell Biology and Anatomy, University of South Florida College of Medicine, Tampa.)

of ion channels and transporters. Adjacent to the macula densa, the tunica media of the afferent arteriole is also modified. The smooth muscle cells are modified as **juxtaglomerular granular (JG) cells**, with a secretory phenotype including more rounded nuclei, rough ER, Golgi complexes, and granules with the protease **renin** (Figures 19–5 and 19–12). Also, at the vascular pole are **lacis cells** (Fr. *lacis*, lacework), which are extraglomerular mesangial cells that have many of the same supportive, contractile, and defensive functions as these cells inside the glomerulus.

Basic functions of the JGA in the autoregulation of the GFR and in controlling blood pressure include the following activities. Elevated arterial pressure increases glomerular capillary blood pressure, which increases the GFR. Higher GFR leads to higher luminal concentrations of Na^+ and Cl^- in the TAL of the nephron, which are monitored by cells of the macula densa. Increased ion levels in the lumen cause these cells to release ATP, adenosine, and other vasoactive compounds

that trigger contraction of the afferent arteriole, which lowers glomerular pressure and decreases the GFR. This lowers tubular ion concentrations, which turns off the release of vasoconstrictors from the macula densa.

Decreased arterial pressure leads to increased autonomic stimulation to the JGA as a result of baroreceptor function, including local baroreceptors in the afferent arteriole, possibly the JG cells themselves. This causes the JG cells to release renin, an aspartyl protease, into the blood. There renin cleaves the plasma protein **angiotensinogen** into the inactive decapeptide **angiotensin I**. Angiotensin-converting enzyme (ACE) on lung capillaries clips this further to **angiotensin II**, a potent vasoconstrictor that directly raises systemic blood pressure and stimulates the adrenals to secrete **aldosterone**. Aldosterone promotes Na^+ and water reabsorption in the distal convoluted and connecting tubules, which raises blood volume to help increase blood pressure. The return of normal blood pressure turns off secretion of renin by JG cells.

FIGURE **19–12**   Juxtaglomerular apparatus.

The **JGA** forms at the point of contact between a nephron's distal tubule (**D**) and the vascular pole of its glomerulus (**G**). At that point cells of the distal tubule become columnar as a thickened region called the macula densa (**MD**). Smooth muscle cells of the afferent arteriole's (**AA**) tunica media are converted from a contractile to a secretory morphology as juxtaglomerular granule cells (**JG**).

Also present are lacis cells (**L**), which are extraglomerular mesangial cells adjacent to the macula densa, the afferent arteriole, and the efferent arteriole (**EA**). In this specimen, the lumens of proximal tubules (**P**) appear filled and the urinary space (**US**) is somewhat swollen. (×400; Mallory trichrome)

Collecting Ducts

The last part of each nephron, the **connecting tubule**, carries the filtrate into a collecting system that transports it to a minor calyx and in which more water is reabsorbed if needed by the body. As shown in Figure 19–13, a connecting tubule extends from each nephron and several join together in the cortical medullary rays to form **collecting ducts** of simple cuboidal epithelium and an average diameter of 40 μm. In the medulla these merge further, forming larger and straighter collecting ducts with increasingly columnar cells and overall diameters reaching 200 μm (Figures 19–11 and 19–14). Approaching

the apex of each renal pyramid, several medullary collecting ducts merge again to form each **papillary duct** (or duct of Bellini), which deliver urine directly into the minor calyx (Figure 19–13). Running parallel with the descending and ascending limbs of the loops of Henle and vasa recta, medullary collecting ducts lie in the area with very high interstitial osmolarity (Figures 19–2 and 19–11).

Collecting tubules and ducts are composed mainly of pale-staining **principal cells** with few organelles, sparse microvilli, and unusually distinct cell boundaries (Figure 19–14). Ultrastructurally the principal cells can be seen to have basal membrane infoldings, consistent with their role in ion transport, and a primary cilium among the microvilli. The medullary collecting ducts are the final site of water reabsorption from the filtrate. Principal cells are particularly rich in **aquaporins**, the integral membrane pore proteins functioning as specific channels for water molecules, but here most aquaporins are sequestered in membranous cytoplasmic vesicles.

Antidiuretic hormone (ADH), released from the posterior pituitary gland as the body becomes dehydrated, makes collecting ducts more permeable to water and increases the rate at which water molecules are pulled osmotically from the filtrate. Upon binding, ADH receptors on the basolateral cell surface stimulate the movement and insertion of vesicles with aquaporins into the apical (luminal) membranes, increasing the number of membrane channels and water movement through the cells. The high osmolarity of the interstitium draws water passively from the collecting ducts, concentrating the filtrate. The water thus saved immediately enters the blood in the vasa recta.

Scattered among the principal cells are variably darker **intercalated cells** with more abundant mitochondria and projecting apical folds. Intercalated cells, some of which also occur in the DCTs, help maintain acid-base balance by secreting either H^+ (from type A or α intercalated cells) or HCO_3^- (from type B or β intercalated cells).

Table 19–1 summarizes the histologic features and major functions of the nephron's parts and collecting ducts.

〉〉 MEDICAL APPLICATION

A common problem involving the ureters is their obstruction by **renal calculi (kidney stones)** formed in the renal pelvis or calyces, usually from calcium salts (oxalate or phosphate) or uric acid. While urate stones are usually smooth and small, calcium stones can become large and irritate the mucosa. Most kidney stones are asymptomatic, but besides causing an obstruction that can lead to renal problems, movement of stones from the renal pelvis into the ureter can cause extreme pain on the affected side of the body. Problems caused by such stones can be corrected by either surgical removal of the stone or its disintegration using focused ultrasonic shock waves in a procedure called **lithotripsy**, although this treatment can cause significant renal damage.

FIGURE **19–13** Fluid transport in the urinary system.

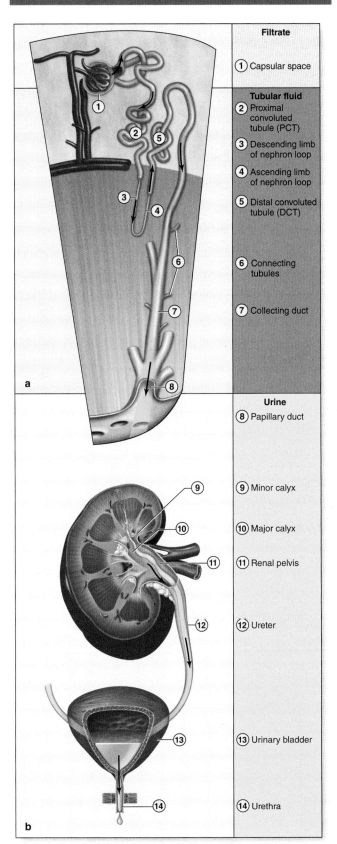

Filtrate

1. Capsular space

Tubular fluid

2. Proximal convoluted tubule (PCT)
3. Descending limb of nephron loop
4. Ascending limb of nephron loop
5. Distal convoluted tubule (DCT)
6. Connecting tubules
7. Collecting duct

Urine

8. Papillary duct
9. Minor calyx
10. Major calyx
11. Renal pelvis
12. Ureter
13. Urinary bladder
14. Urethra

FIGURE **19–14** Collecting ducts.

Pale-staining columnar **principal cells**, in which ADH-regulated aquaporins of the cell membrane allow more water reabsorption, are clearly seen in these transversely sectioned collecting ducts (**CD**), surrounded by interstitium with vasa recta (**VR**). (×600; PT)

» URETERS, BLADDER, & URETHRA

Urine is transported by the **ureters** from the renal pelvis to the **urinary bladder** where it is stored until emptying by micturition via the **urethra**. The walls of the ureters are similar to that of the calyces and renal pelvis, with mucosal, muscular, and

(Left) (a) Diagram of a **nephron and collecting system** shows the flow of filtrate. **(b)** Upon delivery at a **minor calyx**, filtrate is no longer modified by reabsorption or secretion and is called **urine**. It flows passively into the **renal pelvis** but moves by peristalsis along the **ureters** for temporary storage in the **urinary bladder**, which is emptied through the **urethra**.

FIGURE **19–15** Renal papilla, collecting ducts, and minor calyx.

A sagittal section of a **renal papilla** shows numerous **collecting ducts** (also called the **ducts of Bellini** at this level) converging at the end of the renal papilla (**RP**) where they empty into the minor calyx (**MC**). The mucosa of the calyx contains dense connective tissue stained blue here and adipose tissue (**A**). The ducts are embedded in interstitial tissue, which also contains thin limbs of the nephron loops (×50; Mallory trichrome).

Inset: An enlarged area shows the columnar epithelium of the collecting ducts (**CD**), the interstitium (**I**) and thin limbs (**T**), and the protective urothelium (**U**) that lines the minor calyx. (×200; Mallory trichrome)

adventitial layers and becoming gradually thicker closer to the bladder. The mucosa of these organs is lined by the uniquely stratified **urothelium** or transitional epithelium introduced in Chapter 4 (Figures 19–15 and 19–16). Cells of this epithelium are organized as three layers:

- A single layer of small basal cells resting on a very thin basement membrane;
- An intermediate region containing from one to several layers of cuboidal or low columnar cells; and
- A superficial layer of large bulbous or elliptical **umbrella cells**, sometimes binucleated, which are highly differentiated to protect the underlying cells against the potentially cytotoxic effects of hypertonic urine.

The thick muscularis of the ureters moves urine toward the bladder by peristaltic contractions and produces prominent mucosal folds when the lumen is empty (Figure 19–16).

> > **MEDICAL APPLICATION**

Bacterial infections of the urinary tract can lead to inflammation of the renal pelvis and calyces, or **pyelonephritis**. In acute pyelonephritis, bacteria often move from one or more minor calyx into the associated renal papilla, causing accumulation of neutrophils in the collecting ducts.

Umbrella cells are especially well developed in the bladder (Figure 19–17) where contact with urine is greatest. These cells, up to 100 μm in diameter, have extensive intercellular junctional complexes surrounding unique apical membranes. Most of the apical surface consists of **asymmetric unit membranes** in which regions of the outer lipid layer appear ultrastructurally to be twice as thick as the inner leaflet. These regions are composed of lipid rafts containing mostly integral membrane proteins called **uroplakins** that assemble into paracrystalline arrays of stiffened plaques 16 nm in diameter. The abundant membranous plaques, together with the tight junctions, allow this epithelium to serve as an osmotic barrier protecting its cells and the cells of surrounding tissues from hypertonic urine and preventing dilution of the stored urine.

Plaques are hinged together by more narrow regions of typical membrane. When the bladder is emptied, not only does the mucosa fold extensively, but individual umbrella cells decrease their apical surface area by folding the membrane at the hinge regions and internalizing the folded plaques in discoidal vesicles. As the bladder fills again these vesicles rejoin the apical membrane, increasing its surface area as the tight junctions are reorganized and the cells become less bulbous. The thickness of the full bladder's urothelium is half that of the empty bladder (2–3 cell layers vs 5–7 layers), apparently the result of the intermediate cells being pushed and pulled laterally to accommodate the increased volume of urine.

Urothelium is surrounded by a folded lamina propria and submucosa, followed by a dense sheath of interwoven smooth muscle layers and adventitia (Figures 19–16 and 19–17). Urine is moved from the renal pelvises to the bladder by peristaltic contractions of the ureters.

The bladder's lamina propria and dense irregular connective tissue of the submucosa are highly vascularized. The bladder in an average adult can hold 400–600 mL of urine, with the urge to empty appearing at about 150–200 mL. The muscularis consists of three poorly delineated layers, collectively called the **detrusor muscle**, which contract to empty the bladder (Figure 19–17). Three muscular layers are seen most distinctly at the neck of the bladder near the urethra (Figure 19–17). The ureters pass through the wall of the bladder obliquely, forming a valve that prevents the backflow of urine into the ureters as the bladder fills. All the urinary passages are covered

FIGURE **19–16** Ureters.

(a) Ureter cross section

(b)

(a) Diagram of a **ureter** in cross section shows a characteristic pattern of longitudinally folded **mucosa**, surrounded by a thick **muscularis** that moves urine by regular waves of peristalsis. The lamina propria is lined by a unique stratified epithelium called

transitional epithelium or **urothelium** that is resistant to the potentially deleterious effects of contact with hypertonic urine.

(b) Histologically the muscularis (**Mu**) is much thicker than the mucosa (**M**) and adventitia (**A**). (×18; H&E)

FIGURE **19–17** Bladder wall and urothelium.

(a) In the neck of the **bladder**, near the urethra, the wall shows four layers: the mucosa with urothelium (**U**) and lamina propria (**LP**); the thin submucosa (**S**); inner, middle, and outer layers of smooth muscle (**IL**, **ML**, and **OL**); and the adventitia (**A**). (×15; H&E)

(b) When the bladder is empty, the **mucosa** is highly folded and the urothelium (**U**) has bulbous umbrella cells. (×250; PSH)

(c) When the bladder is full, the **mucosa** is pulled smooth, the urothelium (**U**) is thinner, and the umbrella cells are flatter. (×250; H&E)

externally by an adventitial layer, except for the upper part of the bladder that is covered by serous peritoneum.

The **urethra** is a tube that carries the urine from the bladder to the exterior (Figure 19–18). The urethral mucosa has prominent longitudinal folds, giving it a distinctive appearance in cross section. In men, the two ducts for sperm transport during ejaculation join the urethra at the prostate gland (see Chapter 21). The male urethra is longer and consists of three segments:

- The **prostatic urethra**, 3–4 cm long, extends through the prostate gland and is lined by urothelium.

- The **membranous urethra**, a short segment, passes through an **external sphincter** of striated muscle and is lined by stratified columnar and pseudostratified columnar epithelium.

- The **spongy urethra**, about 15 cm in length, is enclosed within erectile tissue of the penis (see Chapter 21) and is lined by stratified columnar and pseudostratified columnar epithelium (Figure 19–18), with stratified squamous epithelium distally.

In women, the urethra is exclusively a urinary organ. The female urethra is a 3- to 5-cm-long tube, lined initially with transitional epithelium which then transitions to nonkeratinized stratified squamous epithelium continuous with that of the skin at the labia minora. The middle part of the urethra in both sexes is surrounded by the external striated muscle sphincter.

FIGURE **19–18** Urethra.

The **urethra** is a fibromuscular tube that carries urine from the bladder to the exterior of the body.

(a) A transverse section shows that the **mucosa** has large **longitudinal folds** around the lumen (**L**). (×50; H&E)

(b) A higher magnification of the enclosed area shows the unusual **stratified columnar** nature of the urethral epithelium (**E**). This thick epithelial lining varies between stratified columnar in some areas and pseudostratified columnar elsewhere, but it becomes stratified squamous at the distal end of the urethra. (×250; H&E)

The Urinary System SUMMARY OF KEY POINTS

Kidney

- Each kidney has a thick outer **cortex**, surrounding a **medulla** that is divided into 8-12 renal pyramids; each pyramid and its associated cortical tissue comprises a **renal lobe**.
- The apical papilla of each renal pyramid inserts into a **minor calyx**, a subdivision of two or three **major calyces** extending from the **renal pelvis**.
- The **ureter** carries urine from the renal pelvis and exits the **renal hilum**, where the **renal artery and vein** are also located.

Renal Vasculature

- Renal arteries branch to form smaller arteries between the renal lobes, with **interlobular arteries** entering the cortex to form the microvasculature; venous branches parallel the arterial supply.
- In the cortex, **afferent arterioles** enter capillary clusters called **glomeruli**, which are drained by **efferent arterioles**, instead of venules, an arrangement that allows higher hydrostatic pressure in the capillaries.
- The **efferent arterioles** from cortical glomeruli branch diffusely as **peritubular capillaries**, while those from juxtamedullary glomeruli branch as long microvascular loops called **vasa recta** in the medulla.

Nephrons

- Functional units of the kidney are the **nephrons**, numbering about 1.25 million, each with a **renal corpuscle** and a long **renal tubule**, and a system of **collecting ducts**.
- The renal corpuscle has a simple squamous parietal layer of the **glomerular (Bowman) capsule**, continuous with the proximal tubule, and a specialized visceral layer of **podocytes** surrounding the glomerular capillaries.
- **Podocytes** extend large primary processes that curve around a capillary and extend short, interdigitating secondary processes or **pedicels**, between which are narrow spaces called **slit pores**.
- The elevated pressure in the capillaries forces water and small solutes of blood plasma through the **glomerular filter** into the **capsular (or urinary) space** inside the glomerular capsule.
- In each glomerulus the filter has three parts: the finely **fenestrated capillary endothelium**; the thick (330 nm) **fused basal laminae** of type IV collagen and other proteins produced by the endothelial cells and podocytes; and the **slit pores** between the pedicels, covered by thin filtration **slit diaphragms**.
- From the renal corpuscle, filtrate enters the long **nephron tubule** that extends through both the cortex and medulla, with epithelial cells for both **reabsorption** and **secretion** of substances into the filtrate.

- The first tubular part, the **PCT**, is mainly cortical, has **simple cuboidal** cells with **long microvilli** in the lumen, **abundant mitochondria**, and large, interdigitating **basolateral folds**.
- In the **PCT**, all glucose and other organic nutrients, all small proteins and peptides (which are degraded to amino acids), and much water and electrolytes are reabsorbed from the filtrate and transferred to the peritubular capillaries.
- From the PCT filtrate flows into the **loop of Henle**, located in the medulla, which has squamous **thin descending** and **ascending limbs**; the latter extends as a **TAL** back into the cortex.
- In the cortex, the **TAL** (also known as the **distal straight tubule**) contacts the arterioles at the vascular pole of its parent renal corpuscle and there thickens focally as the **macula densa**.
- Tall epithelial cells of the **macula densa** and specialized smooth muscle cells in the adjacent afferent arteriole called **juxtaglomerular cells**, which secrete **renin**, comprise a JGA that is an important regulator of blood pressure.
- Beyond the macula densa, the tubule continues as the **DCT**, where electrolyte levels of the filtrate are adjusted further, and which lead to short **connecting tubules**.
- **Connecting tubules** from several nephrons join to form the cortical **collecting ducts**, of simple cuboidal epithelium, which enter the medulla in parallel with the loops of Henle and vasa recta and become larger with more columnar cells.

Urinary Tract

- **Principal cells** of the **collecting ducts** are pale-staining, with relatively few mitochondria and distinct cell membranes that are rich in **aquaporins** (water channels) for passive water reabsorption.
- The largest collecting ducts deliver filtrate into the **minor calyces**, where it undergoes no further modification and is called **urine**.
- The calyces, renal pelvis, ureters, and urinary bladder are lined by **urothelium**, or transitional epithelium, which protects underlying cells from hypertonic, potentially toxic effects of urine.
- Large, bulbous superficial cells of the urothelium, called **umbrella cells**, have apical membranes consisting of hinged regions with dense plaques of **uroplakin** proteins that protect the cytoplasm.
- As the **urinary bladder** fills its highly folded mucosa unfolds, the urothelium gets somewhat thinner by cell movements, and the hinged membrane plaques of umbrella cells partially unfold.
- The **urethra** drains the bladder and in both genders is lined initially by urothelium, followed (in males) by alternating **stratified columnar** and **pseudostratified columnar epithelium** and distally by stratified squamous epithelium.
- In males, the urethra has three regions: the **prostatic urethra** in the prostate gland, the short **membranous urethra** passing through the urogenital diaphragm, and the long **penile urethra**.

The Urinary System   ASSESS YOUR KNOWLEDGE

1. Blood in the renal arcuate arteries flows next into which vessels?
   a. Afferent arterioles
   b. Efferent arterioles
   c. Glomerular capillaries
   d. Interlobar arteries
   e. Interlobular arteries

2. Which cell type comprises the visceral layer of Bowman capsule?
   a. Endothelial cells
   b. Juxtaglomerular cells
   c. Mesangial cells
   d. Podocytes
   e. Extraglomerular mesangial (or Lacis) cells

3. Which type of epithelium lines the thick ascending limb of the loop of Henle?
   a. Pseudostratified columnar
   b. Simple columnar
   c. Simple cuboidal
   d. Simple squamous
   e. Transitional (urothelium)

4. Which cell is a modified smooth muscle cell that secretes renin?
   a. Macula densa cells
   b. Mesangial cells
   c. Podocytes
   d. Juxtaglomerular cells
   e. Endothelial cells

5. Epithelial cell membrane domains containing many stiffened plaques of protein are an important feature in which part of the urinary system?
   a. Juxtaglomerular apparatus
   b. Bladder mucosa
   c. Collecting ducts
   d. Renal pyramids
   e. Membranous urethra

6. An immunohistochemical technique using antibodies against aquaporins to stain a section of kidney would be expected to stain cells in which structures most intensely?
   a. Collecting ducts
   b. Lining of the major and minor calyces
   c. Proximal convoluted tubules
   d. Distal convoluted tubules
   e. Glomeruli

7. What type of epithelium lines the prostatic urethra?
   a. Simple columnar
   b. Pseudostratified columnar
   c. Stratified squamous
   d. Simple squamous
   e. Transitional (urothelium)

8. A 14-year-old patient presents in the nephrology clinic with fatigue, malaise, anorexia, abdominal pain, and fever. She reports a loss of 6 lb in the past 2 months. Serum gamma globulin and the immunoglobulins IgG, IgA, and IgM are all elevated. Her serum creatine is 1.4 mg/dL (normal 0.6–1.2 mg/dL) and urinalysis of glucose and protein are 2+ on a dipstick test, confirmed by laboratory at 8.0 g/dL and 0.95 g/dL, respectively. A renal biopsy is prepared for light microscopy, and an infiltrate containing lymphocytes, plasma cells, and eosinophils is found among tubules having cells with prominent brush borders. Which one of the following statements correctly pertains to these epithelial cells?
   a. Impermeable to water despite presence of ADH
   b. The primary site for the reduction of the tubular fluid volume
   c. The site of the countercurrent multiplier
   d. The site of action of aldosterone
   e. Indirectly involved in the release of renin

9. A 45-year-old man presents with nephrolithiasis or kidney stones. The process of calcium oxalate stone formation as seen in this patient begins with Randall plaques found in the basement membranes of which one of the following structures found only in the renal medulla?
   a. Proximal convoluted tubules
   b. Distal convoluted tubules
   c. Thin limbs in the loops of Henle
   d. Afferent arterioles
   e. Collecting tubules

10. A 15-year-old boy presents with hematuria, hearing loss, lens dislocation, and the onset of cataracts. Genetic analysis reveals a mutation in the *COL4A5* gene. Transmission EM examination of a renal biopsy confirms that the disorder has affected a component of the renal corpuscles in which damage disrupts normal glomerular filtration. Which one of the following structures would most likely be abnormal in the TEM of this patient's biopsy?
   a. Pedicels
   b. Filtration slits
   c. Slit diaphragms
   d. Glomerular basement membranes
   e. Fenestrated endothelium of glomerular capillaries

Answers: 1e, 2d, 3c, 4d, 5b, 6a, 7e, 8b, 9c, 10d

20 Endocrine Glands

Secretory cells of endocrine glands release their products, signaling molecules called **hormones**, into neighboring vascularized compartments for uptake by capillaries and distribution throughout the body. Unlike exocrine gland secretions, hormone release does not involve secretory ducts. Most endocrine cells are typically epithelial, at least in origin, and aggregated as cords or clusters. Besides the specialized endocrine glands discussed in this chapter, many other organs specialized for other functions, such as the heart, thymus, gut, kidneys, testis, and ovaries, contain various endocrine cells (Figure 20–1). As described in earlier chapters, release of hormone-like factors also occurs in certain cells developing and functioning also as neurons, smooth and cardiac muscle fibers, leukocytes, and fibroblasts.

Distribution by the circulatory system allows hormones to act on target cells with their cognate receptors at a distance from the site of their secretion. As discussed briefly in Chapter 2, some endocrine cells produce hormones that act on target cells only a short distance away. This may involve **paracrine** secretion, with localized dispersal in interstitial fluid or through short loops of blood vessels, as when gastrin made by pyloric G cells reaches target cells in the fundic glands, or **juxtacrine** secretion in which signaling molecules remain on the secreting cell's surface or adjacent extracellular matrix and affect target cells when the cells make contact. Juxtacrine signaling is particularly important in embryonic and regenerative tissue interactions. In **autocrine** secretion cells produce molecules that act on themselves or on cells of the same type. For example, insulin-like growth factor (IGF) produced by several cell types may target the same cells that produced it. Endocrine glands are often also target organs for other hormones that can establish feedback mechanisms controlling hormone secretion that keep blood hormonal levels within strict limits.

Hormones, like neurotransmitters, are frequently hydrophilic molecules such as proteins, glycoproteins, peptides, or modified amino acids with receptors on the surface of target cells. Alternatively, hydrophobic steroid and thyroid hormones circulate bound to transport proteins but can diffuse through the cell membrane bilayer to be taken up and activate cytoplasmic receptors in target cells (see Chapter 2).

❯ PITUITARY GLAND (HYPOPHYSIS)

The **pituitary gland**, or **hypophysis** (Gr. *hypo*, under + *physis*, growth), weighs about 0.5 g in adults and has dimensions of about 10 × 13 × 6 mm. As described below, this bit of secretory tissue represents the body's "master gland," as well as the connector between the brain and most of the body's endocrine system. It lies below the brain in a small cavity on the sphenoid bone, the sella turcica (Figure 20–2). The two-part pituitary arises in the embryo from two developing regions, the brain and the oral cavity (Figure 20–3). The neural component consists of the neurohypophyseal bud growing down from the floor of the future diencephalon as a stalk (or infundibulum) that remains attached to the brain. The oral component arises as an outpocketing of ectoderm from the roof of the embryonic mouth and grows cranially, forming a structure called the **hypophyseal (Rathke) pouch**. The base of this pouch eventually constricts and separates from the pharynx and its anterior wall thickens greatly, developing as the bulk of the anterior pituitary (Figure 20–3).

FIGURE **20–1** Locations of the major endocrine glands and the hormones they release.

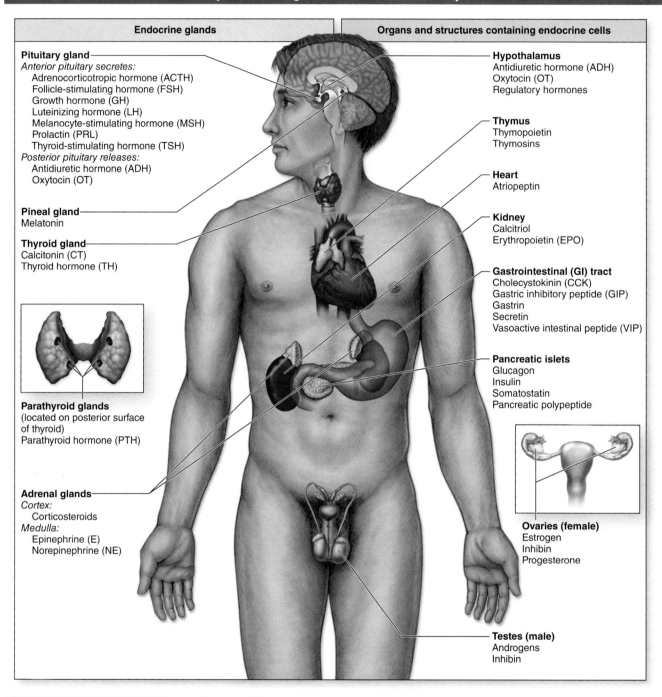

Endocrine glands	Organs and structures containing endocrine cells

Pituitary gland
Anterior pituitary secretes:
  Adrenocorticotropic hormone (ACTH)
  Follicle-stimulating hormone (FSH)
  Growth hormone (GH)
  Luteinizing hormone (LH)
  Melanocyte-stimulating hormone (MSH)
  Prolactin (PRL)
  Thyroid-stimulating hormone (TSH)
Posterior pituitary releases:
  Antidiuretic hormone (ADH)
  Oxytocin (OT)

Pineal gland
Melatonin

Thyroid gland
Calcitonin (CT)
Thyroid hormone (TH)

Parathyroid glands
(located on posterior surface
of thyroid)
Parathyroid hormone (PTH)

Adrenal glands
Cortex:
  Corticosteroids
Medulla:
  Epinephrine (E)
  Norepinephrine (NE)

Hypothalamus
Antidiuretic hormone (ADH)
Oxytocin (OT)
Regulatory hormones

Thymus
Thymopoietin
Thymosins

Heart
Atriopeptin

Kidney
Calcitriol
Erythropoietin (EPO)

Gastrointestinal (GI) tract
Cholecystokinin (CCK)
Gastric inhibitory peptide (GIP)
Gastrin
Secretin
Vasoactive intestinal peptide (VIP)

Pancreatic islets
Glucagon
Insulin
Somatostatin
Pancreatic polypeptide

Ovaries (female)
Estrogen
Inhibin
Progesterone

Testes (male)
Androgens
Inhibin

In addition to the **major endocrine glands** shown at the (left), there are widely **distributed endocrine cells** as well as various other tissues in organs throughout the body with endocrine functions (right), which are discussed in the chapters on those organ systems. Not shown here are adipocytes, which exert important endocrine functions, and the many tissues in which paracrine signaling is important.

Because of its dual origin, the pituitary actually consists of two glands—the posterior neurohypophysis and the anterior adenohypophysis—united anatomically but with different functions. The **neurohypophysis** retains many histologic features of brain tissue and includes a large part, the **pars nervosa**, and a smaller **infundibulum** or stalk attached to the hypothalamus (Figures 20–2 and 20–4). The **adenohypophysis**, derived from the oral ectoderm and retaining

FIGURE **20–2** Pituitary gland.

The **pituitary gland** is composed of an **anterior part** and a **posterior part** that is directly attached to the **hypothalamus** region of the brain by an infundibular stalk. The gland occupies a fossa of the sphenoid bone called the sella turcica (L. Turkish saddle).

FIGURE **20–3** Formation of the pituitary gland.

(a) Week 3: Hypophyseal pouch and neurohypophyseal bud form

(b) Late second month: Hypophyseal pouch loses contact with roof of pharynx

(c) Fetal period: Anterior and posterior parts of pituitary have formed

The **pituitary gland** forms from two separate embryonic structures.

(a) During the third week of development, a **hypophyseal pouch** (or Rathke pouch, the **future anterior pituitary**) grows from the roof of the pharynx, while a **neurohypophyseal bud (future posterior pituitary)** forms from the diencephalon.

(b) By late in the second month, the **hypophyseal pouch** detaches from the roof of the pharynx and merges with the **neurohypophyseal bud**.

(c) During the fetal period, the anterior and posterior parts of the **pituitary** complete development.

FIGURE 20–4   Pituitary gland.

Histologically the two parts of the **pituitary gland** reflect their origins, as seen in this low-magnification section of an entire gland. The infundibular stalk (**IS**) and pars nervosa (**PN**) of the neurohypophysis resemble CNS tissue, while the adenohypophysis' pars distalis (**PD**), pars intermediate (**PI**), and pars tuberalis (**PT**) are typically glandular in their level of staining. (×30; H&E)

more typically secretory cells, comprises three parts: a large **pars distalis** or **anterior lobe**; the **pars tuberalis**, which wraps around the infundibulum; and the thin **pars intermedia** adjacent to the posterior pars nervosa (Figures 20–2 and 20–4).

The Hypothalamic-Hypophyseal Tract & Blood Supply

The pituitary gland's neural connection to the brain and its blood supply, diagrammed in Figure 20–5, are both of key importance for its function. Embryologically, anatomically, and functionally, the pituitary gland is connected to the median eminence of the hypothalamus at the base of the brain. In addition to the vascular portal system carrying small regulatory peptides from the hypothalamus to the adenohypophysis, a bundle of axons called the **hypothalamic-hypophyseal tract** courses into the neurohypophysis from two important

hypothalamic nuclei. The peptide hormones ADH (antidiuretic hormone) and oxytocin are synthesized within large neurons in the **supraoptic** and the **paraventricular nuclei**, respectively. Both hormones undergo axonal transport and accumulate temporarily in the axons of the hypothalamic-hypophyseal tract before their release and uptake by capillaries branching from the inferior arteries.

The blood supply derives from two groups of vessels coming off the internal carotid artery and drained by the hypophyseal vein. The **superior hypophyseal arteries** supply the median eminence and the infundibular stalk; the **inferior hypophyseal arteries** provide blood mainly for the neurohypophysis. The superior arteries divide into a **primary plexus** of fenestrated capillaries that irrigate the stalk and median eminence. These capillaries then rejoin to form venules that branch again as a larger secondary capillary plexus in the adenohypophysis (Figure 20–5). These vessels make up the **hypothalamic-hypophyseal portal system** which has great

FIGURE 20–5 **The hypothalamic-hypophyseal tract and portal system.**

Hypothalamus

Paraventricular nucleus
(produces oxytocin)

Supraoptic nucleus
(produces ADH)

Optic chiasm

Hypothalamic-hypophyseal
tract

Posterior pituitary
Infundibulum

Pars nervosa
(With axons storing
oxytocin and ADH)

(a)

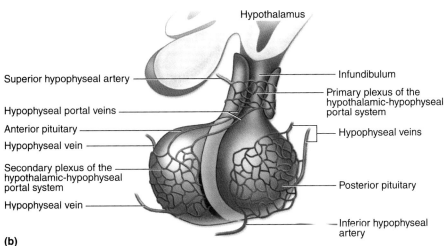

Hypothalamus

Superior hypophyseal artery

Hypophyseal portal veins

Anterior pituitary

Hypophyseal vein

Secondary plexus of the
hypothalamic-hypophyseal
portal system

Hypophyseal vein

Infundibulum

Primary plexus of the
hypothalamic-hypophyseal
portal system

Hypophyseal veins

Posterior pituitary

Inferior hypophyseal
artery

(b)

(a) The **hypothalamic-hypophyseal tract** consists of **axons** extending from the hypothalamic supraoptic and paraventricular nuclei, through the infundibulum and into the pars nervosa of the posterior pituitary, where peptide hormones they carry are released for capillary uptake.

(b) The **hypothalamic-hypophyseal portal system**, with **blood** from the superior hypophyseal artery, consists of two capillary networks connected by the hypophyseal portal vein. The primary plexus surrounds the infundibulum and median eminence, and the second is throughout the pars distalis and drains into the hypophyseal veins.

importance because it carries neuropeptides from the median eminence the short distance to the adenohypophysis where they either stimulate or inhibit hormone release by the endocrine cells there.

Adenohypophysis (Anterior Pituitary)

All three parts of the adenohypophysis develop from the embryonic hypophyseal pouch.

Pars Distalis

The **pars distalis** accounts for 75% of the adenohypophysis, all covered by a thin fibrous capsule. The main components are cords of well-stained endocrine cells interspersed with fenestrated capillaries and supporting reticular connective tissue (Figures 20–4 and 20–6). Routine staining revealed two broad groups of cells in the pars distalis with different staining affinities: chromophils and much less common chromophobes. Chromophils are secretory cells with hormone stored in cytoplasmic granules and can be further distinguished as

basophils and **acidophils**, based on their affinities for basic and acidic dyes, respectively (Figure 20–6).

TEM uncovered specific basophilic and acidophilic cell subtypes based on their granular morphology, subtypes now most easily identified by immunohistochemistry (Figure 20–7). As listed in Table 20–1, specific chromophils now usually have names that refer to their hormone's function or target cells. Acidophils secrete either growth hormone (somatotropin) or prolactin and are called **somatotrophs** and **lactotrophs** (or somatotropic cells and lactotropic cells), respectively. The basophilic cells called **corticotrophs, gonadotrophs, and thyrotrophs**, have target cells in the adrenal cortex, gonads, and thyroid gland, respectively. Somatotrophs typically constitute about half the cells of the pars distalis in humans, with thyrotrophs the least abundant chromophils.

With two exceptions, each type of anterior pituitary cell makes one kind of hormone (Table 20–1). Gonadotrophs secrete two different glycoproteins: **follicle-stimulating hormone (FSH)** and **luteinizing hormone (LH)** (called

FIGURE 20–6 Pars distalis: Acidophils, basophils, and chromophobes.

(a) Hematoxylin & eosin staining and most other general staining methods simply allow the parenchymal cells of the **pars distalis** to be subdivided into acidophil cells (**A**), basophils (**B**), and chromophobes (**C**) in which the cytoplasm is poorly stained. Also shown are capillaries and sinusoids (**S**) in the second capillary plexus of the portal system. Cords of acidophils and basophils vary in distribution and number in different regions of the pars distalis, but are always closely associated with microvasculature that carries off secreted hormones into the general circulation. (×400; H&E)

(b) Another micrograph of H&E stained pars distalis shows the variability of staining of acidophil cells (**A**), basophils (**B**), and chromophobes (**C**). Sinusoids (**S**) of the second capillary plexus of the portal system are also shown. Cords of acidophils and basophils are closely associated with the microvasculature flushing secreted anterior pituitary hormones into the general circulation. (×400; H&E)

(c) A similar area of **pars distalis** shown here after Gomori trichrome staining, which renders acidophils (**A**) orange, basophils (**B**) violet, and chromophobes (**C**) poorly stained. All are close to sinusoids (**S**). (×400)

interstitial cell-stimulating hormone [ICSH] in males). The main protein synthesized in corticotrophs is proopiomelanocortin (POMC), which is cleaved posttranslationally into the polypeptide hormones **adrenocortical trophic hormone (ACTH)** and **β-lipotropin (β-LPH)**. Hormones produced by the pars distalis have widespread functional activities. They regulate almost all other endocrine glands, ovarian function and sperm production, milk production, and the metabolism of muscle, bone, and adipose tissue (Table 20–1; Figure 20–8).

As shown in Figure 20–6 **chromophobes** stain weakly, with few or no secretory granules, and comprise another

heterogeneous group, including stem and undifferentiated progenitor cells along with degranulated cells.

Pars Tuberalis

The **pars tuberalis** consists of a smaller funnel-shaped region surrounding the infundibulum of the neurohypophysis (Figures 20–2 and 20–4). Gonadotrophs make up most of the cells of the pars tuberalis.

Pars Intermedia

A narrow zone lying between the pars distalis and the pars nervosa, the **pars intermedia** contains corticotrophs,

FIGURE **20–7** Ultrastructure and immunohistochemistry of somatotropic cells.

(a) Ultrastructurally, cytoplasm of all chromophil cells is shown to have well-developed Golgi complexes (**G**), euchromatic nuclei (**N**), and cytoplasm filled with secretory granules, as seen here in a **somatotroph**, the most common acidophil. The **arrow** near the top of the photo indicates the cell membrane. Specific

chromophils are more easily identified using immunohistochemistry and antibodies against the hormone products. (×10,000)

(b) This light micrograph shows **somatotrophs** stained using an antibody against somatotropin. (×400; IHC, with hematoxylin counterstain)

chromophobes, and small, colloid-filled cysts derived from the lumen of the embryonic hypophyseal pouch (Figure 20–9). Best-developed and active during fetal life, corticotrophs of the pars intermedia express POMC but cleave it differently from cells in the pars distalis, producing mainly smaller peptide hormones, including γ-LPH, β-endorphin, and two forms of melanocyte-stimulating hormone (MSH). MSH increases melanocyte activity, but

TABLE **20–1**	Major cell types of the anterior pituitary and their major functions.		
Cell Type	**% of Total Cells**	**Hormone Produced**	**Major Function**
Somatotrophs	50	Somatotropin (growth hormone, GH), a 22-kDa protein	Stimulates growth in epiphyseal plates of long bones via insulin-like growth factors (IGFs) produced in liver
Lactotrophs (or mammotrophs)	15–20	Prolactin (PRL), a 22.5-kDa protein	Promotes milk secretion
Gonadotrophs	10	Follicle-stimulating hormone (FSH) and luteinizing hormone (LH; interstitial cell-stimulating hormone [ICSH] in men), both 28-kDa glycoprotein dimers, secreted from the same cell type	FSH promotes ovarian follicle development and estrogen secretion in women and spermatogenesis in men; LH promotes ovarian follicle maturation and progesterone secretion in women and interstitial cell androgen secretion in men
Thyrotrophs	5	Thyrotropin (TSH), a 28-kDa glycoprotein dimer	Stimulates thyroid hormone synthesis, storage, and liberation
Corticotrophs	15–20	Adrenal corticotropin (ACTH), a 4-kDa polypeptide	Stimulates secretion of adrenal cortex hormones
		Lipotropin (LPH)	Helps regulate lipid metabolism

FIGURE 20–8 Hormones of the pars distalis, their releasing/inhibiting hormones, and targets.

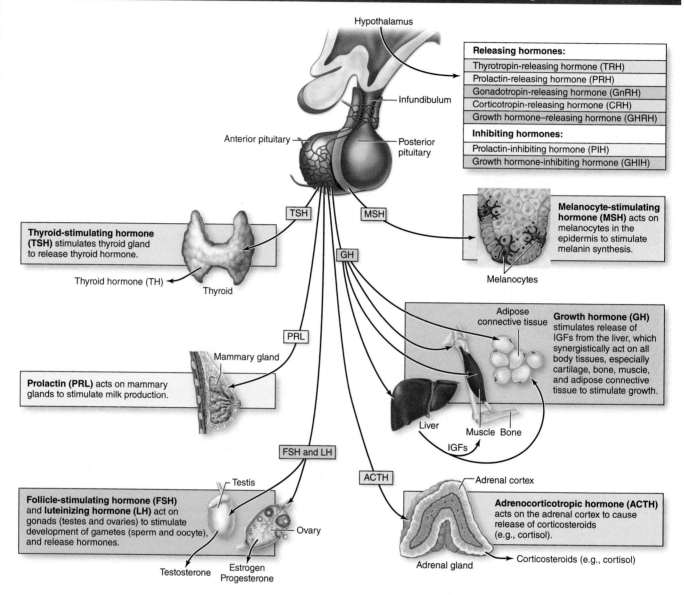

Releasing hormones:
| Thyrotropin-releasing hormone (TRH) |
| Prolactin-releasing hormone (PRH) |
| Gonadotropin-releasing hormone (GnRH) |
| Corticotropin-releasing hormone (CRH) |
| Growth hormone–releasing hormone (GHRH) |

Inhibiting hormones:
| Prolactin-inhibiting hormone (PIH) |
| Growth hormone-inhibiting hormone (GHIH) |

Hypothalamus
Infundibulum
Anterior pituitary
Posterior pituitary

TSH — **Thyroid-stimulating hormone (TSH)** stimulates thyroid gland to release thyroid hormone.
Thyroid hormone (TH)
Thyroid

MSH — **Melanocyte-stimulating hormone (MSH)** acts on melanocytes in the epidermis to stimulate melanin synthesis.
Melanocytes

GH — **Growth hormone (GH)** stimulates release of IGFs from the liver, which synergistically act on all body tissues, especially cartilage, bone, muscle, and adipose connective tissue to stimulate growth.
Adipose connective tissue
Liver   Muscle Bone
IGFs

PRL — **Prolactin (PRL)** acts on mammary glands to stimulate milk production.
Mammary gland

FSH and LH — **Follicle-stimulating hormone (FSH)** and **luteinizing hormone (LH)** act on gonads (testes and ovaries) to stimulate development of gametes (sperm and oocyte), and release hormones.
Testis
Ovary
Testosterone
Estrogen
Progesterone

ACTH — **Adrenocorticotropic hormone (ACTH)** acts on the adrenal cortex to cause release of corticosteroids (e.g., cortisol).
Adrenal cortex
Adrenal gland
Corticosteroids (e.g., cortisol)

Release of the six major tropic hormones from the **anterior pituitary** (all except MSH) is promoted by specific **peptide releasing hormones**. Release of PRL and GH is further regulated by **specific inhibiting peptide hormones**. These regulatory peptides are all secreted by specific **hypothalamic neurons** and then carried to the anterior pituitary by the **hypothalamic-hypophyseal blood supply** shown in the upper diagram. Organs throughout the body targeted specifically by the seven tropic hormones are also shown here.

the overall functional significance of the pars intermedia in adults remains uncertain.

Control of Hormone Secretion in the Anterior Pituitary

Cellular activities in the anterior pituitary occur primarily under the control of **hypothalamic hormones**, peptides produced by small neurons near the third ventricle, discharged from axons in the median eminence, and transported by capillaries of the portal system throughout the anterior pituitary. As shown in Table 20–2 most of these hormones serve as **releasing hormones** stimulating secretion in specific anterior pituitary cells. Two hypothalamic factors, however, act as **inhibiting hormones**, which block hormone secretion in specific cells of the adenohypophysis (Table 20–2). Because of the strategic position of the hypothalamic neurons and the control they exert on the adenohypophysis and therefore on many bodily functions, many sensory stimuli coming to the brain or arising within the central nervous system (CNS) can

FIGURE 20–9 Pars intermedia.

The **pars intermedia** (**PI**) is a narrow region lying between the pars distalis (**PD**) and the pars nervosa (**PN**), with many of its basophils (**B**) often invading the latter. Remnants of the embryonic hypophyseal pouch's lumen are usually present in this region as colloid-filled cysts (**C**) of various sizes. Function of this region in humans is not clear. (×56; H&E)

affect pituitary function and then also quickly influence activities of many other organs and tissues.

Additional important controls on anterior pituitary activity occur as **negative feedback** by hormones from the target organs on secretion of the relevant hypothalamic factors and on hormone secretion by the related pituitary cells. Figure 20–10 illustrates this mechanism, using the thyroid as an example, and shows the complex chain of events that begins with the action of neural stimuli in the hypothalamus and ends with the effects of hormones from the pituitary's target organs.

Finally, hormone secretion in the anterior pituitary is affected by other polypeptide hormones from outside the feedback loops or even outside the major target tissues. Examples include the "hunger hormone" ghrelin produced mainly in the stomach mucosa, which also acts as a releasing hormone for somatotropin secretion, and oxytocin, released in the posterior pituitary during breast-feeding, which increases prolactin secretion.

All these mechanisms allow the fine tuning of hormone secretion by anterior pituitary cells with conditions throughout the body.

❯❯ MEDICAL APPLICATION

Benign **pituitary adenomas** often produce excessive numbers of functional acidophils or basophils. Adenomas involving somatotropic cells can cause **gigantism** if occurring in children before closure of the long bones' epiphyseal plates or **acromegaly** in adults, with musculoskeletal, neurologic, and other medical consequences.

Neurohypophysis (Posterior Pituitary)

The neurohypophysis consists of the pars nervosa and the infundibular stalk (Figures 20–2 and 20–4) and, unlike the adenohypophysis, does not contain the cells that synthesize its two hormones. It consists of neural tissue, containing some 100,000 unmyelinated axons of large secretory neurons with cell bodies in the supraoptic and paraventricular nuclei of

TABLE 20–2	Hypothalamic hormones regulating cells of the anterior pituitary.	
Hormone	**Chemical Form**	**Functions**
Thyrotropin-releasing hormone (TRH)	3-amino acid peptide	Stimulates release of thyrotropin (TSH)
Gonadotropin-releasing hormone (GnRH)	10-amino acid peptide	Stimulates the release of both follicle-stimulating hormone (FSH) and luteinizing hormone (LH)
Somatostatin	14-amino acid peptide	Inhibits release of both somatotropin (GH) and TSH
Growth hormone-releasing hormone (GHRH)	40- or 44-amino acid polypeptides (2 forms)	Stimulates release of GH
Dopamine	Modified amino acid	Inhibits release of prolactin (PRL)
Corticotropin-releasing hormone (CRH)	41-amino acid polypeptide	Stimulates synthesis of pro-opiomelanocortin (POMC) and release of both β-lipotropic hormone (β-LPH) and corticotropin (ACTH)

FIGURE 20–10 Negative feedback loops affecting anterior pituitary secretion.

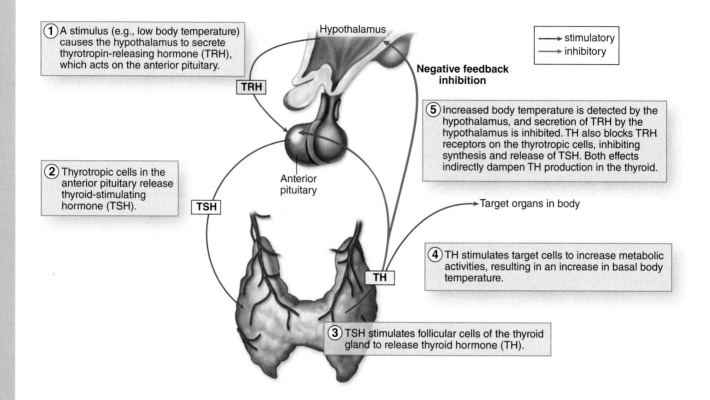

① A stimulus (e.g., low body temperature) causes the hypothalamus to secrete thyrotropin-releasing hormone (TRH), which acts on the anterior pituitary.

Hypothalamus

→ stimulatory
→ inhibitory

Negative feedback inhibition

TRH

⑤ Increased body temperature is detected by the hypothalamus, and secretion of TRH by the hypothalamus is inhibited. TH also blocks TRH receptors on the thyrotropic cells, inhibiting synthesis and release of TSH. Both effects indirectly dampen TH production in the thyroid.

② Thyrotropic cells in the anterior pituitary release thyroid-stimulating hormone (TSH).

Anterior pituitary

TSH

Target organs in body

④ TH stimulates target cells to increase metabolic activities, resulting in an increase in basal body temperature.

TH

③ TSH stimulates follicular cells of the thyroid gland to release thyroid hormone (TH).

Relationship between the **hypothalamus**, the **anterior pituitary**, and its **target organs** is shown, using the thyroid as an example. Hypothalamic thyrotropin-releasing hormone (**TRH**) stimulates secretion of thyroid-stimulating hormone or thyrotropin (**TSH**), which stimulates synthesis and secretion of thyroid hormone (**TH**). In addition to their effects on target organs, TH inhibits TSH secretion from the pars distalis and TRH secretion from the hypothalamus by negative feedback.

the hypothalamus (Figure 20–5). Highly branched glial cells resembling astrocytes but called **pituicytes** make up the most abundant cell type in the posterior pituitary (Figure 20–11).

The secretory neurons have all the characteristics of typical neurons, including the ability to conduct an action potential, but have larger diameter axons and well-developed synthetic components related to the production of the 9-amino acid peptide hormones **antidiuretic hormone** (**ADH**, also called arginine vasopressin) and **oxytocin**. Transported axonally into the pars nervosa, these hormones accumulate in axonal dilations called **neurosecretory bodies** or **Herring bodies**, visible in the light microscope as faintly eosinophilic structures (Figure 20–11). The neurosecretory bodies contain membrane-enclosed granules with either oxytocin or ADH bound to 10-kDa carrier proteins called **neurophysin** I and II, respectively. The hormone-neurophysin complex is synthesized as a single protein and then cleaved to produce the peptide hormone and its binding protein. Nerve impulses along the axons trigger the release of the peptides from the neurosecretory bodies for uptake by the fenestrated capillaries of the pars nervosa, and the hormones then get distributed in the general circulation. Axons from the supraoptic and paraventricular nuclei mingle in the neurohypophysis but carry out ADH and oxytocin secretion, respectively.

ADH release occurs in response to increased blood tonicity, sensed by osmoreceptor cells in the hypothalamus, which then stimulates ADH synthesis in supraoptic neurons. ADH increases the permeability of the renal collecting ducts to water (see Chapter 19) so that these ducts reabsorb more water from the filtrate and osmotic balance of body fluids is restored (Table 20–3).

››MEDICAL APPLICATION

Posterior pituitary function can be adversely affected by heritable mutations in the gene for vasopressin (ADH)-neurophysin, by compression from a tumor in adjacent tissues, and by **head trauma**. By lowering levels of vasopressin, such conditions can produce diabetes insipidus, a disorder characterized by inability to concentrate urine, which leads to frequent urination (**polyuria**) and increased thirst (**polydipsia**).

FIGURE **20–11** Pars nervosa: neurosecretory bodies and pituicytes.

The **pars nervosa** of the posterior pituitary consists of modified neural tissues containing unmyelinated axons supported and ensheathed by glia cells called **pituicytes** (**P**), the most numerous cell present. The axons run from the supraoptic and paraventricular hypothalamic nuclei, and have swellings called **neurosecretory** (**Herring**) **bodies** (**NB**) from which either oxytocin or vasopressin is released upon neural stimulation. The released hormones are picked up by capillaries (**C**) for distribution. (×400; H&E)

Oxytocin stimulates contraction of uterine smooth muscle during childbirth and the myoepithelial cells in the mammary gland (Table 20–3). A nursing infant induces oxytocin secretion by stimulating sensory tracts that act on the

hypothalamus in a neurohormonal reflex causing rapid ejection of milk. Oxytocin also produces psychological effects, such as promotion of pair-bonding behavior.

ADRENAL GLANDS

The adrenal (or suprarenal) **glands** are paired organs lying near the superior poles of the kidneys, embedded in the pararenal adipose tissue and fascia (Figures 20–1 and 20–12). They are flattened structures with a half-moon shape, about 4-6-cm long, 1–2-cm wide, and 4–6-mm thick in adults. Together, they weigh about 8 g, but their weight and size vary with the age and physiologic condition of the individual. Adrenal glands are each covered by a dense connective tissue capsule that sends thin trabeculae into the gland's parenchyma. The stroma consists mainly of reticular fibers supporting the secretory cells and microvasculature. Each gland has two concentric regions: a yellowish **adrenal cortex** and a reddish-brown central **adrenal medulla**.

FIGURE **20–12** Location and blood supply of the adrenal glands.

Left inferior
phrenic artery

Left superior
suprarenal arteries

Left middle
suprarenal artery

Left adrenal gland

Left inferior
suprarenal arteries

Left suprarenal vein

Abdominal
aorta

The paired **adrenal glands** are located at the superior pole of each **kidney** and each consists of an outer cortex producing a variety of steroid hormones and an inner medulla producing epinephrine and norepinephrine. This anterior view of the left adrenal gland and kidney shows the **blood vessels** supplying these glands.

TABLE **20–3**	Hormones of the posterior pituitary.
Hormone	**Function**
Vasopressin/antidiuretic hormone (ADH)	Increases water permeability of renal collecting ducts
Oxytocin	Stimulates contraction of mammary gland myoepithelial cells and uterine smooth muscle

The adrenal cortex and medulla can be considered two different organs with distinct embryonic origins, functions, and morphologic characteristics that become united during embryonic development. The cortex arises from mesoderm and the medulla from the neural crest. The general histologic appearance of the adrenal gland is typical of an endocrine gland in which cells of both cortex and medulla are grouped in cords along wide capillaries.

The adrenal gland lacks a hilum; superior, middle, and inferior suprarenal arteries arising from larger abdominal arteries penetrate the capsule independently (Figure 20–12) and branch immediately to form a subcapsular arterial plexus. From this plexus arterioles for the adrenal cortex and medulla emerge separately to form rich networks of fenestrated capillaries and sinusoids. Cortical capillaries irrigate endocrine cells of the cortex and then drain into the microvasculature of the medulla. The adrenal medulla thus has a dual blood supply: arterial blood from the medullary arterioles and venous blood from capillaries of the cortex. Venous drainage from the glands occurs via the suprarenal veins (Figure 20–12).

Adrenal Cortex

Cells of the **adrenal cortex** have characteristic features of steroid-secreting cells: acidophilic cytoplasm rich in lipid droplets, with central nuclei. Ultrastructurally their cytoplasm shows an exceptionally profuse smooth ER (SER) of interconnected tubules, which contain the enzymes for cholesterol synthesis and conversion of the steroid prohormone pregnenolone into specific active steroid hormones. The mitochondria are often spherical, with tubular rather than shelflike cristae (Figure 20–13). These mitochondria not only synthesize ATP but also contain the enzymes for converting cholesterol to pregnenolone and for some steps in steroid synthesis. The function of steroid-producing cells involves close collaboration between SER and mitochondria.

Steroid hormones are not stored in granules like proteins nor undergo exocytosis. As small lipid-soluble molecules, steroids diffuse freely from cells through the plasma membrane.

The adrenal cortex has three concentric zones in which the cords of epithelial steroid-producing cells are arranged somewhat differently, and which synthesize different classes of steroid hormones (Figure 20–14):

- The **zona glomerulosa**, immediately inside the capsule and comprising about 15% of the cortex, consists of closely packed, rounded or arched cords of columnar or pyramidal cells with many capillaries (Figure 20–15). The steroids made by these cells are called **mineralocorticoids** because they affect uptake of Na⁺, K⁺, and water by cells of renal tubules. The principal product is **aldosterone**, the major regulator of salt balance, which acts to stimulate Na⁺ reabsorption in the distal convoluted tubules (see Chapter 19). Aldosterone secretion

FIGURE 20–13 Ultrastructure of cortical adrenalocytes.

TEM of two adjacent steroid-secreting cells from the zona fasciculata shows features typical of steroid-producing cells: lipid droplets (**L**) containing cholesterol esters, mitochondria (**M**) with tubular and vesicular cristae, abundant **SER**, and autophagosomes (**A**), which remove mitochondria and SER between periods of active steroid synthesis. Also seen are the euchromatic nuclei (**N**), a Golgi apparatus (**G**), RER, and lysosomes. (×25,700)

is stimulated primarily by angiotensin II and also by an increase in plasma K⁺ concentration, but only weakly by ACTH.

- The middle **zona fasciculata**, occupies 65%–80% of the cortex and consists of long cords of large polyhedral cells, one or two cells thick, separated by fenestrated sinusoidal capillaries (Figure 20–15). The cells are filled with lipid droplets and appear vacuolated in routine histologic preparations. These cells secrete **glucocorticoids**, especially **cortisol**, which affect carbohydrate metabolism by stimulating gluconeogenesis in many cells and glycogen synthesis in the liver. Cortisol also suppresses many immune functions and can induce fat mobilization and muscle proteolysis. Secretion is controlled by ACTH with negative feedback proportional to the concentration of circulating glucocorticoids (Figure 20–10). Small amounts of weak androgens are also produced here.

- The innermost **zona reticularis** comprises about 10% of the cortex and consists of smaller cells in a network of irregular cords interspersed with wide capillaries (Figure 20–15). The cells are usually more heavily stained than those of the other zones because they contain fewer

FIGURE 20–14 Adrenal gland.

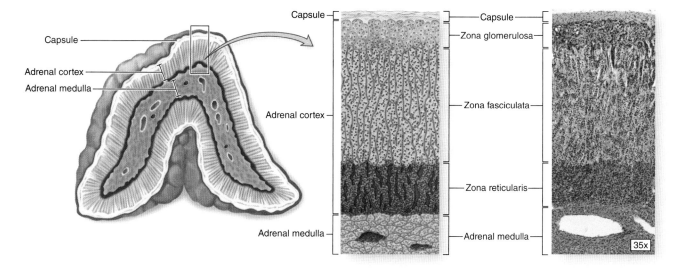

Inside the capsule of each **adrenal gland** is an **adrenal cortex**, formed from embryonic mesodermal cells, which completely surrounds an innermost **adrenal medulla** derived embryologically from neural crest cells. Both regions are very well vascularized with fenestrated sinusoidal capillaries.

Cortical cells are arranged as three layers: the **zona glomerulosa** near the capsule, the **zona fasciculata** (the thickest layer), and the **zona reticularis**.

lipid droplets and more lipofuscin pigment. Cells of the zona reticularis also produce cortisol but primarily secrete the **weak androgens**, including **dehydroepiandrosterone (DHEA)** that is converted to testosterone in both men and women. Secretion by these cells is also stimulated by ACTH with regulatory feedback.

>> **MEDICAL APPLICATION**

Addison disease or **adrenal cortical insufficiency** is a disorder, usually autoimmune in origin, which causes degeneration in any layer of adrenal cortex, with concomitant loss of glucocorticoids, mineralocorticoids, or androgen production.

Adrenal Medulla

The **adrenal medulla** is composed of large, pale-staining polyhedral cells arranged in cords or clumps and supported by a reticular fiber network (Figure 20–16). A profuse supply of sinusoidal capillaries intervenes between adjacent cords and a few parasympathetic ganglion cells are present. Medullary parenchymal cells, known as **chromaffin cells**, arise from neural crest cells, as do the postganglionic neurons of sympathetic and parasympathetic ganglia. Chromaffin cells can be considered modified sympathetic postganglionic neurons, lacking axons and dendrites and specialized as secretory cells.

>> **MEDICAL APPLICATION**

In the adrenal medulla, benign pheochromocytomas periodically secrete high levels of catecholamines that cause swings in blood pressure between hypertension and hypotension.

Unlike cells of the adrenal cortex, chromaffin cells contain many electron-dense granules, 150–350 nm in diameter, for storage and secretion of catecholamines, either **epinephrine** or **norepinephrine**. The granules of epinephrine-secreting cells are less electron-dense and generally smaller than those of norepinephrine-secreting cells (Figure 20–16). Both catecholamines, together with Ca^{2+} and ATP, are bound in granular storage complexes with 49-kDa proteins called **chromogranins**.

Norepinephrine-secreting cells are also found in paraganglia (collections of catecholamine-secreting cells adjacent to the autonomic ganglia) and in various viscera. The conversion of norepinephrine to epinephrine (adrenalin) occurs only in chromaffin cells of the adrenal medulla. About 80% of the catecholamine secreted from the adrenal medulla is epinephrine.

Medullary chromaffin cells are innervated by preganglionic sympathetic neurons, which trigger epinephrine and norepinephrine release during stress and intense emotional reactions. Epinephrine increases heart rate, dilates

FIGURE **20–15** Adrenal cortex.

The steroid-secreting cells of the **adrenal cortex** are arranged differently to form three distinct concentric layers, the zonae glomerulosa (**G**), fasciculata (**F**), and reticularis (**R**), surrounding the medulla (**M**). As with all endocrine glands, the layers of the adrenal cortex all contain a rich microvasculature.

Shown here are sections from two adrenal glands, stained with H&E (left) and Mallory trichrome, in which the sparse collagen appears blue (right).

(**a** and **b**) Immediately beneath the capsule (**C**), the **zona glomerulosa** consists of rounded clusters of columnar or pyramidal cells

principally secreting the mineral corticoid aldosterone. Blood-filled regions are parts of the subcapsular arterial plexus.

(**c** and **d**) The thick middle layer, the **zona fasciculata**, consists of long cords of large, spongy-looking cells mainly secreting gluco-corticoids such as cortisol.

(**e** and **f**) Cells of the innermost **zona reticularis**, next to the medulla (**M**), are small, have fewer lipid droplets and are therefore better stained, arranged in a close network and secrete mainly sex steroids, including the androgen precursor DHEA. Cells of all the layers are closely associated with **capillaries** and **sinusoids**.
Left photo: (×20); a–f: (×200)

FIGURE **20–16** Adrenal medulla.

The hormone-secreting cells of the **adrenal medulla** are **chromaffin cells**, which resemble sympathetic neurons.

(a) The micrograph shows that **chromaffin cells** are large pale-staining cells, arranged in cords interspersed with wide capillaries. Faintly stained cytoplasmic granules can be seen in most of these cells. (×200; H&E)

(b) TEM reveals that the granules of norepinephrine-secreting cells (**NE**) are more electron-dense than those of cells secreting epinephrine (**E**), which is due to the chromogranins binding the catecholamines. Most of the hormone produced is epinephrine, which is only made in the **adrenal medulla**. (×33,000)

bronchioles, and dilates arteries of cardiac and skeletal muscle. Norepinephrine constricts vessels of the digestive system and skin, increasing blood flow to the heart, muscles, and brain. Both hormones stimulate glycogen breakdown, elevating blood glucose levels. Together these effects augment the capability for defensive reactions or escape of stressors, the fight-or-flight response. During normal activity, the adrenal medulla continuously secretes small quantities of these hormones.

▷ PANCREATIC ISLETS

The **pancreatic islets** (islets of Langerhans) are compact spherical or ovoid masses of endocrine cells embedded within the acinar exocrine tissue of the pancreas (Figure 20–17). Most islets are 100–200 μm in diameter and contain several hundred cells, but some have only a few cells. The pancreas has more than 1 million islets, mostly in the gland's narrow tail region, but they only constitute 1%–2% of the organ's total volume. A very thin reticular capsule surrounds each islet, separating it from the adjacent acinar tissue. Pancreatic islets have the same embryonic origin as the pancreatic acinar tissue: in epithelial outgrowths from endoderm of the developing gut.

The cells of islets are polygonal or rounded, smaller, and more lightly stained than the surrounding acinar cells, arranged in cords separated by fenestrated capillaries (Figure 20–17).

Routine stains or trichrome stains show that most islet cells are acidophilic or basophilic with fine cytoplasmic granules (Figure 20–17). Ultrastructural features are those of active polypeptide-secreting cells, with secretory granules that vary in size, morphology, and electron density from cell to cell. The major human islet cells are most easily identified and localized by immunohistochemical staining of their major products:

- **α or A cells** secrete primarily **glucagon** and are abundant and scattered through most islets.
- **β or B cells** produce **insulin** (L. *insula*, island), are about twice as abundant as α cells and also usually scattered.
- **δ or D cells**, secreting **somatostatin**, are much less abundant than the other major cell types.

The scattered cellular distribution within human islets allows contact of most cells with cells of another type, suggesting paracrine effects on hormone secretion.

FIGURE **20–17** Pancreatic islets.

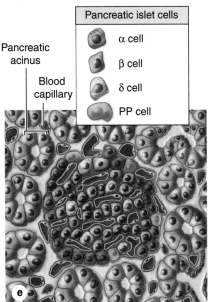

Pancreatic islets are clumped masses of pale-staining endocrine cells embedded in the exocrine acinar tissue of the pancreas.

(a) The islets are clusters of cells smaller and lighter staining than cells of the surrounding tissue. (×12.5; H&E)

(b) At higher magnification, an islet's capillary system can be seen. Several arterioles enter each islet, branch into fenestrated capillaries (**C**) among the peripheral islet cells, then converge centrally before leaving the islet as efferent capillaries carrying blood to the acini surrounding the islet. This **local vascular system** allows specific islet hormones to help control secretion of other islet cells and the neighboring acini. (×40; H&E)

(c) With H&E staining all cells of an islet appear similar, although differences in cell size and basophilia may be apparent. Capillaries (**C**) are also apparent. (×55; H&E)

(d) A murine islet prepared with a modified aldehyde fuchsin stain shows that granules in the **peripheral α cells** are a deep brownish purple and the **central β cells** granules are brownish orange. Reticulin connective tissue of the islet capsule and along the capillaries stains green in this preparation. Immunohistochemistry with antibodies against the various islet polypeptide hormones allows definitive identification of each islet cell type. (×300; Modified aldehyde fuchsin and light green)

(e) The diagram shows the four major islet cells, each colored differently. The products of these cells are: α cells secrete glucagon, β cells secrete insulin, δ cells secrete somatostatin, and PP cells secrete pancreatic polypeptide.

(Figure 20–17d, reproduced with permission from Dr Arthur A. Like, Department of Pathology, University of Massachusetts Medical School, Worcester.)

>> **MEDICAL APPLICATION**

Diabetes mellitus is characterized by loss of the insulin effect and a subsequent failure of cells to take up glucose, leading to elevated blood sugar or **hyperglycemia. Type 1 diabetes** or **insulin-dependent diabetes mellitus (IDDM)** is caused by loss of the β cells from autoimmune destruction and is treated by regular injections of insulin. In **type 2 diabetes** or **non–insulin-dependent diabetes mellitus (NIDDM)**, β cells are present but fail to produce adequate levels of insulin in response to hyperglycemia, and the peripheral target cells "resist" or no longer respond to the hormone. Type 2 diabetes commonly occurs with obesity, and poorly understood, multifactorial genetic components are also important in this disease's onset.

A minor fourth cell type, more common in islets located within the head of the pancreas, are **PP cells**, which secrete **pancreatic polypeptide**. Table 20–4 summarizes the types, quantities, and main functions of the major pancreatic hormones. Pancreatic islets also normally contain a few enterochromaffin cells, like those of the digestive tract, which are also scattered in the pancreatic acini and ducts, and which secrete other hormones affecting the digestive system.

Activity of α and β cells is regulated largely by blood glucose levels above or below the normal level of 70 mg/dL. Increased glucose levels stimulate β cells to release insulin and inhibit α cells from releasing glucagon; decreased glucose levels stimulate α cells to release glucagon. Opposing actions of these hormones help to precisely control blood glucose concentration, an important factor in homeostasis (Table 20–4).

These hormones and somatostatin from the δ cells also act in a paracrine manner to affect hormone release within an islet as well as activity of the neighboring acinar cells. Sympathetic

and parasympathetic nerve endings are closely associated with about 10% of α, β, and δ cells and can also function as part of the control system for insulin and glucagon secretion. Gap junctions transfer the autonomic neural stimulus to the other cells. Sympathetic fibers increase glucagon release and inhibit insulin release; parasympathetic fibers increase secretion of both glucagon and insulin.

> **DIFFUSE NEUROENDOCRINE SYSTEM**

The enterochromaffin cells scattered in both the islets and small ducts of the pancreas are similar to those of the digestive tract (see Chapter 15). Collectively these dispersed cells, as well as similar cells in the respiratory mucosa, make up the **diffuse neuroendocrine system (DNES)**. Like the pancreatic islets, most of these cells are derived from endodermal cells of the embryonic gut or bronchial buds. These secretory cells are considered neuroendocrine because they produce many of the same polypeptides and neurotransmitter-like molecules, such as serotonin (5-hydroxytryptamine), also released by neurosecretory cells in the CNS. Several such cells, along with their hormones and major functions, are summarized in Table 15–1 with the digestive system. Most of these hormones are polypeptides and act in a paracrine manner, affecting primarily the activities of neighboring contractile cells and secretory cells (both exocrine and endocrine). Enteroendocrine cells of the stomach and small bowel are shown ultrastructurally in Figures 15–20, 15–24c, and 15–27.

Many cells of the DNES are stained by solutions of chromium salts and have therefore been called **enterochromaffin cells**, while those staining with silver nitrate are sometimes called **argentaffin cells**. DNES cells secreting serotonin or certain other amine derivatives demonstrate amine precursor uptake and decarboxylation and are often referred to

TABLE **20–4**	Major cell types and hormones of pancreatic islets.			
Cell Type	**Quantity (%)**	**Hormone Produced**	**Hormone Structure and Size**	**Hormone Function**
α	~30	Glucagon	Polypeptide; 3500 Da	Acts on several tissues to make energy stored in glycogen and fat available through glycogenolysis and lipolysis; increases blood glucose content
β	~60	Insulin	Dimer of α and β chains with S-S bridges; 5700–6000 Da	Acts on several tissues to cause entry of glucose into cells and promotes decrease of blood glucose content
δ or D	5–10	Somatostatin	Polypeptide; 1650 Da	Inhibits release of other islet cell hormones through local paracrine action; inhibits release of GH and TSH in anterior pituitary and HCl secretion by gastric parietal cells
PP	Rare	Pancreatic polypeptide	Polypeptide; 4200 Da	Stimulates activity of gastric chief cells; inhibits bile secretion, pancreatic enzyme and bicarbonate secretion, and intestinal motility

acronymically as **APUD cells**. Such names are still widely used, but, as indicated in Table 15–1, they have been largely replaced by letter designations like those used for pancreatic islet cells. Whatever name is used, cells of the DNES are highly important due to their role in regulating motility and secretions of all types within the digestive system.

› THYROID GLAND

The **thyroid gland**, located anterior and inferior to the larynx, consists of two lobes united by an isthmus (Figure 20–18). It originates in early embryonic life from the foregut endoderm near the base of the developing tongue. It synthesizes the thyroid hormones **thyroxine** (tetraiodothyronine or **T4**) and **triiodothyronine (T3)**, which help control the basal metabolic rate in cells throughout the body, as well as the polypeptide hormone **calcitonin**.

The parenchyma of the thyroid is composed of millions of rounded epithelial **thyroid follicles** of variable diameter, each with simple epithelium and a central lumen densely filled with gelatinous acidophilic **colloid** (Figure 20–19). The thyroid is the only endocrine gland in which a large quantity of secretory product is stored. Moreover, storage is outside the cells, in the colloid of the follicle lumen, which is also unusual. There is sufficient hormone in follicles to supply the body for up to 3 months with no additional synthesis. Thyroid colloid contains the large glycoprotein **thyroglobulin** (660 kDa), the precursor for the active thyroid hormones.

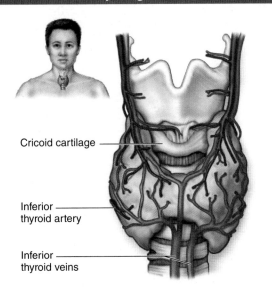

FIGURE **20–18** Thyroid gland.

Cricoid cartilage

Inferior thyroid artery

Inferior thyroid veins

The **thyroid** is a highly vascular, butterfly-shaped gland surrounding the anterior surface of the trachea just below the larynx.

The thyroid gland is covered by a fibrous capsule from which septa extend into the parenchyma, dividing it into lobules and carrying blood vessels, nerves, and lymphatics. Follicles are densely packed together, separated from one another only by sparse reticular connective tissue (Figure 20–19), although this stroma is very well vascularized with fenestrated capillaries for transfer of released hormone to the blood.

The follicular cells, or **thyrocytes**, range in shape from squamous to low columnar (Figure 20–19), their size and other features varying with their activity, which is controlled by thyroid-stimulating hormone (TSH) from the anterior pituitary. Active glands have more follicles of low columnar epithelium; glands with mostly squamous follicular cells are hypoactive.

Thyrocytes have apical junctional complexes and rest on a basal lamina (Figure 20–20). The cells exhibit organelles indicating active protein synthesis and secretion, as well as phagocytosis and digestion. The nucleus is generally round and central. Basally the cells are rich in rough ER and apically, facing the follicular lumen, are Golgi complexes, secretory granules, numerous phagosomes and lysosomes, and microvilli.

Another endocrine cell type, the **parafollicular cell**, or **C cell**, is also found inside the basal lamina of the follicular epithelium or as isolated clusters between follicles (Figure 20–20). Derived from the neural crest, parafollicular cells are usually somewhat larger than follicular cells and stain less intensely. They have a smaller amount of rough ER, large Golgi complexes, and numerous small (100-180 nm in diameter) granules containing calcitonin (Figure 20–20). Secretion of calcitonin is triggered by elevated blood Ca^{2+} levels, and it inhibits osteoclast activity, but this function in humans is less important than the roles of parathyroid hormone and vitamin D in the regulation of normal calcium homeostasis.

›› MEDICAL APPLICATION

Chronic dietary iodine deficiencies inhibit thyroid hormone production, causing thyrotropic cells of the anterior pituitary gland to produce excess TSH. This leads to excessive growth of thyroid follicles and enlargement of the thyroid gland, a condition known as **goiter**.

Production of Thyroid Hormone & Its Control

Production, storage, and release of **thyroid hormones** involve an unusual, multistage process in the thyrocytes, with both an exocrine phase and an endocrine phase. Both phases are promoted by TSH and occur in the same cell, as summarized in Figure 20–21. The major activities of this process include the following:

1. The **production of thyroglobulin**, which is similar to that in other glycoprotein-exporting cells, with synthesis in the rough ER and glycosylation in the Golgi apparatus.

FIGURE **20–19** Thyroid follicular cells and parafollicular cells.

(a) A low-power micrograph of **thyroid gland** shows the thin capsule (**C**), from which septa (**S**) with the larger blood vessels, lymphatics, and nerves enter the gland. The parenchyma of the organ is distinctive, consisting of **colloid-filled epithelial follicles** of many sizes. The lumen of each follicle is filled with a lightly staining colloid of a large gelatinous protein called **thyroglobulin**. (×12; H&E)

(b) The lumen (**L**) of each follicle is surrounded by a simple epithelium of **thyrocytes** in which the cell height ranges from squamous to low columnar. Also present are large pale-staining parafollicular

or C cells (**C**) secreting **calcitonin**, a polypeptide involved with calcium metabolism. (×200; H&E)

(c–e) C cells may be part of the follicular epithelium or present singly or in groups outside of follicles. Thyrocytes (**T**) can usually be distinguished from parafollicular C cells (**C**) by their smaller size and darker staining properties. Unlike thyrocytes, C cells seldom vary in their size or pale staining characteristics. C cells are somewhat easier to locate in or between small follicles. c and d: (×400; H&E); e: (×400; Mallory trichrome)

Thyroglobulin has no hormonal activity itself but contains 140 tyrosyl residues critical for thyroid hormone synthesis. The glycoprotein is released as an exocrine product from apical vesicles of thyrocytes into the follicular lumen.

2. The **uptake of iodide** from blood by Na/I symporters (NIS) in the thyrocytes' basolateral cell membranes, which allows for 30-fold concentration of dietary iodide in thyroid tissue relative to plasma. Decreased levels of circulating iodide trigger synthesis of NIS, increasing iodide uptake and compensating for the lower plasma concentration. An apical iodide/chloride transporter (also called **pendrin**) pumps I⁻ from thyrocytes into the colloid.

3. **Iodination of tyrosyl residues** in thyroglobulin with either one or two atoms occurs in the colloid after oxidation of iodide to iodine by membrane-bound thyroid peroxidase on the microvilli surfaces of thyrocytes.

4. **Formation of T$_3$ and T$_4$** (also called thyroxine) occurs as two iodinated tyrosines, still part of colloidal thyroglobulin, which are covalently conjugated in coupling reactions.

5. **Endocytosis of iodinated thyroglobulin** by the thyrocytes involves both fluid-phase pinocytosis and receptor-mediated endocytosis. The endocytic vesicles fuse with lysosomes, and the thyroglobulin is thoroughly degraded by lysosomal proteases, freeing active thyroid hormone as both T$_3$ and T$_4$.

FIGURE **20–20** Ultrastructure of thyroid follicular and parafollicular cells.

(a) TEM of the **follicular epithelium** shows pseudopodia and microvilli extending from the follicular thyrocytes (**T**) into the colloid of the lumen (**L**). The cells have apical junctional complexes, much RER, well-developed Golgi complexes, and many lysosomes. Inside the basement membrane (**BM**) of the follicle, but often not contacting the colloid in the lumen, are occasional C cells (**C**).

To the left and right of the two C cells seen here are capillaries intimately associated with the follicular cells, but outside the basement membrane. (×2000)

(b) A TEM of a **C cell**, with its large Golgi apparatus (**G**), extensive RER, and cytoplasm filled with small secretory granules containing calcitonin. (×5000)

6. **Secretion of T$_4$ and T$_3$** at the basolateral domains of thyrocytes occurs in an endocrine manner: both molecules are immediately taken up by capillaries.

Nearly all of both thyroid hormones are carried in blood tightly bound to thyroxine-binding globulin or albumen. T$_4$ is the more abundant compound, constituting 90% of the circulating thyroid hormone. Both molecules bind the same intracellular receptors of target cells, but T$_3$ is 2- to 10-fold more active than T$_4$. The half-life of T$_3$ is 1.5 days in comparison with a week for T$_4$. Both thyroid hormones increase the number and size of mitochondria and stimulate mitochondrial protein synthesis, helping to enhance metabolic activity.

The major regulator of the anatomic and functional state of thyroid follicles is TSH (thyrotropin) from the anterior pituitary (Figure 20–8). With TSH receptors abundant on the basal cell membrane of thyrocytes, this tropic hormone increases cell height in the follicular epithelium and stimulates all stages of thyroid hormone production and release. Thyroid hormones inhibit the release of TSH, maintaining levels of circulating T$_4$ and T$_3$ within the normal range (Figure 20–10). Secretion of TSH in the pituitary is also increased by exposure to cold and decreased by heat and stressful stimuli.

›› MEDICAL APPLICATION

Graves disease is an autoimmune disorder in which antibodies produce chronic stimulation of the follicular cells and release of thyroid hormones (**hyperthyroidism**), which causes a hypermetabolic state marked by weight loss, nervousness, sweating, heat intolerance, and other features. **Hypothyroidism**, with reduced thyroid hormone levels, can be caused by local inflammation (**thyroiditis**) or inadequate secretion of TSH by the anterior pituitary gland and is often manifested by tiredness, weight gain, intolerance of cold, and decreased ability to concentrate.

› PARATHYROID GLANDS

The parathyroid glands are four small ovoid masses—each 3 × 6 mm—with a total weight of about 0.4 g. They are located on the back of the thyroid gland, usually embedded in the larger gland's capsule (Figure 20–22). The microvasculature of each arises from the inferior thyroid arteries. Each parathyroid gland is contained within a thin capsule from which septa extend into the gland. A sparse reticular stroma supports dense elongated clusters of secretory cells.

FIGURE **20–21** Thyrocyte activities in thyroid hormone synthesis.

The diagram shows the multistep process by which thyroid hormones are produced via the stored thyroglobulin intermediate. In an exocrine phase of the process, (1) the glycoprotein **thyroglobulin** is made and secreted into the follicular lumen and (2) iodide is pumped across the cells into the lumen. In the lumen (3) iodide is converted to iodine by membrane-bound **thyroid peroxidase** and added to **tyrosine residues** of thyroglobulin (4) to form monoiodotyrosine (MIT) or diiodotyrosine (DIT), which are then covalently coupled to form T_3 and T_4 still within the glycoprotein, as shown at the right. The iodinated thyroglobulin is then (5) endocytosed by the thyrocytes and degraded by lysosomes, (6) releasing free **active T_3 and T_4** to the adjacent capillaries in an endocrine manner. Detailed steps are given in the text. Both phases are promoted by TSH and may occur simultaneously in the same cell.

The parathyroid glands are derived from the embryonic pharyngeal pouches—the superior glands from the fourth pouch and the inferior glands from the third pouch. Their migration to the developing thyroid gland is sometimes misdirected so that the number and locations of the glands are somewhat variable. Up to 10% of individuals may have parathyroid tissue attached to the thymus, which originates from the same pharyngeal pouches.

The endocrine cells of the parathyroid glands, called **principal (chief) cells**, are small polygonal cells with round nuclei and pale-staining, slightly acidophilic cytoplasm (Figure 20–23). Irregularly shaped cytoplasmic granules contain the polypeptide **parathyroid hormone (PTH)**, an important regulator of blood calcium levels. PTH has three major targets:

- Osteoblasts respond to PTH by producing an osteoclast-stimulating factor, which increases the number and activity of osteoclasts. The resulting resorption of the calcified bone matrix and release of Ca^{2+} increase the

FIGURE **20–22** Parathyroid glands.

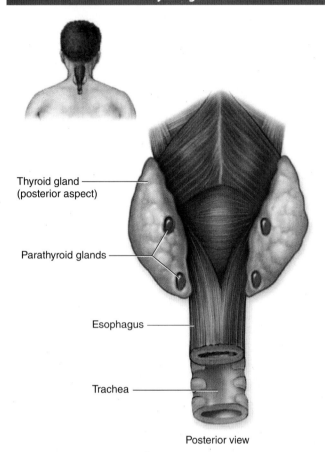

Thyroid gland
(posterior aspect)

Parathyroid glands

Esophagus

Trachea

Posterior view

The **parathyroid glands** are four small nodules normally embedded in the capsule on the posterior surface of the thyroid gland.

FIGURE **20–23** Parathyroid principal cells.

(a) A small lobe of **parathyroid gland**, surrounded by connective tissue septa (**S**), shows mainly densely packed cords of small principal cells (**P**). Older parathyroid glands show increasing numbers of much larger and acidophilic nonfunctional oxyphil cells (**O**) that may occur singly or in clumps of varying sizes. (×60; H&E)

(b) Higher magnification shows that **principal cells** have round central nuclei and pale-staining cytoplasm. Cords of principal cells secreting PTH surround capillaries (**C**). (×200; H&E)

concentration of circulating Ca^{2+}, which suppresses PTH production. The effect of PTH on blood levels of Ca^{2+} is thus opposite to that of calcitonin.

■ In the distal convoluted tubules of the renal cortex, PTH stimulates Ca^{2+} reabsorption (and inhibits phosphate reabsorption in the proximal tubules).

■ PTH also indirectly increases the Ca^{2+} absorption in the small intestine by stimulating vitamin D activation.

With increasing age, many secretory cells are replaced with adipocytes, which may constitute more than 50% of the gland in older people.

Much smaller populations of **oxyphil cells**, often clustered, are sometimes also present in parathyroid glands, more commonly in older individuals. These are much larger than the principal cells and are characterized by very acidophilic cytoplasm filled with abnormally shaped mitochondria. Accumulating with age, oxyphil cells are degenerated derivatives of principal cells, with some still exhibiting low levels of PTH synthesis.

❯❯ MEDICAL APPLICATION

In **hypoparathyroidism**, diminished secretion of PTH can cause bones to become more mineralized and denser and striated muscle to exhibit abnormal contractions due to inadequate calcium ion concentrations. Excessive **PTH** produced in **hyperparathyroidism** stimulates osteoclast number and activity, leading to increased levels of blood calcium that can be deposited pathologically in cartilage, arteries, or the kidneys.

» PINEAL GLAND

The **pineal gland**, also known as the **epiphysis cerebri**, regulates the daily rhythms of bodily activities. A small, pine cone-shaped organ, approximately 5–8 mm by 3–5 mm, the pineal gland develops from neuroectoderm in the posterior wall of the third ventricle and remains attached to the brain by a short stalk. The pineal gland is covered by connective tissue of the pia mater, from which septa-containing small blood vessels emerge and subdivide variously sized lobules.

Prominent and abundant secretory cells called **pinealocytes** have slightly basophilic cytoplasm and irregular euchromatic nuclei (Figure 20–24). Ultrastructurally pinealocytes are seen to have secretory vesicles, many mitochondria, and long cytoplasmic processes extending to the vascularized septa,

where they end in dilatations near capillaries, indicating an endocrine function. These cells produce **melatonin**, a low-molecular-weight tryptophan derivative. Unmyelinated sympathetic nerve fibers enter the pineal gland and end among pinealocytes, with some forming synapses.

Melatonin release from pinealocytes is promoted by darkness and inhibited by daylight. The resulting diurnal fluctuation in blood melatonin levels induces rhythmic changes in the activity of the hypothalamus, pituitary gland, and other endocrine tissues that characterize the circadian (24 hours, day/night) rhythm of physiological functions and behaviors. In humans and other mammals, the cycle of light and darkness is detected within the retinas and transmitted to the pineal via the retinohypothalamic tract, the suprachiasmatic nucleus, and the tracts of sympathetic fibers entering

---

FIGURE 20–24 Pineal gland.

(a) The micrograph shows a group of **pinealocytes** surrounded by septa (**S**) containing venules (**V**) and capillaries (arrows). Also seen is an extracellular mineral deposit called a **corpus arenaceum** (**CA**) of unknown physiologic significance but an excellent marker for the pineal. (×200; H&E)

(b) At higher magnification the numerous large pinealocytes (**P**) with euchromatic nuclei can be compared to much fewer astrocytes (**A**) that have darker, more elongated nuclei and are located mainly within septa and near small blood vessels (**V**). Capillaries

(arrow) are not nearly as numerous as in other endocrine glands. At the lower left is a part of a very large corpus arenaceum (**CA**), the calcified structures also known as **brain sand**. Along the septa run unmyelinated tracts of sympathetic fibers, associated indirectly with photoreceptive neurons in the retinas and running to the pinealocytes to stimulate **melatonin** release in periods of darkness. Levels of circulating melatonin are one factor determining the diurnal rhythms of hormone release and physiologic activities throughout the body. (×400; H&E)

the pineal. The pineal gland acts, therefore, as a neuroendocrine transducer, converting sensory input regarding light and darkness into variations in many hormonal functions.

The pineal gland also has interstitial glial cells that are modified **astrocytes**, staining positively for glial fibrillary acidic protein, which represent about 5% of the cells. These have elongated nuclei more heavily stained than those of pinealocytes and are usually found in perivascular areas and between the groups of pinealocytes.

A characteristic feature of the pineal gland is the presence of variously sized concretions of calcium and magnesium salts called **corpora arenacea**, or brain sand, formed by mineralization of extracellular protein deposits. Such concretions may appear during childhood and gradually increase in number and size with age, with no apparent effect on the gland's function.

❯❯ MEDICAL APPLICATION

Densely calcified corpora arenacea can be used as landmarks for the midline location of the pineal gland in various **radiological examinations** of the brain. **Tumors** originating from pinealocytes are very rare, but they can be either benign or highly malignant.

Table 20–5 summarizes the major endocrine cells, hormones, and functions of the adrenal gland, pancreatic islets, thyroid, parathyroid, and pineal glands.

TABLE **20–5**	Cells, important hormones, and functions of other major endocrine organs.		
Gland	**Endocrine Cells**	**Major Hormones**	**Major Functions**
Adrenal glands: Cortex	Cells of zona glomerulosa	Mineralocorticoids	Stimulate renal reabsorption of water and Na⁺ and secretion of K⁺ to maintain salt and water balance
	Cells of zona fasciculata	Glucocorticoids	Influence carbohydrate metabolism; suppress immune cell activities
	Cells of zona reticularis	Weak androgens	Precursors for testosterone or estrogen
Adrenal glands: Medulla	Chromaffin cells	Epinephrine	Increases heart rate and blood pressure
		Norepinephrine	Constricts vessels; increases heart rate and blood pressure
Pancreatic islets	α Cells	Glucagon	Raises blood glucose levels
	β Cells	Insulin	Lowers blood glucose levels
	δ Cells	Somatostatin	Inhibits secretion of insulin, glucagon, and somatotropin
	PP cells	Pancreatic polypeptide	Inhibits secretion of pancreatic enzymes and HCO_3^-
Thyroid glands	Follicular cells	Thyroid hormones (T_3 and T_4)	Increases metabolic rate
	Parafollicular or C cells	Calcitonin	Lowers blood Ca^{2+} levels by inhibiting osteoclast activity
Parathyroid glands	Chief cells	Parathyroid hormone (PTH)	Raises blood Ca^{2+} levels by stimulating osteoclast activity
Pineal gland	Pinealocytes	Melatonin	Regulates circadian rhythms

Endocrine Glands SUMMARY OF KEY POINTS

Pituitary Gland

- The **pituitary gland** has two major parts: the **posterior** part called the **pars nervosa** develops as a downgrowth of the developing brain and is attached in the **hypothalamus** by the **infundibulum**.
- The anterior pituitary includes the large **pars distalis**, the **pars tuberalis** that surrounds the infundibulum, and the thin **pars intermedia** adjacent to the pars nervosa.
- Blood vessels of the **hypothalamic hypophyseal portal system** are important in carrying peptide factors from hypothalamic neurons to cells of the anterior pituitary where they control cell secretion.
- This portal system includes a **primary capillary plexus** in the infundibulum and lower hypothalamus and a **secondary plexus** in the pars distalis, connected by **portal veins** and draining to the **hypophyseal vein**.
- Endocrine cells of the anterior pituitary can be called **acidophils**, **basophils**, or **chromophobes** based on their general staining properties; the latter lack secretory granules and stain poorly.
  - Acidophils and basophils can be identified as to which pituitary hormone they produce using **immunohistochemistry** and antibodies against specific hormones.
  - Acidophils are primarily **somatotrophs** producing **somatotropin** (**growth hormone**), or **lactotrophs** (or mammotrophs) producing **prolactin (PRL)**.
  - Basophils include **gonadotrophs** producing **FSH** and **LH** and **thyrotrophs** making **TSH**.
  - A third type of basophil is the **corticotroph**, synthesizing **POMC** that is cleaved by proteases to make **ACTH** and **β-LPH**.
- The **hypothalamic hypophyseal tract** includes bundles of nerve axons that run from **supraoptic nucleus** (**SON**) and **paraventricular nucleus** (**PVN**) in the hypothalamus to the posterior pituitary.
- Hypothalamic neurons in the SON synthesize **vasopressin/ADH** and those of the PVN synthesize **oxytocin**, both of which are stored in axonal dilations called **Herring bodies** before release to capillaries in the posterior pituitary.

Adrenal Glands

- The **adrenal cortex** of each adrenal gland consists of three concentric zones, all histologically distinct but with cells producing steroid hormones and all drained by the same system of capillaries.

- The most superficial **zona glomerulosa** has round clusters of cells producing **mineralocorticoids** such as **aldosterone** regulating electrolyte levels.
- The wider, middle **zona fasciculata** has elongated strands of cells producing **glucocorticoids** such as **cortisol**, which regulates several aspects of carbohydrate metabolism.
- The innermost **zona reticularis** has a network of cells making the weak androgen **DHEA** that is converted to **testosterone** in men and women.
- The **adrenal medulla** contains neural crest-derived **chromaffin cells** synthesizing either **epinephrine** or **norepinephrine** that regulate the stress response.

Pancreatic Islets

- **Pancreatic islets of Langerhans** are small clusters of pale cells embedded within the exocrine tissue; they have primarily **β cells making insulin**, **α cell** (**glucagon**), and **δ cells** (**somatostatin**).

Thyroid Gland

- The **thyroid gland** consists mainly of spherical **follicles** composed of simple epithelium of **thyrocytes** surrounding a lumen with **thyroglobulin**.
- **Thyroglobulin** is a large glycoprotein in which tyrosine residues are **iodinated** as precursors of the thyroid hormones **thyroxine** and **triiodothyronine**, which are released when the precursor is degraded.
- Thyroid follicles also contain a few smaller and paler cells called **parafollicular cells**, or **C cells**, which produce the polypeptide hormone **calcitonin**.

Parathyroid Glands

- On the posterior side of the thyroid glands are four small **parathyroid glands**, each consisting primarily of **principal cells** that secrete **PTH** that raises blood Ca^{2+} levels.

Pineal Gland

- The **pineal gland** develops from embryonic neuroectoderm, remains attached to the brain, and contains modified neurons called **pinealocytes** that secrete the amine **melatonin**.
- Pineal landmarks are the concretions called **corpora arenacea** (brain sand); neural connections from the retina to **pinealocytes** allow diurnal secretion of melatonin and rhythms in physiological activities.

Endocrine Glands ASSESS YOUR KNOWLEDGE

1. Which of the following accurately describes glucocorticoids?
   a. Include the steroid hormone aldosterone
   b. Are produced in response to stimulation by ACTH
   c. Are produced primarily by the zona glomerulosa
   d. Typically enhance the immune response
   e. Include the steroid hormone DHEA

2. Pregnant women who have begun labor but in whom this process is no longer progressing are often given an IV injection of Pitocin to stimulate uterine contractions and facilitate parturition. Pitocin is a trade name of a hormone produced in what endocrine tissue?
   a. Pars distalis
   b. Ovarian follicles
   c. Pars nervosa
   d. Placenta
   e. Pars tuberalis

3. What hormone is produced in response to decreased blood calcium levels?
   a. Pancreatic polypeptide
   b. β-Endorphin
   c. Somatostatin
   d. Calcitonin
   e. PTH

4. Addison disease (or adrenal cortex insufficiency) is a disorder, usually autoimmune in origin, which can cause degeneration and cell loss in the adrenal glands. Fludrocortisone is a mineralocorticoid used to treat Addison patients. Response to this drug indicates which region of the adrenal glands was involved in the disease?
   a. Medulla
   b. Zona glomerulosa
   c. Zona reticularis
   d. Macula densa
   e. Zona fasciculate

5. A glucagonoma is a malignant tumor consisting of what cells?
   a. A or α cells
   b. B or β cells
   c. Chromophils
   d. D or δ cells
   e. Mucous cells

6. Secretion, chemical modification and storage, reuptake, and digestion of a protein occur in epithelial cells of what endocrine tissue?
   a. Neurohypophysis
   b. Adrenal medulla
   c. Adenohypophysis
   d. Thyroid gland
   e. Neuroendocrine cells in the duodenum

7. Secretion in what neuroendocrine cell is controlled directly by neural activity and involves a hormone that generally slows metabolic activity at night?
   a. Pituicyte
   b. Melanocyte
   c. Herring body of the neurohypophysis
   d. Chromaffin cell
   e. Pinealocyte

8. Some mammalian endocrine tissues or cells can be experimentally transplanted to other well-vascularized sites (such as the oral mucosa) in genetically similar hosts and the tissue's function continues normally and with proper regulation. The pars distalis is not a good candidate for such transplantation studies for which one of the following reasons?
   a. More severe rejection of neurally related tissue occurs compared with other endocrine organs.
   b. Its hormonal source is unavailable after its axonal connections to the hypothalamus are disrupted.
   c. Its cells stop functioning when separated from the hypothalamo-hypophyseal portal system.
   d. Neogenesis of blood vessels into this tissue will not occur at the transplant site.
   e. The vascular wall of the superior hypophyseal arteries is unique.

9. A 45-year-old corporate executive presents with the primary complaint of "always being tired." She comments that she has been tired for 4 months even though she is sleeping more. She complains of being unable to finish chores at home and "dragging at work." She indicates that she is often constipated and is intolerant of cold. She is continuously turning the thermostats in the house and office to higher temperatures, to the dismay of family and coworkers. She also complains that her skin is very dry; use of lotions and creams have not helped the dryness. A biopsy of her thyroid gland shows dense lymphocytic infiltration with germinal centers throughout the parenchyma and a battery of further tests is carried out, which also suggest thyroiditis. Which of the following results of blood tests would be most likely in this patient?
   a. Elevated TSH levels
   b. Elevated T_3 and T_4 levels
   c. Autoantibodies to the thyroid hormone receptor
   d. Elevated calcitonin levels
   e. Elevated glucocorticoid levels

10. A 9-year-old girl, the youngest of four daughters, is taken to the pediatrician by her mother, who indicates that for at least 4 months the child has seemed "hyperactive," unable to sleep soundly because "she says her room is too hot," and no longer able to concentrate in school. Upon questioning, the mother also remembers that her daughter's periods also began within the past few months. Blood tests indicate high levels of estrogen-related hormones and cortisol. Which of the following tentative diagnoses is consistent with all of these symptoms?
   a. Graves disease, caused by antibodies stimulating the TSH receptor
   b. A defect in the PVN
   c. Excessively active cells of the adrenal cortex zona glomerulosa
   d. A benign tumor involving cells in the adenohypophysis
   e. A disabling mutation in the gene for thyroglobulin

21 The Male Reproductive System

The male reproductive system consists of the testes, genital ducts, accessory glands, and penis (Figure 21–1). Testes produce sperm but also contain endocrine cells secreting testosterone, which drives many aspects of male reproductive physiology. Testosterone influences sexual differentiation during embryonic and fetal development, activates spermatogenesis, and controls gonadotropin secretion in the pituitary. A metabolite of testosterone, dihydrotestosterone, also begins to act on many tissues during puberty, including the male accessory glands and hair follicles.

The genital ducts and accessory glands produce secretions required for sperm activity and contract to propel spermatozoa and the secretions from the penile urethra. These secretions also provide nutrients for spermatozoa while they are confined to the male reproductive tract. Spermatozoa and the secretions of the accessory glands make up the **semen** (L. seed), which is introduced into the female reproductive tract by the penis.

❯ TESTES

Each **testis** (or testicle) has a dense connective tissue capsule, the **tunica albuginea**, which thickens on the posterior side to form the **mediastinum testis**. From this fibrous region, septa penetrate the organ, dividing it into about 250 pyramidal compartments or **testicular lobules** (Figures 21–2 and 21–3). Each lobule contains sparse connective tissue with endocrine

interstitial cells (or **Leydig cells**) for testosterone synthesis, and one to four highly convoluted **seminiferous tubules** in which sperm production occurs.

The testes develop retroperitoneally in the dorsal wall of the embryonic abdominal cavity and descend during fetal development to become suspended at the ends of the spermatic cords in the two halves of the scrotal sac, or **scrotum** (Figure 21–2). During migration from the abdominal cavity, each testis brings along a serous sac, the **tunica vaginalis**, derived from the peritoneum. This tunic consists of an outer parietal layer lining the scrotum and an inner visceral layer, covering the tunica albuginea on the anterior and lateral sides of the testis (Figure 21–2).

Having evolved in cold-blooded animals, certain molecular events during sperm formation cannot occur at the core body temperature of 37°C. Within the scrotum a permissive temperature of about 34°C normally occurs, maintained by a combination of mechanisms. As in the integument generally, evaporation of sweat from the scrotal skin cools local blood and tissues. In the spermatic cord the testicular artery is surrounded by a network of veins, the **pampiniform plexus**, carrying blood already cooled in the testis, which draws heat from the arterial blood by a countercurrent heat-exchange system. The thin dartos muscle of the scrotum and the cremaster muscle of the spermatic cord relax or contract to move the testes away from or closer to the body, respectively, allowing further control on testicular temperature.

FIGURE **21–1** **The male reproductive system.**

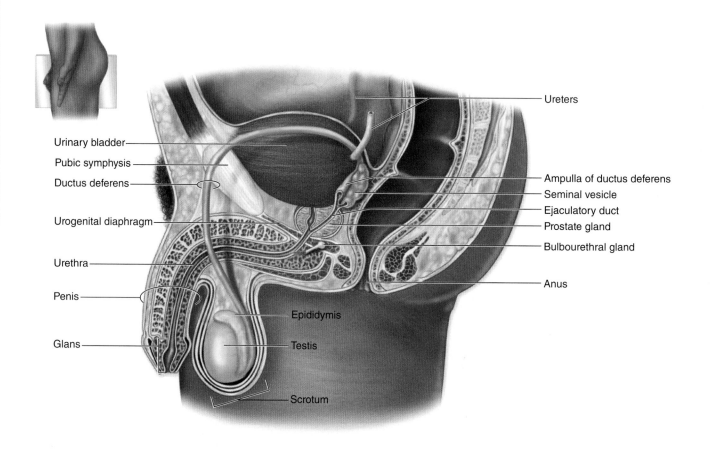

Urinary bladder

Pubic symphysis

Ductus deferens

Urogenital diaphragm

Urethra

Penis

Glans

Ureters

Ampulla of ductus deferens

Seminal vesicle

Ejaculatory duct

Prostate gland

Bulbourethral gland

Anus

Epididymis

Testis

Scrotum

The diagram shows the locations and relationships of the **testes, epididymis, glands,** and the **ductus deferens** running from the scrotum to the urethra. The ductus deferens is located along the anterior and superior sides of the bladder as a result of the testes descending into the scrotum from the abdominal cavity during fetal development.

›› MEDICAL APPLICATION

An excessive accumulation of serous fluid in one or both sides of the scrotal sac, termed a **hydrocele**, represents the most common cause of scrotal swelling and a condition easily corrected surgically.

Cryptorchidism (Gr. *Kryptos*, hidden + *orchis*, testis), the failure of one or both testes to descend from the abdomen, occurs in about 4% of male neonates, but in most of these individuals, the testes move to the scrotum during the first year. Bilateral cryptorchidism causes infertility if not surgically corrected by 2–3 years of age.

Interstitial Tissue

Sparse interstitial tissue among the seminiferous tubules consists of connective tissue containing fibroblasts, lymphatics, and blood vessels including fenestrated capillaries. During puberty **interstitial cells** (**Leydig cells**) develop singly or in small groups as large polygonal cells with central nuclei and eosinophilic cytoplasm rich in mitochondria, smooth endoplasmic reticulum (SER), and small lipid droplets (Figures 21–2b and 21–4). Interstitial cells produce the steroid hormone **testosterone**, which promotes development of the secondary male sex characteristics. Testosterone synthesis here involves the same system of enzymes in the SER and mitochondria used by adrenal cortical cells.

Unlike that in the adrenals, interstitial cell testosterone secretion is triggered by the pituitary gonadotropin, **interstitial cell-stimulating hormone (ICSH)**, known as luteinizing hormone in females. Testosterone synthesis here thus begins at puberty when the hypothalamus starts producing gonadotropin-releasing hormone. In the late embryonic testes, gonadotropin from the placenta stimulates interstitial cells to synthesize sufficient testosterone for development of the ducts and glands of the male reproductive system. These fetal

FIGURE **21–2** Testes and seminiferous tubules.

Spermatic cord

Blood vessels and nerves

Ductus deferens

Head of epididymis
Duct of epididymis
Seminiferous tubule
Straight tubule

Efferent ductule

Mediastinum testis (housing rete testis)

Septum

Lobule

Body of epididymis

Visceral layer of tunica vaginalis

Parietal layer of tunica vaginalis

Tunica albuginea

Tail of epididymis

a

(a) The diagram shows a partially cutaway sagittal section of the **testis**. **(b)** A **seminiferous tubule** cross section shows spermatogonia (**SG**) near the periphery, near nuclei of Sertoli cells (**SC**), primary spermatocytes (**PS**), and late spermatids (**LS**) near the lumen, with interstitial cells (**IC**) in the surrounding connective tissue. (×400; H&E)

interstitial cells remain very active during the third and fourth months of pregnancy, then become quiescent cells resembling fibroblasts until puberty when they resume testosterone synthesis in response to the pituitary gonadotropin.

Seminiferous Tubules

Sperm are produced in the **seminiferous tubules** of young men at a rate of about 200 million per day. Each testis has from 250 to 1000 such tubules in its lobules, each tubule measuring 150–250 μm in diameter and 30–70 cm in length. The combined length of the tubules of one testis totals about 250 m. Each tubule develops as a loop linked by a very short, narrower segment, the **straight tubule**, to the **rete testis**, a labyrinth of epithelium-lined channels embedded in the mediastinum testis (Figures 21–2a and 21–3). Between 10 and 20 **efferent ductules** then connect the rete testis to the head of the **epididymis** (Figure 21–2a).

Each seminiferous tubule consists of a complex, specialized stratified epithelium called **germinal** or **spermatogenic epithelium** (Figure 21–2b). The basement membrane of this epithelium is covered by a very thin connective tissue layer containing flattened, smooth muscle-like **myoid cells** (Figure 21–2b), which allow weak contractions of the tubule. The germinal epithelium consists of two types of cells:

- Large nondividing **Sertoli cells** (Figure 21–4), which physically and metabolically support developing sperm cell precursors, and
- Dividing cells of the **spermatogenic lineage** (Figure 21–5a).

The cells of the spermatogenic lineage, comprising four or more concentric layers of cells in the germinal epithelium, develop from progenitor cells to fully formed sperm cells over

FIGURE 21–3 Lobules converging at rete testis.

The dense capsule of the **testis**, the tunica albuginea, thickens on the posterior side as the mediastinum (**M**) testis, from which many thin septa (**S**) subdivide the organ into about 250 **lobules**. Each lobule contains one to four convoluted seminiferous tubules (**ST**) in a sparse connective tissue interstitium. Each **tubule** is a loop attached by means of a short **straight tubule** to the rete testis (**RT**), a maze of channels embedded in the mediastinum testis. From the **rete testis**, the sperm move into the **epididymis**. (×60; H&E)

approximately 10 weeks. As shown in Figure 21–5 **spermatogenesis**, the first part of sperm production involves mainly mitosis and meiosis; the resulting haploid cells then undergo **spermiogenesis** or differentiation as mature sperm cells.

Spermatogenesis

Spermatogenesis begins at puberty with proliferation of spermatogenic progenitor cells called **spermatogonia** (Gr. *sperma* + *gone*, generation). These are small round cells about 12 μm in diameter, occupying a basal niche in the epithelial wall of the tubules, next to the basement membrane, and all closely associated with Sertoli cell surfaces (Figures 21–5 and 21–6).

Different stages of spermatogonia development can be recognized by subtle changes in shape and staining properties of their nuclei. Spermatogonia with dark, ovoid nuclei act as stem cells, dividing infrequently and giving rise both to new stem cells and to cells with more pale-staining, ovoid nuclei that divide more rapidly as transit amplifying (progenitor) cells (Figure 21–7). These **type A spermatogonia** each

undergo several unique clonal divisions that leave most of the cells interconnected as a syncytium. These become **type B spermatogonia**, which have more spherical and pale nuclei.

Each type B spermatogonium then undergoes a final mitotic division to produce two cells that increase in size and become **primary spermatocytes**, which are spherical cells with euchromatic nuclei (Figures 21–6 and 21–7). Primary spermatocytes replicate their DNA, so each chromosome consists of duplicate chromatids, and enter meiosis, during which homologous chromosomes come together in synapsis, DNA recombination occurs, and two rapid cell divisions produce haploid cells (see Chapter 3).

The primary spermatocyte has 46 (44 + XY) chromosomes, the diploid number, and a DNA content of 4N. (The letter *N* denotes either the haploid number of chromosomes, 23 in humans, or the amount of DNA in this set.) Soon after their formation, these cells enter the first meiotic prophase that lasts about 3 weeks. Most spermatocytes seen in sections of testis are in this phase of meiosis. The primary spermatocytes are the largest cells of the spermatogenic lineage and are characterized

FIGURE **21–4** Interstitial cells and Sertoli cells.

(a) Seminiferous tubules (**ST**) are surrounded by stroma containing many interstitial cells (**IC**), typically located near capillaries, which secrete androgens. The **seminiferous tubule wall** consists of a unique **germinal epithelium** composed of columnar **Sertoli cells** and dividing **spermatogenic stem cells**. Seen around the seminiferous tubules are myoid cells (**M**) with elongated nuclei, the contractions of which help move fluid and mature sperm in the tubules. (×400; H&E)

(b) A plastic section shows lipid droplets filling the cytoplasm of the clumped interstitial cells (**IC**), or **Leydig cells**, in the connective tissue (**CT**) between tubules. Such cytoplasm is typical of steroid-secreting endocrine cells and here indicates cells actively secreting **testosterone**. The epithelium of a nearby seminiferous tubule is immediately surrounded by myoid cells (**M**). (×400; PT)

(c) Immunohistochemistry of a seminiferous tubule wall with antibodies against prosaposin, a glycoprotein abundant in **Sertoli cells**. The yellow fluorescent stain indicates the tall columnar shape of Sertoli cells (**S**) and the dendritic nature of their apical

ends. Sertoli cells support all spermatogenic cells physically and metabolically, phagocytize debris, and have endocrine roles affecting spermatogenesis and fetal development of the male reproductive tract. (×400; Immunofluorescence)

(d) Immunohistochemistry of the seminiferous tubule with the same antibodies labeled with peroxidase shows the tall **Sertoli cells** in brown. This bright-field preparation also shows the close association of the Sertoli cells with the numerous spermatogenic cells, whose nuclei are stained with hematoxylin. (×400; Immuno-peroxidase & hematoxylin)

(e) Lower magnification of the same preparation as part **c** shows the distribution and density of Sertoli cells (**S**) in the **seminiferous tubules**. (×200; Immunofluorescence)

(Figure 21–4c-e, reproduced with permission from Dr Richard Sharpe and Chris McKinnell, University of Edinburgh, MRC Centre for Reproductive Health, UK.)

FIGURE **21–5** Spermatogenesis and spermiogenesis.

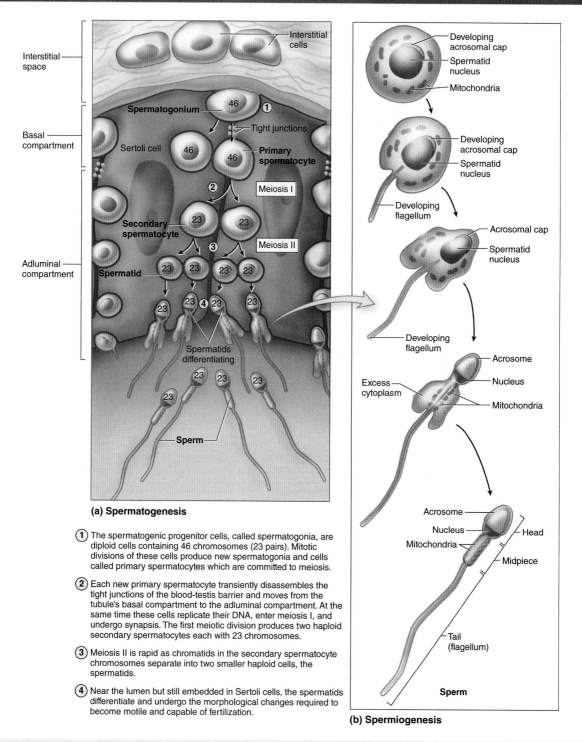

(a) Spermatogenesis

① The spermatogenic progenitor cells, called spermatogonia, are diploid cells containing 46 chromosomes (23 pairs). Mitotic divisions of these cells produce new spermatogonia and cells called primary spermatocytes which are committed to meiosis.

② Each new primary spermatocyte transiently disassembles the tight junctions of the blood-testis barrier and moves from the tubule's basal compartment to the adluminal compartment. At the same time these cells replicate their DNA, enter meiosis I, and undergo synapsis. The first meiotic division produces two haploid secondary spermatocytes each with 23 chromosomes.

③ Meiosis II is rapid as chromatids in the secondary spermatocyte chromosomes separate into two smaller haploid cells, the spermatids.

④ Near the lumen but still embedded in Sertoli cells, the spermatids differentiate and undergo the morphological changes required to become motile and capable of fertilization.

(b) Spermiogenesis

(a) The diagram shows two large, columnar Sertoli cells with their surfaces binding many germ cells in various stages of **spermatogenesis**. Near the basement membrane are **spermatogonia,** which divide by mitosis to produce both more spermatogonia and also **primary spermatocytes** undergoing meiosis to produce secondary spermatocytes and then haploid spermatids differentiating as sperm. Newly formed spermatocytes temporarily disassemble the tight junctions between Sertoli cells comprising the "blood-testis barrier" in order to move from the **basal compartment** to the **adluminal compartment** of the tubule.

(b) Spermiogenesis is the process of cell differentiation by which spermatids become sperm. The major changes that occur during spermiogenesis are shown here. These involve flattening of the nucleus, formation of an **acrosome** resembling a large lysosome, growth of a **flagellum** (tail) from the basal body, reorganization of the mitochondria in the **midpiece** region, and shedding of unneeded cytoplasm.

FIGURE **21–6** Seminiferous tubules: Sertoli cells and spermatogenesis.

(a, b) In these cross sections of **seminiferous tubules**, most of their cell types can be seen. Outside the tubules are myoid cells **(M)** and fibroblasts **(F)**. Inside near the basement membrane are many prominent spermatogonia **(SG)**, small cells that divide mitotically but give rise to a population that enters meiosis. The primary spermatocytes **(PS)** remain for 3 weeks in prophase of the first meiotic division during which recombination occurs. **Primary spermatocytes** are the largest spermatogenic cells and are usually abundant at all levels between the basement membrane and the lumen. Each divides to form two secondary spermatocytes, which are rarely seen because they undergo the second meiotic division almost immediately to form two haploid **spermatids**. Newly formed round, early spermatids **(ES)** differentiate and lose volume in becoming late spermatids **(LS)** and finally highly specialized sperm cells. All stages of **spermatogenesis** and **spermiogenesis** occur with the cells intimately associated with the surfaces of adjacent Sertoli cells **(SC)** that perform several supportive functions. (Both ×750; H&E)

by the presence of partially condensed chromosomes in various stages of synapsis and recombination (Figure 21–6).

Homologous chromosomes separate in the first meiotic division, which produces smaller cells called **secondary spermatocytes** (Figures 21–5a and 21–7) with only 23 chromosomes (22 + X or 22 + Y), but each still consists of two chromatids so the amount of DNA is 2N (see Chapter 3). Secondary spermatocytes are rare in testis sections because they are very short-lived cells that remain in interphase only briefly and quickly undergo the second meiotic division.

Division of each secondary spermatocyte separates the chromatids of each chromosome and produces two haploid cells called **spermatids** each of which contains 23 chromosomes (Figures 21–5a, 21–6, and 21–7). Because no S phase (DNA replication) occurs between the first and second meiotic divisions, the amount of DNA per cell is reduced by half when the chromatids separate and the cells formed are haploid (1N). With fertilization, a haploid ovum and sperm produced by meiosis unite and the normal diploid chromosome number is restored.

FIGURE **21–7** Clonal nature of spermatogenesis.

A subpopulation called **type A spermatogonia** act as **stem cells**, dividing to produce new stem cells and other type A spermatogonia that undergo transit amplification as **progenitor cells**. Mitosis in these cells occurs with incomplete cytokinesis, leaving the cytoplasm of most or all of these cells connected by cytoplasmic bridges. Type A spermatogonia divide mitotically two or three more times, then differentiate as **type B spermatogonia** that undergo a final round of mitosis to form the cells that then enter meiosis and become **primary spermatocytes** (only two are shown), still interconnected. The intercellular bridges persist during the **first and second meiotic divisions**, but they are lost as the haploid **spermatids** differentiate into **sperm** (spermiogenesis) and shed excess cytoplasm as **residual bodies**. The interconnections of the cells allow free cytoplasmic communication among the cells and help coordinate their progress through meiosis and spermiogenesis.

The Clonal Nature of Male Germ Cells

The stem cells produced by mitotic divisions of spermatogonia remain as separate cells. However, all subsequent divisions of the daughter cells, which become transit amplifying progenitor cells, have incomplete cytokinesis after telophase and the cells remain attached to one another by **intercellular bridges** of cytoplasm (Figure 21–7). These allow free cytoplasmic communication among the cells during their remaining mitotic and meiotic divisions. Although some cells degenerate without completing spermatogenesis and some cells may separate, clones of approximately a hundred cells may remain linked through meiosis. The complete significance of this **spermatogenic syncytium** is not clear, but the cytoplasmic bridges allow the haploid cells to be supplied with products of the complete diploid genome, including proteins and RNA encoded by genes on the X or Y chromosome missing in their haploid nuclei. The germ cells finally become separated from one another during differentiation (Figure 21–7).

The cellular events and changes between the final mitoses of spermatogonia and the formation of spermatids take about 2 months. The spermatogenic cells are not randomly distributed in the spermatogenic epithelium. Cells at different stages of development are typically grouped together along the tubule, with the intercellular bridges helping to coordinate their divisions and differentiation.

Spermiogenesis

Spermiogenesis, the final phase of sperm production, is the temperature-sensitive process by which spermatids differentiate into **spermatozoa**, which are highly specialized to deliver male DNA to the ovum. No cell division occurs during this process, and as with spermatogenesis the cells involved remain associated with Sertoli cells.

The haploid spermatids are small (7-8 μm in diameter) cells near the lumen of the seminiferous tubules (Figures 21–5a and 21–6b). Spermiogenesis includes formation of the **acrosome** (Gr. *akron*, extremity + *soma*, body), condensation and elongation of the nucleus, development of the **flagellum** (L, whip), and the loss of much of the cytoplasm. The end result is the mature spermatozoon, which is released from the Sertoli cell surface into the tubule's lumen. Spermiogenesis is commonly divided into four phases:

- In the **Golgi phase** the cytoplasm contains a prominent Golgi apparatus near the nucleus, mitochondria, paired centrioles, and free ribosomes. Small **proacrosomal vesicles** from the Golgi apparatus coalesce as a single membrane-limited **acrosomal cap** close to one end of the nucleus (Figures 21–5b and 21–8). The centrioles migrate to a position farthest from the acrosomal cap and one acts as a basal body, organizing the axoneme of the flagellum which is structurally and functionally similar to that of a cilium (see Chapter 2).

FIGURE 21–8 Differentiating spermatid.

The head of a late **spermatid** during spermiogenesis is completely enclosed by **Sertoli cell** cytoplasm. As shown by TEM, the sperm nucleus (**N**) is half covered by the thin Golgi-derived acrosomal cap (**A**). The flagellum (**F**) can be seen emerging from a basal body near the nucleus on the side opposite the acrosome. A perinuclear bundle of microtubules and actin filaments called the **manchette** (**M**) transports vesicles, mitochondria, and keratins into position as the spermatid elongates. (×7500)

- In the **cap phase**, the acrosomal cap spreads over about half of the condensing nucleus (Figures 21–5b and 21–8). The acrosome is a specialized type of lysosome containing hydrolytic enzymes, mainly hyaluronidase and a trypsin-like protease called **acrosin**. These enzymes are released when a spermatozoon encounters an oocyte and the acrosomal membrane fuses with the sperm's plasma membrane. They dissociate cells of the corona radiata and digest the zona pellucida, both structures that surround the egg (see Chapter 22). This process, the **acrosomal reaction**, is one of the first steps in fertilization.

- In the **acrosome phase**, the **head** of the developing sperm, containing the acrosome and the condensing nucleus, remains embedded in the Sertoli cell while the growing axoneme extends into the lumen of the tubule (Figure 21–6b). Nuclei become more elongated and very highly condensed, with the histones of nucleosomes replaced by small basic peptides called **protamines**. Flagellum growth continues distally in the tail and mitochondria aggregate around it proximally to form a thickened **middle piece** where the ATP for flagellar movements is generated (Figure 21–5).

- In the **maturation phase** of spermiogenesis, unneeded cytoplasm is shed as a **residual body** from each spermatozoon and remaining intercellular bridges are lost. Fully formed, but not yet functional or mobile, sperm (Figure 21–5) are released into the lumen of the seminiferous tubule.

❯❯ MEDICAL APPLICATION

Decreased semen quality, which is frequently idiopathic (arising from unknown causes), is a major cause of **male infertility**. Common features of poor semen quality include **oligospermia** (ejaculate volume >2 mL), sperm cell density less than 10–20 million/mL, abnormal sperm morphology, and flagellar defects that impair sperm motility.

Sertoli Cells

The **Sertoli cells**, named after Enrico Sertoli (1842–1910) who first demonstrated their physiologic significance, are tall "columnar" epithelial cells, which nourish the spermatogenic cells and divide the seminiferous tubules into two (basal and adluminal) compartments (Figure 21–4c to e). All cells of the spermatogenic lineage are closely associated with the extended surfaces of Sertoli cells and depend on them for metabolic and physical support.

Sertoli cells adhere to the basal lamina and their apical ends extend to the lumen, as shown immunohistochemically in Figure 21–4c to e. In routine preparations, the outlines of Sertoli cells surrounding the spermatogenic cells are very poorly defined (Figures 21–6 and 21–8). Each Sertoli cell supports 30–50 developing germ cells. Ultrastructurally Sertoli cells are seen to contain abundant SER, some rough ER, well-developed Golgi complexes, numerous mitochondria, and lysosomes (Figure 21–8). Their nuclei are typically ovoid or triangular, euchromatic, and have a prominent nucleolus, features that allow Sertoli cells to be distinguished from the neighboring germ cells (Figure 21–6).

Important in Sertoli cell function are elaborate tight occluding junctions between their basolateral membranes, which form a **blood-testis barrier** within the seminiferous epithelium (Figure 21–5a). The tightest blood-tissue barrier in mammals, this physical barrier is one part of a system preventing autoimmune attacks against the unique spermatogenic cells, which first appear after the immune system is mature and central self-tolerance is well established.

Spermatogonia lie in a **basal compartment** of the tubule, below the tight junctions and not sealed off from the vascularized interstitial tissue containing lymphocytes and other immune cells. Newly formed primary spermatocytes temporarily disassemble the adhesion molecules of the local occluding junctions and move into the tubule's **adluminal compartment** while still adhering to Sertoli cells (Figure 21–5a). Like the spermatogonia, all spermatocytes and spermatids lie within invaginations of the Sertoli cells surfaces. Adluminal migration occurs without compromising the blood-testis barrier, which is all the more impressive when one remembers that the germ cells remain linked by intercellular bridges. Sertoli cells are also connected and coupled ionically by gap junctions, which may help regulate the transient changes in the occluding junctions and synchronize activities in the spermatogenic cells. As the flagellar tails of the spermatids develop, they appear as tufts extending from the apical ends of the Sertoli cells.

Related to their role in establishing the blood-testis barrier, Sertoli cells have three general functions:

- **Support, protection, and nutrition of the developing spermatogenic cells**: Because spermatocytes, spermatids, and developing sperm are isolated from plasma proteins and nutrients by the blood-testis barrier, they depend on Sertoli cells for production or transport into the lumen of metabolites and nutritive factors such as the iron-transport protein transferrin. Thus, while protecting spermatogenic cells from circulating immune components, Sertoli cells supply many plasma factors needed for cell growth and differentiation.

- **Exocrine and endocrine secretion**: Sertoli cells continuously release into the seminiferous tubules water that carries new sperm out of the testis. Production of nutrients and **androgen-binding protein (ABP)**, which concentrates testosterone to a level required for spermiogenesis, is promoted by follicle-stimulating hormone (FSH). As endocrine cells, they secrete the 39-kDa glycoprotein **inhibin**, which feeds back on the anterior pituitary gland to suppress FSH synthesis and release.

In the fetus, Sertoli cells also secrete a 140-kDa glycoprotein called **müllerian-inhibiting substance (MIS)** that causes regression of the embryonic müllerian (paramesonephric) ducts; in the absence of MIS, these ducts persist and become parts of the female reproductive tract.

- **Phagocytosis**: During spermiogenesis, excess cytoplasm shed as residual bodies is phagocytosed and digested by Sertoli cell lysosomes. No proteins from sperm normally pass back across the blood-testis barrier.

›› MEDICAL APPLICATION

Acute or chronic inflammation of the testis, **orchitis**, frequently involves the ducts connecting this organ to the epididymis. Common forms of orchitis are produced by infective agents and occur secondarily to a **urinary tract infection** or a **sexually transmitted pathogen** such as *Chlamydia* or *Neisseria gonorrhoeae* entering the testis from the epididymis or via the lymphatics.

Acute **epididymitis** is a result of **sexually transmitted infections** such as gonorrhea or *Chlamydia* infection and causes intrascrotal pain and tenderness. Persistent inflammation of the epididymis, such as that associated with **gonorrhea** infections, includes massive invasion by leukocytes into the infected duct, stimulating fibrosis that obstructs the epididymis and is a common cause of **male infertility**.

› INTRATESTICULAR DUCTS

The intratesticular ducts are the **straight tubules** (or tubuli recti), the **rete testis**, and the **efferent ductules** (Figure 21–2), all of which carry spermatozoa and liquid from the seminiferous tubules to the duct of the epididymis (Table 21–1).

The loops of seminiferous tubules join the rete testis by the short straight tubules, which are lined initially only by Sertoli cells (Figure 21–9). These empty into the rete testis, an interconnected network of channels lined with cuboidal epithelium and supported by connective tissue of the mediastinum (Figure 21–9).

The rete testis drains into about 20 efferent ductules lined by an unusual epithelium in which groups of nonciliated cuboidal cells alternate with groups of taller ciliated cells and give the tissue a characteristic scalloped appearance (Figure 21–10). The nonciliated cells absorb some of the fluid secreted by the Sertoli cells of seminiferous tubules. This absorption and the ciliary activity create a fluid flow, which carries sperm passively out of the testis toward the epididymis. A thin layer of circularly oriented smooth muscle cells in the walls of efferent ductules aids the movement of sperm into the duct of the epididymis.

› EXCRETORY GENITAL DUCTS

The excretory genital ducts are those of the **epididymis**, the **ductus (or vas) deferens**, and the **urethra**. They transport sperm from the scrotum to the penis during ejaculation.

TABLE **21–1**	Summary of histology and functions of male genital ducts.			
	Location	Epithelium	Support Tissues	Function(s)
Seminiferous tubules	Testicular lobules	Spermatogenic, with Sertoli cells and germ cells	Myoid cells and loose connective tissue	Produce sperm
Straight tubules (tubuli recti)	Periphery of the mediastinum testis	Sertoli cells in proximal portions, simple cuboidal in distal portions	Connective tissue	Convey sperm into the rete testis
Rete testis	In mediastinum testis	Simple cuboidal cells with microvilli and single cilia	Dense irregular connective tissue	Channels with sperm from all seminiferous tubules
Efferent ductules	From rete testis to head of epididymis	Alternating patches of simple cuboidal nonciliated and simple columnar ciliated	Thin circular layer of smooth muscle and vascular loose connective tissue	Absorb most fluid from seminiferous tubules; convey sperm into the epididymis
Epididymal duct	Head, body, and tail of the epididymis	Pseudostratified columnar, with small basal cells and tall principal cells bearing long stereocilia	Circular smooth muscle initially, with inner and outer longitudinal layers in the tail	Site for sperm maturation and short-term storage; expels sperm at ejaculation
Ductus (vas) deferens	Extends from epididymis to ejaculatory ducts in prostate gland	Pseudostratified columnar, with fewer stereocilia	Fibroelastic lamina propria and three very thick layers of smooth muscle	Carries sperm by rapid peristalsis from the epididymis to the ejaculatory ducts
Ejaculatory ducts	In prostate, formed by union of ductus deferens and ducts of the seminal vesicles	Pseudostratified and simple columnar	Fibroelastic tissue and smooth muscle of the prostate stroma	Mix sperm and seminal fluid; deliver semen to urethra, where prostatic secretion is added

FIGURE **21–9** Seminiferous tubules, straight tubules, and rete testis.

Micrographs here show the transition of a **seminiferous tubule** into a **straight tubule**, and then into the **rete testis**.

(a) The seminiferous tubules (**S**) drain into short, much narrower straight tubules (**T**), which connect to the rete testis (**R**), a network of channels embedded along with blood vessels (**V**) in the connective tissue (**CT**) of the mediastinum testis. (×120; H&E)

(b) At higher magnification the enclosed portion of part **a** shows the transition from wide seminiferous tubule (**S**) to the straight tubule (**T**). Initially, the straight tubule wall has only tall Sertoli cells devoid of germ cells. The wall becomes a simple cuboidal epithelium near its connection to the rete testis (**R**), which is also lined with simple cuboidal epithelium. (×300; H&E)

Epididymis

The long, highly coiled duct of the **epididymis**, surrounded by connective tissue, lies in the scrotum along the superior and posterior sides of each testis (Figure 21–2). Nearly 6 m in length, the epididymis includes a **head** region where the efferent ductules enter, a **body** where sperm cells undergo further subtle modifications, and a **tail** where sperm are stored until ejaculation.

The epididymal duct is lined with pseudostratified columnar epithelium consisting of columnar **principal cells**, with characteristic long **stereocilia** and small round stem cells (Figure 21–11). The principal cells remove most of the water and residual bodies entering the epididymis with the

sperm and secrete various products, greatly changing the fluid in which sperm are suspended. In addition to the secretion of many proteins and glycoproteins by exocytosis, these epithelial cells release abundant 25–300-nm-diameter exosomes and other vesicles from multivesicular bodies and by apocrine secretion. These contain many different proteins, glycoproteins, glycolipids, and lipids, their composition varying along the epididymis. Passage of sperm through the duct of the epididymis normally takes 2–4 weeks, during which time the spermatozoa cell membranes bind and integrate many components secreted by the principal cells and released from their exosomes. Without these modifications, sperm cannot participate in fertilization, but the significance of most factors involved is not well-understood. In general, changes within

FIGURE **21–10** Rete testis and efferent ductules.

(a) Rete testis (**R**) channels have simple cuboidal epithelium and are usually embedded in dense connective tissue. (×350; Mallory trichrome)

(b) The efferent ductules (**E**) draining the **rete testis** have a lining with a characteristic scalloped appearance in section, consisting of patches of simple cuboidal cells with water-absorbing microvilli alternating with patches of taller cells with cilia (**arrows**). (×350; H&E)

spermatozoa while passing through the epididymis include the following:

- Development of competence for forward motility,
- Final modifications within the acrosome, and
- Importantly, reorganization of the cell membrane surrounding the sperm head, including the addition of cholesterol and other "decapacitation factors," which block the acrosomal reaction, a key event in fertilization. The fertilizing ability of spermatozoa is inhibited until their cell membranes are modified again as part of the **capacitation** process, which occurs in the female reproductive tract.

The epididymal duct is surrounded by a thin, circular layer of smooth muscle cells, supplemented in the tail region with the addition of inner and outer longitudinal layers. At ejaculation, peristaltic contractions of these muscle layers rapidly empty stored sperm from this tail region, which is continuous with the ductus deferens.

Ductus or Vas Deferens

Each **ductus** (or **vas**) **deferens**, a long straight tube with a thick, muscular wall and a relatively small lumen, leaves the scrotum and continues toward the prostatic urethra where it empties (Figure 21–1). As shown in Figure 21–12, its mucosa is slightly folded longitudinally, the lamina propria contains many elastic fibers, and the epithelial lining is pseudostratified with some cells having sparse stereocilia. The very thick muscularis consists of longitudinal inner and outer layers and a middle circular layer. The muscles produce strong peristaltic contractions during ejaculation, which rapidly move sperm along this duct from the epididymis.

The ductus (vas) deferens forms part of the spermatic cord, which also includes the testicular artery, the pampiniform plexus, and nerves (Figure 21–2). Following the general path along which the embryonic testes descend, each ductus passes over the urinary bladder where it enlarges as an **ampulla** (L. a small bottle) where the epithelium is thicker and more extensively folded (Figure 21–13). Within the prostate gland, the ends of the two ampullae merge with the ducts of the two seminal vesicles, joining these ducts to form the **ejaculatory ducts** which open into the **prostatic urethra**.

Table 21–1 summarizes the locations, histological features, and main functions of the intratesticular and excretory genital ducts.

›› MEDICAL APPLICATION

The accessibility of the ductus (vas) deferens in the spermatic cords allows for the most common surgical method of male contraception: **vasectomy**. In this procedure, a very small incision is made through the scrotal skin near the two ducts and each vas is exposed, cut, and the two ends (or only the end leading to the abdomen) are cauterized and tied.

After vasectomy sperm are still produced, they degenerate and are removed by macrophages in the epididymis (and in the scrotal sac if the short portion of the vas is left open-ended). Inflammatory and other changes occur in the mucosa of the epididymis, but serious adverse effects of vasectomy are usually minimal. A vasectomy may be reversed by surgically reconnecting the two ends of each ductus deferens. However, even successful surgery very often fails to restore fertility, due to incomplete sperm maturation in the epididymis changed by postvasectomy inflammation.

› ACCESSORY GLANDS

The accessory glands of the male reproductive tract produce secretions, which become mixed with sperm during ejaculation to produce semen and are essential for reproduction.

FIGURE **21–11** Epididymis.

(a) The long, coiled duct of the epididymis (**DE**), where sperm undergo maturation and short-term storage, is enclosed by connective tissue with many blood vessels (**V**) and covered by a capsule and the tunica vaginalis (**TV**). The duct is lined by a **pseudostratified columnar epithelium** with long **stereocilia** (**arrows**). (×140; H&E)

(b) The columnar epithelium of the **epididymal duct** is surrounded by a thin circular layer of smooth muscle (**SM**) cells

and its lumen contains sperm (**S**). The **smooth muscle** becomes thicker and a longitudinal layer develops in the body and tail of the epididymis. (×400; H&E)

(c) The inset photo shows the epithelium with tall principal cells (**P**) with **stereocilia** and fewer small basal stem cells (**B**). Intraepithelial lymphocytes are also commonly seen in the epididymal duct. (×500; H&E)

The accessory genital glands are the **seminal vesicles** (or glands), the **prostate gland**, and the **bulbourethral glands** (Figure 21–13).

Seminal Vesicles

The two **seminal vesicles** consist of highly tortuous tubes, each about 15-cm long, enclosed by a connective tissue capsule. The unusual mucosa of the tube displays a great number of thin, complex folds, which fill much of the lumen (Figure 21–14). The folds are lined with simple or pseudostratified columnar epithelial cells rich in secretory granules. The lamina propria contains elastic fibers and is surrounded by

smooth muscle with inner circular and outer longitudinal layers, which empty the gland into the ejaculatory ducts during ejaculation. Dependent on testosterone, the seminal vesicles produce a viscid, yellowish secretion. Fluid from seminal vesicles typically makes up about 70% of the ejaculate and its components include the following:

- **Fructose**, a major energy source for sperm, as well as inositol, citrate, and other metabolites,
- **Prostaglandins**, which stimulate activity in the female reproductive tract, and
- **Fibrinogen**, which allows semen to coagulate after ejaculation.

FIGURE **21–12** Ductus deferens.

(a) A cross section of the **vas deferens** shows the mucosa (**M**), a thick muscularis with inner and outer layers of longitudinal smooth muscle (**L-SM**) and an intervening layer of circular smooth muscle (**C-SM**), and an external adventitia (**A**). The **muscularis** is specialized for powerful peristaltic movement of sperm at ejaculation. (×60; H&E)

(b) The lamina propria (**LP**) is rich in elastic fibers and the thick epithelial lining (**E**) shows longitudinal folds (×150; Mallory trichrome).

(c) Higher magnification of the mucosa shows that the epithelium is pseudostratified with basal cells and many columnar cells, some with stereocilia. (×400; H&E)

Prostate Gland

The **prostate gland** is a dense, somewhat conical organ just below the bladder surrounding the urethra and distal ends of the ejaculatory ducts. With a normal adult weight of approximately 20 g, the prostate consists of 30–50 tubuloacinar glands embedded in a dense fibromuscular stroma in which smooth muscle contracts at ejaculation (Figure 21–13b). Ducts from individual glands may converge but all empty into the prostatic urethra, which runs through the center of the prostate. As shown in Figure 21–15, the normal prostate gland is often divided most simply into three major zones surrounding the urethra:

- The **peripheral zone**, with about 70% of the organ's tissue, contains the prostate's **main glands** with the longest ducts into the prostatic urethra (Figure 21–16).
- The **central zone** comprises 25% of the gland's tissue and contains the periurethral **submucosal glands** with somewhat shorter ducts.
- The **transition zone** occupies about 5% of the prostate volume, contains the periurethral **mucosal glands**, and like the central zone surrounds only the superior portion of the urethra.

The tubuloacinar glands of the prostate are lined by simple or pseudostratified columnar epithelium and produce a fluid

FIGURE 21–13 Accessory glands of the male reproductive tract.

(a) Posterior view

(b) Seminal vesicle

(c) Prostate gland

(d) Bulbourethral gland

(a) Three sets of glands connect to the ductus deferens or urethra: the paired **seminal vesicles**, the **prostate**, and the paired **bulbourethral glands**. The first two types of glands contribute the major volume to semen and the latter produces a secretion that lubricates the urethra before ejaculation.

(b) **Seminal vesicles** have a large number of characteristically thin mucosal folds (**F**) with a large surface area.

(c) The **prostate gland** has many individual tubuloacinar glands (**G**), some containing concretions called corpora amylacea (**CA**).

(d) The small, paired **bulbourethral glands** consist mainly of mucous acini (**M**). (b,c,d: ×80; H&E)

that contains a complex mixture of exosomes, various glycoproteins, enzymes, and small molecules, such as prostaglandins, and is stored until ejaculation. One clinically important product of the prostate is prostate-specific antigen (PSA), a 34-kDa serine protease, which helps liquefy coagulated semen for the slow release of sperm after ejaculation. Small amounts of PSA also leak normally into the prostatic vasculature; elevated levels of circulating PSA indicate abnormal glandular mucosa typically due to prostatic carcinoma or inflammation.

Small spherical concretions, up to 2 mm in diameter and often partially calcified, are normally present in the lumens of many prostatic tubuloacinar glands (Figure 21–16).

FIGURE **21–14** Seminal vesicles.

a b c

The **seminal vesicles** are paired exocrine glands, which secrete most **seminal fluid**, including sperm nutrients.

(a) A low-power micrograph shows that each consists of a coiled duct with a mucosa organized with many thin folds (**arrows**) in

the lumen (**L**) and surrounded by two layers of smooth muscle (**SM**). (×20; H&E)

(b, c) The mucosal folds include smooth muscle (**SM**), a thin lamina propria (**LP**), and a simple columnar epithelium of principal secretory cells. (Both: ×300. b: H&E; c: PSH)

FIGURE **21–15** Organization of the prostate gland.

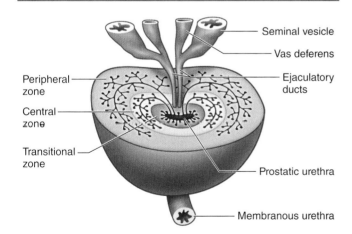

The **prostate** consists of 30–50 **branched tubuloacinar glands** organized into **three zones**, shown here schematically at a level just above the junction of the ejaculatory ducts with the urethra. Around the prostatic urethra is the **transition zone** containing mucosal glands. Surrounding most of that zone is the intermediate **central zone**, which contains the submucosal glands. The outermost and largest layer is the **peripheral zone**, which contains the most numerous main glands.

These concretions, called **corpora amylacea**, containing primarily deposited glycoproteins and keratan sulfate, may become more numerous with age but seem to have no physiologic or clinical significance. The prostate is surrounded by a fibroelastic capsule, from which septa extend and divide the gland into indistinct lobes. Like the seminal vesicles, the prostate's structure and function depend on the level of testosterone.

▶▶ MEDICAL APPLICATION

The prostate gland is prone to three common problems: (1) **chronic prostatitis**, usually involving bacteria or other infectious agents; (2) **nodular hyperplasia** or **benign prostatic hypertrophy**, occurring mainly in the periurethral mucosal glands where it often leads to compression of the urethra and problems with urination; and (3) **prostate cancer** (adenocarcinoma), the most common cancer in nonsmoking men, occurring mainly in glands of the peripheral zone.

Bulbourethral Glands

The paired round **bulbourethral glands** (or Cowper glands), 3-5 mm in diameter, are located in the urogenital diaphragm (Figure 21–13) and empty into the proximal part of the penile urethra. Each gland has several lobules with tubuloacinar secretory units surrounded by smooth muscle cells and lined

FIGURE **21–16** Prostate gland.

(a) The **prostate** has a dense fibromuscular stroma (**S**) in which are embedded a large number of small tubuloacinar glands (**G**). (×20; H&E)

(b) A micrograph of **one prostatic gland**, showing a corpus amylaceum (**CA**) concretion and the secretory epithelium (**E**)

surrounded by a thin lamina propria (**LP**) and thick smooth muscle (**M**). (×122; H&E)

(c) Higher magnification shows the lamellar nature of a corpus amylaceum (**CA**) and the pseudostratified columnar epithelium underlain by lamina propria (**LP**). (×300; Mallory trichrome)

by a mucus-secreting simple columnar epithelium that is also testosterone-dependent (Figure 21–13d). During erection, the bulbourethral glands, as well as numerous, very small, and histologically similar urethral glands along the penile urethra, release a clear mucus-like secretion, which coats and lubricates the urethra in preparation for the imminent passage of sperm.

❱ PENIS

The penis consists of three cylindrical masses of erectile tissue, plus the penile urethra, surrounded by skin (Figure 21–1). Two of the erectile masses—the **corpora cavernosa**—are dorsal; the ventral **corpus spongiosum** surrounds the urethra (Figure 21–17). At its end the corpus spongiosum expands, forming the **glans** (Figure 21–13a). Most of the penile urethra is lined with pseudostratified columnar epithelium. In the glans, it becomes stratified squamous epithelium continuous with that of the thin epidermis covering the glans surface. Small mucus-secreting **urethral glands** are found along the length of the penile urethra. In uncircumcised men, the glans is covered by the **prepuce** or foreskin, a retractable fold of thin skin with sebaceous glands on the internal surface.

The corpora cavernosa are each surrounded by a dense fibroelastic layer, the **tunica albuginea** (Figures 21–17 and 21–18). All three erectile tissues consist of many venous

cavernous spaces lined with endothelium and separated by trabeculae with smooth muscle and connective tissue continuous with the surrounding tunic (Figure 21–19).

Central arteries in the corpora cavernosa branch to form nutritive arterioles and small coiling **helicine arteries**, which

FIGURE **21–17** Structure of the penis.

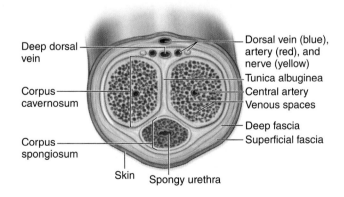

A diagram of the **penis** in transverse section shows the relationships of the three **erectile bodies**, the **tunica albuginea**, and **major blood vessels**. Compare this section to the longitudinal diagram in Figure 21–13.

FIGURE 21–18 Penis.

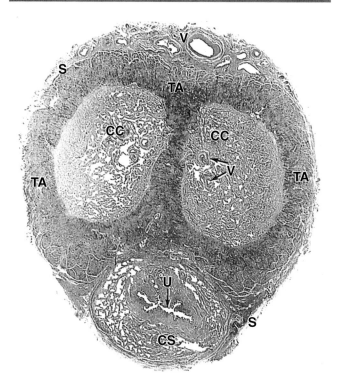

The corpus spongiosum (**CS**) is on the ventral side of the **penis** and surrounds the urethra (**U**). Two corpora cavernosa (**CC**) occupy most of the dorsal side and are surrounded by dense, fibrous tunica albuginea (**TA**). Along the dorsal side run the major blood vessels (**V**) and deep in each corporal mass of erectile tissue are smaller blood vessels (**V**), including the **central arteries**. The penis is covered loosely by skin (**S**), which distally forms the large **foreskin** fold and becomes thin over the **glans**. (×15; H&E)

lead to the cavernous vascular spaces of erectile tissue. Arteriovenous shunts are present between the central arteries and the dorsal veins.

Penile **erection** involves blood filling the cavernous spaces in the three masses of erectile tissue. Triggered by external stimuli to the CNS, erection is controlled by autonomic nerves in these vascular walls. Parasympathetic stimulation relaxes the trabecular smooth muscle and dilates the helicine arteries, allowing increased blood flow and filling the cavernous spaces. This enlarges the corpora cavernosa and causes them to compress the dorsal veins against the dense tunica albuginea, which blocks the venous outflow and produces tumescence and rigidity in the erectile tissue. Beginning at ejaculation, sympathetic stimulation constricts the helicine arteries and trabecular muscle, decreasing blood flow into the spaces, lowering the pressure there, and allowing the veins to drain most blood from the erectile tissue.

❯❯ MEDICAL APPLICATION

At the beginning of an erection, acetylcholine from parasympathetic nerves in the penis causes the vascular endothelial cells of the helicine arteries and cavernous tissue to release nitric oxide (NO). Diffusing into the adjacent smooth muscle cells, NO activates guanylate cyclase to produce cyclic GMP, which causes these cells to relax, resulting in increased blood flow, filling of the cavernous spaces, and penile erection.

Erectile dysfunction, or **impotence**, can result from diabetes, anxiety, vascular disease, or nerve damage during prostatectomy. The drug **sildenafil** may alleviate the problem by inhibiting the phosphodiesterase degrading cyclic GMP in the smooth muscle cells of helicine arteries and erectile tissue. The subsequent higher level of cGMP promotes relaxation of these cells and enhances the neural effect to produce or maintain an erection.

The male reproductive System SUMMARY OF KEY POINTS

Testes

- In each **testis** approximately each of 250 **lobules** contains one or more very long, convoluted **seminiferous tubules** in a sparse, vascular stroma containing testosterone-producing **interstitial cells (of Leydig)**.
- **Seminiferous tubules** consist of spermatogenic epithelium containing columnar **Sertoli cells**, each of which supports and nourishes many germ cells embedded at its surface.
- **Tight junctions** between Sertoli cells establish two compartments within seminiferous tubules: a **basal compartment** with spermatogonia and an **adluminal compartment** with spermatocytes and spermatids.
- **Sertoli cells** also produce **androgen-binding protein**, which concentrates testosterone, **phagocytose** shed debris from differentiating spermatids, and **secrete fluid**, which carries sperm along the tubules.

- Progenitor cells called **spermatogonia** undergo mitosis and give rise to **primary spermatocytes**, which undergo a first meiotic division to form haploid **secondary spermatocytes**.
- After a very short interval, **secondary spermatocytes** undergo the second meiotic division to produce small, round **spermatids**, which differentiate while still associated with Sertoli cells.
- A spermatid undergoes **spermiogenesis** by greatly condensing its **nucleus**, forming a long **flagellum** with a surrounding mitochondrial **middle piece**, and forming a perinuclear **acrosomal cap**.
- From the seminiferous tubules, sperm enter the short **straight tubules**, which lead to channels of the **rete testis** in the mediastinum testis, then move via 15 or 20 **efferent ductules** where some fluid is absorbed.

(a) The corpus spongiosum (**CS**) surrounds the longitudinally folded wall of the penile urethra (**PU**). Small urethral glands (**UG**) with short ducts to the urethra release mucus during erection, supplementing the similar secretion from the bulbourethral glands. The two dorsal corpora cavernosa (**CC**) are ensheathed by dense, fibrous tunica albuginea (**TA**) and in one here a small helicine artery (**HA**) is shown. (×100; H&E)

(b) A higher magnification of erectile tissue is shown with a small portion of tunica albuginea (**TA**) and fibrous, elastic connective tissue containing smooth muscle (**SM**) and many small, cavernous spaces (**CS**) lined by vascular endothelium. Very little blood normally passes through this vasculature due to constriction of the helicine arteries (**HA**) serving them. During erection the vascular smooth muscle relaxes, allowing rapid blood flow into the cavernous spaces, filling them and causing compression of their venous drainage, which makes the masses of erectile tissue much larger and turgid. (×200; H&E)

Excretory Genital Ducts

- From efferent ductules sperm move into and through **epididymal ducts** in the head, body, and tail of **epididymis**, also located in the scrotum, for their final maturation and short storage prior to ejaculation.
- The **epididymis** is lined by **pseudostratified columnar epithelium** containing **principal cells**, which have long **stereocilia**; along its length the number of surrounding **smooth muscle** layers increases.
- At ejaculation, the body and tail of the **epididymis** are emptied into the **ductus (vas) deferens**, also lined by **pseudostratified columnar epithelium** with three thick layers of **smooth muscle** for peristalsis.

Accessory Glands

- Most semen is produced by the paired **seminal vesicles** (glands), characterized by numerous thin folds of secretory mucosa; a duct from each seminal vesicle joins a ductus deferens as an **ejaculatory duct**.
- Inside the medial **prostate gland**, the two **ejaculatory ducts** and dozens of ducts from **tubuloacinar prostatic glands** merge with the **urethra** that transports semen through the penis.

- **Semen** components from the seminal vesicles nourish sperm (eg, **fructose**), activate ciliary and muscle activity in the female reproductive tract (**prostaglandins**), and gradually decrease semen viscosity for better sperm movement.

Penis

- The **penis** contains two dorsal **corpora cavernosa** and a periurethral **corpus spongiosum**, all composed of vascular **cavernous tissue** and small amounts of surrounding **smooth muscle** and **helicine arteries**.
- For erection **parasympathetic** stimulation relaxes muscle of the small **helicine arteries** and adjacent tissues, allowing vessels of the **cavernous tissue** to fill with blood; the enlarging corpora compress the venous drainage, producing further enlargement and turgidity in the three corpora masses.
- The **sympathetic** stimulation at ejaculation constricts blood flow through the **helicine** arteries, allowing blood to empty from the cavernous tissues.

The male reproductive System ASSESS YOUR KNOWLEDGE

1. Which of the following accurately describes spermiogenesis?
   a. Occurs before puberty
   b. Involves stem cells, meiosis, and spermatogenesis
   c. Involves cytodifferentiation of early spermatids
   d. Occurs in diploid cells
   e. Results in the formation of primary spermatocytes

2. A man with a pituitary gonadotrophic tumor causing hyposecretion of FSH is most likely to exhibit which condition?
   a. No symptoms, since he has no ovarian follicles
   b. Loss of libido (sex drive)
   c. Low serum testosterone levels
   d. Low sperm count
   e. Prostatic hypertrophy

3. Interstitial cells of Leydig have an important function in male gamete production. Because of this function, which of the following organelles is abundant within these cells?
   a. Lysosomes
   b. Smooth endoplasmic reticulum
   c. Peroxisomes
   d. Polyribosomes
   e. Golgi complexes

4. While studying a germ cell line developed from a patient's testicular biopsy, the researcher notes that colchicine-treated cells blocked in metaphase have 46 chromosomes. From which of the following regions of the male genital tract would you expect these cells to have originated?
   a. Within the rete testis
   b. At the basal lamina of the seminiferous tubule
   c. In the middle region of the germinal epithelium
   d. Within the adluminal compartment of the seminiferous tubule
   e. Within the straight tubules

5. Which of the following organs is normally characterized by the accumulation of corpora amylacea with increasing age?
   a. Prostate
   b. Seminal vesicles
   c. Bulbourethral (Cowper) glands
   d. Epididymis
   e. Ductus (vas) deferens

6. Within the male reproductive tract, stereocilia project from cells lining which of the following regions?
   a. Rete testis
   b. Seminiferous tubules
   c. Ampulla of the ductus deferens
   d. Epididymis
   e. Penile urethra

7. As sperm pass through the male genital ducts, proteins and low-molecular-weight products are added from several sources producing semen. Which of the following provides a nutritive, fructose-rich secretion?
   a. Interstitial cells of Leydig
   b. Bulbourethral (Cowper) glands
   c. Prostate gland
   d. Epididymis
   e. Seminal vesicles

8. A 20-year-old man contracts cholera during a long tour of military duty in a remote, completely undeveloped region. After a 5-day period of severe diarrhea and treatment, he gradually recovers and slowly returns to work. He is married 3 years later but after a few years of trying to conceive a child, semen analysis reveals that his sperm are few in number and malformed, and blood tests show a high titer of antibodies against sperm antigens. The causative agent of cholera, *Vibrio cholera*, secretes a toxin that interferes with tight (occluding) junctions. What cells in the gonad are the likely target of this toxin in the male reproductive system?
   a. Spermatogonia
   b. Sertoli cells
   c. Myoid cells
   d. Interstitial cells of Leydig
   e. Differentiating spermatozoa

9. A 29-year-old man presents with testicular pain and a burning sensation during urination. Tests reveal the presence of *Neisseria gonorrhea*, and penicillin is prescribed. Gonorrhea often produces acute or chronic inflammation of the testes and frequently involves the channels that connect the testis to the epididymis. What is the name of these channels?
   a. The mediastinum testis
   b. The rete testis
   c. Efferent ductules
   d. The straight tubules (tubuli recti)
   e. The seminiferous tubules

10. A 39-year-old man undergoing an extensive series of tests for infertility is found to have a genetic mutation preventing formation of a functional synaptonemal complex during meiosis, causing almost complete failure of sperm formation. Which cells would be directly affected by this mutation?
    a. Primary spermatocytes
    b. Spermatogonia
    c. Secondary spermatocytes
    d. Spermatids
    e. Cells undergoing spermiogenesis

Answers: 1c, 2d, 3b, 4b, 5a, 6d, 7e, 8b, 9c, 10a

22 The Female Reproductive System

The female reproductive system consists of the paired ovaries and uterine tubes (or oviducts/fallopian tubes), the uterus, the vagina, and the external genitalia (Figure 22–1). This system produces the female gametes (**oocytes**), provides the environment for fertilization, and holds the embryo during its complete development through the fetal stage until birth. As with male gonads, the ovaries produce steroidal sex hormones that control development and function of the reproductive organs and influence other tissues. Beginning at **menarche**, when the first menses occurs, the reproductive system undergoes monthly changes in structure and function, under the control of neurohormonal mechanisms. **Menopause** represents a variably timed period during which the cyclic changes become irregular and eventually disappear. In the postmenopausal period the reproductive organs slowly involute. Although the mammary glands do not belong to the genital system, they are included here because they undergo changes directly connected to the functional state of the reproductive organs.

› OVARIES

Ovaries are almond-shaped bodies approximately 3-cm long, 1.5-cm wide, and 1-cm thick. Each ovary is covered by a simple cuboidal epithelium, the **surface** (or germinal) epithelium, continuous with the mesothelium and overlying a capsule of dense connective tissue, the **tunica albuginea**, like that of the testis. Most of the ovary consists of the **cortex**, a region of highly cellular connective tissue stroma containing many **ovarian follicles** that vary greatly in size after menarche (Figure 22–1). The most internal part of the ovary, the **medulla**, encompasses loose connective tissue and blood vessels entering the organ through the hilum from the mesenteries suspending the ovary (Figures 22–1 and 22–2). No distinct border delineates the ovarian cortex and medulla.

Early Development of the Ovary

In the first month of embryonic life, a population of gamete stem cells, referred to as "primordial germ cells" or gonocytes, migrates from the yolk sac to the two developing gonads. As the ovaries develop in chromosomal females, gonocytes there differentiate as progenitor cells called **oogonia**. These proliferate to produce ~600,000 oogonia, each associated with somatic support cells, by the end of the second gestational month. After this point the number of oogonia depends on three ongoing activities: continued mitosis, the onset of meiosis, and an apoptotic process in the female gametes called **atresia**. The number of gametes in the ovaries peaks at ~7 million around the fifth month of gestation, by which time mitotic division has ceased

FIGURE 22–1 The female reproductive system and overview of ovary.

(a) Posterior view

(b) Lateral sectional view

(c)

(a) The diagram shows the internal organs of the **female reproductive system**, which includes as the principal organs: the **ovaries, uterine tubes, uterus,** and **vagina.**

(b) A lateral sectional view of an **ovary** shows the ovary and the relationship of its main supporting mesenteries, the mesovarium, and the mesosalpinx of the broad ligament.

(c) A sectioned **ovary**, indicating the **medulla** and **cortex**, with follicles of several different sizes in the cortex. (×15; H&E)

and the oogonia have entered prophase of the first meiotic division (see Chapter 3). Most of these cells undergo apoptotic cell death, but others complete synapsis, genetic recombination, and arrest in meiotic prophase I. These cells are now **primary oocytes** (Gr. *oon*, egg + *kytos*, cell) and each is surrounded by flattened, supportive **follicular cells** in a nongrowing primordial follicle, the total number of which constitutes the "ovarian reserve." About 2–2.5 million such follicles are present at birth and ~400,000 remain at puberty, the others having been lost through atresia. Because generally only one oocyte completes meiosis and ovulation during each 28-day menstrual cycle and the reproductive life of a woman averages about 30–35 years, only about 450 oocytes are typically liberated from the ovaries in a lifetime. All others undergo atresia, which itself ceases with menopause.

Ovarian Follicles

An **ovarian follicle** consists of one oocyte surrounded by one or more layers of epithelial cells within a basal lamina. Follicles that develop during fetal life—**primordial follicles**—do so without gonadotrophin input, form mainly in the superficial ovarian cortex, and consist of primary oocytes each enveloped by a single layer of squamous follicular cells form mainly in the superficial ovarian cortex (Figures 22–2b, 22–3, and 22–4). The oocyte in the primordial follicle is large and spherical, about 25–30 μm in diameter, with a proportionately

FIGURE 22–2 Follicle development and changes within the ovary.

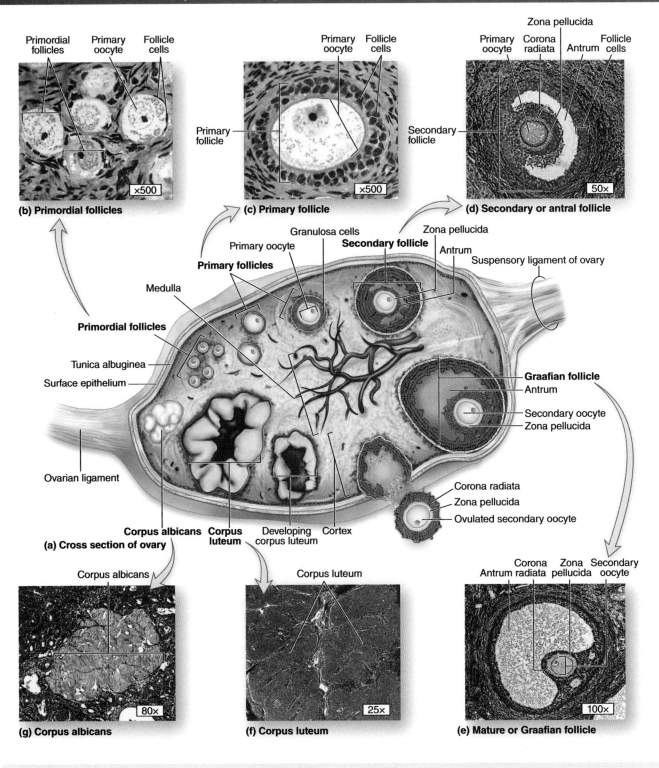

(b) Primordial follicles

(c) Primary follicle

(d) Secondary or antral follicle

(a) Cross section of ovary

(g) Corpus albicans

(f) Corpus luteum

(e) Mature or Graafian follicle

The **ovary** produces both **oocytes** and **sex hormones**. A diagram of a sectioned **ovary (a)** shows the **different stages of follicle maturation**, **ovulation**, and **corpus luteum formation and degeneration**. All of the stages and structures shown in this diagram actually would appear at different times during the ovarian cycle and do not occur simultaneously. Follicles are arranged here for easy comparisons. The **primordial follicles** shown are greatly enlarged.

The histologic sections identify **primordial follicles (b)**, a **primary follicle (c)**, a secondary or **antral follicle (d)**, and a mature **vesicular follicle (e)**. After ovulation, the portion of the follicle left behind forms the **corpus luteum (f)**, which then degenerates into the **corpus albicans (g)**. (All H&E)

FIGURE **22–3** Stages of ovarian follicles, from primordial to mature.

Primordial follicle
— Oocyte
— Stromal cells
— Follicular cell

Unilaminar primary follicle
— Basal lamina
— Zona pellucida forming

Multilaminar primary follicle
— Zona pellucida
— Granulosa cells
— Theca interna

Secondary or antral follicle
— Antrum
— Theca interna
— Theca externa
— Granulosa cells

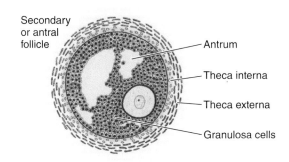

Mature or Graafian follicle
— Theca externa
— Theca interna
— Antrum
— Granulosa cells
— Corona radiata
— Cumulus oophorus

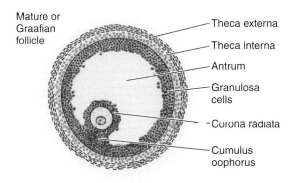

Diagrams of sectioned **ovarian follicles** show the changing size and morphology of **follicular/granulosa cells** at each stage and the disposition of the surrounding thecal cells. However, the series of drawings does not maintain the relative proportions of the follicles: mature follicles are much larger relative to the early follicles. Through all these stages the follicle harbors a single large, growing **primary oocyte** with a large nucleus and prominent nucleolus. Follicular or granulosa cells around the oocyte nourish that cell's rapid growth.

FIGURE **22–4** Primordial follicles.

The surface epithelium (**SE**), a mesothelium with usually cuboidal cells, covers the cortex of the ovary and is sometimes called the germinal epithelium. Underlying the epithelium is a connective tissue layer, the tunica albuginea (**TA**). Groups of **primordial follicles**, each formed by an oocyte (**O**) surrounded by a layer of flat epithelial follicular cells (**arrows**), are present in the ovarian connective tissue (stroma). (×200; H&E)

sized nucleus containing chromosomes in the first meiotic prophase. The organelles tend to concentrate near the nucleus and include numerous mitochondria, extensive RER, and several Golgi complexes. The basal lamina surrounding the follicular cells marks a clear boundary between the follicle and the vascularized stroma and acts as a blood-follicle barrier.

Follicular Growth & Development

Beginning in puberty with the release of follicle-stimulating hormone (FSH) from the pituitary, several primordial follicles each month begin to grow and develop further. This involves more enlargement of the oocyte, mitoses and thickening of the follicular cells, as well as proliferation and differentiation of the stromal fibroblasts immediately around each follicle. Selection of the primordial follicles recruited to begin growth early in each monthly cycle and choice of the dominant follicle destined to ovulate that month both involve complex hormonal balances and subtle differences among follicles in FSH receptor numbers, aromatase activity, estrogen synthesis, and other variables.

Prompted by FSH, an oocyte grows rapidly during the first part of follicular development, reaching a diameter of about 120 μm. Oocyte differentiation includes the following:

■ Great growth of the cell and its nucleus;
■ Mitochondria becoming more numerous and uniformly distributed;
■ RER becoming much more extensive and Golgi complexes enlarging and moving peripherally; and

FIGURE **22–5** Primary follicles: unilaminar and multilaminar.

(a) A micrograph of **ovarian cortex** shows several primordial follicles (**PF**) and their flattened **follicle cells** (**arrows**), and two unilaminar primary follicles (**UF**) in which the follicle cells (**F**) form a single cuboidal layer around the large primary oocyte (**O**). (×200; PT)

(b) This micrograph taken at the same magnification shows a larger multilayered **primary follicle**. Follicle cells are now active granulosa cells (**G**) and have proliferated to form several layers. Between them and the oocyte (**O**) is the 5- to 10-μm-thick zona pellucida (**ZP**), a glycoprotein layer produced by the oocyte that is required for sperm binding and fertilization. The **primary oocyte** is now a very large cell. With this stain, the basement membrane (**BM**) separating the follicle from the surrounding stroma can also be seen. (×200; PSH)

■ Formation of small secretory granules called **cortical granules** containing various proteases. These become densely distributed just inside the oocyte's plasma membrane and undergo exocytosis during fertilization.

Follicular cells divide and enlarge, making a simple cuboidal epithelium around the growing oocyte in the expanding **unilaminar primary follicle** (Figures 22–3 and 22–5a). Follicular proliferation continues, creating a stratified epithelium, the **granulosa**, in which abundant gap junctions allow cellular coordination and transfer of materials. The follicular cells are now termed **granulosa cells**, in a still avascular **multilaminar primary follicle** surrounded by a basement membrane (Figures 22–3 and 22–5b).

Between the rapidly growing oocyte and the first layer of granulosa cells of the growing primary follicle, proteins secreted from both cell types assemble into a layer of extracellular matrix 5–10 μm thick known as the **zona pellucida** (Figures 22–5b and 22–6). Zona pellucida glycoproteins ZP1, ZP2, and ZP3, all synthesized in the oocyte, represent components of sperm-binding receptors that attach specific proteins on capacitated sperm and begin acrosomal activation, allowing sperm to progress through this ECM. Maintaining contact through the zona pellucida, gap junctions between abundant processes of the granulosa cells and the oocyte allow rapid transfer of small molecules from the former into the latter.

FIGURE 22–6 Ultrastructure of primary follicle and zona pellucida.

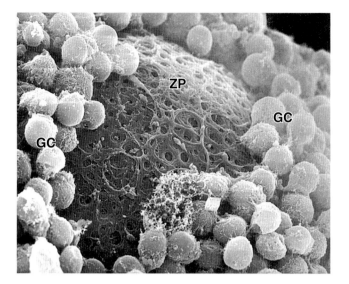

An SEM of a fractured **primary follicle** shows the **oocyte** surrounded by granulosa cells (**GC**) of the **corona radiata**. Between the very large oocyte surface and the granulosa cells is a layer of extracellular material, the zona pellucida (**ZP**), which contains four related glycoproteins that bind sperm and form an irregular meshwork. (×3000)

❯❯ MEDICAL APPLICATION

Growing primary follicles can become involved in **polycystic ovary syndrome (PCOS)** that is characterized by enlarged ovaries with numerous cysts and an anovulatory state (with no follicles completing maturation successfully). The clinical presentation of this disorder is variable, and the etiology is unclear, although increased androgen production by the ovaries or adrenals is likely involved. PCOS is a common cause of **infertility** in women.

Stromal cells immediately outside each growing primary follicle differentiate to form the vascularized **follicular theca** (Gr. *theca*, outer covering), which subsequently develops further as two distinct tissues around the follicle (Figures 22–3, 22–7, and 22–8).

- A well-vascularized endocrine tissue, the **theca interna**, consists of fibroblasts, capillaries, and typical steroid-producing cells which in response to luteinizing hormone (LH) secrete androstenedione. This steroid diffuses into the follicle through the basement membrane to the granulosa cells, where the enzyme aromatase converts it to estradiol, an FSH-dependent activity. This estrogen disperses back into the thecae, enters capillaries, and is distributed throughout the body, inducing changes that characterize puberty and the monthly reproductive cycle. Estrogen concentrations required to drive such

systemic changes are achieved as many follicles develop into functional multilaminar follicles concurrently.

- A more fibrous **theca externa** with fibroblasts, capillaries, and smooth muscle merges gradually with the surrounding stroma.

As the primary follicles grow, they move deeper in the ovarian cortex. Within such follicles, small spaces gradually appear among the granulosa layers as the cells secrete **follicular fluid** (or **liquor folliculi**). This fluid accumulates, the spaces enlarge and gradually coalesce, and the granulosa cells reorganize themselves around a larger cavity called the **antrum** (Figures 22–3 and 22–7a), producing follicles now called **secondary** or **antral follicles**. Follicular fluid contains the large GAG hyaluronic acid, growth factors, plasminogen, fibrinogen, the anticoagulant heparan sulfate proteoglycan, and high concentrations of steroids (progesterone, androstenedione, and estrogens) with binding proteins.

As the antral follicle develops, the oocyte and granulosa cells immediately around it form a small hillock, the **cumulus oophorus** (L. *cumulus*, heap + Gr. *oo*, egg + *phorus*, carrying) protruding into the largest antrum (Figures 22–3 and 22–7b). The granulosa cells tightly adhering to the oocyte through the zona pellucida comprise the **corona radiata** and accompany the oocyte when it leaves the ovary at ovulation.

Each month typically only one antral follicle that began developing 2 or 3 months earlier becomes a **mature** or **Graafian follicle** (named after the 17th-century reproductive biologist Regnier De Graaf) with a single large antrum that rapidly accumulates more follicular fluid and expands to a diameter of 2 cm. A mature follicle can create a bulge at the ovary surface visible with ultrasound imaging. The granulosa layer becomes thinner at this stage, its cells no longer multiplying in proportion to the growth of the antrum. A mature follicle has thick thecal layers and normally develops from a primordial follicle over a period of about 90 days.

Follicular Atresia

Most ovarian follicles undergo the degenerative process called **atresia**, in which follicular cells and oocytes undergo apoptosis and removal by phagocytic cells. Follicles at any stage of development, including antral follicles nearing maturity, may become atretic (Figure 22–9). Atresia involves detachment of the apoptotic granulosa cells, autolysis of the oocyte, and collapse of the zona pellucida. Macrophages invade the degenerating follicle and remove the apoptotic bodies and other debris. Typically, during a woman's fourth decade, menopause begins when atresia and ovulation have reduced the ovarian reserve to fewer than about 1000 follicles.

During a typical menstrual cycle, one antral follicle becomes the **dominant follicle**, developing farther than the others, reaching the most developed stage and undergoing ovulation, while most of the other primary and antral follicles undergo atresia. Although the oocytes of follicles destined for atresia never complete meiosis, these growing and developing follicles under the influence of the pituitary gonadotrophins

FIGURE **22–7**   Antral follicle and mature follicle.

(a) An **antral follicle** shows the large, fluid-filled antral cavities or vesicles (**A**) forming within the **granulosa layer** as the cells produce **follicular fluid**. The oocyte (**O**) is surrounded by the zona pellucida (**ZP**) and granulosa cells (**G**), which also line the wall of the follicle. Fibroblastic cells immediately outside the growing follicles have developed as a steroid-secreting theca interna (**TI**) and a covering theca externa (**TE**). A follicle developing antral cavities is sometimes called a secondary follicle, a potentially misleading name since it still contains a **primary oocyte**. (X100; H&E)

(b) A more developed **preovulatory follicle** shows a single, very large antrum (**A**) filled with **follicular fluid** with proteins that formed a thin film during fixation. The oocyte (**O**) now projects into this cavity, still surrounded by tightly adherent **granulosa cells**, which make up the corona radiata (**CR**). The **corona radiata and oocyte** are attached to the side of the follicle within a larger mass of granulosa cells called the **cumulus oophorus** (**CO**), which is continuous with the cells of the granulosa layer (**G**). Thecae interna (**TI**) and externa (**TE**) surround the whole follicle. (×100; PT)

produce much estrogen before becoming atretic. As described later, this estrogen stimulates the reproductive tract to transport and sustain the early embryo if fertilization of the oocyte from the dominant follicle occurs.

and lead to menstrual irregularities. If cyst formation disrupts blood vessels, blood enters the fluid, often rapidly, and produces a **hemorrhagic cyst**.

Ovulation & Its Hormonal Regulation

Ovulation is the hormone-stimulated process by which the oocyte undergoes release from the ovary. Ovulation normally occurs midway through the menstrual cycle, that is, around the 14th day of a typical 28-day cycle. Shortly before ovulation, the mature dominant follicle bulges against the ovary's tunica albuginea sufficiently

FIGURE 22–8 Wall of antral follicle.

A   G BM   TI   TE   S

At higher magnification, a small part of the wall of an **antral follicle** shows the cell layers of the granulosa (**G**) next to the antrum (**A**), in which proteins have aggregated on cells in contact with the **follicular fluid**. The theca interna (**TI**) surrounds the follicle, its cells appearing vacuolated and lightly stained because of their cytoplasmic lipid droplets, a characteristic of steroid-producing cells. The overlying theca externa (**TE**) contains fibroblasts and smooth muscle cells and merges with the surrounding ovarian stroma (**S**). A basement membrane (**BM**) separates the **theca interna** from the **granulosa**, blocking vascularization of the latter tissue. (×400; PT)

FIGURE 22–9 Atresia.

O   A

G

Atresia or degeneration of a follicle can begin at any stage of follicular development and is shown here in a follicle that had already developed a large antrum. Atresia involves **apoptosis** of follicle or granulosa cells (**G**) and **autolysis** of the oocyte, with **macrophages** entering the degenerating structure to clean up debris. Many **apoptotic bodies** are seen loose in the antrum (**A**) here and the cells of the corona radiata have already disappeared, leaving the degenerative oocyte (**O**) free within the antrum. (×200; PT)

to block local blood flow and produce an elevated, ischemic area, the **stigma**, below the germinal epithelium.

Just before ovulation, the oocyte completes the first meiotic division, which began and arrested in prophase during fetal life (Figure 22–10). The chromosomes undergo equal division between two daughter cells, but one of these retains almost all the cytoplasm. That cell now becomes a **secondary oocyte** and the other cell becomes the **first polar body**, a very small nonviable structure with a nucleus but hardly any cytoplasm. Immediately after expulsion of the first polar body, the nucleus of the secondary oocyte begins the second meiotic division but arrests again at metaphase and never completes meiosis unless it gets fertilized (Figure 22–10).

As mentioned before, follicular development depends on FSH from pituitary gonadotrophs, whose secretion is stimulated by gonadotropin-releasing hormone (GnRH) from the hypothalamus. Figure 22–11 summarizes the main hormonal interactions that regulate follicular growth as well as the ovulation and formation of the corpus luteum. Note that negative feedback of estrogen and progesterone on the hypothalamus and anterior pituitary is reinforced by a polypeptide hormone, **inhibin**, also produced by granulosa and luteal cells. In the days preceding ovulation, the dominant follicle releases higher levels of estrogen that stimulate more rapid pulsatile secretion of GnRH from the hypothalamus.

This causes the pituitary gland to release a surge of **luteinizing hormone (LH)** that rapidly triggers a sequence of major events in and around the dominant follicle:

- **Meiosis I is completed** by the primary oocyte, yielding a secondary oocyte and the first short-lived polar body (Figure 22–10).
- Granulosa cells are stimulated to produce more follicular fluid containing **prostaglandins**, proteoglycans, and proteases that break down the surrounding blood-follicle barrier. The granulosa cells in the cumulus oophorus also release **hyaluronan**, which increases fluid viscosity and swells to greatly increase the extracellular volume within this structure, loosening its outer cells, and dissociating it from the follicle wall.
- At the stigma, the **ovarian wall weakens** as activated plasminogen (plasmin) from broken capillaries degrades collagen in the tunica albuginea and surface epithelium.
- **Smooth muscle contractions** begin in the theca externa, triggered by prostaglandins diffusing from follicular fluid.

The increasing pressure within the follicle and weakening of the ovary wall locally combine to rupture the ovarian surface at the stigma. The oocyte and its surrounding corona radiata, along with follicular fluid, are expelled by thecal smooth muscle contractions and adhere loosely to the ovarian surface in that viscous fluid. As described later, the ovulated structures get drawn into the opening of the uterine tube where fertilization may occur. If not fertilized within about 24 hours, the secondary oocyte begins to degenerate. Cells of the now empty follicle remaining in the ovary redifferentiate

FIGURE 22–10 Summary of Oogenesis and Follicle Development.

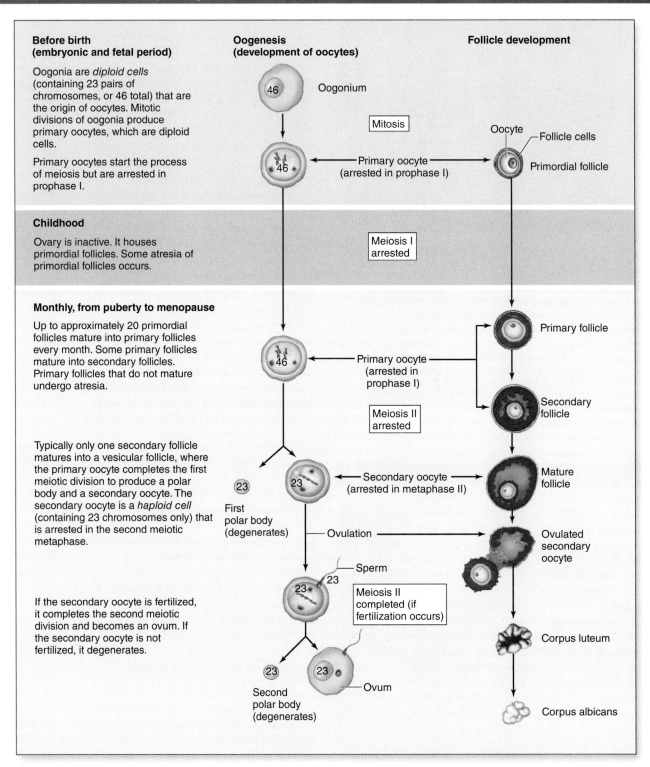

Before birth (embryonic and fetal period)

Oogonia are *diploid cells* (containing 23 pairs of chromosomes, or 46 total) that are the origin of oocytes. Mitotic divisions of oogonia produce primary oocytes, which are diploid cells.

Primary oocytes start the process of meiosis but are arrested in prophase I.

Childhood

Ovary is inactive. It houses primordial follicles. Some atresia of primordial follicles occurs.

Monthly, from puberty to menopause

Up to approximately 20 primordial follicles mature into primary follicles every month. Some primary follicles mature into secondary follicles. Primary follicles that do not mature undergo atresia.

Typically only one secondary follicle matures into a vesicular follicle, where the primary oocyte completes the first meiotic division to produce a polar body and a secondary oocyte. The secondary oocyte is a *haploid cell* (containing 23 chromosomes only) that is arrested in the second meiotic metaphase.

If the secondary oocyte is fertilized, it completes the second meiotic division and becomes an ovum. If the secondary oocyte is not fertilized, it degenerates.

Oogenesis (development of oocytes)

Oogonium

Mitosis

Primary oocyte (arrested in prophase I)

Meiosis I arrested

Primary oocyte (arrested in prophase I)

Meiosis II arrested

First polar body (degenerates)

Secondary oocyte (arrested in metaphase II)

Ovulation

Sperm

Meiosis II completed (if fertilization occurs)

Second polar body (degenerates)

Ovum

Follicle development

Oocyte — Follicle cells

Primordial follicle

Primary follicle

Secondary follicle

Mature follicle

Ovulated secondary oocyte

Corpus luteum

Corpus albicans

Oogenesis begins in the female **fetus**, with **primary oocytes arresting at prophase** I in **primordial follicles**, which remain inactive during childhood. Chapter 3 describes meiosis in general, but important aspects specific to oogenesis, importantly the arrest points of primary and secondary oocytes and the formation of the first and second polar bodies, are illustrated here.

At puberty, a population of **primordial follicles** begins to develop each month, with their **primary oocytes** increasing in size and the surrounding **follicular cells** first proliferating to produce several cell layers (so-called **multilaminar primary follicles**) and then developing fluid-filled antral cavities among these layers (called **antral or secondary follicles**). Typically, one **mature follicle** per month produces a female gamete (a secondary oocyte) and undergoes ovulation.

FIGURE **22–11** Hormonal regulation of ovarian function.

The **ovarian cycle** of follicular growth, followed by **ovulation** and **luteal formation**, is initiated when the hypothalamus secretes gonadotrophin releasing hormone (GnRH). This stimulates the anterior pituitary to secrete **FSH and LH**, in the cycle depicted here.

under the influence of LH and develop into the corpus luteum (Figure 22–11).

Corpus Luteum

After ovulation cells of the ovulated follicle's granulosa and theca interna reorganize to form a larger temporary endocrine gland, the **corpus luteum** (L., yellowish body), in the ovarian cortex. The granulosa and thecal layers of the follicle's wall immediately collapse and fold, with blood from disrupted capillaries often clotting in the former antrum (Figure 22–12). The granulosa is now invaded by capillaries, which bring in cholesterol, the major precursor of steroid hormones, and under the influence of LH cells of both the granulosa and theca interna change histologically and functionally, becoming specialized for extensive production of progesterone in addition to estrogens.

Granulosa cells increase in size to 20–35 μm in diameter, without dividing, and eventually comprise about 80% of the corpus luteum, mostly centrally located. Now called **granulosa lutein cells** (Figure 22–12), they still release some inhibin while losing many features of protein synthesis and

greatly expanding the SER, the site of progesterone synthesis and aromatase conversion of androstenedione into estrogens. The former theca interna comprises the rest of the corpus luteum as **theca lutein cells** (Figure 22–12). Half the size of the granulosa lutein cells, the theca lutein cells synthesize androstenedione and typically aggregate in the peripheral folds of the now well-vascularized corpus luteum. LH drives cells of the corpus luteum for their cooperative and copious production of progesterone and estrogens.

The short-term fate of the corpus luteum depends on whether a pregnancy occurs. The ovulatory LH surge causes the corpus luteum to secrete progesterone for 10–12 days. Without further LH stimulation and in the absence of pregnancy, both cell types of the corpus luteum cease hormone production and undergo apoptosis, with regression of the tissue. Reduction in the circulating levels of progesterone leads to menstruation, the shedding of the thickened, richly vascularized part of the uterine mucosa. As shown in Figure 22–11, decreased levels of progesterone, estrogens, and inhibin lead to greatly renewed pituitary secretion of FSH, stimulating the growth of another group of follicles and beginning the next reproductive cycle. The short-term corpus luteum that

FIGURE 22–12 Corpus luteum.

The **corpus luteum** develops as a large endocrine structure from the remains of a dominant follicle after it undergoes ovulation.

(a) A low-power micrograph shows the corpus luteum (**CL**), characterized by folds of the former granulosa, which collapses as the theca externa contracts at ovulation. The former antrum often contains a blood clot (**BC**) from vessels in the thecal layers disrupted during ovulation. Cells of the **granulosa and theca interna** become reorganized under the influence of pituitary **LH** and their names are changed. (×15; H&E)

(b) Granulosa lutein cells (**GL**), seen at higher magnification here, undergo significant hypertrophy, producing most of the corpus luteum's increased size, and begin producing **progesterone**. The theca lutein cells (**TL**) increase only slightly in size, are somewhat darker staining than the granulosa lutein cells and continue to produce **estrogens**. Theca lutein cells, derived from the theca interna, typically become located within the folds that comprise the bulk of this tissue. (×100; H&E)

persists for only part of one menstrual cycle represents a **corpus luteum of menstruation**. Remnants from its regression are removed by macrophages, and fibroblasts invade the area and produce a scar of dense connective tissue called a **corpus albicans** (L., white body) (Figure 22–13).

If pregnancy occurs, the uterine mucosa must not be allowed to undergo menstruation because the embryo would be lost. To prevent the drop in circulating progesterone, trophoblast cells outside the implanting 7-day embryo begin secreting a glycoprotein called **human chorionic gonadotropin (hCG)** functionally similar to LH. Human chorionic gonadotropin maintains the corpus luteum and promotes its further growth, continuing and increasing progesterone secretion for sustained support of the uterine mucosa. This **corpus luteum of pregnancy** becomes very large with hCG support for 4–5 months, by which time the placenta itself produces progesterone (and estrogens) at levels adequate to maintain

the uterine mucosa. The corpus luteum then degenerates and becomes a large corpus albicans.

› UTERINE TUBES

The paired **uterine tubes** or **oviducts**, supported by ligaments and mesenteries that allow considerable mobility, each measure about 10–12 cm in length. Each uterine tube opens distally into the peritoneal cavity very near the paired ovaries. As shown in Figure 22–14, from that opening each tube has the following regions:

- The **infundibulum**, a funnel-shaped segment with its opening fringed with fingerlike extensions called **fimbriae** (L., fringes) next to the ovary;
- The **ampulla**, the longest and expanded region where fertilization normally occurs;

FIGURE **22–13** Corpus albicans.

CA

A corpus albicans (**CA**) represents the remnant scar of **connective tissue** formed at the site of a **corpus luteum** during its involution. It contains mostly collagen, with few fibroblasts or other cells, and gradually becomes very small and lost in the ovarian stroma. Involution of the corpus luteum does not involve atresia; the two processes are very different. (×60; H&E)

- The **isthmus**, a narrow portion adjoining the uterus; and
- The **uterine** or **intramural part**, which passes through the wall of the uterus and opens into the interior of that organ.

The wall of the oviduct consists of a folded mucosa, a thick, well-defined muscularis with interwoven circular (or spiral) and longitudinal layers of smooth muscle (Figure 22–15a), and a thin serosa covered by visceral peritoneum with mesothelium.

The numerous branching, longitudinal folds of the mucosa develop most prominently in the ampulla, which in cross section resembles a labyrinth (Figure 22–14b). The mucosal folds become smaller in the regions closer to the uterus and disappear in the intramural portion of the tube.

Along its entire length the mucosa consists of simple columnar epithelium on a lamina propria of loose connective tissue (Figure 22–15b). The epithelium contains two interspersed, functionally important cell types:

- **Ciliated cells** in which ciliary movements sweep fluid toward the uterus, and
- **Secretory peg cells**, nonciliated and often darker staining, often with an apical bulge into the lumen, which secrete glycoproteins of a nutritive mucus film that covers the epithelium.

Triggered primarily by estrogens, the cilia elongate and both cell types undergo hypertrophy during the follicular growth phase of the ovarian cycle and undergo atrophy with loss of cilia during the late luteal phase.

At the time of ovulation mucosal hypertrophy and increased local blood flow have enlarged and moved the uterine tubes. The fringed infundibulum lies very close to the ovary and the fimbriae partially surround that organ. This favors the transport of the ovulated secondary oocyte into the tube. Promoted by sweeping muscular contractions of the fimbriae and ciliary activity, the oocyte enters the infundibulum and moves to the ampulla. The secretion covering the mucosa has nutritive and protective functions for both the oocyte and the sperm, including **capacitation factors** that activate sperm and make those cells able to fertilize an oocyte.

❯ MAJOR EVENTS OF FERTILIZATION

Fertilization, in humans the union of a secondary oocyte and a spermatozoan, normally occurs in the tube's ampulla, a region usually reached by only a few hundred of the millions of ejaculated sperm. Sperm that have undergone capacitation by immersion in female reproductive tract fluid have the capacity to fertilize the oocyte. Fertilization itself involves the following major steps.

- Upon contact with cells of the corona radiata sperm release **hyaluronidase** by exocytosis, which allows sperm to move more easily between the coronal cells to the zona pellucida.
- At the zona pellucida, specific enzymes on the sperm surface interact with the multimeric sperm-binding receptors, in which the ZP3 component then activates the **acrosomal reaction**. This causes rapid exocytosis of the main acrosomal protease **acrosin** and other hydrolytic enzymes at multiple sites across the broad acrosomal surface, leading to localized degradation of the zona pellucida.
- The cell membrane of the first sperm to completely penetrate the zona pellucida fuses with the plasmalemma of the oocyte, producing weak membrane depolarization that triggers a fast wave of Ca^{2+} release from vesicles in the oocyte. This then triggers exocytosis of proteases from the oocyte's cortical granules, the **cortical reaction**, which quickly spreads like a wave across the entire surface of the oocyte. Proteases released from the granules very rapidly hydrolyze ZP3 and other sperm-binding components throughout the zona pellucida, converting it to the impenetrable **perivitelline barrier** that constitutes a permanent block to polyspermic fertilization.
- The rise of $[Ca^{2+}]$ in the secondary oocyte causes its nucleus to immediately complete meiosis II, producing a second polar body and the **female pronucleus** of the haploid **ovum**. Leaving the flagellum and midpiece behind, the haploid nucleus of the single penetrating sperm head is drawn into the ovum toward its pronucleus, losing protamines, loosening its chromatin compaction, and becoming the **male pronucleus**. Fusion of the two pronuclei yields a new diploid cell, the **zygote** (Gr. *zygotos*, yoked together).

FIGURE 22–14 Uterine tubes and uterus.

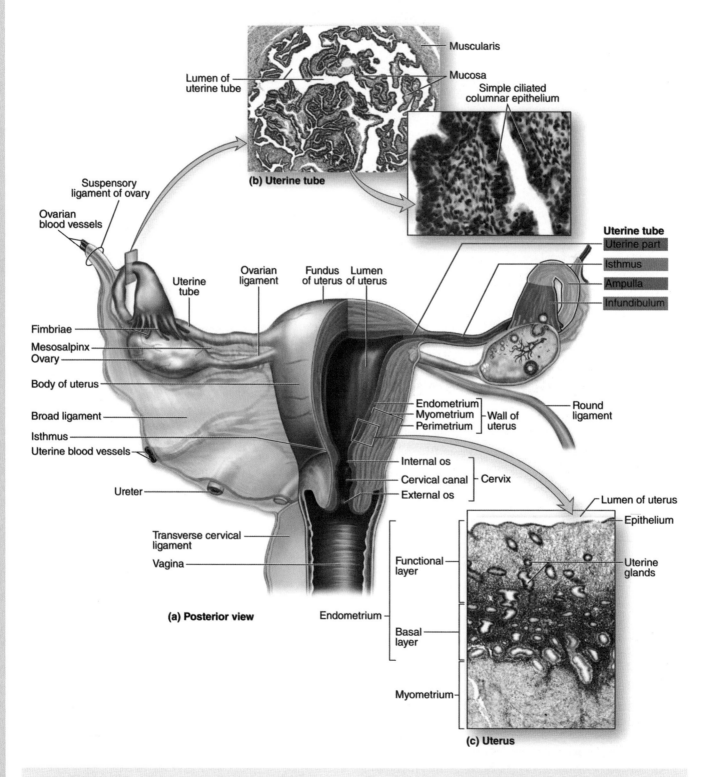

Muscularis

Lumen of uterine tube

Mucosa

Simple ciliated columnar epithelium

(b) Uterine tube

Suspensory ligament of ovary

Ovarian blood vessels

Uterine tube

Uterine part

Isthmus

Ampulla

Infundibulum

Uterine tube

Ovarian ligament

Fundus of uterus

Lumen of uterus

Fimbriae

Mesosalpinx

Ovary

Body of uterus

Broad ligament

Isthmus

Uterine blood vessels

Ureter

Endometrium
Myometrium
Perimetrium

Wall of uterus

Round ligament

Internal os

Cervical canal

External os

Cervix

Transverse cervical ligament

Vagina

Lumen of uterus

Epithelium

Functional layer

Uterine glands

Endometrium

Basal layer

Myometrium

(a) Posterior view

(c) Uterus

The **uterine tubes or oviducts** are paired ducts that catch the ovulated secondary oocyte, nourish both the oocyte and sperm, provide the microenvironment for fertilization, and transport the embryo undergoing cleavage to the uterus.

(a) The diagram shows the relationship between the **uterine tubes and the uterus** in an intact posterior view (left) and in a cutaway view (right).

(b) A cross section of **uterine tube** with a high magnification of the intricately folded mucosa. (×35 and 400; H&E)

(c) A section of the wall of the **uterus** showing the **myometrium** and the two layers of the **endometrium**. (×45; H&E)

FIGURE **22–15** Mucosa of the uterine tube wall.

(a) A cross section of the **uterine tube** at the **ampulla** shows the interwoven circular (**C**) and longitudinal (**L**) layers of smooth muscle in the **muscularis** and in the complex of **folded mucosa**, the lamina propria (**LP**) underlying a **simple columnar epithelium** (arrows). (×140; H&E)

(b) The **oviduct mucosa**, with folds projecting into the lumen (**L**), has simple columnar epithelium (**E**) on the lamina propria (**LP**). (×200; PT)

(c, d) Higher magnification shows **two epithelial cell types**: ciliated cells (**CC**) interspersed with the secretory peg cells (**PC**), which produce the nutritive fluid covering the epithelium. These cells' histologic and functional features vary during the ovarian cycle due to hormonal fluctuations. In **(d)**, the **peg cells** shown are at their most developed and most active state in the period shortly after ovulation when an embryo might be present. (c: ×400, PT; d: ×400, Mallory trichrome)

Cell division within the zygote/embryo gets underway as ciliary movements and contractions of the oviduct muscularis transport it to the uterus, which takes about 5 days. This transport occurs normally in women with immotile ciliary syndrome, indicating a more important role for muscle contractions here.

›› MEDICAL APPLICATION

Tubal ligation is a common surgical type of contraception. The uterine tube mucosa can become inflamed if infectious agents ascend from the lower genital tract, producing a condition named **salpingitis** after another name for these tubes, the **salpinges**. Mucosal damage or adhesions caused by chronic salpingitis can lead to **infertility** or an **ectopic (tubal) pregnancy** if there is blockage of oocyte or embryo transport to the uterus.

In tubal pregnancies, the lamina propria may react like the uterine endometrium and form decidual cells. But because of its small diameter and inability to expand, the tube cannot contain the growing embryo and will rupture, causing potentially fatal hemorrhage.

› UTERUS

As shown in Figure 22–14, the **uterus** develops as a medial, pear-shaped organ with thick, muscular walls. The two uterine tubes enter its largest part, the uterine **body**, and the curved, superior area between the tubes represents the **fundus**. The uterus narrows in the **isthmus** and ends in a lower cylindrical structure, the **cervix**. The lumen of the cervix, the **cervical canal**, has constricted openings at each end: the **internal os** (L. *os*, mouth) opens to the lumen of the isthmus and the **external os** to the vagina (Figure 22–14).

Supported by the set of ligaments and mesenteries also associated with the ovaries and uterine tubes (Figure 22–1), the uterine wall has three major layers (Figure 22–14):

- An outer connective tissue layer, the **perimetrium**, continuous with the ligaments, which is adventitial in some areas, but largely a serosa covered by mesothelium;
- A thick middle tunic of highly vascularized smooth muscle, the **myometrium** (Figure 22–16a); and
- A mucosa, the **endometrium**, lined by simple columnar epithelium (Figure 22–16).

FIGURE 22–16 Uterine myometrium and endometrium.

(a) The basal layer (B) of the **endometrium**, bordering the myometrium (M), contains the **basal ends** of the uterine glands (G) and many small arteries (A) embedded in a distinctive connective tissue **stroma** with many fibroblasts, ground substance, and primarily fine type III collagen, but no adipocytes. (×100; Mallory trichrome)

(b) Superficial to the basal layer of the endometrium is its **functional layer**, the part that changes histologically and functionally

depending on **estrogen levels**. This micrograph shows only the **functional layer** and includes parts of the long uterine glands (G) as well as one spiral artery (A). (×100; Mallory trichrome)

(c) The surface epithelium (SE) lining the endometrium is simple columnar, with many cells having cilia. The underlying stroma (S) has an extensive **microvasculature**, much ground substance, and **fibroblastic cells** with large, active nuclei. (×400; Mallory trichrome)

All three layers have continuity with their counterparts in the uterine tubes, but the thickness and structure of the endometrium undergoes much greater cyclic changes with the shifting levels of ovarian hormones than the mucosa of the uterine tubes (Figure 22–17).

Myometrium

The **myometrium** (Gr. *myo*, muscle + *metra*, uterus), the thickest uterine tunic, shows bundles of smooth muscle fibers separated by connective tissue containing venous plexuses and lymphatics (Figure 22–16a). The smooth muscle forms interwoven layers, with fibers of the inner and outer layers disposed generally parallel to the long axis of the organ.

During pregnancy the myometrium goes through a period of extensive growth involving both **hyperplasia** (increasing the number of smooth muscle cells), cell hypertrophy, and increased collagen production by the muscle cells, all of which strengthen the uterine wall. This well-developed uterine myometrium contracts very forcefully during **parturition** to expel the infant through the cervix. After pregnancy uterine smooth muscle cells shrink and many undergo apoptosis, with removal of unneeded collagen, and the uterus returns almost to its size before pregnancy.

Endometrium

The **endometrium's** lamina propria or stroma consists primarily of nonbundled type III collagen with abundant fibroblasts and ground substance. Its simple columnar epithelial lining has both ciliated and secretory cells, and the latter line the numerous tubular **uterine glands**, which penetrate the full thickness of the endometrium (Figures 22–16 and 22–18).

The endometrium has two concentric zones:

- The **basal layer** adjacent to the myometrium has a more highly cellular lamina propria and contains the deep basal ends of the uterine glands (Figure 22–16a) and
- The superficial **functional layer** has a spongier lamina propria, richer in ground substance, and includes most of the length of the glands, as well as the surface epithelium (Figure 22–16b, c).

The functional layer undergoes profound changes and loss during the menstrual cycles, but the basal layer remains relatively unchanged (Figure 22–17).

Blood vessels supplying the endometrium have special significance in the periodic sloughing of the functional layer during menses. Arcuate arteries in the myometrium send two sets of smaller radial arteries into the basal layer of the

FIGURE **22–17** Correlation of ovarian and menstrual cycles with levels of their controlling hormones.

The cyclic development of **ovarian follicles** and the **corpus luteum**, controlled by the pituitary **gonadotropins** FSH and LH, lead to cyclic shifts in the levels of the major ovarian hormones: steroidal **estrogens and progesterone**.

Estrogen stimulates the proliferative phase of the uterine cycle and its level peaks near the day of ovulation, which marks the midpoint of the ovarian cycle.

After ovulation the corpus luteum forms and produces both progesterone and estrogens, which together promote growth and development of the endometrial **functional layer**.

Unless fertilization and implantation of an embryo occur, regression of the corpus luteum leads to declining levels of the steroid hormones and failure of the new endometrial tissue to be maintained. This tissue sloughs off as the menstrual flow, the first day of which is taken to mark day 1 of both the ovarian cycle and the uterine cycle. The **basal layer** of endometrium is **not sensitive** to the loss of progesterone and is retained during menstruation, serving to **regenerate** the functional layer during the ensuing proliferative phase.

FIGURE **22–18** Arterial supply to the endometrium.

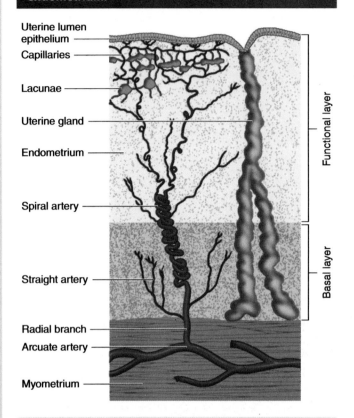

Uterine lumen epithelium
Capillaries
Lacunae
Uterine gland
Endometrium
Spiral artery
Straight artery
Radial branch
Arcuate artery
Myometrium

Functional layer
Basal layer

The **basal and functional layers** of the endometrium are supplied by different sets of small arteries emerging from the uterine arcuate arteries in the myometrium: the **straight arteries** and **spiral arteries**, respectively.

The spiral arteries are uniquely sensitive to progesterone, growing rapidly in a spiral fashion as the functional layer thickens under the influence of that luteal steroid and providing blood to a microvasculature, which includes many **lacunae** lined by thin endothelium. This blood supply brings oxygen and nutrients to cells of the functional layer and to an embryo implanting itself into that tissue.

If no embryo is present to produce the gonadotropin replacing LH, the corpus luteum undergoes regression 8–10 days after ovulation. The rapid decline in the level of progesterone causes constriction of the spiral arteries and other changes, which quickly lead to local **ischemia** in the functional layer and its separation from the basal layer during **menstruation**.

endometrium (Figure 22–18). These branch further, forming two types of smaller arteries:

- typical **straight arteries**, which supply only the basal layer, and
- long, coiled, progesterone-sensitive **spiral arteries**, which carry blood throughout the functional layer. Spiral arteries branch into numerous arterioles supplying a rich, superficial capillary bed that includes many dilated, thin-walled **vascular lacunae** drained by venules.

Menstrual Cycle

Estrogens and progesterone control growth and differentiation of epithelial cells and associated connective tissue throughout the female reproductive system. After menopause diminished synthesis of these hormones causes a general involution of tissues in the reproductive tract.

❯❯ MEDICAL APPLICATION

Viable endometrial cells frequently undergo menstrual reflux into or through the uterine tubes. In some women, this can lead to **endometriosis**, a disorder with pelvic pain due to endometrial tissue growing on the ovaries, oviducts, or elsewhere. Under the influence of estrogen and progesterone, the ectopic tissue grows and degenerates monthly but cannot be removed effectively from the body. In addition to pain, endometriosis can produce inflammation, ovarian cysts, adhesions, and scar tissue that can cause infertility.

From puberty until menopause, pituitary gonadotropins produce cyclic changes in ovarian hormone levels, causing cyclic endometrial modifications during the menstrual cycle (Figures 22–17 and 22–19). The duration of the menstrual cycle may be variable but averages 28 days. Because menstrual cycles result from ovarian changes related to oocyte production, a woman's fertility coincides with the years punctuated by her menstrual cycles.

Day 1 of the menstrual cycle is usually taken as the day when menstrual bleeding begins. The menstrual discharge consists of degenerating endometrium mixed with blood from its ruptured microvasculature. As shown in Figure 22–17, this **menstrual period** lasts 2–5 days, followed by the endometrium's **proliferative phase** from days 6 to 14 typically. Its **secretory phase** begins at ovulation and lasts about 14 days. The cyclic structural changes occur gradually and the activities characterizing these phases overlap somewhat.

Proliferative Phase

After the menstrual phase the uterine mucosa is relatively thin (~0.5 mm). The beginning of the **proliferative phase**, also called the **follicular phase**, coincides with the rapid growth of a small group of ovarian follicles growing as vesicular follicles. With development of their thecae interna, these follicles actively produce estrogen, increasing its plasma concentrations (Figure 22–17).

Estrogens induce regeneration of the endometrial functional layer lost during menstruation. Epithelial cells in the basal ends of the broken glands proliferate, migrate, and cover the surface exposed by menstruation. Here the endometrial lining comprises a simple columnar surface epithelium and the uterine glands are short and relatively straight tubules with narrow, nearly empty lumens (Figure 22–19a, d). Mitotic activity prevails among both the epithelial cells and fibroblasts of the regenerating functional layer. Spiral arteries

FIGURE **22–19** Proliferative, secretory, and premenstrual phases in the uterus.

The **major phases of the uterine cycle** overlap but produce distinctly different and characteristic changes in the **functional layer** (**F**) closest to the lumen (**L**) with little effect on the **basal layer** (**B**) and myometrium (**M**). Characteristic features of each phase include the following.

During most of the **proliferative phase** (**a, d**), the **functional layer** remains relatively thin, its stroma highly cellular and its glands (**G**) relatively straight, narrow, and empty. Cells of both the stroma and glands undergo very rapid proliferation and growth during this phase.

In the **secretory phase** (**b, e**), the **functional layer** has become less heavily cellular and perhaps four times thicker than the **basal layer**. The **tubular glands** have wider lumens

containing secretory product and **coil tightly** up through the stroma, giving a zigzag or folded appearance histologically. Superficially in the functional layer, lacunae (**La**) develop from the microvasculature, becoming widespread and filled with blood.

The short **premenstrual phase** (**c, f**) begins with constriction of the **spiral arteries**, which produces **hypoxia** that causes swelling and dissolution of the glands (**G**). The stroma of the peripheral functional layer becomes more compact and near the basal layer typically appears more sponge-like. During this time **blood stasis**, **apoptosis**, and **proteolytic** breakdown of the stromal matrix sets the stage for the imminent **menses**.

(a: ×20; b and c: ×12; d, e, and f: ×50. All H&E)

TABLE 22–1	Summary of events of the menstrual cycle.			
	Stage of Cycle			
	Proliferative	**Secretory or Luteal**		**Menstrual**
Main actions of pituitary hormones	Follicle-stimulating hormone stimulates rapid growth of ovarian follicles	Peak of luteinizing hormone at the beginning of secretory stage, secreted after estrogen stimulation, induces ovulation and development of the corpus luteum		
Main events in the ovary	Growth of ovarian follicles; dominant follicle reaches preovulatory stage	Ovulation	Development of the corpus luteum	Degeneration of the corpus luteum
Dominant ovarian hormone	Estrogens, produced by the growing follicles, act on vagina, tubes, and uterus	Progesterone, produced by the corpus luteum, acts mainly on the uterus		Progesterone production ceases
Main events in the endometrium	Growth of the mucosa after menstruation	Further growth of the mucosa, coiling of glands, secretion		Shedding of part of the mucosa about 14 days after ovulation

lengthen (Figure 22–16) and extensive microvasculature begin to develop near the surface of the growing functional layer. At the end of the proliferative phase, the endometrium is 2–3 mm thick.

Secretory Phase

After ovulation, the secretory or **luteal phase** starts because of progesterone secreted by the corpus luteum. Progesterone stimulates additional cell proliferation, and epithelial cells of the new uterine glands begin to secrete and accumulate glycogen, dilating the glandular lumens and causing the glands to become coiled (Figure 22–19b, e). The superficial microvasculature now includes thin-walled, blood-filled lacunae (Figures 22–18 and 22–19e). The endometrium reaches its maximum thickness (5–6 mm) during the secretory phase due to growth, accumulation of secretions, and edema in the stroma.

If fertilization occurred during the day after ovulation, the embryo has been transported to the uterus by about 5 days later and attaches to the uterine epithelium when the endometrial thickness and secretory activity are optimal for embryonic implantation and sustenance. The uterine secretion comprises the embryo's major nutrient source before and during implantation. In addition to promoting this secretion, progesterone inhibits strong contractions of the myometrium that might hinder embryo implantation.

Menstrual Phase

When fertilization or embryonic implantation do not occur, the corpus luteum regresses and circulating levels of progesterone and estrogens begin to decrease 8–10 days after ovulation, soon causing the onset of menstruation (Figure 22–17). With loss of progesterone, the spiral arteries begin to contract and relax intermittently, interrupting normal blood flow, and local release of prostaglandins then produces strong vasoconstriction and local hypoxia. Cells undergoing hypoxic injury release cytokines that increase immigration of leukocytes releasing collagenase and other matrix metalloproteinases that degrade basement membranes and other ECM components (Figure 22–19c, f).

The basal layer of the endometrium, not dependent on the progesterone-sensitive spiral arteries, remains relatively unaffected by these activities. However, major portions of the functional layer, including the surface epithelium, most of each gland, the stroma and blood-filled lacunae, detach from the basal layer and slough away as the menstrual flow or **menses**. Arterial constriction limits blood loss during menstruation, but some blood emerges from the open ends of venules. The amount of endometrium and blood lost in menstruation varies among women and in the same woman at different times.

At the end of the menstrual phase the endometrium is reduced to a thin layer, ready to begin a new cycle as its cells begin dividing to reconstitute the functional mucosa. Table 22–1 summarizes the major events of the menstrual cycle in the pituitary, ovary, and endometrium.

› EMBRYONIC IMPLANTATION, DECIDUA, & THE PLACENTA

The zygote produced by fertilization undergoes mitotic cleavages as it is moved toward the uterus, with its cells called **blastomeres** (Gr. *blastos*, germ + *meros*, part) in a compact aggregate called the **morula** (L. *morum*, mulberry). No growth occurs during the period of cleavages; blastomeres become smaller at each division and the morula remains about the same size as the fertilized oocyte.

About 5 days after fertilization the embryo reaches the uterine cavity, by which time blastomeres have rearranged to form a central cavity in the morula and the embryo enters the **blastocyst** stage of development. The blastomeres then develop as two groups: a peripheral layer called the **trophoblast** surrounding the cavity, and a small cluster of cells just inside this layer, the **embryoblast** or **inner cell mass** (Figure 22–20). The blastocyst remains in the lumen of the uterus for about 2 days, immersed in the endometrial glands' viscous mucosal secretion.

Implantation, or nidation, involves attachment of the blastocyst to the surface epithelial cells of the endometrium and its proteolytic penetration through this epithelium into the underlying stroma (Figure 22–20), a process lasting about 3 days. The trophoblast cells drive the events of implantation, during which time cells of the embryoblast rearrange to form two cavities, the future **amniotic cavity** and the **yolk sac**. Where the cells lining these structures make contact, the **bilaminar embryonic disc** develops with its **epiblast** layer continuous with the amnion and its **hypoblast** layer part of the yolk sac (Figure 22–20).

FIGURE 22–20 Embryo implantation.

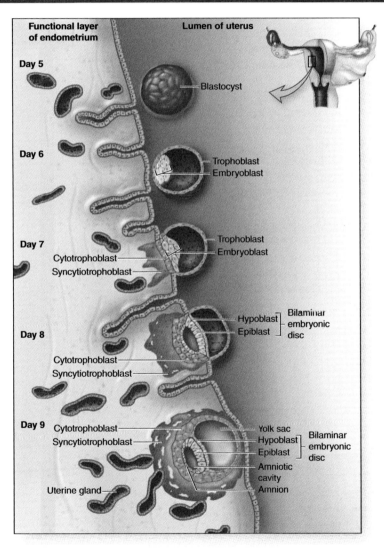

The **embryo** enters the uterus as a **blastocyst** about 5 days after ovulation or fertilization, when the uterus is in the secretory phase and best prepared for **implantation**. To begin implantation, receptors on cells of the outer embryonic **trophoblast** bind glycoprotein ligands on the **endometrial epithelium**. The trophoblast forms an invasive, outer syncytial layer called the **syncytiotrophoblast**.

Proteases are activated and/or released locally to digest stroma components, which allows the developing embryo to **embed** itself within the stroma. The newly implanted embryo absorbs nutrients and oxygen from the endometrial tissue and blood in the **lacunae**. Closer to the embryo, the **cytotrophoblast** contributes nuclei and cytoplasm to the surrounding syncytial layer.

All parts of the embryo develop from this early embryonic disc. The yolk sac and amnion form extraembryonic structures, but only the latter persists throughout pregnancy. As shown in Figure 22–20, the trophoblast develops extensively during implantation to form:

■ The **cytotrophoblast**, a layer of mitotically active cells immediately around the amnion and yolk sac, and

■ The **syncytiotrophoblast**, a more superficial, nonmitotic mass of multinucleated cytoplasm that invades the endometrium and eventually surrounds the developing embryoblast and the cytotrophoblast. It is the developing syncytiotrophoblast layer that produces increasing amounts of hCG, maintaining the corpus luteum and providing the basis for pregnancy tests.

On its side nearest the embryoblast, the trophoblast attaches to the uterine epithelium and the syncytiotrophoblast begins to invade the endometrium and quickly allow the developing embryo and trophoblast both to become embedded in the endometrial stroma.

By about the ninth day after ovulation, the trophoblast and embryo complete implantation into the endometrium and derive nutrients primarily from maternal blood there. Cytotrophoblast cells synthesize anti-inflammatory cytokines to prevent an adverse uterine reaction to the implanted embryo, an activity replaced later by various embryonic factors producing local immune tolerance for the embryo throughout the pregnancy.

The endometrial stroma undergoes histologic changes in the period following implantation. Fibroblasts become enlarged, polygonal, more active in protein synthesis, and are now called **decidual cells**. The whole endometrium now becomes the **decidua** (L. *deciduous*, shedding) and includes three areas shown in Figure 22–21:

■ The **decidua basalis**, the area between the implanted embryo and the myometrium;

■ The **decidua capsularis**, the region immediately around the embryo and the extraembryonic structures that thins as these structures grow; and

■ The **decidua parietalis**, on the side of the uterus away from the embryo.

›› MEDICAL APPLICATION

The initial attachment of the embryo usually occurs on the ventral or dorsal walls of the body of the uterus. Sometimes the embryo attaches close to the internal os. In this case, the placenta will be interposed between the fetus and the vagina, obstructing the passage of the fetus at parturition. This situation, called **placenta previa**, must be recognized by the physician, and the fetus must be delivered by cesarean section. Otherwise, obstructed parturition can lead to death of the fetus.

The **placenta** soon develops as the organ for exchange for nutrients, wastes, O_2 and CO_2 between the mother and the embryo, containing tissues components from each. The **chorion** represents the embryo's contribution, derived from the trophoblast and embryonic mesodermal cells; the maternal part develops from the decidua basalis. Exchange occurs between embryonic blood in chorionic villi outside the embryo and maternal blood in lacunae of the decidua basalis. Chorionic villi of the growing placenta go through three stages of development.

■ **Primary villi** first appear 2 days after implantation as simple cords of proliferating cytotrophoblast cells covered by syncytiotrophoblast that extend into lacunae containing maternal blood.

■ **Secondary villi** begin to form on about the 15th day of embryonic development as the cores of primary villi are invaded by extraembryonic mesenchyme.

■ **Tertiary villi** develop within a few more days as these mesenchymal cells in the secondary villi differentiate as capillary loops continuous with the embryonic circulatory system.

By the end of the first month of the pregnancy, the placenta contains thousands of tertiary chorionic villi, each branching many times and each branch having one or more capillary loops (Figure 22–21c). Suspended in pools of maternal blood in the decidua, the chorionic villi provide an enormous surface area for metabolite exchange (Figure 22–22). Exchange of gases, nutrients, and wastes occurs between fetal blood in the capillaries and maternal blood bathing the villi, with bidirectional diffusion occurring across the trophoblast layer and the capillary endothelium.

The placenta also develops as a multipurpose endocrine organ, producing hCG, a lactogen, relaxin, and various growth factors, in addition to estrogen and progesterone. More detailed information on the developing embryo and placenta should be sought in embryology textbooks.

› CERVIX

As noted earlier, the **cervix** makes up the lower, cylindrical part of the uterus (Figure 22–14). The cervix differs histologically from the rest of the uterus. The **endocervical mucosa** is a simple columnar epithelium on a thick lamina propria, with many large, branched, mucus-secreting **cervical glands**. It lacks spiral arteries, does not change its 2–3 mm thickness during the ovarian cycle or undergo menstruation.

The cervical region around the external os projects slightly into the upper vagina and is covered by the **exocervical mucosa** with nonkeratinized stratified squamous epithelium continuous with that of the vagina. An abrupt change from this squamous epithelium and the mucus-secreting columnar epithelium of the endocervix occurs in a **transformation zone**, an area just outside the external os that shifts slightly with the cyclical changes in uterine size

FIGURE **22–21** Extraembryonic membranes, decidua, and placenta.

(a) The membranous extraembryonic **amnion, chorion,** and **yolk sac** appear during the second week of development, with the embryonic disc between the amnion and yolk sac. As the embryo develops the yolk sac disappears while the fluid-filled amniotic cavity enlarges to surround the growing embryo/fetus entirely. The third extraembryonic structure, the chorion, also filled with fluid initially, develops from the two trophoblastic layers and a lining of mesenchymal cells migrating out of the embryo itself.

(b) Growth of the embryo and amnion gradually eliminate the distance between the amnion with the chorion, leading to the eventual fusion of these two layers to produce the amniotic sac filled with amniotic fluid. Soon after implantation the endometrium begins

to change histologically and is now referred to as the **decidua**. It develops three different regions: **decidua basalis**, the region where implantation occurred; **decidua capsularis**, closely applied to first the chorion and the later the developing amniotic sac; and **decidua parietalis**, which includes all other areas of the pregnant endometrium. **Chorionic villi** develop most profusely in the decidua basalis, which becomes the major portion of the **placenta**.

(c) Each of the many **chorionic tertiary stem villi** in the placenta contains a branch of the umbilical artery and vein, which form loops of microvasculature carrying **embryonic blood** and branching into smaller villus branches. The entire stem villus is bathed in **maternal blood** circulated by endometrial arteries and veins.

FIGURE **22–22** Term placenta.

The **placenta** contains **chorionic villi** of the fetus and a large space for **pooled maternal blood** in the decidua.

(a) A section through a **full-term placenta** showing in cross-section here a single villus stem, containing arteries (**A**) and (**V**) of the **extraembryonic vasculature**, and dozens of smaller **villus branches (arrows)** that consist of connective tissue and microvasculature. Maternal blood (**MB**) normally fills the space around the many villi, which is largely empty here. (×50; H&E)

(b) Higher magnification of villus branches surrounded by maternal blood (**MB**) each containing capillaries (**C**) or sinusoids (**S**) with fetal blood. By the end of pregnancy cytotrophoblast cells have greatly decreased in number in many areas, leaving only a thin **syncytiotrophoblast** and basement membrane covering the villus in these regions (**arrows**). The extraembryonic blood vessels become closely associated with these areas of thin trophoblast for maximal diffusion of material between the two pools of blood. (×400; H&E)

(Figure 22–23). Periodic exposure of this squamous-columnar junction to the vaginal environment can stimulate reprogramming of epithelial stem cells, which occasionally leads to intraepithelial neoplasia at that site.

Under the influence of progesterone, the consistency of **cervical mucus** changes cyclically and plays a significant role in fertilization and early pregnancy. Around ovulation abundant, watery mucus facilitates sperm movements into the uterus. In the luteal phase, more viscous mucus hinders sperm passage. During pregnancy the cervical glands proliferate and secrete highly viscous mucus that forms a plug in the cervical canal (Figure 22–21b).

The deeper wall of the cervix consists mainly of dense connective tissue, with much less smooth muscle than the rest of the uterus (Figure 22–23). The cervix becomes relatively rigid during pregnancy, helping to retain the fetus in the uterus. Before parturition a process of **cervical effacement** occurs in which its connective tissue undergoes extensive remodeling and significant collagen dissolution, mediated in part by macrophages. As a result, the cervix softens, the cervical canal dilates, and birth occurs more easily.

›› MEDICAL APPLICATION

The incidence of **cervical cancer** worldwide has been greatly reduced by widespread, routine screening by **exfoliative cytology** to examine for dysplasia of the cervical epithelium (Figure 22–23c). The test called the **Pap smear** after its developer George Papanicolaou, who introduced this diagnostic technique in the 1920s, uses cells that have been lightly scraped from cervix. Abnormal cells suggestive of precancerous changes in the epithelium are then detected microscopically. The epithelial dysplasia, which precedes **squamous cell neoplasia**, the most common type of cervical cancer, occurs in metaplastic cells of the transformation zone at a mean age of 54 years. The **human papillomavirus** (HPV) is strongly implicated in the pathogenesis of this cancer.

FIGURE **22–23** Cervix.

(a) The **mucosa** of the cervical canal (**CC**) is continuous with the **endometrium** and like that tissue is lined by simple columnar epithelium (**SC**). This **endocervical mucosa** includes many large branched cervical **mucous glands** (**arrows**). At the external os, the point at which the cervical canal opens into the vagina (**V**), there is an abrupt junction (**J**) between the **columnar epithelium** and the **stratified squamous epithelium** (**SS**) covering the exocervix and vagina. The deeper cervical wall consists primarily of fibromuscular tissue (**F**). (×15; H&E)

(b) The **epithelial junction** (**arrow**) between the endocervical and exocervical mucosae shown at higher magnification. (×50; H&E)

(c) Exfoliative cytology of epithelial cells from the exocervical mucosa in a routine cervical smear. The squamous cells, stained on a slide by the **Papanicolaou procedure** using hematoxylin, orange G, and eosin, stain differently according to their content of keratins. Cells with atypical nuclei or other abnormalities can be detected by this method, which is used routinely to check for cervical carcinoma. (×200; Papanicolaou stain)

(d) The **endocervical mucosa** is exposed to a relatively high population of microorganisms and normally has many **neutrophils** and other leukocytes. Such cells occur in the lamina propria and epithelium (**arrows**), but they are also numerous and readily apparent in the mucus layer (**M**), which was fixed in place here. (×400; H&E)

❯ VAGINA

The wall of the **vagina** (L., *vagina*, sheath, scabbard) lacks glands and is kept moist mainly by cervical gland secretions. The vagina consists of the usual layers: a **mucosa**, a **muscular layer**, and an **adventitia**.

The epithelium of the vaginal mucosa is stratified squamous, with a thickness of 150–200 μm in adults (Figure 22–24).

Stimulated by estrogens, the epithelial cells synthesize and accumulate glycogen. When the cells desquamate, bacteria metabolize glycogen to lactic acid, causing a relatively low pH within the vagina, which helps protect against pathogenic microorganisms. The lamina propria has abundant elastic fibers and forms numerous narrow papillae that project into the overlying epithelium (Figure 22–24). The mucosa normally contains lymphocytes and neutrophils in relatively large quantities.

FIGURE 22–24 Vagina.

The **vagina** has **mucosal, muscular,** and **adventitial layers.**

(a) The highly cellular lamina propria (**LP**) extends narrow **papillae** into the **thick, nonkeratinized stratified squamous** epithelium (**E**). The muscular layer (**M**) has inner circular and outer longitudinal bundles of smooth muscle. (×60; H&E)

(b) Higher magnification of the vaginal **stratified squamous epithelium** and its very scant, underlying lamina propria (**LP**) shows invasion of **leukocytes** (**arrows**) between the epithelial cells from the connective tissue. (×200; PSH)

The muscular layer of the vagina is composed mainly of two indistinct layers of smooth muscle, disposed as circular bundles next to the mucosa and as thicker longitudinal bundles near the adventitial layer (Figure 22–24). The dense connective tissue of the adventitia is also rich in elastic fibers, making the vaginal wall strong and elastic while binding it to the surrounding tissues. This outer layer also contains an extensive venous plexus, lymphatics, and nerves.

≫ MEDICAL APPLICATION

Atrophic vaginitis involves thinning or atrophy of the vaginal epithelium caused by diminished estrogen levels and occurs most often in postmenopausal women. This change allows the more frequent inflammation and infections characteristic of this condition. Primary **squamous cell carcinoma** of the vagina occurs rarely, with most vaginal malignancies having spread secondarily from the cervix or vulva.

❯ EXTERNAL GENITALIA

The female **external genitalia**, or **vulva**, include several structures, all having many Meissner and Pacinian corpuscles and covered by stratified squamous epithelium.

- The paired **labia majora** consist of thick lateral folds of skin, homologous to and similar histologically to the skin of the scrotum.
- The **labia minora** are smaller paired folds, medial and parallel to the labia majora, with richly vascular loose connective tissue, numerous sebaceous glands and melanocytes.
- The **vestibule** occupies the space between the labia minora and encompasses the urethral and vaginal openings. Its wall includes numerous small tubuloacinar vestibular glands and the paired **greater vestibular glands** (of Bartholin), which are homologous to the male bulbourethral glands. During sexual arousal the large glands provide lubricating mucus for the entire vulva and vagina.
- The **clitoris** is a small erectile structure, homologous to the penis with paired corpora cavernosa.

❯ MAMMARY GLANDS

The **mammary glands** of the breasts develop embryologically as invaginations of surface ectoderm along two ventral lines, the milk lines, from the axillae to the groin. In humans, one set of glands resembling highly modified apocrine sweat glands persists on each side of the chest. Each mammary gland consists of 15–20 **lobes** of the compound tubuloacinar type which secrete nutritive milk for newborns. Each lobe, separated from the others by dense connective tissue and much adipose tissue, represents a separate gland with its own excretory **lactiferous duct** that emerge independently at the **nipple** Figure 22-25). The histologic structure of the mammary glands varies greatly according to sex, age, and physiologic status.

Breast Development During Puberty

Before puberty the mammary glands in both sexes consist only of **lactiferous sinuses** near the nipple, with very small, branching ducts emerging from these sinuses. In girls undergoing puberty, higher levels of circulating estrogens cause the breasts to grow with accumulation of new adipocytes and elongation of the duct system.

In nonpregnant adult women each mammary gland lobe develops many smaller **lobules**, sometimes called **terminal duct lobular units (TDLU)** (Figure 22–25). Each lobule has several branching ducts, but the attached acinar secretory units remain very small and rudimentary. The lactiferous sinuses are lined with stratified cuboidal epithelium, but the lining of the lactiferous ducts and terminal ducts is simple cuboidal epithelium with many myoepithelial cells. Sparse fibers of smooth muscle also encircle the larger ducts. The entire duct system develops within loose, vascular connective tissue, with denser tissue separating the lobes. In the premenstrual phase of the reproductive cycle, connective tissue of the breast becomes somewhat edematous, making the breasts slightly larger.

The **areola**, or skin covering the nipple, is continuous with the mucosa of the lactiferous sinuses and contains sebaceous glands and abundant sensory nerves. The areola keratinocytes have much more melanin than those of adjacent skin and darken further during pregnancy. Connective tissue in the nipple is rich in smooth muscle fibers running parallel to the lactiferous sinuses and making the nipple fully erect when they contract.

Breasts During Pregnancy & Lactation

During pregnancy mammary glands undergo growth due to the synergistic action of several hormones, mainly estrogen, progesterone, prolactin, and the placental lactogen. These cause cell proliferation in the secretory **alveoli** of TDLUs (Figures 22–25 and 22–26). The spherical alveoli consist of cuboidal epithelium, with numerous myoepithelial cells. The degree of glandular development varies among lobules and even within a single lobule.

While the alveoli and duct system grow and develop during pregnancy in preparation for lactation, the stroma becomes less prominent (Figures 22–26 and 22–27). The loose connective tissue within TDLUs becomes infiltrated with lymphocytes and plasma cells, the latter becoming more numerous late in pregnancy.

Late in pregnancy the glandular alveoli and ducts dilate with accumulated **colostrum**, a fluid rich in proteins

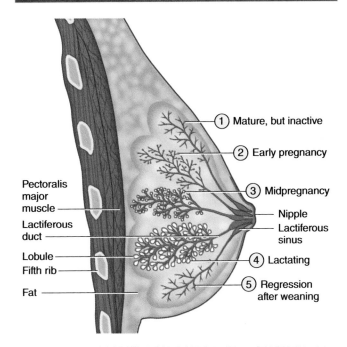

FIGURE 22–25 Mammary gland.

- ① Mature, but inactive
- ② Early pregnancy
- ③ Midpregnancy
- Nipple
- Lactiferous sinus
- ④ Lactating
- ⑤ Regression after weaning

Pectoralis major muscle
Lactiferous duct
Lobule
Fifth rib
Fat

Shown here is the sequence of changes that occur in the **alveolar secretory units**, also known as **terminal duct lobular units or TDLUs**, and the duct system of **mammary glands** before, during, and after pregnancy and lactation.

(1) Before pregnancy, the gland is inactive, with small ducts and only a **few small TDLUs**.

(2) Alveoli develop and begin to grow extensively early in a **pregnancy**.

(3) By the middle of pregnancy the alveoli and ducts have become large and developed dilated lumens.

(4) At **parturition** and during the entire time of **lactation**, the alveoli remain greatly dilated and maximally active in production of all milk components.

(5) After weaning, the TDLUs regress with apoptotic cell death.

produced under the influence of prolactin. The abundant plasma cells secrete IgA antibodies for transfer into colostrum (and into milk for up to 7 months postpartum), conferring passive acquired immunity on the breastfed newborn.

Following parturition, the mammary TDLUs start active milk production, or **lactation**, stimulated primarily by prolactin from the anterior pituitary (see Chapter 20). Epithelial cells of the alveoli enlarge and activate various processes involved in lactation.

- Large amounts of **protein** are synthesized and packaged into secretory vesicles that undergo **merocrine secretion** into the lumen (Figure 22–28). Human milk contains about 1 g of protein per deciliter, including aggregated caseins (44% of the total), as well as soluble α-lactalbumin, epidermal growth factor (EGF), lysozyme, IgA, lactoferrin, all of which are sources of

FIGURE 22–26 Mammary gland alveolar development before, during, and after pregnancy.

(a) The **mammary glands** of **adult, nonpregnant** women are inactive, with **small ducts** and few lobules (**L**) having secretory alveoli that are not well-developed. The structure with the large lumen in each lobule is part of the duct; the smaller structures are the small, undeveloped alveoli. The breasts are composed largely of connective tissue (**CT**), having considerable fat.

(b) The glands become active **during pregnancy**, with the **duct system growing rapidly** and the secretory units of each lobule (**L**) becoming **much larger and more extensively branched**.

Here the connective tissue (**CT**) contains more collagen and adipocytes (**A**) are included, but these are only a small fraction of those present.

(c) During lactation, the **lobules are greatly enlarged** and the lumens of both the numerous glandular alveoli (**A**) and the excretory ducts (**D**) are **filled with milk**. The intralobular connective tissue is sparser and more difficult to see, except for small septa (arrows). (All ×60; H&E)

amino acids for the infant, with the last three also providing antimicrobial activity and EGF promoting gut development in the newborn.

■ **Lipid droplets** form initially from short-chain fatty acids synthesized in the epithelial cells and grow by accretion of longer fatty acids and cholesterol originating from the diet or fat stores. They eventually undergo **apocrine secretion**, during which the droplets become enveloped with a portion of the apical cell membrane (Figure 22–28). Milk contains 4 or 5 g of total fat per deciliter.

■ **Lactose**, the major carbohydrate and energy source in milk, is synthesized by Golgi apparatus enzymes regulated by α-lactalbumin. Human milk contains over 7 g of lactose per deciliter, more than the combined total of proteins and lipids. Lactose also generates the osmotic gradient that draws water and Ca^{2+} into the lumens of TDLUs.

Throughout lactation, secretion of proteins, membrane-bound lipid droplets, lactose, iron, and calcium is ongoing, with the products accumulating as milk in the lumens of the lactiferous ducts and sinuses (Figure 22–27).

>> MEDICAL APPLICATION

When a woman breastfeeds, the nursing action of the child stimulates tactile receptors in the nipple, resulting in liberation of the posterior pituitary hormone **oxytocin**. This hormone not only causes contraction of both the smooth muscle of the lactiferous sinuses and ducts and the myoepithelial cells of TDLUs, resulting in the **milk-ejection reflex**, but also promotes bonding between mother and child. Negative emotional stimuli, such as frustration, anxiety, or anger, can inhibit release of oxytocin and thus prevent the milk-ejection reflex.

Postlactational Regression in the Mammary Glands

When breastfeeding is stopped (weaning), most alveoli that developed during pregnancy and lactation degenerate. Epithelial cells undergo apoptosis, autophagy, or sloughing, with dead cells and debris removed by macrophages. The duct system of the gland returns to its general appearance in the inactive state (Figure 22–25). After menopause, alveoli and ducts of the mammary glands are reduced further in size and there is loss of fibroblasts, adipocytes, collagen, and elastic fibers in the stroma.

FIGURE **22–27** Actively developing and lactating alveoli.

Glandular alveoli develop completely **only during pregnancy** and begin milk production near the end of pregnancy.

(a) Alveoli (**A**) develop as spherical structures composed of cuboidal epithelial cells surrounded by the contractile processes of myoepithelial cells (**M**). **Late in pregnancy lymphocytes** (**L**) leave venules (**V**), accumulate in the intralobular connective tissue, and differentiate as plasma cells (**P**) secreting IgA. Intralobular ducts (**D**) are lined by epithelium containing secretory cells, nonsecretory cells, and plasma cells; larger lumens may show milk (**arrow**). (×400; H&E)

(b) During **lactation,** secretory cells of the mammary gland become more columnar and very active in milk production. Some epithelial cells secrete **milk proteins** by **exocytosis**, while others bulge apically with variously sized **lipid droplets**, which are also visible in the milk (**LD**) having undergone **apocrine secretion**. Connective tissue (**CT**) contains small blood vessels (**V**). Secretory cells in the enclosed area are shown diagrammatically in Figure 22 28. (×400; PT)

FIGURE **22–28** Secretion in the mammary gland.

Alveolar cells in TDLUs of the lactating mammary gland are highly active in **protein synthesis and lipid synthesis**. Most proteins are packaged into secretory vesicles in the Golgi apparatus and secreted at the apical end of the cells by typical **exocytosis or merocrine secretion**. Lipids coalesce as free cytoplasmic droplets and eventually undergo **apocrine secretion**, in which they are extruded from the cell along with a portion of the apical cell membrane (and often a small amount of attached cytoplasm). Both types of secretion are shown here in a sequence moving from left to right.

The alveolar stroma has a very rich **microvasculature** during lactation, providing fluid that undergoes transcytosis into the TDLUs. **Myoepithelial cells** help move secretions from the acini into the TDLU ducts.

Breast cancer almost always originates from epithelial cells in the terminal lobules of the glands. The most common form is invasive **ductal carcinoma** in which neoplastic cells of intralobular ducts or small branches of lactiferous ducts invade the surrounding stroma, forming a fixed, palpable mass. Cell spreading (or metastasizing) from the carcinoma via the circulatory or lymphatic vessels to critical organs such as the lungs or brain is responsible for the mortality associated with breast cancer. If the treatment is

mastectomy, axillary lymph nodes are usually also removed surgically and examined histologically for the presence of metastatic mammary carcinoma cells. Early detection (eg, through self-examination, mammography, ultrasound, and other techniques) and consequent early treatment have significantly reduced the mortality rate.

Bacterial infection of a mammary gland, or acute mastitis, may occur in the lactating or involuting breast, usually after obstruction by milk left within small components of the duct system.

The Female Reproductive System SUMMARY OF KEY POINTS

Ovaries, Follicles, and Oocytes

- The female gonads, the paired **ovaries**, each have an outer **cortex** containing many hundreds of **ovarian follicles** and an inner **medulla** of dense connective tissue and large blood vessels.
- The ovary's cortex is covered by a cuboidal mesothelium, the **surface epithelium** (or germinal epithelium) that overlies a layer of connective tissue, the **tunica albuginea**.
- Before puberty, all follicles are **primordial follicles**, formed in the developing fetal gonad, with each having one **primary oocyte** arrested in **meiotic prophase I** and a surrounding layer of squamous **follicular epithelial cells**.
- After puberty, some primordial follicles develop each month as growing **primary follicles**, with an enlarging primary oocyte surrounded by larger epithelial cells now called **granulosa cells**.
- During follicular growth, the **granulosa cells**, surrounded by a basement membrane, become stratified and actively engage in fluid secretion and steroid hormone metabolism.
- Between the oocyte and the granulosa cells, a thin layer forms called the **zona pellucida**, which contains glycoproteins (**ZO proteins**) to which the sperm surface must bind to reach the oocyte at fertilization.
- **Antral** or **vesicular follicles** are larger than younger primary follicles, but still avascular, and have developed fluid-filled spaces among their granulosa cells, but the growing oocyte remains in prophase I.
- While the primary follicle grows, mesenchymal cells immediately around it form the highly vascular layer, the **theca interna**, and a more fibrous **theca externa** with smooth muscle cells.
- Endocrine cells of the **theca interna** secrete both **progesterone** and estrogen precursors, which are converted by **granulosa cells** into **estrogen**.
- Antral follicles continue developing as **mature, graafian follicles**, which have a large antrum filled with fluid, with the large primary oocyte enclosed by granulosa cells of the **cumulus oophorus**.
- Each month only one graafian follicle becomes a **dominant follicle** and undergoes **ovulation**; most other developing follicles arrest and degenerate with apoptosis in a process called **atresia**.

Ovulation and the Corpus Luteum

- **Ovulation** involves movement of a very large, dominant graafian follicle to the ovary surface to form a bulge, completion of meiosis I, and release of a **polar body** from the oocyte.
- Rupture of the follicle and ovarian coverings releases the **secondary oocyte**, arrested now in **metaphase II**, and a layer of attached granulosa cells that make up the **corona radiata**.
- Cells of the granulosa and thecal layers left in the ovary after ovulation reorganize under the influence of **LH** to form the endocrine gland called the **corpus luteum**.

- The cells of the **corpus luteum** are **granulosa lutein cells**, producing estrogen and comprising 80% of the gland, and **theca lutein cells** producing progesterone.
- LH levels drop about 2 weeks after ovulation, causing the **corpus luteum** to lose activity, degenerate, and be removed by macrophages, leaving a temporary collagen-filled region called a **corpus albicans**.

Uterine Tubes or Oviducts

- The **ovulated secondary oocyte** is swept into the large open **infundibulum** of the **uterine tube**, or **oviduct**, and enters that organ's **ampulla** region where it degenerates if it is not fertilized.
- **Fertilization** involves **sperm capacitation** in the oviduct, **acrosomal activation**, and sperm penetration of the corona radiata, and the following events at the oocyte surface:
  - Surface ligands on one sperm first attach to **zona pellucida** proteins around the oocyte, allowing penetration.
  - **Cortical granules** of the oocyte undergo exocytosis, releasing proteases that convert the zona pellucida to the **vitelline barrier** that prevents **polyspermic fertilization**.
  - The oocyte only now completes meiosis II, producing the second **polar body** and the female pronucleus of the haploid **ovum**.
  - The **female pronucleus** and the **male pronucleus** from the sperm fuse, yielding a diploid cell, the **zygote**.
- The **oviduct mucosa** becomes **highly folded** in the ampulla region, lined by **simple columnar epithelium** with **ciliated cells** and **secretory cells** producing nutritive mucus bathing sperm (and zygote).
- The thick oviduct **muscularis**, organized for peristaltic contractions of the tube, provides the main activity moving the developing embryo to the **uterus**.

Uterus

- The **uterine mucosa** or **endometrium** is lined by **simple columnar epithelium**, from which numerous large **uterine glands** extend into underlying connective tissue.
- This connective tissue is vascular, lacks fat, and consists of a highly cellular **basal layer** next to the uterine muscularis or **myometrium**, and a more superficial **functional layer**.
- Changing levels of estrogen and progesterone from the **ovarian follicles** and **corpus luteum** produce cyclic changes in the thickness, glandular activity, and vascular status of the endometrial **functional layer**.
- A **blastocyst** stage embryo arriving in the uterus attaches to the endometrial surface and implants itself into the **functional layer** when that layer's secretory activity and vascular supply are maximal.
- If no embryo implants, degeneration of the **corpus luteum** causes collapse of the progesterone-dependent **spiral arteries** that bring blood to the **functional layer**.
- Spiral artery degeneration produces ischemia in the **functional layer**, causing this layer to be sloughed off during **menses**, after which it regenerates from the **basal layer** under the influence of estrogen.

- The **placenta** consists mainly of **chorionic villi**, which form as highly vascularized projections of the extraembryonic **trophoblast** into the **vascular lacunae** of the endometrium.
- **Placental exchange** of nutrients, wastes, O_2, and CO_2 occurs between **fetal blood** in the **chorionic villi** and **maternal blood** bathing the villi in the **lacunae**.

Cervix, Vagina, and Mammary Glands

- The mucosa of the narrow, inferior end of the uterus, the **cervix**, does not change cyclically under hormone influence; at its **external os**, columnar epithelium changes abruptly to stratified squamous.

- The mucosa of the **vagina** and the **external genitalia (vulva)** is covered by **stratified squamous epithelium** and is rich in sensory receptors, with a muscularis best-developed in the vagina.
- In the **mammary glands**, **alveolar secretory units** develop after puberty on a branching duct system with **lactiferous sinuses** converging at the **nipple**.
- **Milk secretion** (lactation), which begins in late pregnancy and continues until weaning, involves both protein exocytosis and apocrine secretion of lipid droplets.

The Female Reproductive System ASSESS YOUR KNOWLEDGE

1. Which stage of ovarian follicle development is characterized by an initial period of follicular fluid accumulation?
   a. Graafian follicle
   b. Mature follicle
   c. Primordial follicle
   d. Oocyte
   e. Secondary follicle

2. Which of the following is characteristic of granulosa lutein cells?
   a. Are a minor cell type in the corpus luteum
   b. Derive from the theca interna
   c. Contain abundant rough endoplasmic reticulum
   d. Are small and dark-staining
   e. Secrete progesterone

3. Which of the following hormones is primarily responsible for inducing ovulation?
   a. Relaxin
   b. LH
   c. Progesterone
   d. FSH
   e. Estrogen

4. Which feature is characteristic of the corpora albicans but not of atretic follicles?
   a. May contain degenerating granulosa cells floating in remnants of follicular fluid
   b. Resemble large collagenous scars
   c. Eventually removed by macrophages and replaced by stroma
   d. Are remnants of follicles that degenerate before maturation
   e. May contain degenerating oocytes

5. Endometrial glands are typically most fully developed and filled with product during which day(s) or phase of a woman's menstrual cycle?
   a. Menstrual phase
   b. Days 1–4
   c. The day ovulation occurs
   d. Proliferative phase
   e. Days 15–28

6. Which feature is characteristic of the endometrium's basal layer but not of its functional layer?
   a. Includes the uterine surface epithelium
   b. Includes connective tissue
   c. Contains cells that replace the surface epithelium after menstruation
   d. Relies solely on spiral arteries for its blood supply
   e. Undergoes cyclic thickening and shedding

7. Most lipid in milk is released from cells by which mechanism?
   a. Apocrine secretion
   b. Paracrine secretion
   c. Holocrine secretion
   d. Merocrine secretion
   e. Autocrine secretion

8. A 33-year-old woman with an average menstrual cycle of 28 days comes in for a routine Pap smear. It has been 35 days since the start of her last menstrual period, and a vaginal smear reveals clumps of basophilic cells. As her physician, you suspect which of the following?
   a. She will begin menstruating in a few days.
   b. She will ovulate within a few days.
   c. Her serum progesterone levels will be found to be very low.
   d. There will be detectable levels of hCG in her serum and urine.
   e. She is undergoing early menopause.

9. A 17-year-old girl with a history of pelvic inflammatory disease presents at the emergency department with severe pain in her lower right side that came on fairly quickly. Upon questioning, she replies that her last menstrual period was 6 weeks ago and that she has never missed a period before. The doctor suspects she has an ectopic pregnancy and this is quickly confirmed by ultrasound testing. The surgeon removes her right uterine tube that is inflamed, scarified, and contains the implanted embryonic tissue in the region where fertilization normally occurs. Where is this?
   a. The uterine part of the oviduct
   b. The ampulla region with highly folded mucosa
   c. The only oviduct region attached to the mesosalpinx
   d. The infundibulum region with fimbriae
   e. The isthmus region

10. A 42-year-old woman visits her physician complaining of recurrent vaginal yeast infections. The doctor explains the likelihood that the woman's vaginal lining is temporarily out of proper acid-base balance, leading to the increased susceptibility to yeast infections. The normally low pH in the vagina is maintained by which of the following?
    a. A proton pump in the epithelial cells similar to that in osteoclasts and parietal cells
    b. Secretions derived from intracellular carbonic acid
    c. Secretion of lactic acid by cells of the stratified squamous epithelium
    d. Bacterial metabolism of glycogen to produce an organic acid
    e. Synthesis and accumulation of acid hydrolases in the epithelium

Answers: 1e, 2e, 3b, 4b, 5e, 6c, 7a, 8d, 9b, 10d

23 The Eye & Ear: Special Sense Organs

Sensory receptors convey information about the external world to the brain. Chemoreceptive cells for the senses of taste and smell were discussed with the digestive and respiratory system (Chapters 15 and 17, respectively) and various mechanoreceptors mediating the sense of touch were presented with the skin (Chapter 18). This chapter describes the eye, both its photoreceptors and auxiliary structures, and the ear, which mediates both the sense of equilibrium and hearing via mechanoreceptors in the vestibulocochlear apparatus.

› EYES: THE PHOTORECEPTOR SYSTEM

Eyes (Figure 23–1) provide the sense of sight, having developed as highly sensitive organs for analyzing the form, intensity, and color of light reflected from objects. Protected by adipose cushions within the orbits of the skull, each eyeball consists externally of a tough, fibrous globe, which maintains an eye's overall shape. Internally the eye contains transparent tissues that refract light to focus the image, a layer of photosensitive cells, and a system of neurons that collect, process, and transmit visual information to the brain.

As indicated in Table 23–1, an eye has three concentric tunics or layers:

- A tough external **fibrous layer** consisting of the **sclera** and the transparent **cornea**;
- A middle **vascular layer** consisting of the **choroid, ciliary body**, and **iris**; and
- An inner sensory layer, the **retina**, which communicates with the cerebrum through the posterior **optic nerve** (Figure 23–1).

Not part of these layers, the **lens** represents a perfectly transparent biconvex structure held in place by a circular system of **zonular fibers** that attach it to the thick region of the middle layer, the **ciliary body**, and by close apposition, to the posterior vitreous body (Figure 23–1). Partly covering the anterior surface of the lens, the **iris** develops as an opaque pigmented extension of the middle layer which surrounds a central opening, the **pupil** (Figure 23–1).

Located in the anterior portion of the eye, the iris and lens are bathed in clear **aqueous humor** filling both the **anterior chamber** between the cornea and iris and the **posterior chamber** between the iris and lens (Figure 23–1). Aqueous humor flows through the pupil that connects these two chambers.

The posterior **vitreous chamber**, surrounded by the retina, lies behind the lens and its zonular fibers and contains a large gelatinous mass of transparent connective tissue called the **vitreous body**.

Figure 23–2 depicts important aspects of eye formation in the embryo, including the following:

- In the 4-week embryo epithelial **optic vesicles** bulge bilaterally from the forebrain, then elongate as the optic stalks bearing the **optic cups** (Figure 23–2a).
- Inductive interactions between an optic cup and the overlying surface ectoderm cause the latter to invaginate and eventually detach as the initially hollow **lens vesicle** (Figure 23–2b).
- The optic stalk develops as the **optic nerve** and in an inferior groove called the **choroid fissure** encloses the **hyaloid vessels**, which supply blood for the developing lens and optic cup (Figure 23–2c).
- In the ensuing weeks, head mesenchyme differentiates to form most of the tissue in the eye's two outer layers and the vitreous. Ectoderm of the optic cup differentiates as the retina and surface ectoderm forms the corneal epithelium (Figure 23–2d). When the lens is fully formed,

FIGURE 23–1 Internal anatomy of the eye.

A schematic hemisected **eye** shows the interrelationships among the major ocular structures, the **three major layers** or tunics of the posterior wall (**sclera**, **choroid**, and **retina**), important regions within those layers, and the **refractive elements** (**cornea**, **lens**, and **vitreous**). Note that the art depicts most components in three dimensions to better explain their interrelationships. For example, the large, scalloped structure at the anterior portion of the **vitreous chamber** is the **ciliary body**, whose parts are labeled in section at the upper right. The **ora serrata** represents the anterior boundary of the **retina**.

the distal hyaloid artery and vein disappear, leaving only the blood supply to the retina.

Fibrous Layer

This layer includes two major regions, the posterior **sclera** and the anterior **cornea**, joined at the **limbus**.

Sclera

The fibrous, external layer of the eyeball protects the more delicate internal structures and provides sites for muscle insertion (see Table 23–1). The posterior five-sixths of this layer is the **sclera** (Figure 23–1), which encloses a portion of the adult eyeball about 22 mm in diameter. The opaque, whitish sclera averages 0.5 mm in thickness and consists mainly of dense connective tissue, with flat bundles of type I collagen parallel to the organ surface but intersecting in various directions. Microvasculature occurs mainly near the outer surface, or episclera.

Tendons of **extraocular muscles** which move the eyes insert into the anterior region of the sclera. Posteriorly the sclera thickens to approximately 1 mm and joins with the epineurium covering the optic nerve. Where it surrounds the choroid, the sclera includes an inner suprachoroid lamina, with less collagen, more fibroblasts, elastic fibers, and melanocytes.

Cornea

In contrast to the sclera, the anterior one-sixth of the eye—the **cornea**—is transparent and completely avascular (Figure 23–1). A section of the cornea shows five distinct layers:

- An external **corneal epithelium**, consisting of a stratified squamous epithelium;
- A thick **anterior limiting membrane (Bowman membrane)**, the basement membrane beneath the corneal epithelium;
- The thick **stroma**;
- A **posterior limiting membrane (Descemet membrane)**, the basement membrane of the endothelium; and
- An inner, simple squamous **endothelium**.

TABLE 23–1	Tunics of the eye.		
	Structures	**Components**	**Function**
Fibrous Tunic (External Layer)			
	Sclera	Dense irregular connective tissue	Supports eye shape
			Protects delicate internal structures
			Extrinsic eye muscle attachment site
	Cornea	Two layers of epithelium with organized connective tissue in between	Protects anterior surface of the eye
			Refracts (bends) incoming light
Vascular Tunic or Uvea (Middle Layer)			
	Choroid	Areolar connective tissue; highly vascularized	Supplies nourishment to retina
			Pigment absorbs extraneous light
	Ciliary body	Ciliary smooth muscle and ciliary processes; covered with a secretory epithelium	Holds suspensory ligaments that attach to the lens and change lens shape for far and near vision
			Epithelium secretes aqueous humor
	Iris	Two layers of smooth muscle (sphincter pupillae and dilator pupillae) and connective tissue, with a central pupil	Controls pupil diameter and thus the amount of light entering the eye
Retina (Internal Layer)			
	Pigmented layer	Pigmented epithelial cells	Absorbs extraneous light
			Provides vitamin A for photoreceptor cells
	Neural layer	Photoreceptors, bipolar neurons, ganglion cells, and supporting Müller cells	Detects incoming light rays; light rays are converted to nerve signals and transmitted to the brain

Diagram labels:
Fibrous tunic — Sclera, Cornea
Vascular tunic — Iris, Ciliary body, Choroid
Retina — Pigmented layer, Neural layer

The **corneal epithelium** is nonkeratinized, five or six cell layers thick, and comprises about 10% of the corneal thickness (Figure 23–3). The basal cells have a high proliferative capacity important for renewal and repair of the corneal surface and emerge from stem cells in the **corneoscleral limbus** that encircles the cornea. The flattened surface cells have microvilli protruding into a protective tear film of lipid, glycoprotein, and water. As another protective adaptation, the corneal epithelium also has one of the richest sensory nerve supplies of any tissue.

The basement membrane of this epithelium, often called **Bowman membrane**, develops considerable thickness (8–10 μm) and contributes to the stability and strength of the cornea, helping to protect against infection of the underlying stroma.

The **stroma**, or substantia propria, makes up 90% of the cornea's thickness and consists of approximately 60 layers of parallel collagen bundles aligned at approximately right angles to each other and extending almost the full diameter of the cornea. The uniform orthogonal arrays of collagen fibrils contribute to the transparency of this avascular tissue. Between the collagen, lamellae are cytoplasmic extensions of flattened fibroblast-like cells called **keratocytes** (Figure 23–3). The ground substance around these cells contains proteoglycans such as lumican, bearing keratan sulfate and chondroitin sulfate sidechains, which help maintain the precise organization and spacing of the collagen fibrils.

❯❯ MEDICAL APPLICATION

The shape or curvature of the cornea can be changed surgically to improve certain visual abnormalities involving the ability to focus. In the common ophthalmologic procedure, laser-assisted in-situ keratomileusis (LASIK) surgery, the corneal epithelium is displaced as a flap and the stroma reshaped by an excimer laser which vaporizes collagen and keratocytes in a highly controlled manner with no damage to adjacent cells or ECM. After reshaping the stroma, the epithelial flap is repositioned, and a relatively rapid regenerative response reestablishes normal corneal physiology.

FIGURE 23–2 Development of eye.

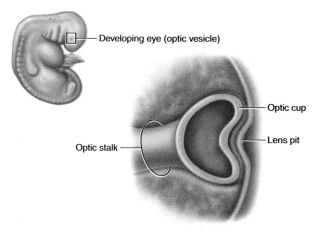

(a) Early week 4: Optic vesicle forms a two-layered optic cup; overlying ectoderm forms a lens pit.

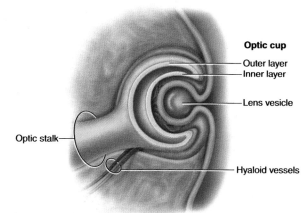

(b) Late week 4: Optic cup deepens and forms inner and outer layers; lens pit forms lens vesicle.

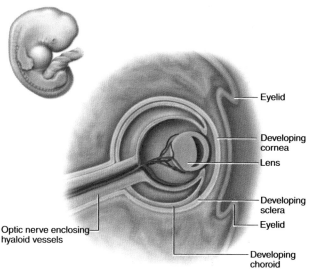

(c) Week 6: Lens becomes an internal structure; corneas, sclera, and choroid start to form.

(d) Week 20: Three tunics of the eye have formed.

Eyes begin to form early in development as the two **optic vesicles** bulge bilaterally from the **forebrain** (prosencephalon). These grow, remaining connected to the developing brain by the **optic stalks**, and approach the surface ectoderm. At this point, each vesicle folds in on itself to form the inner and outer layers of the **optic cup** and inducing surface ectoderm to invaginate into the cup as the **lens vesicle**, which soon detaches from the surface and lies in the opening of the optic cup.

Blood vessels, called the **hyaloid vessels**, grow along the optic stalk, enter the optic cup, and grow toward the developing lens.

Head mesenchyme associates with the developing optic cup as it forms the two major layers of the **retina**. The mesenchymal cells differentiate around the pigmented layer of the developing retina as the **iris**, **ciliary body** and **choroid** of the vascular layer, and as the more external fibrous layer. The hyaloid vessels regress, leaving a space called the **hyaloid canal**, in the vitreous body. Folds of skin develop features of the eyelids and **conjunctiva**, the latter developing in continuity with the surface epithelium of the **cornea** and **sclera**.

LASIK surgery is used to correct myopia (near-sightedness), hyperopia (far-sightedness), or astigmatism (irregular curvature of the cornea). Corneal grafts (transplants) between unrelated individuals can usually be accomplished successfully

without immune rejection due in part to this tissue's lack of both a vascular supply and lymphatic drainage and to local immune tolerance produced by ocular antigen-presenting cells and immunomodulatory factors in aqueous humor.

FIGURE 23–3 Cornea.

The most anterior structure of the eye, the **cornea** has five layers, counting two prominent **basement membranes**.

(a) The external stratified squamous epithelium (**E**) is nonkeratinized, five or six cells thick, and densely supplied with sensory-free nerve endings that trigger the blinking reflex. The stroma (**S**) comprises approximately 90% of the cornea's thickness, consisting of some 60 layers of long type I collagen fibers arranged in a precise orthogonal array and alternating with flattened cells called **keratocytes**. The **stroma** is lined internally by endothelium (**EN**). (×100; H&E)

(b) The corneal epithelium (**E**) attaches to the thick homogeneous Bowman's membrane (**B**). The stroma (**S**) is completely avascular, and nutrients reach keratocytes by diffusion from the surrounding **limbus** and **aqueous humor** behind the cornea. (×400; H&E)

(c) The posterior surface of the **cornea** is covered by simple squamous epithelium (**EN**) that rests on another thick layer called Descemet membrane (**D**) adjacent to the stroma (**S**). (×400; H&E)

The posterior surface of the stroma involves another thick basement membrane, called **Descemet membrane**, which supports the internal simple squamous endothelium (Figure 23–3).

This **corneal endothelium** maintains Descemet membrane and includes the most metabolically active cells of the cornea. Na⁺/K⁺ ATPase pumps in the basolateral membranes of these cells are largely responsible for regulating the proper hydration state of the corneal stroma, highly important for maximal transparency and optimal light refraction.

Limbus

Encircling the cornea, the **limbus** forms a transitional area where the transparent cornea merges with the opaque sclera (Figures 23–1 and 23–4). Here the thickened Bowman membrane ends, and the surface epithelium becomes more stratified as the **conjunctiva** that covers the anterior part of the

sclera (and lines the eyelids). Epithelial stem cells located in the limbus give rise to rapidly dividing progenitor cells, which then move centripetally into the corneal epithelium. The stroma becomes less well-organized and vascularized at the limbus, as the collagen bundles merge with those of the sclera.

Also at the limbus, the Descemet membrane and its simple endothelium are replaced by a **trabecular meshwork** (Figure 23–5), a loose, collagenous network of small, irregular channels lined by specialized endothelial cells promoting slow, continuous filtration and drainage of aqueous humor from the anterior chamber. This fluid moves from these channels into the adjacent larger space of the **scleral venous sinus**, or **canal of Schlemm** (Figures 23–1, 23–4, and 23–5), which encircles the anterior eye. From this sinus, aqueous humor drains into small blood vessels (veins) of the sclera.

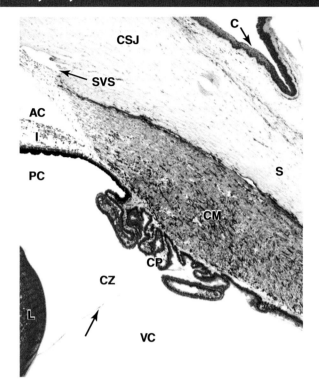

FIGURE 23–4 Corneoscleral junction (limbus) and ciliary body.

At the circumference of the cornea is the **limbus** or corneoscleral junction (**CSJ**), where the transparent corneal stroma merges with the opaque, vascular sclera (**S**). The epithelium of the limbus is slightly thicker than the corneal epithelium, containing stem cells for the latter, and is continuous with the conjunctiva (**C**) covering the anterior sclera and lining the eyelids. The stroma of the **limbus** contains the scleral venous sinus (**SVS**), or **canal of Schlemm**, which receives **aqueous humor** from an adjacent **trabecular meshwork** at the surface of the anterior chamber (**AC**).

Internal to the limbus, the middle layer of the eye consists of the **ciliary body** and its anterior extension, the iris (**I**). The thick ring of the ciliary body includes loose connective tissue containing melanocytes, highly organized fibers of smooth ciliary muscle (**CM**), numerous extensions called ciliary processes (**CP**) at its surface covered by a bilaminar epithelium, and the ciliary zonule (**CZ**), a system of fibrillin-rich microfibrils that attach to the capsule of the lens (**L**) in the center of the ciliary body. Pieces of one **zonular fiber** can be seen (**arrow**). Projecting into the posterior chamber (**PC**), the **ciliary processes** produce **aqueous humor**, which then flows into the **anterior chamber** through the **pupil**. Behind the ciliary zonule and lens, a thin, transparent membrane (not shown) surrounds the vitreous body and separates the **posterior chamber** from the vitreous chamber (**VC**). (×12.5; H&E)

Vascular Layer

The eye's more **vascular middle layer**, known as the **uvea**, comprises three parts, from posterior to anterior: the **choroid**, which lines the sclera, the **ciliary body**, and the **iris** (Table 23–1).

Choroid

Located in the posterior two-thirds of the eye between the sclera and retina, the **choroid** consists of well-vascularized connective tissue with numerous large, flattened melanocytes (Figure 23–6). These form a characteristic heavily pigmented choroidal layer that blocks very bright light that may penetrate the sclera. Two main layers make up the choroid (Figure 23–6):

- The inner **choroidocapillary lamina** has a rich microvasculature important for nutrition of the neighboring retinal layers, and
- A basal complex usually called **Bruch's membrane**, comprising a layer of elastin sandwiched between two thinner sheets of collagen fibers continuous with the basement membranes of both the capillaries of the inner lamina and the retinal epithelium.

Ciliary Body

The **ciliary body**, the anterior expansion of the uvea that encircles the lens, lies posterior to the limbus (Figures 23–1 and 23–4). Like the choroid, most of the ciliary body rests on the sclera. Two simple cuboidal epithelia, derived from the inner and outer layers of embryonic optic cup (Figure 23–2), comprise a bilaminar cover for the ciliary body. Important features associated with the well-vascularized ciliary body include the following.

- **Ciliary muscle** makes up most of the ciliary body's stroma and consists of smooth muscle fibers developing in three complementary orientations. Importantly, contracting and relaxing these muscle fibers changes the shape of the lens, regulating its focal plane (see below).
- **Ciliary processes** comprise a radially arranged series of about 75 ridges extending from the inner highly vascular region of the ciliary body. These provide a large surface area covered by the bilaminar ciliary epithelium (Figure 23–7). The epithelial cells on a basement membrane directly over the stroma contain much melanin and correspond to the anterior extension of the pigmented retina epithelium. The superficial cell layer lacks pigment and has continuity with the retina's sensory layer.
- Cells of this dual epithelium become specialized for secretion of **aqueous humor**, having extensive basolateral folds with Na^+/K^+-ATPase activity. Fluid from the stromal microvasculature moves across this epithelium as aqueous humor, with an inorganic ion composition like that of plasma but almost no protein. As shown in Figure 23–8, aqueous humor is secreted by ciliary processes into the posterior chamber, flows through the pupil into the anterior chamber, and drains at the angle formed by the cornea and the iris into the channels of the trabecular meshwork and the scleral venous sinus, from which it enters venules of the sclera.
- The **ciliary zonule** represents a system of many radially oriented fibrillin microfibrils produced by the superficial, nonpigmented ciliary epithelial cells. The microfibrils extend from between the ciliary processes and attach to the surface of the lens, serving as the suspensory ligament for that structure (Figures 23–8 and 23–9).

FIGURE **23–5** Trabecular meshwork and scleral venous sinus.

(a) The **limbus**, or corneoscleral junction (**CSJ**), encircles the cornea, and here the posterior endothelium is replaced by an extensive trabecular meshwork (**TM**). This is a network of small, irregular channels lined by variously specialized endothelial cells supported by trabeculae of connective tissue continuous with that of muscle in the ciliary body (**CB**). At the iridocorneal (filtration) angle between the limbus and iris (**I**), **aqueous humor** moves from the anterior chamber (**AC**) into this meshwork where it is filtered and transported to the adjacent scleral venous sinus (**SVS**) by actions of the lining endothelial cells. (×50; H&E)

(b) In a surface view of the tissues covering the **scleral venous sinus**, scanning electron microscopy better reveals the transition from the posterior corneal endothelium (**CE**) surface to the endothelial cell-lined collagenous channels of the trabecular meshwork (**TM**). (×300)

(Figure 23–5b reproduced with permission from Prof. Piera Versura, Laboratory of Ocular Surface Analysis and Translational Research, Alma Mater Studiorum University of Bologna, Italy.)

❯❯ MEDICAL APPLICATION

Aqueous humor is produced continuously. If its drainage from the anterior chamber is impeded, typically by obstruction of the trabecular meshwork or scleral venous sinus, intraocular pressure can increase, causing the condition called **glaucoma**. Untreated glaucoma can cause pressing of the vitreous body against the retina, affecting visual function and possibly leading to neuropathy in that tissue.

When the iridocorneal angle is more narrow than usual, the thickening of the peripheral iris that occurs with dilation of the pupil can occlude the angle and obstruct drainage of aqueous humor at the trabecular meshwork. This can result in the rapid development of intraocular hypertension known as **angle closure glaucoma**, **acute glaucoma**, or **closed (narrow) angle glaucoma**. This condition usually affects both eyes and causes blurred vision, eye pain, and headache. Treatment of this type of glaucoma usually includes some form of surgical intervention.

Iris

The **iris** is the most anterior extension of the middle uveal layer and covers part of the lens, leaving a round central opening, the **pupil** (Figure 23–1). The anterior surface of the iris, exposed to aqueous humor in the anterior chamber, consists of a dense layer of fibroblasts and melanocytes with interdigitating processes and is unusual for its lack of an epithelial covering (Figure 23–10). Deeper in the iris the stroma consists of loose connective tissue with melanocytes and sparse microvasculature.

The posterior surface of the iris has a bilaminar epithelium continuous with that covering the ciliary body, but here both epithelia contain melanin. The highly pigmented posterior epithelium of the iris blocks all light from entering the eye except that passing through the pupil. The less-pigmented layer adjacent to the stroma consists of myoepithelial cells, which extend contractile processes radially to comprise the very thin **dilator pupillae muscle** (Figure 23–10). In contrast, smooth muscle fibers form a circular bundle near the pupil as the **sphincter**

FIGURE **23–6** Sclera, choroid, and retina.

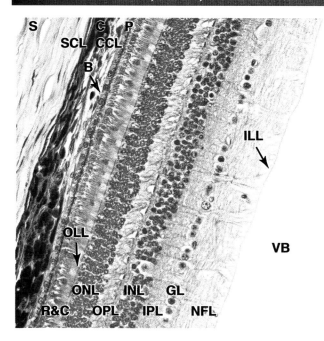

The **lateral wall** of an eye includes dense connective tissue of the sclera (**S**) and the loose, vascular connective tissue of the choroid (**C**). **Melanocytes** are prominent in the **choroid**, especially in its outer region, the suprachoroidal lamina (**SCL**). The choroid's inner region, the choroidocapillary lamina (**CCL**), has a rich **microvasculature** that helps provide O₂ and nutrients to the adjacent **retina**. Between the **choroid** and the **retina** is a thin layer of extracellular material known as Bruch's membrane or layer (**B**).

The outer layer of the retina is the pigmented layer (**P**) of **cuboidal epithelium** containing **melanin**. Adjacent to this are the packed **photoreceptor components** of the rods and cones (**R&C**), whose cell bodies make up the outer nuclear layer (**ONL**). **Junctional complexes** between these cells and glia are aligned and can be seen as a thin line called the outer limiting layer (**OLL**). **Axons** of the rods and cones extend into the outer plexiform layer (**OPL**) forming synapses there with **dendrites** of the **neurons** in the inner nuclear layer (**INL**). These neurons send axons into the inner plexiform layer (**IPL**), where they synapse with dendrites of cells in the ganglionic layer (**GL**). Axons from these cells fill most of the **NFL**, which is separated by the inner limiting layer (**ILL**) from the gelatin-like connective tissue of the vitreous body (**VB**). (×200; H&E)

FIGURE **23–7** Epithelium of ciliary processes.

The **bilaminar epithelium** covering the **ciliary processes** consists of two simple cuboidal epithelia: one heavily pigmented (**PE**) and adjacent to the stroma, and one nonpigmented (**NE**) and superficial. The two epithelia derive developmentally from the folded rim of the **embryonic optic cup**, so that the exposed side of the nonpigmented layer represents the cells' basal surface. No true basal lamina is present, but instead these cells produce the components that give rise to the **microfibrils** of the **ciliary zonule** in the embryo. Beneath the double epithelium is a core of connective tissue with many small blood vessels (**V**). Fluid from these vessels is pumped by the epithelial cells out of the ciliary processes as **aqueous humor**. (×200; PT)

Lens

The lens develops as a transparent, biconvex structure suspended immediately behind the iris, which focuses light on the retina (Figure 23–1). Derived from an invagination of the embryonic surface ectoderm (Figure 23–2), the lens consists of unique avascular tissue with an elastic property that normally decreases with age. The lens has three principal components:

- A very thick (10–20 μm), homogeneous lens capsule composed of proteoglycans and type IV collagen surrounds the lens (Figure 23–11). Originating as the basement membrane of the invaginating lens vesicle, the capsule provides the place of attachment for the microfibrils of the ciliary zonule (Figure 23–9b).
- A subcapsular lens epithelium consists of a single layer of cuboidal cells present only on the anterior surface of the lens (Figure 23–11). The epithelial cells attach basally to the lens capsule and their apical surfaces bind to the internal lens fibers. At the posterior edge of this epithelium, near the equator of the lens, the epithelial

pupillae muscle. The dilator and sphincter muscles of the iris have sympathetic and parasympathetic innervation respectively for enlarging and constricting the pupil.

Melanocytes of the iris stroma are major determinants of eye color. In individuals with few slightly pigmented cells in the stroma, light with a blue color is reflected from the black pigmented epithelium on the posterior iris surface. Eye color ranges from green to brown as the number of melanocytes and density of melanin or other components increase in the iris stroma. Individuals with albinism lack iris pigment almost completely in both the stroma and epithelium; their pink eye color results from light reflection by blood vessels of the iris and retina.

FIGURE 23–8 Production and removal of aqueous humor.

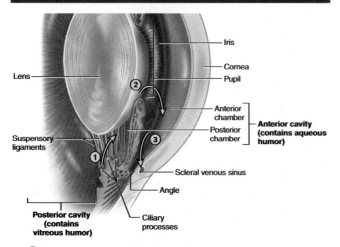

(1) Aqueous humor is secreted by the ciliary processes into the posterior chamber.

(2) Aqueous humor moves from the posterior chamber, through the pupil, to the anterior chamber.

(3) Excess aqueous humor is resorbed via the scleral venous sinus.

A slow, continuous flow of **aqueous humor** carries metabolites to and from cells around the **anterior cavity** of the eye and helps maintain an optimally refractile microenvironment for the cornea and lens. As shown here, aqueous humor is released from **ciliary processes** into the **posterior chamber** of the anterior cavity, flows into the **anterior chamber** of that cavity through the **pupil**, and drains into the **scleral venous sinus (canal of Schlemm)**.

FIGURE 23–9 Ciliary zonule fibers.

The structure of the **ciliary zonule** is best studied by SEM.
(a) The surface of the ciliary body **(CB)** has projecting **ciliary processes**, between which emerge delicate zonular fibrils **(ZF)**. An array of these microfibrils constitutes the **zonule** that anchors the **lens** in the center of the **ciliary body**. (×400)

(b) At the **lens** the bundled zonular fibrils **(ZF)** subdivide and fuse tangentially with the fibrous ECM of the lens capsule **(LC)**. (×500)

(Figure 23-9a,b, reproduced with permission from Prof. Piera Versura, Laboratory of Ocular Surface Analysis and Translational Research, Alma Mater Studiorum University of Bologna, Italy.)

cells divide to provide new cells, which differentiate as lens fibers. This process allows for growth of the lens and continues at a slow, decreasing rate throughout life.

▪ **Lens fibers** represent highly elongated cells, terminally differentiated as thin, flattened structures (Figure 23–11). Developing from lens epithelial cells, lens fibers typically become 7–10 mm long, with 2 by 8 μm cross-section dimensions. The cytoplasm becomes filled with a group of proteins called **crystallins**, followed by autophagy of the fiber's organelles and nucleus. Packed tightly together, lens fibers comprise a perfectly transparent tissue highly specialized for light refraction.

The microfibrils at its capsule suspend the lens centrally within the **ciliary zonule** (Figures 23–1 and 23–12). Together with the ciliary muscles, this structure allows the process of visual **accommodation**, which permits focusing on objects at any distance by changing the curvature of the lens (Figure 23–12). When the eye is at rest or gazing at distant objects, ciliary muscles relax and change the form of the ciliary body, putting tension on the zonule and pulling the lens into a flatter shape. To focus on a close object the ciliary muscles contract, causing forward displacement of the ciliary body, which relieves some of the tension on the zonule and allows the lens to return to a more rounded shape and keep the object in focus. In the fourth decade of life **presbyopia**

(Gr. *presbyter*, elder + L. *opticus*, relating to eyes) normally causes the lenses to lose elasticity, decreasing their ability to undergo accommodation.

›› MEDICAL APPLICATION

Presbyopia is corrected by wearing glasses with convex lenses (reading glasses). In older individuals, denaturation of crystallins commonly begins to occur in lens fibers, making them less transparent. When areas of the lens become opaque or cloudy and vision is impaired, the condition is termed a **cataract**. Causes of cataract include excessive exposure to ultraviolet light or other radiation, trauma, and as secondary effects in diseases such as diabetes mellitus and hypertension.

In modern cataract surgery, the lens is removed by aspiration of the lens substance while it is emulsified by a vibrating probe. The posterior side of the lens capsule and its inserted zonular fibers are left in place at the posterior chamber. The concave posterior capsule, or capsular bag, is then used as the site for implantation of an acrylic intraocular lens (IOL) prosthesis. Research is underway to develop IOLs capable of natural accommodation.

FIGURE **23–10** Iris.

The **iris** regulates the amount of light to which the **retina** is exposed. **(a)** The low-power micrograph shows a section of the **central iris**, near the pupil (**P**). The **anterior surface**, exposed to aqueous humor in the anterior chamber (**AC**), has **no epithelium** and consists only of a matted layer of interdigitating fibroblasts and melanocytes. Cells of the external pigmented epithelium (**PE**) are very rich in **melanin granules** to protect the eye's interior from an excess of light. Cells of the other layer are **myoepithelial**, less heavily pigmented, and comprise the dilator pupillae muscle (**DPM**) that extends along most of the iris. Near the pupil, fascicles of **smooth muscle** make up the sphincter pupillae muscle (**SPM**).

The underlying stroma (**S**) contains many **melanocytes** with varying amounts of melanin. (×140; H&E)

(b) SEM reveals the dense layer of **stromal fibroblasts**, not epithelial cells, covering the **anterior surface** of the iris. (×900).

(c) The deep stroma also is richly **vascularized** (**arrows**). The **myoepithelial** dilator pupillae muscle (**DPM**) is more easily seen here, in relation to the sphincter pupillae muscle (**SPM**) and posterior pigmented epithelium (**PE**). (×100; PT)

Figure 23-10b, reproduced with permission from Prof. Piera Versura, Laboratory of Ocular Surface Analysis and Translational Research, Alma Mater Studiorum University of Bologna, Italy.)

Vitreous Body

The **vitreous body** occupies the large vitreous chamber behind the lens (Figure 23–1). It consists of transparent, gel-like connective tissue that is 99% water (vitreous humor), with collagen fibrils and hyaluronate, contained within an external lamina called the vitreous membrane. Sparse, peripherally located mesenchymal cells called **hyalocytes** synthesize collagen and hyaluronate and represent the only cells in the vitreous body, along with a few macrophages.

FIGURE **23–11** Lens.

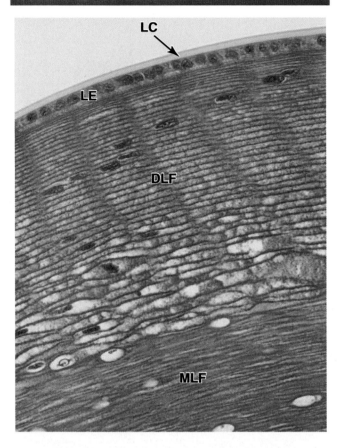

The **lens** is a transparent, elastic tissue that focuses light on the retina. Surrounding the entire lens is a thick, homogenous **external lamina** called the **lens capsule (LC)**. The anterior surface of the lens, beneath the capsule, is covered by a simple cuboidal lens epithelium (**LE**). Because of its origin as an embryonic vesicle pinching off surface ectoderm, the basal ends of the lens epithelial cells rest on the capsule and the apical regions are directed into the lens interior.

At the equator of the lens, near the **ciliary zonule**, the **epithelial cells** proliferate and give rise to cells that align parallel to the epithelium and become the **lens fibers**. Differentiating lens fibers (**DLF**) still have their nuclei but are greatly elongating and filling their cytoplasm with proteins called **crystallins**. The mature lens fibers (**MLF**) have lost their nuclei and become densely packed to produce a unique **transparent** structure. The lens is difficult to process histologically and sections usually have cracks or blisters among the lens fibers. (×200; H&E)

Retina

The **retina**, the innermost tunic of the eye, develops with two fundamental sublayers from the outer and inner layers of embryonic optic cup (Figure 23–2 and Table 23–1):

■ The outer **pigmented layer** attaches through Bruch's membrane to the choroidocapillary lamina of the choroid (Figure 23–6). This heavily pigmented layer, derived from the outer surface of the optic cup, extends

FIGURE **23–12** Accommodation of the lens.

(a)

(b)

Continuous changes in the shape of the **lens** keep images **focused** on the retina. **(a)** The lens flattens for **distant** vision when the **ciliary muscles** are **relaxed**, and the shape of the ciliary body holds the ciliary zonule taut.

(b) To see **closer** objects the **ciliary muscle** fibers **contract**, changing the shape of the ciliary body, relaxing tension on the ciliary zonule, and allowing the lens to assume the more rounded shape.

anteriorly and becomes the outer part of the dual epithelium that covers the ciliary body and posterior iris.

■ The inner retinal region, the **neural layer**, is much thicker and stratified with various neurons and photoreceptors. Its neural structure and visual function extend anteriorly only as far as the **ora serrata** (Figure 23–1), beyond which this layer continues as the nonpigmented part of the dual epithelium attached to the stroma of the ciliary body and posterior iris.

›› MEDICAL APPLICATION

The pigmented epithelium and the photoreceptor layer of the retina, derived from the two layers of the optic cup, are not firmly joined to each other. Head trauma or other conditions can cause the two layers to separate with an intervening space. In such regions of **detached retina**, the photoreceptor cells no longer have access to metabolic support from the pigmented layer and choroid and will eventually die. Prompt repositioning of the retina and reattaching it with laser surgery is an effective treatment.

Retina Pigmented Epithelium

The pigmented epithelial layer consists of cuboidal or low columnar cells and surrounds the neural layer of the retina. The cells have well-developed junctional complexes, gap junctions, and numerous invaginations of the basal membranes associated with mitochondria. The apical ends of the cells extend processes and sheath-like projections surrounding the tips of the photoreceptors. Melanin granules are numerous in these extensions and in the apical cytoplasm (Figure 23–13). This cellular region also contains numerous phagocytic vacuoles and secondary lysosomes, peroxisomes, and abundant smooth ER (SER) specialized for **retinal** (vitamin A) isomerization. The diverse functions of the retinal pigmented epithelium include the following.

- The pigmented layer **absorbs scattered light** that passes through the neural layer, supplementing the choroid in this regard.
- With many tight junctions, cells of the pigmented epithelium form an important part of the protective **blood-retina barrier** isolating retina photoreceptors from the highly vascular choroid and regulating **ion transport** between these compartments.
- The cells play key roles in the visual cycle of **retinal regeneration**, having enzyme systems that isomerize all-*trans*-retinal released from photoreceptors and produce 11-*cis*-retinal that is then transferred back to the photoreceptors.
- **Phagocytosis** of shed components from the adjacent photoreceptors and degradation of this material occurs in these epithelial cells.
- Pigmented epithelial cells **remove free radicals** by various protective antioxidant activities and **support the neural retina** by secretion of ATP, various polypeptide growth factors, and immunomodulatory factors.

Neural Retina

True to its embryonic origin, the neural retina functions as an outpost of the CNS with glia and several interconnected neuronal subtypes in well-organized strata. Nine distinct layers comprise the neural retina, described here with their functional significance.

Three major layers contain mostly cell bodies and nuclei of interconnected neurons (Figures 23–14 and 23–15):

- Near the pigmented epithelium, the **outer nuclear layer (ONL)** contains cell bodies of photoreceptors (the rod and cone cells). These cells, like the pigmented epithelial cells, receive O_2 and nutrients by diffusion from the choroidocapillary lamina of the choroid.
- The **inner nuclear layer (INL)** contains the nuclei of the retina's principal glial cells and various interneurons, notably the bipolar cells, amacrine cells, and horizontal cells (Figure 23–14b), all of which make specific connections with other neurons and integrate signals from rods and cones over a wide area of the retina.

FIGURE 23–13 Pigmented epithelium of retina.

The two distinct layers of the **retina** are the **pigmented epithelium** and the **photosensitive neural layer**, which are derived from the outer and inner layers of the optic cup, respectively. Shown here is the interface between the two layers. The pigmented epithelium (**PE**) is of simple cuboidal cells resting on Bruch membrane inside the choroid (**C**). **Rod cells and cone cells** are **neurons** with their nuclei collected in the outer nuclear layer (**ONL**) and with axons of one end forming synapses in an area called the outer plexiform layer (**OPL**) and modified dendrites at the other end serving as photosensitive structures. These structures have mitochondria-rich inner segments (**IS**) and photosensitive outer segments (**OS**) with stacks of folded membranes where the visual pigments are located.

The inner segments of the rod and cone cells are attached to elongated glial cells called **Müller cells**, which are modified **astrocytes** of the **retina**. The **junctional complexes** of these attachments can be seen in light micrographs as the outer limiting layer (**OLL**). (×500; H&E)

- Near the vitreous body, the **ganglionic layer (GL)** has neurons (ganglion cells) with much longer axons. These axons comprise the **nerve fiber layer (NFL)** and converge to form the **optic nerve**, which leaves the eye and passes to the brain. The GL becomes thickest near the central, macular region of the retina (Figure 23–15), but thins peripherally to only one layer of cells (Figure 23–6).

FIGURE 23–14 General organization and specialized areas of the retina.

The **retina** is the thick layer of the eye immediately inside the choroid. **(a)** The central **retinal artery and vein** pass through the **optic nerve** and enter the eye at the **optic disc** where they divide to form smaller lateral branches in the **retina's nerve fiber layer**. Capillaries extend as deep as the inner nuclear layer. (Nutrients and O_2 for the **outer retinal layers** diffuse from capillaries in the **choroid**.)

(b) The **major layers** and **neurons** of the **retina** and their general organization are depicted schematically here; the supporting Müller cells which penetrate all the neural layers are not included.

(c) The optic disc **(OD)** at the head of the optic nerve **(ON)** is the point at which **ganglion cell axons** from all regions of the retina **(R)** converge, penetrate the choroid and sclera **(S)**, and leave the eye as the **optic nerve** to enter the brain. Blood vessels **(BV)** in the

ganglionic and nerve fiber layers also converge at the optic disc to form the central artery **(CA)** and vein of the retina within the optic nerve. (×40; H&E)

(d) The fovea **(F)** is a small, specialized spot in the retina where cell bodies and axons of the ganglionic and inner nuclear layer become dispersed peripherally, thinning this retinal area and allowing light to hit the cones with very little light scattering. The **fovea** contains **no rods** and a greatly **increased density of cones**, causing the layer with their cell bodies to be slightly thicker here than elsewhere. These and other structural modifications at the fovea provide this area of the retina with the **greatest visual acuity** or sharpness of detail, but only when adequate light is present. The adjacent choroid **(C)** and sclera **(S)** are also shown. (×100; H&E)

FIGURE 23–15 Layers of the retina.

VB

ILM
NFL
GL
IPL
INL
OPL
ONL
OLL
RCL
PL

C

Between the vitreous body (**VB**) and the choroid (**C**), the **retina** can usually be seen to consist of **nine neural layers** and a **pigmented layer**. Following the path of the light, these are

- the inner limiting membrane (**ILM**), a basement membrane covered by expanded processes of **Müller cells**, which are not distinguishable in routine preparations.
- the nerve fiber layer (**NFL**), containing the **ganglionic cell axons**, which converge at the optic disc and form the **optic nerve**.
- the ganglionic layer (**GL**), containing cell bodies of the **ganglion cells** and thicker near the retina's center than its periphery.
- the inner plexiform layer (**IPL**), containing **fibers and synapses** of the ganglion cells and the bipolar neurons of the next layer.
- the inner nuclear layer (**INL**), with the cell bodies of several types of **bipolar neurons**, which begin to integrate signals from the rod and cone cells.
- the outer plexiform layer (**OPL**), containing **fibers and synapses** of the bipolar neurons and rod and cone cells.
- the outer nuclear layer (**ONL**), with the **cell bodies and nuclei of the photosensitive rod and cone cells**.
- the outer limiting layer (**OLL**), a line formed by **junctional complexes** holding the rod and cone cells to the intervening **Müller cells**.
- the rod and cone layer (**RCL**), which contains the **outer segments** of these cells where the photoreceptors are located.
- the non-neural pigmented layer (**PL**), which has several supportive functions important for the function and maintenance of the neural retina. (×150; H&E)

Between those three layers with cell bodies are two "plexiform" regions containing only axons and dendrites connected by synapses (Figure 23–15):

- The **outer plexiform layer (OPL)** includes axons of the photoreceptors and dendrites of interneurons in the INL.
- The **inner plexiform layer (IPL)** consists of axons and dendrites connecting neurons of the INL with the ganglion cells.

The rod and cone cells, named for the shape of their outer segments, represent polarized neurons with their photosensitive portions aligned in the retina's **rod and cone layer (RCL)** and their axons in the OPL (Figure 23–15).

All retina neurons receive metabolic and physical support from elongated, regularly arranged glial cells called **Müller cells**. With their perikarya in the INL, Müller cells extend processes that span the entire thickness of the neural retina, as visualized by immunofluorescent staining (Figure 23–16). From these major Müller cell processes, smaller lateral extensions ramify in each layer and sheath virtually all neuronal processes, cell bodies, and blood vessels. Müller cells are critical for retinal function, providing neurotrophic substances, removing waste products, regulating ion and water homeostasis, regulating blood flow, and maintaining a blood-inner retina barrier.

Müller cells also organize two physical boundaries that appear as very thin retinal "layers."

- The **outer limiting layer (OLL)** is a poorly stained but well-developed series of anchoring adherent junctions (zonulae adherens) between the photoreceptors and Müller cells (Figures 23–15 through 23–17).
- The **inner limiting membrane (ILM)** consists of terminally expanded Müller cell processes, which cover the collagenous membrane of the vitreous body and form this inner surface of the retina.

All these layers of the retina can be seen by routine light microscopy, as shown in Figures 23–6 and 23–15. It is important to note that light must pass through all the layers of the neural retina before reaching the layer of rods and cones. Branches of the central retinal artery and vein (Figure 23–1) run mainly within the nerve fiber and ganglionic layers, surrounded by perivascular feet of Müller cells and astrocytes located there. In some retina regions capillaries extend as deeply as the INL. A few scattered microglial cells occur throughout the neural retina.

Rod Cells

A human retina contains on average 92 million **rod cells**. Extremely sensitive to light, rods can respond to single photons, allowing some vision even with low light levels, such as at dusk or nighttime. Rod cells are thin, elongated cells (50 μm × 3 μm), composed of two functionally distinct segments (Figure 23–17a). The **outer segment** represents a modified primary cilium, photosensitive, and shaped like a short rod. It connects to the inner segment, part of the cell body with glycogen, mitochondria, and polyribosomes for the cell's biosynthetic activity.

FIGURE **23–16** Müller cells.

NFL
GL

IPL

INL

OPL

ONL

OLL

RCL

Müller cells are large **glial cells** unique to the **retina**, which are critical for retinal function by providing trophic and metabolic support for adjacent neurons, regulating homeostasis and synaptic activity, and helping to organize retinal components structurally. The attenuated and **diffuse nature** of Müller cells makes these cells difficult to study microscopically in most routine preparations of retina.

This **confocal light microscope image** of a section of living guinea pig retina, with its layers named as in the previous figure, shows the large **Müller cells in red**. Axons and dendrites, abundant in the plexiform layers, and the outer segments of the photoreceptor cells appear **green**.

Müller cells extend through the full thickness of the retina, with fine lateral processes contacting all adjacent neuronal cell bodies, synapses, and blood vessels. At a level just beyond the layer of photoreceptor cell nuclei, Müller cells are sealed to the photoreceptor cells by **zonula adherens junctions**, forming the outer limiting layer (**OLL**). A few long Müller cell processes extend beyond this layer, into the layer of rods and cones (**RCL**). The NFL is very thin in the area shown here and the pigmented epithelium is not stained. (×400; Vital dyes Mitotracker Orange [red] & FM-43 for synaptic membranes [green])

(Reproduced with permission from Dr Andreas Reichenbach, Paul Flechsig Institute of Brain Research, University of Leipzig, Germany.)

The rod-shaped outer segment consists mainly of 600–1000 flattened **membranous discs** stacked like coins and surrounded by the plasma membrane (Figure 23–17). Proteins on the cytoplasmic surface of each disc include abundant **rhodopsin** (or **visual purple**) which is bleached by light and initiates the visual stimulus (see below). Between this outer segment and the cell's inner segment is a constriction, the **connecting stalk**, which is part of the modified primary cilium arising from a basal body (Figure 23–17).

The membranous discs form by repetitive in-folding of the plasma membrane near the connecting stalk and insertion of rhodopsin and other proteins transported there from the inner segment. In rod cells, the newly assembled discs detach from the plasma membrane and are displaced distally as new discs form. Eventually, the discs arrive at the end of the rod, where they are shed, phagocytosed, and digested by the cells of the pigmented epithelium (Figure 23–13). Each day approximately 90 membranous discs are lost and replaced in each rod, with the process of assembly, distal movement, and apical shedding taking about 10 days.

Cone Cells

Less numerous and less light-sensitive than rods, the 4.6 million **cone cells** in a typical human retina produce color vision in adequately bright light. There are three morphologically similar classes of cones, each containing one type of the visual pigment **iodopsin** (or photopsins). Each of the three iodopsins has maximal sensitivity to light of a different wavelength, in the red, blue, or green regions of the visible spectrum, respectively. By mixing neural input produced by these visual pigments, cones produce a color image.

Like rods, cone cells (Figure 23–17a) are elongated, with outer and inner segments, a modified cilium connecting stalk, and an accumulation of mitochondria and polyribosomes. The outer segments of cones differ from those of rods in their shorter, more conical form and in the structure of their stacked membranous discs, which in cones remain as continuous invaginations of the plasma membrane along one side (Figure 23–17a). Also, newly synthesized iodopsins and other membrane proteins get distributed uniformly throughout the cone outer segment and, although iodopsin turns over, discs in cones are shed much less frequently than in rods.

❯❯ MEDICAL APPLICATION

Partial **color blindness** is normally an inherited disorder due to recessive mutations in genes for one or more iodopsins or other genes required for cone function. The most common form, **red-green** color blindness, affects the cones responsible for detecting light at these two wavelengths and occurs much more frequently in men than women because many key genes for the color sensitivity of cones are on the X chromosome. With two X chromosomes, women do not show the disability but can be carriers of the mutation.

FIGURE 23–17 Rod and cone photoreceptor cells.

External plexiform layer. Synapses with bipolar cells.

Metabolic region. Protein and phospholipid synthesis plus ATP production.

Outer limiting layer

Inner segment

Mitochondria

Cilium

Photosensitive region. Generation of the receptor potential.

Outer segments

(a)

b

IS

CS

OS

Rod and cone cells are the two types of **photoreceptors** of the **outer retina**, sensitive to low levels of light and higher levels of light with a broader spectrum of wavelengths respectively. Both are elongated, parallel structures consisting of **inner and outer segments**, with the **outer segments** consisting largely of stacked **membranous discs**.

(a) Rod cells (right) and **cone cells** (left) all have the general shapes and important cytoplasmic features shown diagrammatically here. The membranous discs of cone outer segments are continuous with the cell membrane; those of rods are not. The line of **adherent junctions** attaching the rod and cone inner segments to the distal ends of the Müller glial cells (not shown) comprises the **outer limiting layer** which helps anchor the

photoreceptors and separates the matrix surrounding the rod and cone cell bodies from that around their metabolically unique outer segments.

(b) TEM of a sectioned **retina** shows two rod cell inner segments **(IS)** with mitochondria and the outer photosensitive segment **(OS)** consisting of flat, parallel membranous discs. The cell in the middle of the figure shows the connecting stalk **(CS)** between the two segments. This connection contains a basal body with a primary cilium that expands distally as the outer segment. The connecting stalks of cone cells are structurally similar. The **stacked membranes** of the **discs** in the outer segments are very distinct and electron-dense due to the high density of proteins they contain. (×24,000)

Specialized Areas of the Retina

The **optic disc**, or blind spot, occurs at the posterior of the retina where the axons in the retina's NFL converge at the optic nerve head and leave the eye as the optic nerve. The optic disk is approximately 1.7 mm in diameter and lacks photoreceptors and other retinal layers except the NFL from ganglion cells (Figure 23–14c). A paired central artery and vein in the

optic nerve branches at the optic disc to produce microvasculature that runs through the NFL to supply the neurons and glial cells of the inner layers in all quadrants of the retina (Figure 23–14a).

Near the optic disc and directly opposite the pupil, lies a specialized retinal area about 1.5 mm in diameter called the **fovea centralis** (Figure 23–14a, d) where visual acuity or sharpness is maximal. The fovea (L. *fovea*, small pit) is a shallow depression within the retina where cells bodies of the ganglionic and INLs become dispersed peripherally, leaving primarily cone cells (Figure 23–14d). Cone cells in the fovea are longer, narrow, and closely packed. Devoid of most conducting neurons as well as capillaries, the fovea allows light to fall directly on its cones with very little scatter. The locations and structural adaptations of the fovea centralis together account for the extremely precise visual acuity of this region.

Surrounding the fovea centralis is the macula lutea (L. *macula*, spot; *lutea*, yellow), or simply macula, about 2 mm in diameter, where axons of the cone cells contain various carotenoids, giving this area its yellowish color. The carotenoids have antioxidant properties and filter potentially damaging short-wavelength light, thus helping to protect the cone cells of the fovea.

Within the GL of the entire retina a subset of ganglion cells serve as **nonvisual photoreceptors**. These neurons contain 11-*cis*-retinal bound to the protein melanopsin and serve to detect changes in light quantity and quality during each 24-hour dawn/dusk cycle. Signals from these cells pass via axons of the retinohypothalamic tract to the suprachiasmatic nuclei and the pineal gland, where they help establish the body's physiologic circadian rhythms (see Chapter 20).

Phototransduction

The membranous discs of rod and cone outer segments become stacked parallel with the retinal surface, which maximizes their exposure to light. The membranes are very densely packed with rhodopsin or one of the iodopsin proteins; one rod contains about a billion rhodopsin molecules. Each of these visual pigments contains a transmembrane protein, the **opsin**, with a small, light-sensitive **chromophore** molecule bound to it. The vitamin A derivative called **retinal** acts as the chromophore of rhodopsin in rods.

Phototransduction involves a cascade of changes in the cells triggered when light hits and activates the chromophore, a basically similar process in both rods and cones. As diagrammed for a rod in Figure 23–18, in darkness rhodopsin is not active and cation channels in the cell membrane are open. The cell is depolarized and continuously releases neurotransmitter at the synapse with the bipolar neurons. When retinal on rhodopsin absorbs a photon of light, it isomerizes within one picosecond from 11-*cis*-retinal to all-*trans*-retinal. This causes a configuration change in the opsin, which in turn activates the adjacent membrane-associated protein **transducin**, a heterotrimeric G protein to which opsin is coupled. Transducin activity then indirectly closes cGMP-gated Na^+ channels, causing hyperpolarization which reduces the synaptic release of neurotransmitter. This change in turn depolarizes sets of bipolar neurons, which send action potentials to the ganglion cells of the optic nerve.

The conformation change induced by light in *cis*-retinal that initiates this cascade of events also causes the chromophore

to dissociate from the opsin, a process called **bleaching** (Figure 23–18). The free all-*trans*-retinal is transported from the rod into the adjacent pigmented epithelial cell where it is converted back to 11-*cis*-retinal, then transported back into a photoreceptor for reuse. This cycle of retinal regeneration and rhodopsin recovery from bleaching may take a minute or more and is part of the slow adaptation of the eyes that occurs when moving from bright to dim light.

❯❯ MEDICAL APPLICATION

A leading cause of blindness in elderly individuals of developed countries is **age-related macular degeneration**, which causes blindness in the center of the visual field. Degenerative changes in the retina around the macula include depigmentation of the posterior epithelium, focal thickening of the adjacent Bruch membrane, major changes and blood loss in the capillaries in the choroid and retina, and eventual loss of the photoreceptor cells producing blind spots. There appears to be a genetic predisposition to the disorder, along with environmental triggers such as excessive exposure to ultraviolet radiation. Progression of the disease can be slowed by laser surgery to destroy the abnormal and excessive retinal capillaries.

Accessory Structures of the Eye

Conjunctiva

The **conjunctiva** develops as a thin, transparent mucosa that covers the exposed, anterior portion of the sclera and continues as the lining on the inner surface of the eyelids. It consists of a stratified columnar epithelium, with numerous small goblet cells, supported by a thin lamina propria of loose vascular connective tissue (Figure 23–19). Mucous secretions from conjunctiva cells are added to the tear film that coats this epithelium and the cornea.

❯❯ MEDICAL APPLICATION

Conjunctivitis, or **pink eye**, is a condition in which the conjunctiva is inflamed usually due to bacterial or viral infection or due to allergies. The inflammation increases the discharge of mucus and enlarges the microvasculature of the sclera, causing the white sclera to have a reddish appearance. Bacterial and viral conjunctivitis are contagious but have little effect on vision.

Eyelids

Eyelids (Figure 23–19) are pliable, protective structures consisting of skin, muscle, and conjunctiva. The skin is loose and elastic, lacks fat, and has only very small hair follicles and fine hair, except at the distal edge, where large follicles with eyelashes develop. Associated with the follicles

FIGURE **23–18** Rod cell phototransduction.

In the dark:

When light enters:

Phototransduction involves a series of changes in **rod and cone cells** that begins when light hits the stacked **membranous discs**. The main parts of the process are similar in both rods and cones but have been better studied in the more abundant rod cells, as shown here. Membranes of the discs are densely packed with proteins, although only one of each major type is shown here. In the dark, **rhodopsin** and its **11-*cis*-retinal** are inactive and the intracellular concentration of the second messenger cyclic GMP (**cGMP**) is high. One effect of cGMP is to keep open the abundant cGMP-gated **sodium channels** in the cell membrane and therefore the cell is **depolarized**, continuously **releasing** its **neurotransmitter** (glutamate) at the synapse with the bipolar neurons.

When photons of light are absorbed by the retinal of rhodopsin, the molecule isomerizes from 11-*cis*-retinal to **all-*trans*-retinal** and this change activates the opsin. This in turn activates the

adjacent peripheral membrane protein **transducin**, a heterotrimeric **G protein**, allowing it to release its α subunit, which moves laterally and stimulates another membrane protein, **phosphodiesterase**, to hydrolyze cGMP. With less cGMP, many of the sodium channels now close, producing **hyperpolarization** of the cell, which decreases the release of neurotransmitter at the synapses.

This change at the synapse depolarizes sets of bipolar neurons, which then send action potentials to the various ganglion cells of the optic nerve, allowing the brain to produce an image. When retinal is activated by light, it also dissociates from rhodopsin, leaving a more pale-colored (bleached) **opsin**. The free retinal moves into the surrounding **pigmented epithelial cells**, where the all-*trans*-isomer is regenerated. It is then transported back into a rod or cone cell to again bind opsin and be used in another round of phototransduction.

---

of eyelashes are sebaceous glands and modified apocrine sweat glands.

Beneath the skin are striated fascicles of the orbicularis oculi and levator palpebrae muscles, which fold the eyelids. Adjacent to the conjunctiva is a dense fibroelastic plate called the **tarsus** supporting the other tissues. The tarsus surrounds a series of 20-25 large sebaceous glands, each with many acini secreting into a long central duct that opens among the eyelashes (Figure 23–19). Oils in the sebum produced by these **tarsal glands**, also called **Meibomian glands**, form a

surface layer on the tear film, reducing its rate of evaporation, and help lubricate the ocular surface.

›› MEDICAL APPLICATION

Infections near an opening of the tarsal gland ducts, generally caused by *Staphylococcus aureus*, are called **styes**. They are most common in infants but can occur at any age and can be quite painful. Like certain other infections, styes can occur in periods of immunosuppression caused by poor nutrition or stress.

FIGURE 23–19   Eyelid.

a

b

(a) The **eyelid** is a pliable tissue with skin (**S**) covering its external surface and smooth conjunctiva (**C**) lining its inner surface. At the outer rim of the eyelid are a series of large hair follicles (**F**) for the **eyelashes**. Associated with these hair follicles are small **sebaceous glands** and modified **apocrine sweat glands**. Internally eyelids contain fascicles of striated muscle (**M**) comprising the orbicularis oculi muscle and closer to the conjunctiva a thick plate of fibroelastic connective tissue called the tarsus (**T**). This tarsal plate provides structural support for the eyelid and surrounds a series of large **sebaceous glands**, the tarsal glands (**TG**) (aka Meibomian glands), with acini secreting into long central ducts (**D**) emptying at the free edge of the eyelids. (×12.5; H&E)

(b) At higher magnification, only the inner aspect of the **eyelid** is seen, and it shows that the conjunctiva (**C**) is a **mucous membrane** consisting of a **stratified columnar epithelium** with small cells resembling **goblet cells** and resting on a thin lamina propria (**LP**). Large cells undergoing typical **holocrine secretion** are shown in the tarsal gland acini (**TG**), and the fibrous connective tissue in the tarsus (**T**) surrounding the acini. **Sebum** from these glands is added to the tear film and helps lubricate the ocular surface. (×200; H&E)

Lacrimal Glands

The **lacrimal glands** produce fluid continuously for the tear film that moistens and lubricates the cornea and conjunctiva and supplies O_2 to the corneal epithelial cells. Tear fluid also contains various metabolites, electrolytes, and proteins of innate immunity such as lysozyme. The main lacrimal glands develop in the upper temporal portion of the orbit and have

FIGURE **23–20** Lacrimal gland.

Lacrimal glands secrete most components of the **tear film**, which moisturizes, lubricates, and helps protect the eyes. The glands have acini (**A**) composed of secretory cells filled with small, light-staining granules and myoepithelial cells (**M**). Connective tissue surrounding the acini contains blood vessels (**V**) of the microvasculature and intra- and interlobular ducts (**D**) converging as excretory ducts, which empty into the superior **conjunctival fornix** between the **upper eyelid** and the **eye**. (×400; H&E)

several lobes, which drain through individual excretory ducts into the superior fornix, the conjunctiva-lined recess between the eyelids and the eye.

The lacrimal glands have acini composed of large serous cells filled with lightly stained secretory granules and surrounded by well-developed myoepithelial cells and a sparse, vascular stroma (Figure 23–20).

Tear film moves across the ocular surface and collects in other parts of the bilateral **lacrimal apparatus**: flowing through two small round openings (0.5 mm in diameter) to canaliculi at the medial margins of the upper and lower eyelids, then passing into the lacrimal sac, and finally draining into the nasal cavity via the nasolacrimal duct. The canaliculi have a stratified squamous epithelial lining, but the more distal sac and duct are lined by pseudostratified ciliated epithelium like that of the nasal cavity.

› EARS: THE VESTIBULOAUDITORY SYSTEM

Sensory receptors of the ear mediate both the sense of equilibrium and hearing. An ear consists of three major parts (Figure 23–21):

- The **external ear**, which receives sound waves;
- The **middle ear**, in which sound waves are transmitted from air to fluids of the inner ear via a set of small bones; and
- The **inner ear**, in which mechanosensory cells transduce these fluid movements into nerve impulses that pass via the acoustic nerve to the CNS. The internal ear contains the vestibular organ that allows the body to maintain equilibrium and the auditory organ, the cochlea.

Most structures of the middle and internal ear develop within cavities of embryonic temporal bone as it forms from head mesenchyme.

External Ear

The **auricle**, or **pinna** (L. *pinna*, wing) develops as an irregularly concave piece of elastic cartilage, covered by tightly adherent skin, which funnels sound waves into the ear.

Sound waves enter the **external acoustic meatus** (L. *passage*), a canal lined with stratified squamous epithelium that extends from the auricle to the middle ear. Near its opening hair follicles, sebaceous glands, and modified apocrine sweat glands called **ceruminous glands** are found in the submucosa (Figure 23–22). **Cerumen**, the waxy material resulting from ceruminous and sebaceous gland secretions, contains various proteins, saturated fatty acids, and sloughed keratinocytes and has protective, antimicrobial properties. Elastic cartilage supports the outer third of the external acoustic meatus, while the temporal bone encloses the inner part (Figure 23–21).

Across the deep end of the external acoustic meatus lies a thin, somewhat transparent sheet called the **tympanic membrane** or **eardrum**. This membrane consists of fibroelastic connective tissue covered externally with epidermis and internally by the simple cuboidal epithelium of the mucosa lining the middle ear cavity. Directed by the auricle sound waves impinge on the tympanic membrane causing it to vibrate, which transmits mechanical energy to the middle ear (Figure 23–21).

Middle Ear

The **middle ear** contains the air-filled **tympanic cavity**, an irregular space lying within the temporal bone between the tympanic membrane and the bony surface of the inner ear (Figure 23–21). Anteriorly, this cavity communicates with the pharynx via the **auditory tube** (also called the **eustachian** or **pharyngotympanic tube**) and posteriorly with the smaller, air-filled mastoid cavities of the temporal bone. The simple cuboidal epithelium lining the cavity rests on a

FIGURE **23–21** **Major divisions of the ear.**

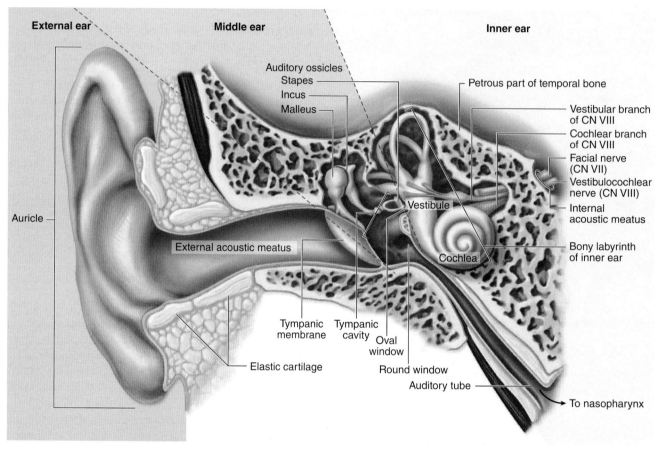

The **external**, **middle**, and **inner regions** of the right **ear** are shown here, along with the major structures within each region. The external ear functions to funnel **sound waves** onto the tympanic membrane. The **auditory ossicles** of the middle ear convert the motion of the **tympanic membrane** into motion of the **fluid** within the inner ear, where it undergoes transduction as neural activity in the **cochlea**. The inner ear also contains **vestibular structures** important for maintaining the body's sense of **equilibrium**.

thin lamina propria continuous with periosteum. Entering the auditory tube, this simple epithelium gradually becomes the ciliated pseudostratified columnar epithelium lining that tube. Below the temporal bone the auditory tube usually remains collapsed; swallowing opens it briefly, which serves to balance the air pressure in the middle ear with atmospheric pressure. In the medial bony wall of the middle ear are two small, membrane-covered regions devoid of bone: the **oval** and **round windows**, with the internal ear behind them (Figure 23–21).

The tympanic membrane connects to the oval window through a series of three small bones, the **auditory ossicles**, which convey that membrane's mechanical vibrations to the vestibule of the inner ear (Figure 23–23). Named for their shapes, the ossicles are the **malleus**, **incus**, and **stapes**, Latin for "hammer," "anvil," and "stirrup," respectively. The malleus attaches to the tympanic membrane and the stapes to the membrane across the oval window, with the stapes connecting the other two. The ossicles articulate with typical synovial joints, which along with their periosteum are also covered with simple squamous epithelium. Two small skeletal muscles, the tensor tympani and stapedius, insert into the malleus and stapes, respectively, restricting ossicle movements and protecting the oval window and inner ear from potential damage caused by extremely loud sound.

> **>> MEDICAL APPLICATION**
>
> The middle ear tympanic cavity may show inflammation **(otitis media)** when viral or bacterial infections extend there from the upper respiratory tract via the auditory tubes. Otitis media is most common in young children, where the short auditory tubes facilitate infection of the tympanic cavity.

Inner Ear

The **inner ear** becomes localized completely within the temporal bone, where an intricate set of interconnected spaces, the **bony labyrinth**, houses the smaller **membranous**

FIGURE **23–22** External acoustic meatus.

The **external acoustic meatus** leads from the opening in the **auricle** to the **tympanic membrane** (or eardrum). This section of the wall in the outer third of the acoustic meatus shows the lining of skin containing small hair follicles (**F**), sebaceous glands (**SG**), and modified apocrine sweat glands called **ceruminous glands** (**CG**). Secretions from these two glands form a yellowish, waxy product called **cerumen** (**C**). (×50; H&E)

labyrinth, a set of continuous fluid-filled, epithelium-lined tubes and chambers (Figure 23–21). The membranous labyrinth develops from an ectodermal vesicle, the otic vesicle, which invaginates into subjacent mesenchyme during the 4th week of embryonic development, loses contact with the surface ectoderm, and becomes embedded in the developing temporal bone.

Table 23–2 lists the three major components of the bony and membranous labyrinths and their functions. The major divisions of the membranous labyrinth include the following:

- Two connected sacs called the **utricle** and the **saccule**;
- Three **semicircular ducts** continuous with the utricle; and
- The **cochlear duct**, which extends from the saccule and provides for hearing.

Mediating the functions of the inner ear, each of these structures contains in its epithelial lining large areas with

FIGURE **23–23** Middle ear.

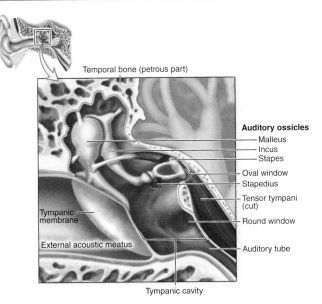

Three **auditory ossicles**, with synovial joints and striated muscles all covered by epithelium, span the **tympanic cavity** of the **middle ear**, an air-filled cavity enclosed by the **temporal bone** and the **tympanic membrane**. The series of ossicles leverage the weak vibrations of the tympanic membrane into more staccato movements of the **oval window** and the fluid beyond it.

columnar mechanoreceptor cells called **hair cells**, in specialized sensory regions consisting of

- Two **maculae** of the utricle and saccule;
- Three **cristae ampullares** in the enlarged ampullary regions of each semicircular duct; and
- The long **spiral organ of Corti** in the cochlear duct.

The entire membranous labyrinth is enclosed within the bony labyrinth, which includes the following regions (Figure 23–24):

- An irregular central cavity, the **vestibule** (L. *vestibulum*, area for entering) housing the saccule and the utricle;
- Behind this, three osseous **semicircular canals** surrounding the semicircular ducts; and
- On the other side of the vestibule, the **cochlea** (L. *cochlea*, snail shell) containing the cochlear duct (Figure 23–24).

The bony and membranous labyrinths contain two different fluids (Figure 23–24), and the separation and ionic differences between these fluids are important for inner ear function.

- **Perilymph** fills all regions of the bony labyrinth and has an ionic composition rather like that of cerebrospinal fluid. Perilymph emerges from the microvasculature of the periosteum and drains via a perilymphatic duct into the adjoining subarachnoid space. Perilymph suspends and supports the closed membranous labyrinth, protecting it from the hard wall of the bony labyrinth.

TABLE 23–2   Structure and function of internal ear components.

Bony Labyrinth Component (Containing Perilymph and the Membranous Labyrinth)	Membranous Labyrinth Component (Within Bony Labyrinth and Containing Endolymph)	Structures With Sensory Receptors	Major Function
Vestibule	Utricle, saccule	Maculae	Detect linear movements and static position of the head
Semicircular canals	Semicircular ducts	Cristae ampullares	Detect rotational movements of the head
Cochlea	Cochlear duct	Spiral organ	Detect sounds

■ **Endolymph** fills the membranous labyrinth and is characterized by a high-K^+ (150 mM) and low-Na^+ (16 mM) content, like that of intracellular fluid. Endolymph is produced in a specialized area in the wall of the cochlear duct (described later) and drains via a small endolymphatic duct into venous sinuses of the dura mater.

Utricle and Saccule

The interconnected, membranous **utricle** and the **saccule** consist of a very thin connective tissue sheath lined with simple squamous epithelium and bound to the periosteum of the bony labyrinth by strands of connective tissue containing microvasculature. The maculae in the walls of the

FIGURE 23–24   Inner ear.

The **inner ear** consists of a cavity in the temporal bone, the **bony labyrinth**, which houses a fluid-filled **membranous labyrinth**. The membranous labyrinth includes the vestibular organs (the **saccule, utricle,** and **semicircular ducts**), which contribute to the sense of **equilibrium and balance**, and the **cochlea** for the sense of **hearing**. Endolymph fills the membranous labyrinth; spaces within the bony labyrinth contain **perilymph**.

utricle and saccule comprise small areas of columnar neuroepithelial cells innervated by branches of the vestibular nerve (Figure 23–25). The macula of the saccule lies in a plane perpendicular to that of the utricle, but each represents a thickening of the wall containing several thousand columnar hair cells and supporting cells.

Hair cells act as mechanoelectrical transducers, converting mechanical energy into nerve action potentials. Each has an apical tuft consisting of one rigid cilium, the **kinocilium**, up to 40 μm long, and 30–50 shorter, rigid, and unbranched **stereocilia** (Figure 23–25). The base of each stereocilium tapers and its microfilaments become bundled before merging

with the actin-rich terminal web, or **cuticular plate**, which returns the stereocilia to a normal upright position after bending at their bases. They are arranged in rows of decreasing length, with the longest adjacent to the kinocilium (Figure 23–26). The stereocilia and kinocilium are embedded in a gelatinous proteoglycan layer called the **otolithic membrane**, which is heavier than endolymph because it contains grain-shaped crystals of protein and $CaCO_3$ called **otoliths** (or statoconia) (Figure 23–25b). Supporting cells surround each hair cell below its apical cuticular plate, along with its synaptic connections to sensory axons, providing metabolic and physical support for all these structures.

FIGURE 23–25 Vestibular maculae.

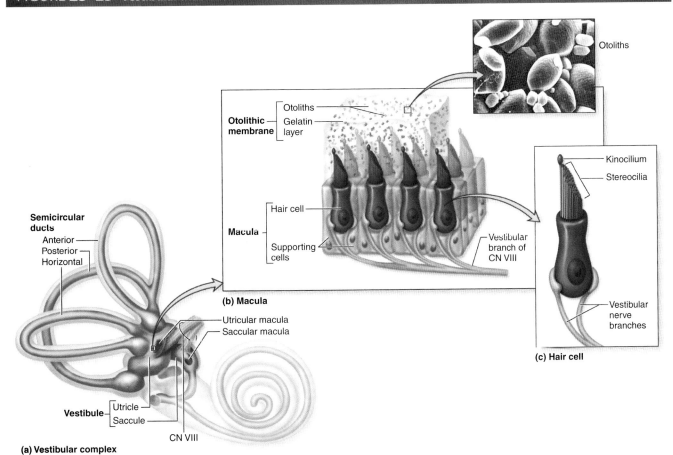

(a) Vestibular complex
(b) Macula
(c) Hair cell

(a) Two sensory areas called **maculae** occur in the **membranous labyrinth** of the vestibular **utricle** and **saccule**, both specialized for detecting gravity and endolymph movements.

(b) A more detailed diagram of a **macular wall** shows that it is composed of **hair cells**, **supporting cells**, and endings of the **vestibular branch** of the eighth cranial nerve. A **gelatinous otolithic layer** or membrane engulfs the apical surface of the hair cells, and the basal ends of the cells have synaptic connections with the nerve fibers. The SEM shows **otoliths** embedded in this external apical layer. These mineralized structures make the otolithic membrane heavier than endolymph alone, which facilitates

bending of the **kinocilia and stereocilia** by gravity or movement of the head.

(c) A diagram of a single generalized **hair cell** shows the numerous straight **stereocilia**, which contain bundled actin, and a longer single **kinocilium**, a modified cilium whose tip may be slightly enlarged.

(Figure 23–25b(inset), reproduced with permission from David J. Lim, House Ear Institute and Department of Cell & Neurobiology, University of Southern California, Los Angeles, CA.)

FIGURE 23–26 Hair cells and details of stereocilia.

(a)

(b)

(a) This diagram shows the two types of **hair cells** in the **maculae** and **cristae ampullares**. Basal ends of **type I hair** cells are rounded and enclosed within a nerve calyx on the afferent fiber. **Type II hair cells** are columnar and associated with typical bouton synaptic connections to their afferents. Both types are also associated with **efferent nerve fibers**.

(b) A more detailed diagram shows that **stereocilia** occur in rows of increasing height, with the tallest next to the single **kinocilium** on one side of the cell. By TEM the end of each stereocilium shows

an electron-dense region containing cation channels and proteins involved in **mechanoelectrical transduction (MET)**, which converts **mechanical activity** of the stereocilia to **electrical activity**. Neighboring stereocilia are connected by proteins of various side links; the best understood of these are the **tip links** connecting the tips of stereocilia and contain very long cadherin proteins. Changes in the tension of the tip links caused by bending of the hair bundle open or close the adjacent **mechanically gated K+ channels** and change the afferent synaptic activity of the hair cells.

Basal synapses with afferent (to the brain) nerve endings occur with all hair cells but are of two types, as shown in Figure 23–26a:

- Type I hair cells with rounded basal ends, each resting within an afferent nerve terminal calyx (L. *calyx*, cup), and
- The more numerous type II hair cells, more cylindrical and having terminal bouton afferent endings.

Synaptic connections with *efferent* (*from* the brain) fibers also occur, either on the afferent nerve calyx or directly on the type II hair cell, to modulate the sensitivity of the mechanoreceptors (Figure 23–26a).

The position and movement of the head determine the nature of the otolithic membranes' contact with hair cells in the maculae and the resulting sensory input from the utricle and saccule allows the brain to monitor the head's position during changing periods of **static equilibrium** and **linear acceleration**. With the head upright and stationary, the hair

cells receive minimal stimulation. Tilting the head up or down moves the otolithic membrane, bending the stereocilia and affecting neuronal activity in the hair cells. Neuronal activity generated within the utricle and saccule helps the body to maintain equilibrium and the eyes to remain fixed on one point while the head moves.

This sensory activity occurs due to hair cells' property of mechanoelectrical transduction, which involves mechanically gated ion channels. Deflection or bending of the stereocilia changes the hair cells' resting potential and their rate of neurotransmitter release to the afferent nerves. As shown in Figure 23–26b, the ends of stereocilia connect via a series of cadherin-based **tip links** that attach to ion channels at each stereocilium tip. When the stereocilia get deflected *toward* the kinocilium, this movement pulls these tip links, opening mechanically gated channels to allow an influx of K+ ions (the major cation in the endolymph). This rapidly depolarizes the hair cell to trigger opening of voltage-gated Ca²⁺ channels in the basolateral membrane, and the entry of Ca^{2+} stimulates release of neurotransmitter that generates an impulse in the afferent nerve (Figure 23–27a).

When the head stops moving, the stereocilia straighten and hair cells quickly repolarize and reestablish the resting potential. Head movements that bend the stereocilia *away from* the kinocilium cause the tip links to be slack, allowing closure of the apical cation channels and hyperpolarization of the cell. This in turn closes Ca^{2+} channels and reduces neurotransmitter release (Figure 23–27b).

FIGURE 23–27 Mechanotransduction in hair cells.

(a)

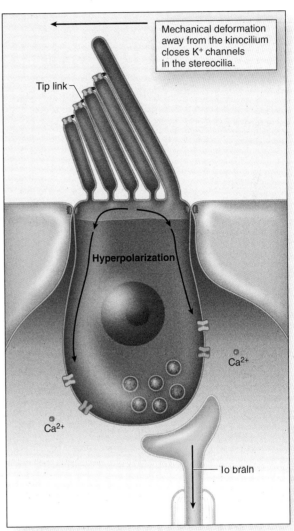

(b)

Hair cells and **supporting cells** are part of an epithelium in which cells are sealed together with tight junctions and which separates **endolymph** from **perilymph**. The *apical* ends of the cells are exposed to endolymph with a high concentration of K^+, and perilymph with a much lower K^+ concentration bathes their *basolateral* surface. At rest, hair cells are **polarized** with a small amount of K^+ entry and a low level of neurotransmitter release to afferent nerve fibers at the basal ends of the cells.

(a) As shown here, head movements that cause the stereocilia bundle to be deflected *toward* **the kinocilium** produce tension in the **tip links**, which is transduced to electrical activity by opening of adjacent cation channels. Entry of K^+ *depolarizes* the cell, opening voltage-gated basolateral Ca^{2+} channels, which stimulates

release of neurotransmitter. When this movement stops, the cells quickly **repolarize**.

(b) Movements in the opposite direction, *away from* **the kinocilium**, produce slackness on the tip links, allowing the mechanically gated apical K^+ channels to close completely, producing *hyperpolarization*, and inhibiting transmitter release. With different numbers of afferent and efferent fibers on the hair cells and with various hair cells responding differently to endolymph movements due to their positions within the maculae and cristae ampullares, the sensory information produced collectively by these cells can be processed by the vestibular regions of the **brain** and used to help maintain **equilibrium**.

>> **MEDICAL APPLICATION**

Problems of the vestibular system can result in vertigo, or dizziness, a sense of bodily rotation and lack of equilibrium. Spinning the body produces **vertigo** due to overstimulation of the cristae ampullares of the semicircular ducts. Over-stimulation of the maculae of the utricle caused by repetitive changes in linear acceleration and directional changes can normally lead to **motion sickness** (seasickness).

The sensation of **vertigo** associated with rapid head movements can also be produced by internal ear inflammation (**vestibular neuritis**) or neurologic conditions that cause dysfunctional activity of the vestibular system. **Ménière disease** involves episodes of vertigo accompanied by hearing loss and ringing in the ears (**tinnitus**) and is caused when increased pressure within the membranous labyrinth (**endolymphatic hydrops**) leads to rupture and leakage of endolymph into the perilymph.

Semicircular Ducts

The three **semicircular ducts** extend from and return to the wall of the utricle, lying in three different spatial planes, at approximately right angles to one another (Figure 23–27).

Each semicircular duct ends in an enlarged ampulla containing hair cells and supporting cells in a crest of its wall called the **crista ampullaris** (Figure 23–28). Each crista ampullaris is perpendicular to the long axis of the duct. These cristae resemble maculae histologically, but the proteoglycan layer called the **cupola** attached to the hair cells apically lacks otoliths and is much thicker, extending completely across the ampulla (Figure 23–28).

The hair cells of the cristae ampullares act as mechano-electrical transducers like those of the maculae in the utricle and saccule, signaling afferent axons by pulsed transmitter release determined by depolarization and hyperpolarization states (Figure 23–27). Here the mechanoreceptors detect **rotational movements** of the head which deflect endolymph in one or more semicircular ducts. These hair cells are oriented with opposite polarity on each side of the head, so that turning the head causes their depolarization on one side and hyperpolarization on the other. Neurons of the **vestibular nuclei** in the CNS receive input from the sets of semicircular ducts on each side simultaneously and interpret head rotation based on the relative transmitter discharge rates of the two sides.

Inputs from the semicircular ducts travel along the eighth cranial nerve to the vestibular nuclei together with those from the utricle and saccule. Collectively the utricle, saccule, and semicircular ducts comprise the **vestibular system**, continuously monitoring and adjusting the body's equilibrium. Along with inputs from the musculoskeletal system mechanoreceptors, this system provides the basis for perceiving the body's movements and orientation in space, as well as maintaining its equilibrium or balance.

FIGURE 23–28 **Ampullae and cristae of the semicircular ducts.**

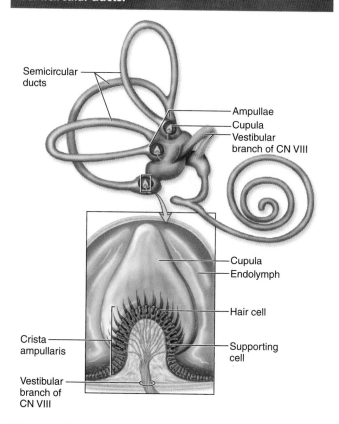

Three **semicircular ducts** lie within the **semicircular canals**, at right angles to one another and connected to the **utricle** at their expanded ends, the **ampullae**. The wall of each ampulla is raised as a ridge called the **crista ampullaris**, a section of which is shown here diagrammatically. **Hair cells** of the crista epithelium resemble the two types found in the **maculae**, each with a **hair bundle of stereocilia** and a **kinocilium** projecting into a dome-shaped overlying layer of proteoglycan called the **cupula**. The cupula attaches to the wall opposite the crista and is moved by **endolymph movement** within the semicircular duct.

>> **MEDICAL APPLICATION**

Brief periods of vertigo produced by sudden changes in position of head, such as standing up quickly or sitting up after lying in bed, may be examples of **benign paroxysmal positional vertigo (BPPV)**. BPPV also results when one or more of the dense otoliths (or otoconia) detach from the otolithic membrane and move into an ampulla of the posterior semicircular duct as **canaliths**, which may also adhere to the cupula. Being heavy, canaliths make the affected crista ampullaris gravity-sensitive. When that semicircular canal is aligned with gravity during head movements, sensory impulses are produced which the brain interprets incorrectly as continuous head rotations. A specific series of slow head movements comprising the **canalith repositioning procedure**, or **Epley maneuver**, can be used to return the otoliths to the utricle and relieve the sensation of dizziness and unsteadiness.

Cochlear Duct

The **cochlear duct** is the part of the membranous labyrinth containing the hair cells and other structures that allow auditory function, and consists of an elongated, spiral chamber held in place along the center of the coiled bony **cochlea** (Figure 23–24). Like other inner ear regions, the bony cochlea develops within the embryonic petrous bone, becoming in this case a canal approximately 35 mm long with 2¾ turns around a bony core called the **modiolus** (L. *modiolus*, hub of wheel). As diagrammed in Figure 23–29 the cochlea comprises three parallel compartments, or scalae (L. *scala*, ramp).

- The cochlear duct itself forms the middle compartment, or **scala media**, filled with endolymph. It connects proximally with the saccule and ends at the apex of the cochlea.
- The larger **scala vestibuli** contains perilymph and is separated from the scala media only by the very thin **vestibular membrane (Reissner membrane)** lined on each side by simple squamous epithelium (Figure 23–30). Extensive tight junctions between cells of this membrane prevent ion diffusion between the perilymph and endolymph.
- On the other side of the middle channel, the **scala tympani** also contains perilymph and is separated from the scala media by the fibroelastic **basilar membrane** (Figure 23–29b).

The scalae tympani and vestibuli communicate with each other at the apex of the cochlea via a small opening called the **helicotrema**. Thus, these two spaces with perilymph comprise one long tube; the scala vestibuli portion begins near the vestibular oval window and the scala tympani ends at the round window (Figure 23–24).

The **stria vascularis**, located in the tall lateral wall of the cochlear duct (scala media) (Figures 23–29b and 23–30), produces the endolymph that fills the entire membranous labyrinth. It has a unique, vascularized stratified epithelium in which cells extend cytoplasmic processes and folds around the capillaries of a dense intraepithelial plexus and transport water and K^+ from capillaries into the endolymph, which bathes the stereocilia of hair cells and produces conditions optimal for these cells' depolarization.

The **organ of Corti**, or **spiral organ**, where sound vibrations of different frequencies are detected, consists of hair cells and other epithelial structures supported by the basilar membrane (Figure 23–29). Each of the sensory hair cells has a precisely arranged, V-shaped bundle with rigid stereocilia only (Figure 23–31), having lost its single kinocilium during development. As shown in Figure 23–29c, d, two major types of hair cells occur in the spiral organ:

- **Outer hair cells**, about 12,000 in total, occurring in three rows near the saccule, increasing to five rows near the apex of the cochlea, each cell with a V-shaped bundle of stereocilia (Figure 23–31), and

- **Inner hair cells** forming a single row of about 3500 cells, each with a single more linear array of shorter stereocilia (Figure 23–31).

❯❯ MEDICAL APPLICATION

Deafness can result from many factors, which usually fall into two categories: (1) **Conductive hearing loss** involves various problems in the middle ear that can reduce conduction of vibrations by the chain of ossicles from the tympanic membrane to the oval window. A common example is otosclerosis, in which scar-like lesions develop on the bony labyrinth near the stapes which inhibit its movement of the oval window. Infection of the middle ear (otitis media) is common in young children and can reduce sound conduction due to fluid accumulation in that cavity. (2) **Sensorineural deafness** can be congenital or acquired and due to defects in any structure or cell from the cochlea to the auditory centers of the brain, but it commonly involves loss of hair cells or nerve degeneration.

Both outer and inner hair cells have synaptic connections with afferent and efferent nerve endings, with the inner row of cells more heavily innervated. The cell bodies of the afferent bipolar neurons make up the **spiral ganglion** located along with blood vessels in the cochlea's bony core, the modiolus (Figures 23–29 and 23–30).

Two major types of columnar supporting cells also develop on the basilar membrane in the organ of Corti (Figure 23–29c):

- Inner and outer **phalangeal cells** extend apical processes, which intimately surround and support the basolateral parts of both the inner and outer hair cells and the synaptic nerve endings. The apical ends of phalangeal cells are joined to those of the hair cells by tight zonulae occludens, forming an apical plate across the spiral organ through which only the stereocilia bundles project into endolymph (Figure 23–31).
- **Pillar cells** are stiffened by heavy bundles of keratin and outline a long triangular space called the inner tunnel, between the outer and inner complexes of hair and phalangeal cells. The stiff inner tunnel also plays a role in sound transmission.

On the outer hair cells the tips of the tallest stereocilia are embedded in the **tectorial membrane**, an acellular layer extending over the organ of Corti from the connective tissue around the modiolus (Figure 23–29). The tectorial membrane consists of various collagens (types II, V, and IX), proteoglycans and tectorin glycoproteins, and develops during the embryonic period from secretions of cells lining this region.

By detecting minute movements of the stereocilia, hair cells in the spiral organ of Corti act as mechanoelectrical transducers very much like those of the vestibular maculae

FIGURE **23–29** Cochlea and spiral organ (of Corti).

(a) Sectioned cochlea

(b) Close-up of cochlea

(c) Organ of Corti

(d) Organ of Corti

(a) The **auditory** portion of the **inner ear**, the **cochlea**, has a snail-like spiral shape in both its bony and membranous labyrinths. A section of the whole cochlea shows its **three parallel compartments** cut in several places.

(b) This diagram shows a more detailed view of one such turn of the **cochlear duct (scala media)**, the **organ of Corti** on the **basilar membrane**, and the adjacent perilymph-filled spaces, the **scala vestibuli** and **scala tympani**. **Endolymph** in the cochlear duct is produced by the stria vascularis (not shown), a capillary-rich area in the lateral wall.

(c) This diagram shows the **organ of Corti** in more detail, including the **tectorial membrane**, the general locations and shape of the **inner and outer hair cells**, their supporting **phalangeal cells**, and the **pillar cells** making the inner tunnel.

(d) The micrograph shows major features of the **organ of Corti** histologically. (×75; H&E)

described previously and mediate the sense of hearing. As shown in Figure 23–32, sound waves collected by the external ear cause the tympanic membrane to vibrate, which moves the chain of middle ear ossicles and the oval window. The large size of the tympanic membrane compared to the oval window and the leverage actions of the ossicles amplify the movements and allow optimal transfer of energy between air and

perilymph, from sound waves to vibrations of the tissues and fluid-filled chambers.

Pressure waves within the perilymph begin at the oval window and move along the scala vestibuli. Each pressure wave causes momentary displacement of the vestibular and/or basilar membranes and the endolymph surrounding the organ of Corti (Figure 23–32).

FIGURE **23–30** Cochlear duct and spiral ganglion.

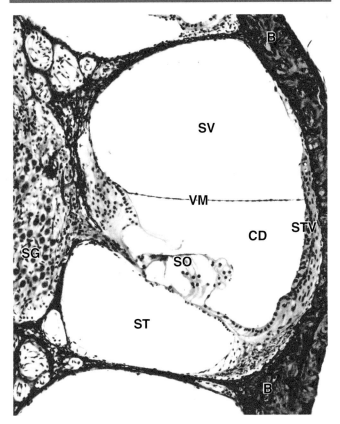

The spiral organ (**SO**) or **organ of Corti** lies within the cochlear duct (**CD**), or **scala media**. This duct is filled with **endolymph** produced in the stria vascularis (**STV**), an unusual association of epithelial cells and intraepithelial capillaries from the periosteum of the bone (**B**). On either side of the cochlear duct are the scala vestibuli (**SV**) and scala tympani (**ST**), both filled with **perilymph** and continuous at the apex of the cochlea. The vestibular membrane (**VM**) separates perilymph in the scala vestibuli from endolymph in the cochlear duct. Cell bodies of **bipolar neurons** in the spiral ganglion (**SG**) send dendrites to the **hair cells** of the spiral organ and axons to the cochlear nuclei of the **brain**. (×25; H&E)

FIGURE **23–31** Stereocilia hair bundles of cochlear hair cells.

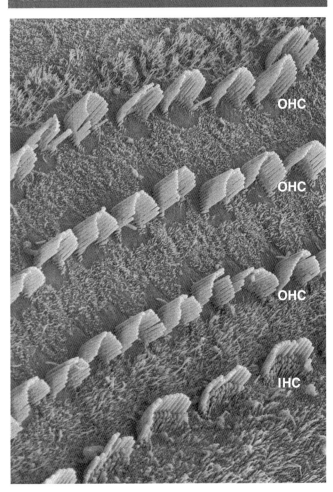

With the tectorial membrane removed, SEM shows the **apical plate** of the rat spiral organ through which rigid **stereocilia bundles** project into **endolymph**. Shown are **hair bundles** from three rows of **outer hair cells** (**OHC**) and the single row of **inner hair cells** (**IHC**) in the middle turn of the cochlea. (×3000)

(Reproduced with permission from Dr Bechara Kachar and Dr Leonardo Andrade, Laboratory of Cell Structure and Dynamics, National Institutes of Health, Bethesda, MD.)

The width, rigidity, thickness, and other physical properties of the basilar membrane and its spiral organ components all vary in precise gradients along its length. This allows the region of maximal displacement to vary with the sound waves' frequency, that is, the number of waves moving past a point per unit of time (measured in *hertz*). High-frequency sounds displace the basilar membrane maximally near the oval window. Sounds of progressively lower frequency produce pressure waves that travel farther along the scala vestibuli and displace the spiral organ at points farther from the oval window (Figure 23–33). The sounds of the lowest detectible frequency move the basilar membrane at the apex or helicotrema of the cochlea. After affecting the cochlear duct (scala media) and organ of Corti, pressure waves are transferred to the scala tympani and exit the inner ear at the round window (Figure 23–32).

The main mechanoreceptors for the sense of hearing are the heavily innervated inner hair cells in the organ of Corti. The outer hair cells, with their stereocilia tips embedded in the tectorial membrane, undergo depolarization when stereocilia are deflected, as described previously for vestibular hair cells (Figure 23–27), but in the organ of Corti hair cell activities are more complex, allowing more finely tuned control on auditory reception.

Depolarization of the outer hair cells causes these columnar cells to shorten very rapidly, an effect mediated

FIGURE **23–32** **Path of sound and pressure waves through the ear.**

1. **Sound waves** enter ear and cause the **tympanic membrane** to vibrate.

2. **Tympanic membrane** vibration moves **auditory ossicles**; sound waves are amplified.

3. The **stapes** at the oval window generates **pressure waves** in the **perilymph** within the **scala vestibuli**.

4. Pressure waves cause the vestibular membrane to **move**, resulting in **pressure wave formation** in the **endolymph** within the **cochlear duct** and displacement of a specific region of the basilar membrane. **Hair cells in the organ of Corti** are distorted, initiating a **nerve signal** in the cochlear branch of CN VIII.

5. **Remaining pressure waves** are transferred to the **scala tympani** and exit the inner ear via the **round window**.

by an unusual 80-kD transmembrane, anion transporter motor protein called **prestin** (It. *presto*, very fast) abundantly expressed in these cells' lateral membranes. Prestin undergoes very fast voltage-dependent conformational changes that deform the cell membrane, shortening the cells slightly upon depolarization and rapidly elongating them again with hyperpolarization. These piston-like movements of the outer hair cells pull the tectorial membrane down against the stereocilia of the inner hair cells (Figure 23–29c) which lack prestin, causing depolarization of these cells and transmission via their afferents of signals to the brain for processing as sounds. This sequential role for outer and inner hair cells produces further cochlear amplification of the sound waves.

FIGURE **23–33** Interpretation of sound waves in the cochlea.

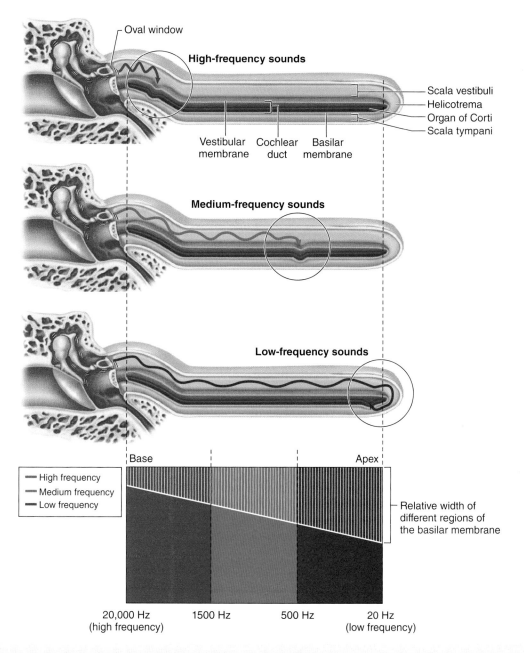

This diagram depicts the **cochlea uncoiled** and straightened to more easily show how **sound waves are interpreted according to their frequency at specific sites along the organ of Corti**. **High-frequency** sound waves (red arrow) generate pressure waves displacing the basilar membrane near the base of the cochlea, close to the oval window. **Medium-frequency** sound waves (green arrow) generate pressure waves that displace the membrane at different points along the central region of the cochlea. **Low-frequency** sound waves (blue arrow) generate waves moving the membrane near the helicotrema, at the apical end of the cochlea.

›› MEDICAL APPLICATION

Some types of sensorineural deafness can be treated by a **cochlear implant**. A small cable with a series of electrodes is threaded into the scala tympani, with the electrodes along the wall containing branches of the cochlear nerve. A device containing a microphone, a speech processor to filter extraneous sounds, and a transmitter is worn behind the external ear. Sounds of various frequencies transmit signals to a receiver implanted in a bone of the skull and attached to the array of electrodes stimulating nerve branches appropriate for those frequencies. The neural impulses are interpreted in the brain as sounds. Cochlear implants do not restore normal hearing but can provide a range of sounds sufficient to allow understanding of speech.

The Eye & Ear: Special Sense Organs SUMMARY OF KEY POINTS

Eye

- The eye has **three tunics**: the **sclera** and **cornea** form the outer **fibrous tunic**; the middle **vascular layer** (or uvea) consists of the **choroid, ciliary body,** and **iris**; and the **retina** forms the **inner tunic**.
- The transparent **cornea** consists of an anterior **stratified squamous epithelium** on Bowman membrane, a thick avascular **stroma**, and an inner **endothelium** on Descemet membrane.
- **Aqueous humor** is secreted by **ciliary processes** into the **posterior chamber**, flows through the **pupil** into the **anterior chamber**, and is drained by the **scleral venous sinus** in the **limbus**.
- The **iris** stroma contains **melanocytes** and posteriorly has smooth muscle fibers of the **sphincter pupillae muscle** and the **myoepithelial cells** forming the **dilator pupillae muscle**.
- The **lens** is a unique avascular tissue composed of long **lens fibers**, covered on its anterior side by cuboidal **lens epithelium**, and surrounded by a thick acellular layer called the **lens capsule**.
- The **lens** is suspended behind the **iris** and its central **pupil** by the **ciliary zonule** of fibrillin microfibrils produced by epithelial cells covering the encircling **ciliary body**.
- The **retina** has the two major parts derived from the embryonic optic cup: the **pigmented epithelium** next to the vascular **choroid** layer and the thicker **neural retina**.
- Cells of the **pigmented epithelium** absorb **scattered light**, form part of a **blood-retina barrier**, regenerate **11-cis-retinal**, **phagocytose** shed discs from rods, and support the rod and cone cells.
- **Rod cells** are **photoreceptors** detecting **light intensity** with short rod-shaped outer segments; less numerous **cone cells**, with conical outer segments, are photoreceptors for the primary **colors** (light of different wavelengths).
- **Rods** have stacked **membrane discs** in which the membranes are densely packed with the protein **rhodopsin** with bound **retinal**.
- Photons of light convert 11-*cis*-retinal to all-*trans*-retinal, causing rhodopsin to release the retinal (**bleaching**), and activate the adjacent G protein **transducin**, which causes a nerve impulse.
- In the **neural retina**, the RCL is nearest to the **retina pigmented epithelium** and near the **ONL** that contains the cell bodies of these photoreceptors.
- An **OPL** contains the photoreceptor's axons connected in synapses with dendrites of various integrating neurons whose cell bodies form the **INL**.
- Axons from cells in the INL form synapses in the **IPL** with neurons of **GL**, which send axons through the **NFL** to the **optic nerve**.
- Eyelids are lined by **conjunctiva**, a stratified columnar epithelium with goblet cells, which also covers the anterior part of the sclera and has continuity with the corneal epithelium.

- **Lacrimal glands** continuously produce the tear film, which drains into the nasal cavity via the ducts of the **lacrimal apparatus**.

Ear

- The **acoustic meatus** of the **external ear** ends at the **tympanic membrane** and its mucosa contains sebaceous and **ceruminous glands** that produce an antimicrobial substance, cerumen.
- The **tympanic cavity** of the **middle ear** opens to the nasopharynx via the **auditory (eustachian) tube**.
- Within the **tympanic cavity**, an articulated series of three small bony **ossicles** (malleus, incus, and stapes) connects the **tympanic membrane** with the **oval window** in the wall of the **internal ear**.
- The **internal ear** consists of a **membranous labyrinth** containing **endolymph**; the membranous labyrinth is enclosed by the temporal bone's **bony labyrinth** that contains perilymph.
- The **membranous labyrinth** has a central **vestibule** with two subdivisions: the **utricle** connects to the three **semicircular ducts** and the **saccule** connects to the **cochlear duct**.
- The walls of the **utricle** and **saccule** each have a thickened area, the **macula**, which contains both sensory **hair cells** with synaptic connections to sensory nerves and **supporting cells**.
- Rigid **stereocilia** and one rigid **kinocilium** project from each **hair cell** into endolymph containing a gel-like matrix with tiny mineralized proteinaceous bodies called **otoliths**.
- Head movements cause **endolymph** and the **otolithic membrane** to move, deforming the rigid apical structures of the **hair cells**, depolarizing them and producing nerve impulses.
- Each of the **semicircular ducts**, oriented 90 degrees from one another, has a terminal **ampulla** region with a thickened **crista ampullaris** containing **hair cells** that contact a gel-like **cupola**.
- **Head movements** displace endolymph and stereocilia of hair cells in the **utricle, saccule,** and **semicircular ducts**, which collectively produce signals that contribute to the sense of equilibrium.
- The **cochlear duct** is the middle compartment (**scala media**) of the **cochlea** and runs between two other long compartments that contain perilymph: the **scala vestibuli** and the **scala tympani**.
- Along the length of the cochlear duct, the **basilar membrane** supports the **spiral organ of Corti**, which consists largely of **hair cells** connected to sensory fibers of cranial nerve VIII.
- The cochlear hair cells include three to five rows of **outer hair cells** with stereocilia embedded in a gel-like **tectorial membrane** and one row of more heavily innervated **inner hair cells**.
- Sound waves transmitted by the **ossicles** move the oval window and produce pressure waves in the cochlear **perilymph** which deflect the **basilar membrane** and **organ of Corti**, causing nerve impulses that the brain interprets as sounds.

The Eye & Ear: Special Sense Organs ASSESS YOUR KNOWLEDGE

1. Which of the following is the thickest component of the cornea?
   a. Corneal epithelium
   b. Stroma
   c. Descemet membrane
   d. Bowman membrane
   e. Corneal endothelium

2. Which description is accurate for lens fibers?
   a. Are terminally differentiated fibroblasts
   b. Consist of specialized type I collagen
   c. Derived from epithelial cells that produce proteins called crystallins
   d. Consist of type III collagen
   e. Have the same embryonic origin as the neural retina

3. Which structure is the most anterior extension of the eye's vascular layer?
   a. Ciliary body
   b. Cornea
   c. Lens
   d. Iris
   e. Zonule

4. Which cells transmit visual signals from the retina to the brain?
   a. Bipolar cells
   b. Amacrine cells
   c. Ganglion cells
   d. Horizontal cells
   e. Müller cells

5. The epithelial cells within the organ of Corti are supported by which of the following structures?
   a. Spiral limbus
   b. Tectorial membrane
   c. Vestibular membrane
   d. Basilar membrane
   e. Spiral ligament

6. The middle ear contains which of the following structures?
   a. The labyrinth
   b. The modiolus
   c. The perilymph
   d. The vestibular apparatus
   e. The ossicles

7. Which structure in the cochlea is analogous in composition and function to the cupola of each semicircular canal?
   a. Tectorial membrane
   b. Pillar cells
   c. Inner tunnel
   d. Saccule
   e. Spiral ganglion

8. A 47-year-old woman is referred to an ophthalmologist after reporting increased difficulty with tasks at night or in dark places for the past 3 or 4 years. She has trouble walking in dimly lit rooms and the movie theater. She has given up driving at night and describes a prolonged adaptation period going from light to dark. She also describes her daylight vision as "tunneled," as she frequently walks into furniture. A family history indicates that her father had a similar condition. In this disease, a single-point mutation in the rhodopsin gene leads to disruption of signal transduction. Visual transduction in the affected cells involves which of the following?
   a. Inactivation of phosphodiesterase
   b. Increase in cGMP levels
   c. Conversion of all-*trans*-retinal to 11-*cis*-retinal
   d. Closing of Na^+ channels
   e. Depolarization of the cell membranes

9. During an eye examination, a 55-year-old man is found to show intraocular pressure exceeding 40 mm Hg and blockage of fluid flow within the eye is suspected. Such a diagnosis would involve a blockage at which of the following sites?
   a. Choroid body
   b. Vessels at the optic disk
   c. Pupillary junction of the posterior and anterior chambers
   d. Choroid layer
   e. Trabecular meshwork

10. During a boxing match, a 23-year-old fighter sustains a direct blow to the right ear. He presents with dizziness, vertigo, imbalance, nausea, vomiting, tinnitus, and fullness in the ears. His vertigo increases with activity and is relieved by rest. He has some hearing loss. The symptoms worsen with coughing, sneezing, or blowing his nose, as well as with exertion. He is diagnosed with perilymphatic fistula, which allows leakage of perilymph. In which of the following structures is perilymph normally found?
    a. Scala media
    b. Scala tympani
    c. Semicircular canals
    d. Saccule
    e. Utricle

Appendix | *Light Microscopy Stains*

Hematoxylin and Eosin (H&E)

Hematoxylin acts as a basic molecule and stains cellular regions rich in acidic macromolecules (DNA or RNA) a purplish blue color. It is the most common stain for demonstrating cell nuclei and cytoplasm rich in rough ER. Usually used as the contrasting "counterstain" with hematoxylin, **eosin** is an acidic stain that binds to basic macromolecules such as collagen and most cytoplasmic proteins, especially those of mitochondria. Eosin stains regions rich in such structures a pinkish red color. Tissue sections showing only structures with shades of purple and pink are most likely stained with H&E.

Pararosaniline–Toluidine Blue (PT)

This dye combination stains chromatin shades of purple and cytoplasm and collagen a lighter violet. These stains penetrate plastic sections more readily than H&E and are used in this atlas primarily with acrylic resin-embedded sections to provide better detail of cell and tissue structures. Toluidine blue is also commonly used for differential staining of cellular components, particularly cytoplasmic granules.

Mallory Trichrome

This procedure employs a combination of stains applied in series that results in nuclei staining purple; cytoplasm, keratin, and erythrocytes staining bright red or orange; and collagen staining bright or light blue. **Mallory trichrome** is particularly useful in demonstrating cells and small blood vessels of connective tissue. Similar stains, such as **Masson trichrome** and Gomori trichrome, yield comparable results except that collagen stains blue-green or green.

Picrosirius-Hematoxylin (PSH)

The dye sirius red in a solution of picric acid stains collagen red and cytoplasm a lighter violet or pink, with nuclei purple if first stained with hematoxylin. Under the polarizing microscope, collagen stained with **picrosirius red** is birefringent and can be detected specifically.

Periodic Acid-Schiff Reaction (PAS)

This histochemical procedure stains complex carbohydrate-containing cell components, which become magenta (shades of purplish pink). **PAS** is used most commonly to demonstrate cells filled with mucin granules, glycogen deposits, or the glycocalyx.

Wright-Giemsa Stain

These are two similar combinations of stains that are widely used on fixed cells of blood or bone marrow smears to demonstrate types of blood cells. Granules in leukocytes are seen to have differential affinity for the stain components. Nuclei stain purple and erythrocytes stain uniformly pink or pinkish orange.

Silver or Gold Stains

Various procedures employing solutions of **silver or gold salts** have been developed to demonstrate filamentous structures in neurons and fibers of reticulin (type III collagen). By these "metal impregnation" techniques these filaments stain dark brown or black. Such stains have been largely replaced now by immunohistochemical procedures.

Stains for Elastin

Several staining methods have been developed to distinguish elastic structures from collagen, most of which stain the elastin-rich structures brown or shades of purple. Examples of such stains are Weigert's **resorcin fuchsin**, **aldehyde fuchsin**, and **orcein**.

Stains for Lipid

When special preparation techniques are used to retain lipids of cells, such as in frozen sections, lipophilic dyes are used to demonstrate lipid droplets and myelin. **Oil red O** and **Sudan black** stains lipid-rich structures as their names suggest. **Osmium tetroxide** (osmic acid), which is used as a fixative for TEM, is reduced to a black substance by unsaturated fatty acids and is also used to demonstrate lipids, including those of myelin and cell membranes.

Other Common Stains

Many basic aniline dyes, including azures, cresyl violet, brilliant cresyl blue, luxol fast blue, and light green, are used because of the permanence and brightness of the colors they impart to cellular and extracellular structures in paraffin sections. Many such stains were initially developed for use in the textile industry.

Figure Credits

Berman I. *Color Atlas of Basic Histology.* 3rd ed. New York, NY: McGraw Hill; 2003.

Eckel CM. *Human Anatomy Lab Manual.* New York, NY: McGraw Hill; 2008.

Fitzpatrick TB, et al. *Dermatology in General Medicine.* New York, NY: McGraw Hill; 1971.

Goldsmith LA, Katz SI, Gilchrest BA, et al: *Fitzpatrick's Dermatology in General Medicine,* 8th ed. New York, NY: McGraw Hill; 2012.

Kaushansky K, Lichtman M, Beutler E, et al. *Williams Hematology.* 8th ed. New York, NY: McGraw Hill; 2010.

Lewis R, Gaffin D, Hoefnagels M, et al. *Life.* 5th ed. New York, NY: McGraw Hill; 2004.

Lichtman MA, Shafer MS, Felgar RE, et al: *Lichtman's Atlas of Hematology.* New York, NY: McGraw Hill; 2016.

McKinley M, O'Loughlin VD. *Human Anatomy.* 3rd ed. New York, NY: McGraw Hill; 2012.

McKinley MP, O'Loughlin VD, Bidle TS. *Anatomy & Physiology: An Integrative Approach.* New York, NY: McGraw Hill; 2013.

McKinley M, O'Loughlin VD, Pennefather-O'Brien EE, et al: *Human Anatomy,* 5th ed. New York, NY: McGraw Hill; 2017.

Raven P, Johnson GB, Losos JB, et al. *Biology.* 7th ed. New York, NY: McGraw Hill; 2005.

Widmaier EP, Raff H, Strang KT. *Vander's Human Physiology.* 11th ed. New York, NY: McGraw Hill; 2008.

Chapter 1

1-3: Nikon Instruments Inc., Melville, NY; **1-14:** McKinley (2013) 1-5.

Chapter 2

2-3: McKinley (2013) 4-5a; **2-6:** McKinley (2012) 2-7; **2-8:** McKinley (2013) 4-19; **2-10a:** McKinley (2012) 2-8a; **2-10b:** Don W. Fawcett/Science Source; **2-13a:** Dennis Kunkel Microscopy/Science Photo Library; **2-13b:** Professors P. Motta and T. Naguro/Science Photo Library; **2-20a:** CNRI/Science Photo Library; **2-21b:** From Fahimi HD. Effect of buffer storage on fine structure and catalase cytochemistry of peroxisomes, *J Cell Biol* 1974 Nov;63(2 Pt 1): 675-683.

Chapter 3

3-2 left: McKinley (2012) 2-17 (left side); **3-2 right:** Don W. Fawcett/Science Source; **3-10:** From Speicher MR, Ward DC. The coloring of cytogenetics, *Nat Med* 1996 Sep;2(9):1046-1048; **3-18:** Lewis 9-10.

Chapter 4

4-4: Raven 7-13; **4-5:** Dennis Kunkel Microscopy/Science Photo Library; **4-15d:** Berman 1-16; **4-21:** McKinley (2012) 4-6; **4-20:** McKinley (2012) 4-4.

Chapter 5

5-2: McKinley (2012) 4-7; **5-3a:** Berman 2-6; **5-8b:** Berman 2-7; **5-12b:** McGraw Hill Education/Al Telser

Chapter 6

6-1c: Berman 2-20.

Chapter 7

7-1a: McKinley (2012) 6-1a.

Chapter 8

8-1: McKinley (2013) 7-7; **8-9:** Berman 4-4; **8-13a:** Berman 5-7; **8-14:** McKinley (2012) 6-11; **8-16a:** Puwadol Jaturawutthichai/stockdevil/123RF; **8-16b:** Alvin Telser, PhD; **8-17a:** Berman 5-3; **8-17b:** Berman 5-4; **8-18:** McKinley (2012) 6-13; **8-19:** McKinley (2012) 6-16.

Chapter 9

9-1: McKinley (2012) 14-1; **9-2:** McKinley (2012) 14-16; **9-3a:** McKinley (2013) 12-2; **9-3b:** Ed Reschke/Getty Images; **9-4:** McKinley (2013) 12-1 (table); **9-5:** Berman 6-8; **9-6a:** McKinley (2012) 14-14b; **9-7 bottom:** McKinley (2012) 14-13c; **9-8b:** Biophoto Associates/Science Photo Library; **9-9:** McKinley (2012) 14-6, 14-7e-f; **9-10a:** Berman 6-9; **9-17 top middle:** Ed Reschke/Getty Images; **9-18a:** McKinley (2012) 16-2b; **9-19:** McKinley (2012) 15-4; **9-20c:** McKinley (2012) 15-7a; **9-21:** McKinley (2012) 14-8; **9-25:** McKinley (2012) 14-10a; **9-26a:** McKinley (2012) 14-12a; **9-26b:** Berman 6-15; **9-26d:** From Ishibe K, Tamatsu Y, Miura M, Shimada K. Morphological study of the vasa nervorum in the peripheral branch of human facial nerve, *Okajimas Folia Anat Jpn* 2011 Nov; 88(3):111-119; **9-28b:** Berman 6-19; **9-28d:** Berman 6-18; **9-29a:** Berman 6-10; **9-29c:** Berman 6-12.

Chapter 10

10-1: Widmaier 9-1; **10-2:** McKinley (2012) 10-4; **10-3:** McKinley (2012) 10-1a; **10-6a:** Berman 7-2; **10-8a-c:** McKinley (2012) 10-6a-c; **10-8d:** Medical Images/Jim Dennis; **10-9:** McKinley (2012) 10-3; **10-12a&b left & middle:** McKinley (2013) 10-12; **10-12a&b right:** Biophoto Associates/Science Source; **10-13b&c:** Widmaier 9-14; **10-14a:** Widmaier 10-4; **10-15:** From Ranatunga KW, Thomas PE. Correlation between shortening velocity, force-velocity relation and histochemical fibre-type composition in rat muscles, *J Muscle Res Cell Motil* 1990 Jun;11(3):240-250; **10-16a:** McKinley (2012) 22-10a; **10-16c:** From Sheikh F, Ross RS, Chen J. Cell-cell connection to cardiac disease, *Trends Cardiovasc Med* 2009 Aug;19(6):182-190; **10-17a:** Berman 7-10; **10-20a:** McKinley (2012) 10-16.

Chapter 11

11-1: McKinley (2017) 23-23; **11-2:** McKinley (2012) 22-11a; **11-5:** Berman 11-2; **11-6:** McKinley (2012) 23-1; **11-7a:** Berman 11-11; **11-7b:** Berman 11-12; **11-13:** McKinley (2013) 20-5; **11-14a:** Berman 11-20; **11-14b:** Berman 11-22; **11-15:** McKinley (2013) 20-8; **11-21c:** Berman 11-21; **11-22b:** Berman 11-18; **11-22c:** Berman 11-13; **11-22d:** Berman 11-19; **11-24b:** McKinley (2012) 24-2b.

Chapter 12

12-1: McKinley (2012) 21-2; **12-4a:** Widmaier 12-67; **12-4b:** McKinley (2012) 21-4a; **12-4c:** Ed Reschke; **12-8:** Lichtman II.A.004; **12-10d:** Lichtman II.E.008; **12-11b:** Berman 8-5; **12-12c:** Berman 8-6; **12-12d:** Berman 8-1; **12-13a:** Berman 8-9; **12-14a:** Steve Gschmeissner/Science Photo Library; **12-14b:** Berman 8-12.

Chapter 13

13-1: Kaushansky 5-1; **13-2:** McKinley (2012) 21-11; **13-5:** McKinley (2013) 18-4b; **13-7a:** Berman 9-6 through 9-9; **13-7b:** Berman 8-8; **13-10:** Berman 9-1, 9-2, 9-4, 9-5; **13-13a:** Berman 9-11; **13-13b:** Berman 9-13; **13-14:** Berman 9-14.

Chapter 14

14-1: McKinley (2013) 21-2; **14-2:** McKinley (2013) 22-17; **14-3:** McKinley (2013) 22-18; **14-5:** McKinley (2013)

22-9; **14-6:** McKinley (2013) 22-15; **14-8a:** McKinley (2013) 21-5a; **14-8c:** Dr. Thomas Caceci, Virginia – Maryland Regional College of Veterinary Medicine; **14-11:** McKinley (2013) 22-14; **14-13a:** Berman 10-5; **14-19c:** From He Y. Scanning electron microscope studies of the rat mesenteric lymph node with special reference to high-endothelial venules and hitherto unknown lymphatic labyrinth, *Arch Histol Jpn* 1985 Feb;48(1):1-15; **14-26a:** SEM of late Prof. Emer. T. Fujita (Courtesy of Prof T. Ushiki, Niigata University).

Chapter 15

15-1: McKinley (2012) 26-1; **15-2:** McKinley (2012) 26-9; **15-4a-c:** McKinley (2013) 16-7a-c; **15-4 d & inset:** Jose Luis Calvo/Shutterstock; **15-5a:** Berman 12-10; **15-5b:** Berman 12-12; **15-6a:** McKinley (2012) 26-6c; **15-6b:** McKinley (2012) 26-5; **15-10a:** Berman 12-1; **15-10b:** Berman 12-4; **15-12a:** Alfred Pasieka/Science Photo Library; **15-13a:** Berman 12-16; **15-14a:** McKinley (2013) 26-9a; **15-14b:** McKinley (2012) 26-13a; **15-14c:** McKinley (2013) 26-10a; **15-15:** Berman 12-22; **15-17d:** McKinley (2013) 26-10c; **15-19:** McKinley (2013) 26-11; **15-22a-c:** McKinley (2013) 26-15; **15-22e:** McKinley (2013) 26-16b; **15-31:** McKinley (2013) 26-22; **15-32a:** McKinley (2013) 26-23a; **15-33a:** Berman 12-41; **15-33b:** Berman 12-43.

Chapter 16

16-1: McKinley (2012) 26-4a; **16-3b:** Berman 13-26; **16-5a:** Berman 13-29; **16-5b:** Berman 13-32; **16-7a:** McKinley (2012) 26-20a; **16-8:** Berman 13-17; **16-9a:** Berman 13-21; **16-11a:** McKinley (2013) 26-19a; **16-11b:** McKinley (2017) 29-19b; **16-12a:** Berman 13-3; **16-12b:** Berman 13-4; **16-18:** From Boron WF, Boulpaep EL. *Medical Physiology: A Cellular and Molecular Approach*. Philadelphia, PA: Saunders Elsevier; 2005; **16-19:** McKinley (2013) 26-17; **16-20a:** Berman 13-15.

Chapter 17

17-1: McKinley (2012) 25-1; **17-2b&c:** From Andrews PM, Porter KR. A scanning electron microscopic study of the nephron, *Am J Anat* 1974 May;140(1):81-115; **17-3a:** McKinley (2013) 16-6; **17-4:** Berman 14-1; **17-6:** McKinley (2012) 25-8; **17-7:** Berman 14-10; **17-8a:** Berman 14-11; **17-8b:** Berman 14-12; **17-9a:** Berman 14-13; **17-9c:** Berman 14-14; **17-11a:** McKinley (2013) 23-11a; **17-11b:** Alvin Telser, PhD; **17-11c:** David Phillips/Science Source; **17-12:** Berman 14-18; **17-13:** McKinley (2013) 23-12; **17-14:** Berman 14-20; **17-18a:** McKinley (2012) 25-11.

Chapter 18

18-1: McKinley (2013) 6-6; **18-2a:** Ed Reschke/Getty Images; **18-2b:** McKinley (2012) 5-2b; **18-3:** Berman 15-4; **18-5:** Berman 15-3; **18-6a:** Berman 15-2; **18-6b:** McKinley (2012) 5-4a; **18-7b:** Fitzpatrick 5-9; **18-8:** From Romani N, Holzmann S, Tripp CH, Koch F, Stoitzner P. Langerhans cells – dendritic cells of the epidermis, *APMIS* Jul-Aug 2003;111(7-8):725-740; **18-9:** Goldsmith 7-6; **18-11:** McKinley (2013) 16-3; **18-12a:** Eckel 17-2a; **18-12b:** Medical Images/Carolina Biological; **18-13b:** Al Telser/McGraw Hill; **18-13c:** SPL/Science Source; **18-14a:** Berman 15-15; **18-14b:** Berman 15-14; **18-14c:** From Jahoda CA, Mauger A, Bard S, Sengel P. Changes in fibronectin, laminin and type IV collagen distribution relate to basement membrane restructuring during the rat vibrissa follicle hair growth cycle, *J Anat* 1992 Aug;181 (Pt 1):47-60; **18-15a&b:** McKinley (2012) 5-8; **18-16:** McKinley (2013) 6-10a; **18-17a:** Berman 15-10; **18-20:** McKinley (2013) 6-12.

Chapter 19

19-2: McKinley (2013) 24-4; **19-3:** McKinley (2013) 24-8; **19-4:** Berman 16-4; **19-5a,c,d:** McKinley (2012) 27-6a,c,d; **19-6c:** McKinley (2013) 24-11b; **19-8a:** Berman 16-8; **19-9a:** McKinley (2012) 27-7a; **19-9b&d:** Alvin Telser, PhD; **19-13:** McKinley (2013) 24-9; **19-16a:** McKinley (2012) 27-8a; **19-17a:** Berman 16-18.

Chapter 20

20-1: McKinley (2017) 20-2; **20-2:** McKinley (2012) 20-4; **20-3:** McKinley (2012) 20-15; **20-4:** Berman 17-1; **20-5a:** McKinley (2012) 20-8; **20-5b:** McKinley (2012) 20-6; **20-6b:** Berman 17-3; **20-8:** McKinley (2017) 20-8; **20-9:** Berman 17-4; **20-12:** McKinley (2012) 20-13a; **20-14 left:** McKinley (2012) 20-13c; **20-14 right:** Alvin Telser/McGraw Hill; **20-17c:** Berman 17-13; **20-19b:** Berman 17-15; **20-21 upper right:** McKinley (2013) 17-18; **20-22:** McKinley (2012) 20-11a; **20-23:** Berman 17-17.

Chapter 21

21-1: McKinley (2012) 28-11; **21-2:** McKinley (2012) 28-13a; **21-3:** Berman 18-2; **21-6a:** Berman 18-7; **21-6b:** Berman 18-8; **21-9a:** Berman 18-10; **21-9b:** Berman 18-11; **21-10b:** Berman 18-13; **21-11a:** Berman 18-14; **21-12a:** Berman 18-16; **21-14a:** Berman 18-18; **21-16a:** Berman 18-20; **21-16b:** Berman 18-21; **21-17:** McKinley (2017) 18-17b; **21-18:** Berman 18-23.

Chapter 22

22-1a&b: McKinley (2012) 28-3a&b; **22-2a:** McKinley (2012) 28-4a; **22-2b&c:** Alvin Telser/McGraw Hill; **22-2d:** Ed Reschke/Stone/Getty Images; **22-2e:** Ed Reschke/Getty Images; **22-2f&g:** Alvin Telser/McGraw Hill; **22-10:** McKinley (2012) 28-5; **22-13:** Berman 19-8; **22-14a:** McKinley (2012) 28-7a; **22-14b&c:** Alvin Telser/McGraw Hill; **22-15a:** Berman 19-16; **22-17:** McKinley (2012) 28-6; **22-19a:** Berman 19-19; **22-19b:** Berman 19-20; **22-19c:** Berman 19-21; **22-20:** McKinley (2012) 3-6; **22-21c:** McKinley (2013) 29-7; **22-23a:** Berman 19-22; **22-24a:** Berman 19-23; **22-26a:** Berman 19-24; **22-26b:** Berman 19-25; **22-26c:** Berman 19-26; **22-27a:** Berman 19-27.

Chapter 23

23-1: McKinley (2012) 19-12; **23-2:** McKinley (2012) 19-19; **23-8:** McKinley (2012) 19-17; **23-10a:** Berman 20-4; **23a&b:** McKinley (2012) 19-14a&b; **23-15:** Berman 20-9; **23-21:** McKinley (2012) 19-20; **23-23:** McKinley (2012) 19-21; **23-24:** McKinley (2012) 19-22; **23-25a-c:** McKinley (2012) 19-23; **23-28:** McKinley (2012) 19-25; **23-29d:** Biophoto Associates/Science Source; **23-32:** McKinley (2013) 16-29; **23-33:** McKinley (2012) 19-29.

Index

Note: Page numbers followed by an "*f*" indicate figures; page numbers followed by a "*t*" indicate tables.